Functional Anatomy
and **Physiology**
of **Domestic Animals**

FOURTH EDITION

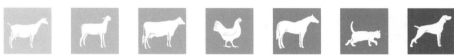

William O. Reece, D.V.M., Ph.D.

Department of Biomedical Sciences

College of Veterinary Medicine

Iowa State University of Science and Technology

Ames, Iowa

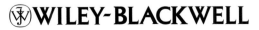
WILEY-BLACKWELL
A John Wiley & Sons, Inc., Publication

Edition first published 2009
© 2009 Blackwell Publishing

Blackwell Publishing was acquired by John Wiley & Sons in February 2007. Blackwell's publishing program has been merged with Wiley's global Scientific, Technical, and Medical business to form Wiley-Blackwell.

Editorial Office
2121 State Avenue, Ames, Iowa 50014-8300, USA

For details of our global editorial offices, for customer services, and for information about how to apply for permission to reuse the copyright material in this book, please see our website at www.wiley.com/wiley-blackwell.

Library of Congress Cataloguing-in-Publication Data

Reece, William O.
    Functional anatomy and physiology of domestic animals / William O. Reece.—4th ed.
        p.   cm.
    Includes bibliographical references and index.
    ISBN 978-0-8138-1451-3 (pbk. : alk. paper)
1. Veterinary physiology.   2. Veterinary anatomy.   I. Title.
SF768.R44 2009
636.089′2–dc22   2008040236

A catalogue record for this book is available from the U.S. Library of Congress.

Set in 10 on 12 Berkeley by SNP Best-set Typesetter Ltd., Hong Kong
Printed in The United States by Sheridan Books, Inc.

2   2010

TO MY DECEASED WIFE
Shirley Ann

AND THE LEGACY OF OUR MARRIAGE,
OUR CHILDREN:
Mary Kay
Kathy Ann
Barbara Jean
Sara Lucinda
Anna Marie
Susan Theresa
William Omar, II

Contents

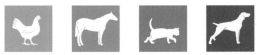

Preface... xi

Acknowledgments... xiii

1 Basics of Structure and Function.............................. 3
   The Cell, Its Structure and Functions 3
   Energy Production 6
   Functions of DNA and RNA....................................7
   Embryology..11
   Tissues..13
   Directional Terms and Planes 19
   Body Cavities 21

2 Body Water: Properties and Functions 28
   Physicochemical Properties of Solutions 28
   Distribution of Body Water...................................36
   Water Balance 37
   Dehydration, Thirst, and Water Intake 39
   Adaptation to Water Lack.....................................41

3 Blood and Its Functions 45
   General Characteristics 45
   Leukocytes...47
   Erythrocytes 55
   Fate of Erythrocytes...60
   Iron Metabolism..61
   Anemia and Polycythemia......................................63
   Hemostasis: Prevention of Blood Loss 64
   Prevention of Blood Coagulation..............................71
   Tests for Blood Coagulation 73
   Plasma and Its Composition 74

4 Nervous System 84
   Structure of the Nervous System 84
   Organization of the Nervous System 87
   The Nerve Impulse and Its Transmission 104
   Reflexes...111
   The Meninges and Cerebrospinal Fluid 114
   Central Nervous System Metabolism 119

5 The Sensory Organs 124
   Classification of Sensory Receptors..........................124
   Sensory Receptor Responses 125

Pain 125
Taste 127
Smell 130
Hearing and Equilibrium 132
Vision 140

6   Endocrine System 160
Hormones 160
Pituitary Gland 161
Thyroid Gland 165
Parathyroid Glands 168
Adrenal Glands 169
Pancreatic Gland 174
Prostaglandins and Their Functions 175

7   Bones, Joints, and Synovial Fluid 179
General Features of the Skeleton 179
Bone Structure 187
Bone Formation 193
Bone Repair 196
Joints and Synovial Fluid 198

8   Muscle 206
Classification 206
Arrangement 208
Skeletal-Muscle Harnessing 209
Microstructure of Skeletal Muscle 210
Skeletal-Muscle Contraction 216
Comparison of Contraction among Muscle Types 222
Changes in Muscle Size 223

9   The Cardiovascular System 228
Heart and Pericardium 228
Blood Vessels 234
Lymphatic System 237
Spleen 242
Cardiac Contractility 245
Electrocardiogram 247
Heart Sounds 251
Heart Rate and Its Control 251
Blood Pressure 254
Blood Flow 256
Capillary Dynamics 260

10   The Respiratory System 269
Respiratory Apparatus 270
Factors Associated with Breathing 275

Respiratory Pressures 282
Pulmonary Ventilation 283
Diffusion of Respiratory Gases 286
Oxygen Transport 287
Carbon Dioxide Transport 290
Regulation of Ventilation 292
Respiratory Clearance 296
Nonrespiratory Functions of the Respiratory System 298
Descriptive Terms and Pathologic Conditions 300
Avian Respiration 301

11 The Urinary System 312
Gross Anatomy of the Kidneys and Urinary Bladder 312
The Nephron 317
Formation of Urine 323
Glomerular Filtration 324
Tubular Reabsorption and Secretion 327
Countercurrent Mechanism 329
Concentration of Urine 333
Extracellular Fluid Volume Regulation 336
Aldosterone 337
Other Hormones with Kidney Association 338
Micturition 339
Characteristics of Mammalian Urine 340
Renal Clearance 341
Maintenance of Acid-Base Balance 344
Avian Urinary System 347

12 Digestion and Absorption 359
Introductory Considerations 360
The Oral Cavity and Pharynx 361
The Simple Stomach 365
Intestines 367
Accessory Organs 376
Composition of Foodstuffs 379
Pregastric Mechanical Functions 384
Gastrointestinal Motility 385
Mechanical Functions of the Stomach and Small Intestine 388
Mechanical Functions of the Large Intestine 391
Digestive Secretions 392
Digestion and Absorption 398
The Ruminant Stomach 400
Characteristics of Ruminant Digestion 404
Chemistry and Microbiology of the Rumen 407
Ruminant Metabolism 408
Avian Digestion 411

13   Body Heat and Temperature Regulation 421
Body Temperature 421
Physiologic Responses to Heat 422
Physiologic Responses to Cold 426
Hibernation 427
Hypothermia and Hyperthermia 428

14   Male Reproduction 432
Testes and Associated Structures 432
Descent of the Testes 437
Accessory Sex Glands and Semen 438
Penis and Prepuce 440
Muscles of Male Genitalia 442
Blood and Nerve Supply 444
Spermatogenesis 445
Erection 450
Mounting and Intromission 451
Emission and Ejaculation 451
Factors Affecting Testicular Function 451
Reproduction in the Avian Male 452

15   Female Reproduction 458
Functional Anatomy of the Female Reproductive System 458
Hormones of Female Reproduction 468
Ovarian Follicle Activity 471
Sexual Receptivity 476
Estrous Cycle and Related Factors 477
Pregnancy 482
Parturition 487
Involution of the Uterus 492
Reproduction in the Avian Female 493

16   Lactation 501
Functional Anatomy of Female Mammary Glands 501
Mammogenesis 506
Lactogenesis and Lactation 507
Composition of Milk 510
Milk Removal and Other Considerations 512

Appendix A. Normal Blood Values 517

Index 524

Preface

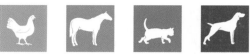

Functional Anatomy and Physiology of Domestic Animals is directed toward undergraduate students seeking a basic understanding of domestic animal anatomy and physiology. It assumes a basic background in biology and a strong interest by students wanting a greater understanding of animal systems. Now in its fourth edition, this text will continue to be of particular interest to preveterinary students, veterinary technician/technology students, and students in animal science and other animal-related majors and is an excellent bridge to other books required for greater depth of understanding. Experience with the first three editions and user comments have guided efforts for this revision.

■ RECOGNITION OF ANATOMY CONTENT

Functional anatomy refers to the concurrent presentation of anatomy (both microscopic and gross) with physiology to achieve a better appreciation of their interconnection. It does not presume in-depth coverage of anatomy nor its coverage preceding the presentation of physiology. Called *Physiology of Domestic Animals* in its first and second editions, this text was renamed with the third edition to provide greater recognition for users of its anatomy content.

The first chapter, Basics of Structure and Function, added in the third edition, has been a useful introduction to the chapters that follow. This chapter includes topics on cell structures and functions, energy production, functions of DNA and RNA, embryology, tissues, directional terms and planes, and body cavities.

■ KEY FEATURES

Contents

In addition to chapter titles, the primary headings for each chapter are now included. This will provide visibility for the focus of each chapter.

Chapter Outline

A further review of the content is provided at the beginning of each chapter in the form of an outline of primary and secondary headings.

Study Aids

Each of the first-order headings within the text is immediately followed by study aids in the form of questions or "take note" statements for which the answers or important concepts are revealed in the text that follows. When students conscientiously approach the chapter content by seeking the answers to these questions or noting the highlights, what may otherwise be difficult reading and comprehension becomes a productive endeavor. These may also provide a focus for quick review.

Self-Evaluation

These exercises are designed to promote teaching effectiveness and are placed at the end of each chapter. The answers immediately follow the questions. They are intended to reinforce meaningful chapter content and provide a thoughtful review of chapter content.

Clinical Correlates

At many locations throughout the chapters, anatomical or physiological topics are extended with a brief mention of a clinical correlation or note of relevance. These are identified in color where they occur.

Key Terms

Key terms that may be new or unfamiliar to the student are highlighted in bold upon first use.

Suggested Reading

Additional resources are listed at the end of each chapter to encourage students in further study of covered material.

Updated Art Program

More than 350 illustrations are included to assist in text presentation. All have been re-evaluated for correctness and simplicity, and new ones have been added to replace those deemed ineffective with more helpful versions.

Appendix

Entitled "Normal Blood Values," the appendix includes nine tables with blood values for each of the domestic species. They are from authoritative sources and can be useful for a reference resource. The content of an appendix in the third edition entitled "Inter-conversion of Units of Measure" has been incorporated into Chapter 2, Body Water: Properties and Functions, where it can be effectively applied.

■ EXPANDED COVERAGE OF AVIAN TOPICS AND BODY WATER

Because poultry are important components of the agricultural industry and pet birds are increasingly more prevalent as components of veterinary medical practices, avian topics are covered in those chapters where their anatomy and physiology are decidedly different. This expanded coverage has been done for the chapters on the kidney, respiration, digestion, and male and female reproduction.

In addition, Chapter 2, Body Water: Properties and Functions, has been expanded. By providing good definitions, examples, and sample problems, students will gain freshness, enthusiasm, and appreciation, which will make applications easier and more meaningful for understanding capillary dynamics, renal dynamics, and fluid replacement therapy.

The study aids, self-evaluation exercises, liberal use of figures and tables, and suggested reading references provide elements needed for independent study. Accordingly, this edition can be valuable support to those courses that teach anatomy and physiology of domestic animals and as a bridge for courses in veterinary medicine.

William O. Reece

Acknowledgments

The first edition of this book was developed from my perceived need while teaching an undergraduate course. My time teaching this course spanned approximately 25 years and involved close to 4,500 students. I am indebted to these students for the inspiration they provided and for assisting me in my personal and professional development. I am also indebted to Dr. Peter Holmes, University of Glasgow, School of Veterinary Medicine, Department of Physiology, for accepting my sabbatical visit and for providing administrative support and a stimulating environment in which to work while I drafted the manuscript for the first edition. Administrative and resource support was continued with the first, second, third, and now the fourth editions by the Biomedical Sciences Department (formerly Physiology and Pharmacology), College of Veterinary Medicine, Iowa State University.

It is humbling to experience the production of a textbook and realize the team effort and friendly cooperation of so many talented people. It is to these people of the fourth edition that I now recognize and extend my sincere appreciation.

Dr. James Bloedel, Chairman, and Dr. Richard Martin, immediate past-Chairman, Department of Biomedical Sciences, College of Veterinary Medicine, Iowa State University, have provided encouragement and consented to diversion of staff time and other resources to this project.

Marilee Eischeid is our talented Department of Biomedical Sciences program assistant. I could not have functioned without her assistance. Her administrative skills allowed for the provision of neat, on-time, error-free manuscripts to the publishers.

Linda Erickson, administrative specialist, Department of Biomedical Sciences, has been in the background as a liaison for my needs for all four editions. Kim Adams, account clerk, provided assistance whenever needed.

Dr. Nani Ghoshal, veterinary anatomist, Department of Biomedical Sciences, willingly provided anatomical expertise in response to my frequent queries.

Kristi Schaaf, Veterinary Medical Library supervisor, was a constant resource for location of publishers and for seeking their permissions for the republishing of images. Lindsey Healey, Veterinary Medical Library assistant, and Andrea Dinkelman, Iowa State University reference librarian, provided help when needed for retrieving publications from various sources.

Ann Staniger, graphic designer, Office of Veterinary Education and Technology Services, provided the expertise for corrections and improvements of images. She was assisted in this effort by Jessica Hamilton, graphic design intern.

Dean Biechler created the animal silhouettes used in the cover design for the first edition when he was employed as an artist by Biomedical Communications. These elegant silhouettes have been continued with pride in the second, third, and fourth editions.

Wiley-Blackwell, my publisher, and their team of experts were involved from the point of acquisition to publication. Antonia Seymour, publishing director, professional, received my proposal for the fourth edition. Her friendly, organized business approach allowed for the decision to publish. Nancy Simmerman, editorial assistant, provided encouragement, recommendations, advice, friendly nudges, and true responsibility for this edition to come forth and to meet high standards. Carrie Sutton, production editor, kept the production on schedule and provided courteous assistance for final correction of oversights.

Many publishers and authors gave permission to use their illustrations. Our thanks to them are conveyed with a credit line to the source.

The memory of my wife, Shirley, was important to me as an incentive for continuation with the third edition. She was a great listener when I "bounced" ideas or problems to her.

Her memory for this has continued during the preparation of the fourth edition.

Above all, I thank God for these people with whom I work and for the privilege of continuing a productive life.

Functional Anatomy and Physiology of Domestic Animals

FOURTH EDITION

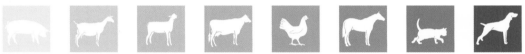

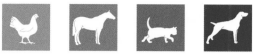

CHAPTER 1

Basics of Structure and Function

CHAPTER OUTLINE

- **THE CELL, ITS STRUCTURE AND FUNCTIONS**
  The Organelles
- **ENERGY PRODUCTION**
- **FUNCTIONS OF DNA AND RNA**
  DNA and Its Replication
  Mitosis
  RNA and Protein Synthesis
- **EMBRYOLOGY**

- **TISSUES**
  Epithelium
  Connective Tissue
- **DIRECTIONAL TERMS AND PLANES**
- **BODY CAVITIES**
  Thoracic Cavity
  The Abdominopelvic Cavity
  The Peritoneum

In general, the study of anatomy refers to the study of the structure of body parts and includes gross anatomy (identification by unaided visual means) and microscopic anatomy (identification by microscopic assistance that usually begins at the cellular level). The study of physiology is a study of the functions of the body, or as sometimes stated, "how the body works," and includes biophysical and biochemical processes and precludes a knowledge of anatomy. Although anatomy and physiology can be taught as separate entities, overlaps are unavoidable and it follows that greater productivity is obtained by integrating the two disciplines.

The study of anatomy and physiology is assisted by prerequisite courses, which include chemistry, physics, biology, and quantitative skills in mathematics. With this in mind, we will rely not only on your previous preparation, but also on the desire to advance your knowledge with application to animal anatomy and physiology. This chapter provides basics of structure and function that should be helpful to you as you study the chapters that follow.

■ THE CELL, ITS STRUCTURE AND FUNCTIONS

1. What separates the cell cytoplasm from interstitial fluid?
2. What are organelles?
3. Define the nuclear membrane.
4. What does chromatin become in dividing cells?
5. Differentiate between granular and agranular endoplasmic reticula and their associated functions.
6. Are the vesicular structures of the endoplasmic reticulum separate or interconnected?
7. What is the function of the Golgi apparatus?
8. What organelle is the site of the citric acid cycle?
9. What is the principal substance of lysosomes?
10. What cellular function are the centrioles associated with? What is their location within the cell known as?

The number of cells in an animal is in the trillions and for the human has been estimated to be about 100 trillion. Each of these cells had their start beginning with fertilization of an oocyte. The appearance of cells varies with the organ of which they are a part and will be shown and described when encountered. Cells are highly organized chemical systems and share many features that are shown schematically in *Figure 1-1*. The basic components of a cell are the **plasma membrane (cell membrane)** that bounds the cell and gives it limits; the **cytoplasm**, which is the homogenous ground substance that forms the background in which the formed elements are suspended; and the nucleus. The **nucleus** is separated from the cytoplasm by a nuclear membrane, and the cytoplasm is separated from the surrounding fluids (interstitial fluid) by a cell membrane. The cell membrane is usually pliable and is composed of phospholipids and proteins. The phospholipid molecules occur in two layers. The protein molecules may be associated with either the outer or inner layer and may penetrate completely or incompletely (see Chapter 2).

Because of cell specialization, no cell can be called typical. The cytoplasm is the location of diverse metabolic activities and is filled with both minute and large dispersed particles and organelles.

The Organelles

The **organelles** are highly organized physical structures represented in Figure 1-1, and in addition to the cell membrane, consist of the nucleus, endoplasmic reticulum, Golgi apparatus, mitochondria, lysosomes, and centrioles. These structures assist the cytoplasm with its metabolic activities by receiving materials into the cell, synthesizing new substances, generating energy, packaging materials for transport to other parts of the cell or to the circulation, excretion of waste products, and reproduction.

Nucleus

The nucleus is the control center of the cell, controlling its chemical reactions and reproduction. It contains large quantities of **DNA**. Nuclear components consist of a nuclear membrane, one or more nucleoli, and chromatin, all bathed in **nuclear sap (nucleoplasm)**. The **nuclear membrane** (also called nuclear envelope) consists of two membranes wherein the outer membrane is continuous with the endoplasmic reticulum, and the space between the two nuclear membranes, the lumen, is also continuous with the lumen of the endoplasmic reticulum. Both layers are penetrated by numerous **nuclear pores**. These pores permit exchange between the nucleoplasm of the nucleus and the cytoplasm outside the nucleus, including movement of **RNA** synthesized in the nucleus, out into the cytoplasm. The **nucleolus** does not have a limiting membrane and is a structure that contains large amounts of RNA and proteins that are found in ribosomes. **Chromatin** appears as dark-staining particles throughout the nucleoplasm in the nondividing cell. In the dividing cell, the chromatin organizes into the chromosomes.

Endoplasmic Reticulum

The **endoplasmic reticulum (ER)** is a network of tubular and flat vesicular (small thin-walled cavity) structures in the cytoplasm that all interconnect with one another. The fluid within the lumen of the ER is continuous with the fluid in the nuclear envelope and is different from the fluid in the cytoplasm. A large number of small granular particles called **ribosomes** are attached to the outer surfaces of many parts of the ER. Where these are present they are called the granular ER, and where they are not present they are called the agranular or smooth ER. Ribosomes are composed of a mixture of RNA and proteins and function in the synthesis of proteins. The agranular ER functions in the synthesis of lipid substances and other enzymatic processes of the cell.

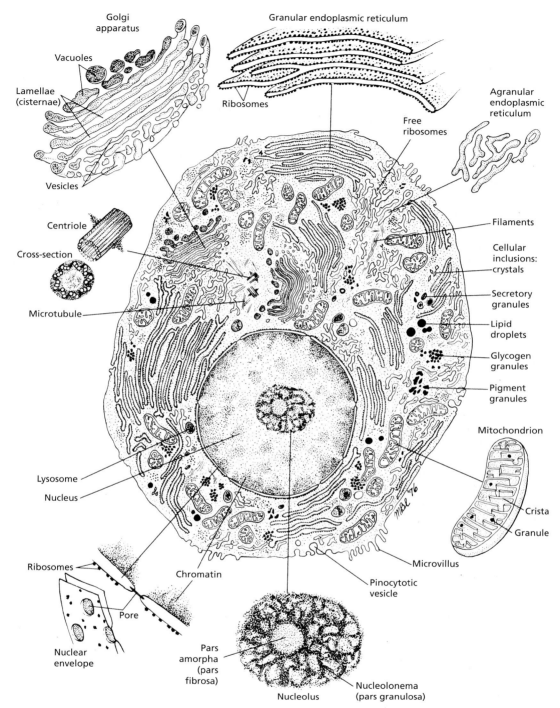

■ FIGURE 1-1 Schematic drawing of a cell and its organelles as seen in electron photomicrographs. (From Crouch, JE. Functional Human Anatomy. 4th Ed. Philadelphia: Lea & Febiger, 1985.)

Golgi Apparatus

The **Golgi apparatus** is closely related to the ER. It is prominent in secretory cells, being well developed in cells secreting enzymes and hormones. It packages materials made in the cell and transforms them into units that are then distributed outside the cell. The packaging begins when vesicles pinch off from the ER and then fuse with the Golgi apparatus. The vesicular substances are then processed in the Golgi apparatus to form lysosomes or other secretory vesicles, which become surrounded by a membrane. They are then released from the Golgi apparatus for storage or use in the cell or are transported to the cell membrane, where they are released into the extracellular fluid as a secretion.

Mitochondria

Mitochondria are the "powerhouses" of the cell because they are the principal sites for energy production. The number in a cell depends on the amount of energy required, and mitochondria increase in number when cellular needs increase. A mitochondrion is composed of an outer and inner membrane. The **inner membrane** has infoldings that provide **shelves** for the attachment of oxidative phosphorylation enzymes (enzymes for production of energy). The **inner cavity** consists of a **matrix** (supporting substance) that contains enzymes and coenzymes (cofactors) required for extracting energy from nutrients. The matrix is the site of the **citric acid cycle** (also known as the tricarboxylic acid cycle and Krebs cycle).

Lysosomes

The vesicular organelles called **lysosomes** are formed by the Golgi apparatus and then become dispersed throughout the cytoplasm. Because lysosomes contain digestive enzymes, their presence in the cytoplasm provides an intracellular digestive system allowing digestion of damaged cellular structures, food particles ingested by the cell, and bacterial cells.

Centrioles

There are typically two centrioles in a cell, and they are located in an area free of ribosomes and endoplasmic reticulum known as the centrosome. Centrioles are involved with cell division. Cells without centrioles cannot replace themselves by cell division. The centrioles are usually oriented at right angles to each other. Each consists of nine groups of three microtubules arranged in a circle. Microtubules constitute the spindle in mitosis.

■ ENERGY PRODUCTION

1. What substance is formed from the catabolism of carbohydrates, lipids, and proteins to begin the aerobic stage of energy production via the citric acid cycle?
2. What are the cofactors involved in the transfer of electrons from the citric acid cycle to the electron transport chain?
3. Where are the electron receptors of the electron transport chain located?
4. What is the energy substance produced by oxidative phosphorylation?
5. What is metabolic water?
6. What is the location for oxygen consumption by the body?

Within mitochondria, energy is released from molecules by controlled metabolic oxidation. The **aerobic** (occurring in the presence of oxygen) **stage** in the catabolism of carbohydrates, lipids, and proteins begins after the formation of **acetyl-Co A** from respective glucose, fatty acids, and some amino acids (*Fig. 1-2*). The acetyl-Co A that has been formed undergoes oxidation via the citric acid cycle within the matrix. Oxidation of the acetyl groups involves the abstraction of electrons and their transfer to the **cofactors nicotinamide adenine dinucleotide (NAD)** and **flavin adenine dinucleotide (FAD)**, wherein the cofactors are reduced to NADH and $FADH_2$.

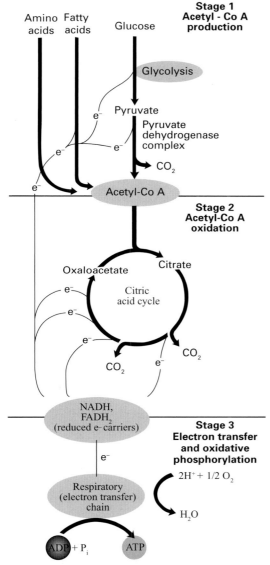

The electrons carried by NADH and $FADH_2$ are funneled to the **electron transfer chain**, a chain of electron acceptors that are an integral part of the inner membrane (the shelf membrane) of the mitochondrion. In the electron flow that follows, **adenosine triphosphate (ATP)**, a high-energy substance, is synthesized from **adenosine diphosphate (ADP)** in the process of **oxidative phosphorylation**. Also, NADH and $FADH_2$ are reoxidized and hydrogen ions (H^+) combine with oxygen (O_2) to form water (H_2O). About 90% of the total ATP formed by glucose metabolism is formed during oxidative phosphorylation described above. The water formed at this location is referred to as metabolic water (see Chapter 2), and also, oxygen consumption for the body occurs at this location (see Chapter 10).

■ FUNCTIONS OF DNA AND RNA

1. What comprises each chromosome?
2. What are the chemical bases that make up the two nucleotide chains of DNA?
3. How are the two nucleotide chains bound together, and what are the complementary positions of the bases?
4. What is the relationship of the histone proteins to the nucleotide chains?
5. Where is the chemical location for the beginning of DNA replication?
6. What is the point of attachment of the two newly formed chromosomes (chromatids) called?
7. Describe a gene as related to the DNA molecule.
8. What are the four stages of mitosis?
9. What is the name of each pair of replicated centrioles?
10. Visualize and describe each of the four stages of mitosis, recognizing interphase as a period between successive sequences.
11. Is DNA in the nucleus able to enter the cytoplasm to initiate the synthesis of protein?

■ **FIGURE 1-2** Catabolism of proteins, fats, and carbohydrates resulting in release of energy. Stage 3, via the electron transfer chain, provides for the oxidative phosphorylation of adenosine diphosphate (ADP) and the production of a high-energy substance, adenosine triphosphate (ATP). This is the location of oxygen consumption by the body and production of metabolic water. (Adapted from Nelson DL, Cox MM. Lehninger Principles of Biochemistry. 3rd Ed. New York: Worth Publishers, 2000.)

12. What are the separate functions of mRNA, tRNA, and rRNA?
13. How is protein synthesis related to allergies and tissue rejection by individual animals?

DNA and Its Replication

The nucleus is composed mostly of the **chromosomes**, those structures providing for inherited and individual characteristics of an animal. Each chromosome is made up of a large molecule of DNA wrapped in the form of **double helices** (a helix is a spiral form) around a core of histone proteins. DNA is made up of two extremely long **polynucleotide chains** each containing the **purine bases** adenine and guanine and the **pyrimidine bases** thymine and cytosine (*Fig. 1-3*). A **nucleotide** is formed by the combination of one molecule of phosphoric acid, one molecule of deoxyribose, and one of the four bases. The chains are bound together by hydrogen bonding between the bases, with adenine bonding to thymine and guanine to cytosine. The bonding relationship is referred to as **complementary** (i.e., they are not identical). Whenever adenine appears on one strand, thymine will be in the same position on the opposite strand. The **histones** are positively charged proteins that associate strongly with DNA by ionic interactions with its many negatively charged phosphate groups. About half of the mass of chromatin is DNA and half is histones. The whole complex of DNA and histones is called chromatin. Before cell division, the coiling around the histone proteins is loosened and replication of DNA begins by splitting the double helices at the point of junction of complementary bases. The separate strands then serve as a template for the formation of its complementary base when replication (making a facsimile or copy) takes place (*Fig. 1-4*). The result is that each of the two original strands of each chromosome is now paired with a new complementary strand, forming two spiral helix chromosomes wher-

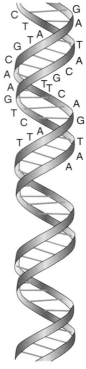

■ **FIGURE 1-3** Two polynucleotide chains constitute the double helix of the DNA molecule. Obligatory base pairing occurs between A (adenine) and T (thymine), and also between G (guanine) and C (cytosine). The chains are held together by hydrogen bonding between bases. Histone proteins (not shown) form a core between the nucleotide chains. (From Cormack DH. Essential Histology. 2nd Ed. Baltimore: Lippincott Williams & Wilkins, 2001.)

ever there was one before. The two newly formed chromosomes remain temporarily attached to each other (until the time for mitosis) at a point called the centromere located near their center. These duplicated but attached chromosomes are called chromatids. The units of heredity are the genes on the chromosomes, and each gene is a portion of the DNA molecule. Large numbers are attached end-on-end on the long, double-stranded, helical molecules of DNA that have molecular weights measured in the billions.

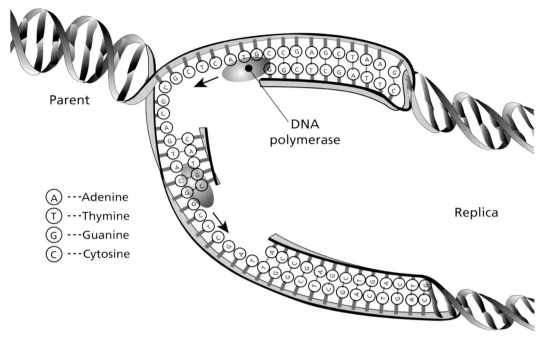

Parent

DNA
polymerase

(A) ---Adenine
(T) ---Thymine
(G) ---Guanine
(C) ---Cytosine

Replica

■ **FIGURE 1-4** Replication of DNA. Coiling around histone proteins is loosened, and the double helices split at point of junction of complementary bases. The separate strands serve as a template for formation of its complementary base. Two new double-helix chromosomes formed where only one was before. (From Frandson RD, Wilke WL, Fails AD. Anatomy and Physiology of Farm Animals. 6th Ed. Baltimore: Lippincott Williams & Wilkins, 2003.)

Mitosis

Mitosis is the division of somatic cells (body cells, as opposed to reproductive cells) in which complex nuclear division precedes cytoplasmic fission and that involves a sequence of four stages: **prophase**, **metaphase**, **anaphase**, and **telophase** (*Fig. 1-5*). The period between successive sequences is called **interphase**. The stages illustrated in Figure 1-5 are not to be considered as stops and starts but rather as an unbroken sequence of events. In the interphase nucleus (nondividing), the chromosomes are in the form of dispersed chromatin. Late in interphase each of the centrioles have replicated so that there are two pairs, each with two centrioles. Each pair is called a centrosome. In early prophase (first step in mitosis), chromatin condenses into chromosomes (the two constituent threads are

called chromatids), and the **mitotic spindle** begins to form, pushing the centrosomes apart. In late prophase, there is further separation of the centrosomes with the development of radiating fibers (microtubules), called **asters**, from each centrosome. The spindle at this point encroaches further into the nucleus as the nuclear membrane gradually disappears. Some of the microtubules become attached to the chromosomes in the area of the centromere. The nucleolus gradually disappears, and the chromosomes shorten and become more visible. In the next step, metaphase, the centrioles are pushed closer to their respective poles by the growing spindle, and the chromatids are aligned at the center of the cell. An early event in anaphase (the next stage) is the separation of the single centromere disc that is common to both chromatids into two so that each chromatid has its own. During anaphase,

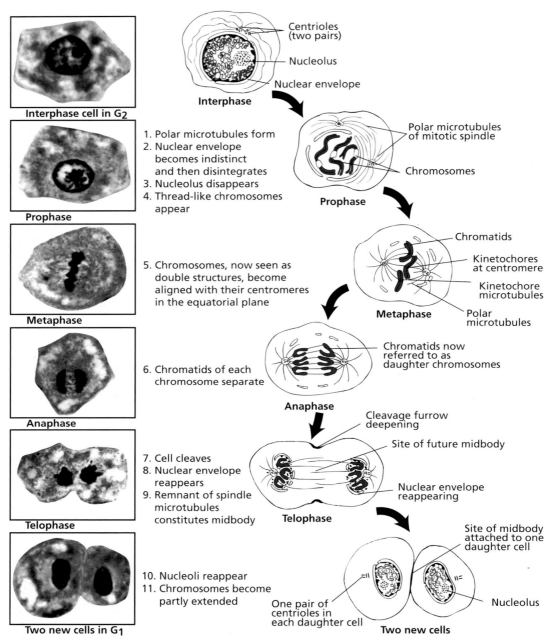

FIGURE 1-5 The stages of mitosis. Until anaphase, the two chromatids of a mitotic chromosome remain joined at a region known as the centromere of the chromosome. At this location, each chromatid has a microtubule attachment site called a kinetochore. (From Cormack DH. Essential Histology. 2nd Ed. Baltimore: Lippincott Williams & Wilkins, 2001.)

separation of the duplicated chromatid takes place (now referred to as **daughter chromosomes**) and they move to opposite poles of the cell, pulled by spindle microtubules attached to the respective centromeres. In telophase, the daughter chromosomes have reached opposite poles of the cell, the mitotic spindles disappear, and a nuclear membrane forms around each set. Two daughter cells form by cell division and then enter early interphase.

RNA and Protein Synthesis

Genes control the formation of cell proteins by a complex process of coding, the so-called **genetic code**. Because of its large size and inability to enter the cytoplasm, DNA in the nucleus is not able to directly control the synthesis of protein that occurs in the cytoplasm. This is accomplished by RNA molecules that are synthesized from DNA. The first of these, **messenger RNA (mRNA)**, moves into the cytoplasm through nuclear pores carrying the code for the synthesis of proteins (**transcription**) and establishes a position with a granular ER ribosome where protein molecules are made. A second, **transfer RNA (tRNA)**, is syn-

thesized by DNA and moves to the cytoplasm, where it picks up an amino acid and carries it to the mRNA. There the amino acid is fitted into the code for the production of a specific protein molecule (**translation**). Each of 20 tRNAs are specific for each of the 20 amino acids. The third type of RNA is **ribosomal RNA (rRNA)**, found in ribosomes. It is believed that it serves as a physical structure on which the protein is formed. The sequence of protein synthesis is shown in *Figure 1-6*. Because of the transfer of information required for protein synthesis from DNA molecules in the nucleus, it can be seen that proteins are specific to each individual animal. Introduction of proteins foreign to an animal results in allergies, tissue rejection, and other incompatibilities.

■ EMBRYOLOGY

1. **Differentiate between diploid and haploid.**
2. **How does meiosis contrast with mitosis?**
3. **What is meiosis accompanied by division of the cells called in the female and in the male?**

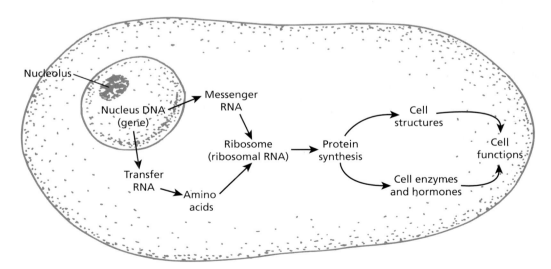

■ **FIGURE 1-6** A schematic summary of genetic coding and its role in protein synthesis and related cell functions.

4. Define embryology.
5. Differentiate among gamete, zygote, morula, and blastocyst.
6. What does the trophoblast contribute to in fetal development?
7. Name the three germ layers established as embryonic development proceeds.
8. What two major events are signified by the development of the germ layers?

Fertilization is the first event of reproduction at the cellular level and requires the joining of the female sex cell (**gamete**), known as the **oocyte**, with the male gamete, known as the **spermatozoon**. So that the fertilized oocyte will have the normal number of chromosomes (**diploid or 2n**), each gamete must be reduced in chromosome numbers by one-half (**haploid or n**) while still in the reproductive systems of the respective female and male. This reduction in chromosomes is called **meiosis**, in contrast to **mitosis**, whereby each cell after division retained the 2n chromosome number. Meiosis accompanied by division of the cells is called **oogenesis** in the female and **spermatogenesis** in the male. The joined gametes now known as a **zygote** will have the proper number of chromosomes (2n) for the species, and further development beyond fertilization will proceed by mitosis. Fertilization and the beginning of mitosis for the formation of a new individual are shown in *Figure 1-7*. For further details of spermatogenesis, oogenesis, and fertilization, see Chapters 14 and 15.

Embryology is the study of prenatal (before birth) development of an individual, and, as indicated above, it begins with the zygote. Mitotic divisions continue and form a cluster of cells known as a **morula** that proceeds to a **blastula** (*Fig. 1-8*). The cavity of the blastula, the **blastocele**, is formed when uterine fluid diffuses into the spaces between the cells of the morula. As the fluid accumulates, it gradually separates the cells into an outer layer of cells called the **trophoblast** and an **inner cell mass** that forms the body of the embryo (*Fig. 1-9A*). The trophoblast contributes to the **fetal placenta (extraembryonic membranes)** that secures the position of the embryo in the uterus and provides for its nutrition from the maternal connection (see Chapter 15).

The portion of the inner cell mass closest to the trophoblast is the **epiblast**, and the portion adjacent to the blastocele is the **hypoblast** (*Fig. 1-9B*). The cavity formed dorsal to the epiblast is the **amniotic cavity** of the embryo (see Chapter 15). Proliferating hypoblast cells migrate to line the blastocele. This lining becomes the **endoderm**. The endoderm grows into the blastocele and generates the lungs, gut, liver, and other visceral organs. The **ectoderm** develops from proliferating outer cells of the inner cell mass (epiblast cells) and migrates toward a longitudinal axis location known as the primitive streak, a thickening of epiblast cells (*Fig. 1-9C*). Skin and all of its derivatives (e.g., hair, hooves, mammary glands) and the entire nervous system are formed from ectoderm. The cells between ectoderm and endoderm become **mesoderm** (*Fig. 1-9D*). The mesoderm grows between the ectoderm and endoderm and splits into two layers that form a cavity between the two layers known as the **coelom (precursor of body cavities)**. The pericardial, pleural, and abdominopelvic cavities are derived from the coelom. Skeletal, smooth, and cardiac muscle, the kidneys, the skeleton, and other connective tissues develop from mesoderm. The establishment of the germ layers is the first segregation of cell groups clearly distinct from one another by way of their definite relations within the embryo. Also, establishment of the germ layers marks the transition between that period of development when an increase in the number of cells was the only outstanding event to one when differentiation and specialization are the dominating aspects of growth. The germ layers are the source of all body structures.

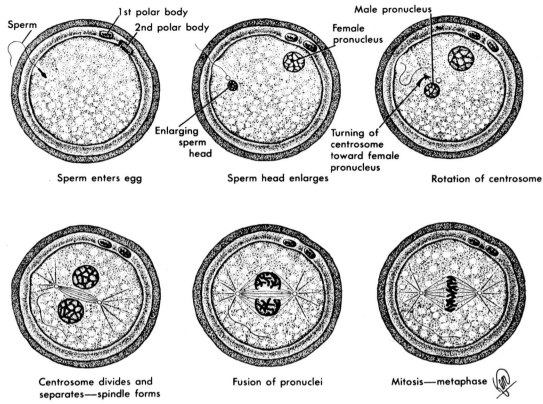

■ FIGURE 1-7 Schematic diagrams of fertilization. Meiosis in spermatozoa and oocytes (division of chromosome numbers by one-half) occurs while in respective male and female reproductive systems. Entrance of a spermatozoon into an oocyte is followed by fusion of respective pronuclei to form a zygote with a proper chromosome number (2n or diploid). Cell division will proceed by mitosis to form a new individual. (From Crouch JE. Functional Human Anatomy. 4th Ed. Philadelphia: Lea & Febiger, 1985.)

■ TISSUES

1. Differentiate among cells, tissues, organs, and systems as units of structure in the body.
2. Name the four basic tissues in the body.
3. Where are the general locations of epithelium?
4. What is the function of a basement membrane?
5. How does epithelium receive nutrition and discharge waste?
6. How is epithelium classified according to the number of cell layers?
7. How is epithelium classified according to shape of the surface cells?
8. Where are the locations of endothelium, mesothelium, and mesenchymal epithelium that are derived from mesoderm and have the appearance of simple squamous epithelium that is derived from ectoderm or endoderm?
9. Know where each of the several classifications of epithelium are located.

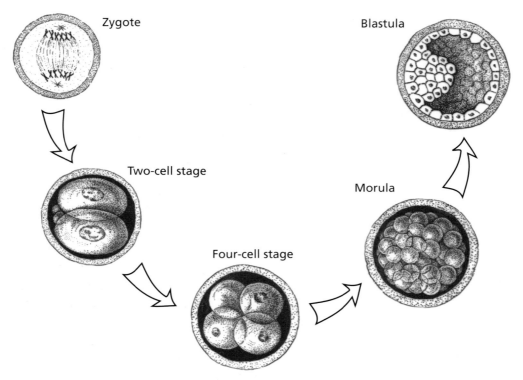

■ **FIGURE 1-8** Continued mitotic division from zygote to blastula. (From Frandson RD, Wilke WL, Fails AD. Anatomy and Physiology of Farm Animals. 6th Ed. Baltimore: Lippincott Williams & Wilkins, 2003.)

10. What is the distinguishing feature between endocrine and exocrine glands?
11. Differentiate among holocrine, merocrine, and apocrine glands.
12. What are the two types of epithelial membranes, and where are they located?
13. What are the chief functions performed by the connective tissue types?
14. What cells produce the intercellular substance of ordinary connective tissue?
15. What are the intercellular substances of loose connective tissue? How do they differ?
16. Differentiate between dense regular and irregular connective tissue.
17. Recognize that cartilage, bone, and blood are other elements of connective tissue.

In considering units of structure within the body, a first consideration involved the cell. The next involves **tissues**, which as a unit, are composed of cells having similar features of structure and function. Two or more tissues, when combined to perform certain functions, are known as **organs** (e.g., the heart and liver are organs). Combinations of organs of similar or related functions, working together as a unit, are represented by **body systems** (e.g., the digestive system and the respiratory system). Most of this book is organized by systems, wherein the cells, tissues, and organs for a system will be studied to recognize the contribution of each in providing for each system's function.

There are four basic tissues in the body, namely: 1) **epithelial tissue (epithelium)**, 2) **connective tissue**, 3) **nervous tissue**, and 4) **muscle tissue**. Unlike nervous and muscle

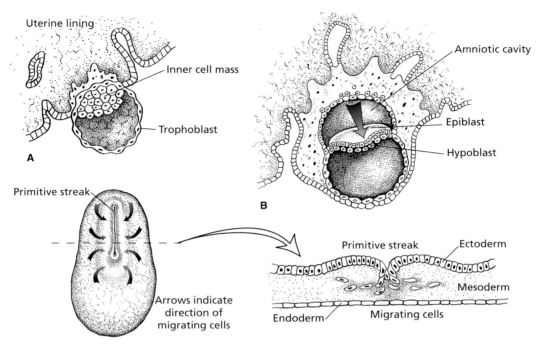

■ FIGURE 1-9 The formation of the germ layers, ectoderm, mesoderm, and endoderm. **A.** Embryo embeds in wall of the uterus. **B.** Formation of epiblast and hypoblast layers. Amniotic cavity is formed dorsal to the epiblast, and the hypoblast cells migrate to line the cavity of the blastula (blastocele), which becomes endoderm. **C.** Embryo viewed from above. The primitive streak is a thickening of epiblast cells on the longitudinal axis that migrate toward the primitive streak and become ectoderm. **D.** Cross-section through the region of the primitive streak showing migration of cells between ectoderm and endoderm that become mesoderm. (From Frandson RD, Wilke WL, Fails AD. Anatomy and Physiology of Farm Animals. 6th Ed. Baltimore: Lippincott Williams & Wilkins, 2003.)

tissues, epithelial and connective tissues are not considered in individual chapters as a system. Therefore, some identifying features will now be given.

Epithelium

Epithelial tissues cover the body surface, line body cavities, and form glands and other structures (e.g., hair, hooves, and horns). With few exceptions, epithelium originates from ectoderm or endoderm, and the cells lie on a noncellular basement membrane. The **basement membrane** serves an adhesive function so that the cells are held closely to the underlying

connective tissue, thereby giving greater strength to the tissue.

Epithelial tissues are not penetrated by blood vessels but rather receive nutrition and discharge waste by diffusion via blood vessels in the underlying or neighboring connective tissue.

Classification

When classified according to the number of layers of cells in the tissue, **simple epithelium** (one layer) and **stratified epithelium** (two or more layers) are recognized. There is also a classification according to shape of the surface cells, namely: 1) **squamous** (thin and plate-like), 2) **cubical**, being about equal in height and width (appear square in a cut perpendicular to the surface), and 3) **columnar**, in which the cells are taller than they are wide and in a perpendicular section are rectangular.

The types of epithelium that commonly exist throughout the body are illustrated in *Figure 1-10*. It will be noted that each is identified according to number of layers and also shape of the cell, and the following are identified:

1. Simple squamous epithelium (*Fig. 1-10A*).

   Simple squamous epithelium consists of a single layer of thin, flat cells of irregular outlines that fit together, with cement substances between their borders, to form a continuous, thin membrane. It is not

adapted to withstanding wear and tear but rather to performing a filtering function (e.g., some portions of kidney tubules).

There are three tissues that have the same appearance as simple squamous epithelium but differ because they are derived from mesoderm rather than ectoderm or endoderm. In these instances they are known as endothelium, mesothelium, and mesenchymal epithelium. **Endothelium** is the simple layer of squamous cells forming the inner lining of the heart, blood vessels, and lymph vessels. **Mesothelium** is the simple squamous epithelium that lines the great body cavities (pleura and peritoneum). **Mesenchymal** epithelium is found in more discreet locations such as the linings of the subarachnoid spaces (in the brain) and chambers of the eye.

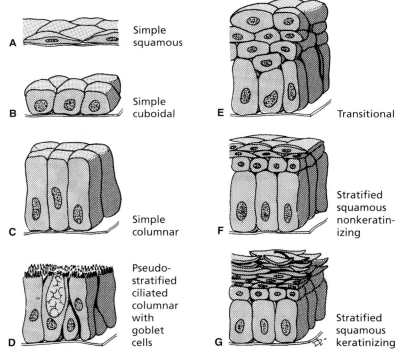

A — Simple squamous
B — Simple cuboidal
C — Simple columnar
D — Pseudo-stratified ciliated columnar with goblet cells
E — Transitional
F — Stratified squamous nonkeratinizing
G — Stratified squamous keratinizing

■ **FIGURE 1-10** Epithelial tissue classifications. The epithelial cells are shown lying on a noncellular basement membrane that serves an adhesive function holding the cells closely to the underlying connective tissue. (From Cormack DH. Essential Histology. 2nd Ed. Baltimore: Lippincott Williams & Wilkins, 2001.)

2. Simple cuboidal epithelium (*Fig. 1-10B*).

    This is a widely distributed tissue, and examples are found in the choroid plexus of the nervous system, the outer covering of the nervous system, the outer covering of the ovary (reproductive system), and the lining of follicles in the thyroid gland (endocrine system).

3. Simple columnar epithelium (*Fig. 1-10C*).

    This tissue provides the lining for the digestive tract. The cells may be absorptive, secretory, or both. A common secretory function of these cells is secretion of mucus on the surface of epithelial membranes, and in this capacity they provide a protective function. There are also simple columnar ciliated tissues. **Cilia** are motile extensions of a cell surface that move tubular contents in a single direction. An example of their presence is in the uterine tubes (oviducts).

4. Pseudostratified ciliated columnar with goblet cells (*Fig. 1-10D*).

    These tissues seem to consist of many layers but actually have only one layer. The one shown is ciliated, but there are also those that are nonciliated. The stratified appearance is caused by some of the cells being short and other taller cells overlapping them. They both share a common basement membrane. The type shown, with cilia and goblet cells, are found in the respiratory tract. The **goblet cells** provide for a wet surface for entrapment of inhaled particles, and the cilia direct the wet surface toward the mouth.

5. Transitional epithelium (*Fig. 1-10E*).

    This tissue is common to the lining of the muscular urinary bladder. It is a stratified epithelium with a varied appearance depending on the fill of the bladder. When the bladder contracts, the epithelium piles up into many layers, but when the bladder fills and is stretched, only two or three layers of cells can be seen.

6. Stratified squamous (*Fig. 1-10, F and G*).

    Stratified membranes serve chiefly to protect. They can withstand more wear and tear than simple membranes. There are dif-ferent kinds and degrees of protection needed at different places in the body, and accordingly, stratified membranes have dis-similarities. The kind shown in the illustra-tion is nonkeratinized stratified squamous epithelium (*Fig. 1-10F*) and is found on wet surfaces subjected to wear and tear. The inside of the mouth and esophagus have this lining, giving protection from coarse foods. Only the surface cells are actually squamous, the deepest layer (on the base-ment membrane) of cells is columnar. As the deep layer cells undergo mitotic divi-sion, the outer cells flatten, die, and finally, slough (separate) from the surface. In this way the tissue renews itself. The epidermis (outer layer) of skin is stratified squamous keratinized tissue (*Fig. 1-10G*). This differs from nonkeratinized epithelium in that the superficial cells are **keratinized (also called cornified)**. The cells of this type are also fused with each other. The cornified and fused layer minimizes fluid loss from the body by evaporation and gives greater pro-tection from wear and tear.

Glands

The glands of the body are classified as exo-crine or endocrine. Both are secretory, but **exocrine glands** are those that have secretions to the outside of the body, and **endocrine glands** are those that secrete within the body. Exocrine glands must be provided with ducts, which are tubes that convey the glandular secretions to a free surface of the body. Because endocrine secretions are those within the body, no ducts are needed and they are often referred to as **ductless glands**.

Development of both glands is shown sche-matically in *Figure 1-11*. It is noted that both originate as a result of surface epithelial cells growing, in the form of either a cord or a tubule, into the connective tissue beneath the membrane. After invasion of the connective tissue, a gland is formed by means of further proliferation and differentiation. The epithelial

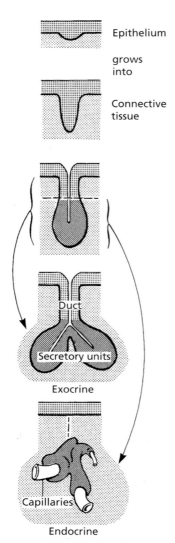

■ FIGURE 1-11 The development of exocrine and endocrine glands. A duct is maintained for exocrine glands, whereas endocrine glands are ductless. (From Cormack DH. Essential Histology. 2nd Ed. Baltimore: Lippincott Williams & Wilkins, 2001.)

connection between the gland and surface is retained for exocrine glands, whereas the connection disappears for endocrine glands. Those cells that form the secretory unit secrete their substances into a central cavity or lumen.

Holocrine, merocrine, and apocrine glands refer to the manner in which the secretory cells of the gland elaborate their secretions. A cell within **holocrine glands** accumulates secretory products in its cytoplasm and then dies and disintegrates. The dead cell and its products constitute the secretion (i.e., the entire cell is secreted). The sebaceous (oily, fatty) glands of the skin are of this type.

Merocrine glands secrete without any part of the cell being lost. Secretory granules are cytoplasmic inclusions, and although produced by the cytoplasm, they are not actually part of the cytoplasm. Therefore, the secretory granules pass into the lumen of the secretory unit without loss of the secretory cells' cytoplasm. The pancreas and salivary glands are in this group.

Apocrine glands are intermediate between holocrine and merocrine glands because their secretions gather at the outer ends of the gland cells and then pinch off to form the secretions. The mammary glands and some sweat glands belong to this group.

Epithelial Membranes

Epithelial membranes consist of a surface layer of epithelium and an underlying layer of connective tissue. Two kinds that are of importance in the body are mucous membranes and serous membranes.

Mucous membranes, referred to as mucosae, line the hollow organs and cavities that open on the skin surface of the body. These membranes line most of the organs of the digestive, respiratory, urinary, and reproductive systems. The surface epithelium may vary in type, but it is always kept moist by mucus. The connective tissue underlying the epithelium is referred to as the lamina propria.

Serous membranes, referred to as **serosae**, line the body cavities and cover the surfaces of related organs. The surface epithelium is mesothelium over a thin layer of loose connective tissue. The mesothelium provides fluid that serves to moisten and lubricate. Pleura (lining the thorax), pericardium (lining the heart), and peritoneum (lining the abdomen) are examples of serous membranes.

Connective Tissue

Connective tissues are represented by a wide range of tissues that share a common origin from mesoderm. The chief functions performed by the various cells of the different types of connective tissue follow: 1) production of intercellular substances, 2) storing fat (adipocytes), and 3) production of the various blood cells, which in turn have specific functions (e.g., phagocytosis of bacteria and production of antibodies). The intercellular substance of chondrocytes and osteocytes (cartilage and bone) are connective tissues specialized for the support of the body. **Cartilage**, **bone**, and **blood** are elements of connective tissue that will be described in separate chapters.

Ordinary Connective Tissues

Ordinary connective tissues connect other tissues and are classified as either loose or dense.

Loose connective tissue contains a variety of different cell types. Loose connective tissue is widely distributed in the body, where it makes up the subcutaneous tissue or superficial fascia. It penetrates between organs to fill space and bind structures together. Because of its loose nature, it allows for movement of muscles relative to one another. **Fibroblasts** are the cells that produce the intercellular substance of ordinary connective tissue. When less active during adult life, fibroblasts are often referred to as **fibrocytes**.

Important intercellular substances of loose connective tissue are 1) collagenous or white fibers, 2) elastic or yellow fibers, 3) reticular fibers, and 4) amorphous ground substance. **Collagenous fibers** appear as wavy ribbons. They are strong and inelastic and are composed of collagen, a family of closely related proteins. **Elastic fibers** are long cylindrical threads or flat ribbons. They tend to regain their original shape after being stretched. They are formed in elastic arteries and are mixed with other tissues wherever elasticity is needed. **Reticular connective tissue fibers** are fine and highly branched. They make up part of the framework of endocrine and lymphatic organs and also form networks where structures are adjacent to connective tissue, as found along the blood vessels, in basement membranes, and around nerve, muscle, and fat cells. Like collagenous fibers, they are inelastic. The above fibers are imbedded in **amorphous** (without form) **ground substance**. The viscosity of amorphous ground substance varies from fluids to gel. *Figure 1-12* illustrates cells and fibers that might be seen in a microscopic section of loose connective tissue.

Dense connective tissues contain essentially the same fiber elements as loose connective tissues. There are two types, **dense regular** and **dense irregular**. The regularity relates to the arrangement of the fiber elements. In dense regular connective tissue, the fibers (especially collagenous fibers) are arranged in parallel bundles forming tendons. In ligaments, the collagenous fibers are not as regularly arranged and may be mixed with elastic fibers. The ligamentum nuchae in the necks of grazing animals has a predominance of elastic fibers. In dense irregular connective tissue, the collagenous fibers are interwoven and compacted to form a dense matting. This type is found in the dermis of the skin. The dermis of the skin is used in the production of leather. It is treated with tannic acid after the epidermis is removed.

Cartilage, bone, and blood are other elements of connective tissue that will be described separately in respective chapters.

■ DIRECTIONAL TERMS AND PLANES

1. **Know the definitions of the directional terms and planes, and visualize the application of these as shown in *Figure 1-13*.**

Throughout this book, descriptive terms will be used when referring to the location of body parts. These frames of reference are in

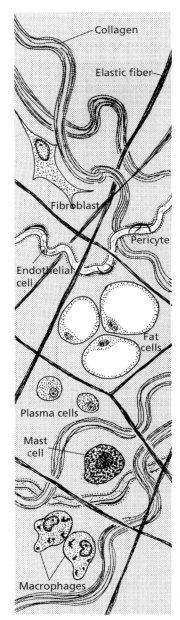

Collagen

Elastic fiber

Fibroblast

Pericyte

Endothelial cell

Fat cells

Plasma cells

Mast cell

Macrophages

■ **FIGURE 1-12** Fibers and cells of loose connective tissue. Mast cells are usually found close to small blood vessels and have granules containing potent inflammatory mediators (e.g., histamine). Macrophages are phagocytic, and plasma cells are the source of circulating antibodies (immunoglobulins). Pericytes are intimately associated with blood capillaries and venules, providing a potential source of new fibroblasts and smooth muscle cells. (From Cormack DH. Essential Histology. 2nd Ed. Baltimore: Lippincott Williams & Wilkins, 2001.)

relation to the animal itself and apply regardless of the position or direction of the animal.

Definitions of the terms that follow are illustrated in Figure 1-13 and apply to quadrupeds (four-footed animals).

1. **Cranial** is a direction toward the head. The lungs are cranial to the intestines (closer to the head).
2. **Caudal** is a direction toward the tail. The intestines are caudal to the lungs (closer to the tail).
3. **Rostral** and **caudal** are terms for direction within the head to mean toward the nose (rostral) or toward the tail (caudal). The cerebrum is rostral to the cerebellum.
4. The **median plane** is one that passes through the body craniocaudally (from head to tail). It divides the body into equal right and left halves.
5. A **sagittal plane** is any plane parallel to the median plane, and except for the midsagittal plane (which is another name for the median plane), it would be either to the right or to the left of the median plane.
6. A **transverse plane** is at right angles to the median plane and divides the body into cranial and caudal parts. A cross-sectional view of the body or part would be made on the transverse plane.
7. A **horizontal plane** is at right angles to both the median and the transverse planes and would divide the body into dorsal (upper) and ventral (lower) segments.
8. **Dorsal** pertains to the back or upper surface of an animal. Often used to indicate the position of one structure of the body relative to another (i.e., nearer the back surface of the body). The kidneys are dorsal to the intestines.
9. **Ventral** pertains to the undersurface of an animal, and as with dorsal, is often used to indicate the position of one structure relative to another. The intestines are ventral to the kidneys.
10. **Medial** relates to the middle or center; nearer to the median or midsagittal plane. The heart is medial to the lungs.

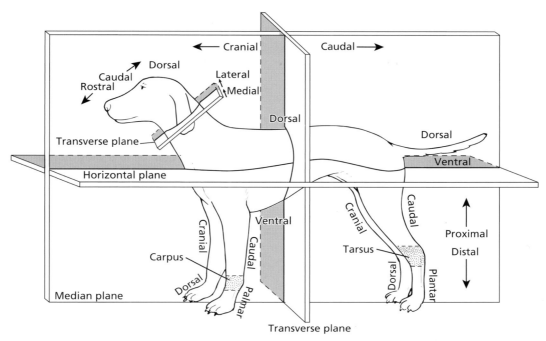

■ **FIGURE 1-13** Directional terms and planes as applied to four-footed animals. The stippled areas represent the carpus and tarsus on the forelimbs and hindlimbs, respectively.

11. **Lateral** is opposite to the meaning of medial (i.e., away from the median plane). The ribs are lateral to the lungs. A lateral radiographic (x-ray) view is one with the animal on its side and the film in the sagittal plane.

12. **Superficial** pertains to the surface or to a structure situated near the surface. The skin is superficial to the muscles.

13. **Deep** refers to a structure situated at a deeper level in relation to a specific reference point. The femur is deep to the quadriceps muscles.

14. **Proximal**, when referring to part of a limb, artery, or nerve, means it is nearest the center of the body or the point of origin.

15. **Distal** means relatively farther from the center of the body. The hoof is distal to the knee.

16. **Palmar** refers to the caudal surface of the forelimb distal to the carpus (joint connecting radius, ulna, and metacarpals).

Dorsal refers to its opposite cranial side.

17. **Plantar** refers to the caudal surface of the hindlimb distal to the tarsus (also known as the hock; joint connecting tibia, fibula, and metatarsals). Dorsal refers to its opposite (cranial) side.

18. **Prone** refers to a position in which the dorsal aspect of the body or any extremity is uppermost. A radiograph from this position with the film on the ventral aspect is identified as a dorsal-ventral view.

19. **Supine** refers to a position in which the ventral aspect of the body or palmar or plantar aspect of an extremity is uppermost. A radiograph from this position with the film on the dorsal aspect is identified as a ventral-dorsal view.

■ BODY CAVITIES

1.   **What are the subdivisions of the ventral body cavity?**

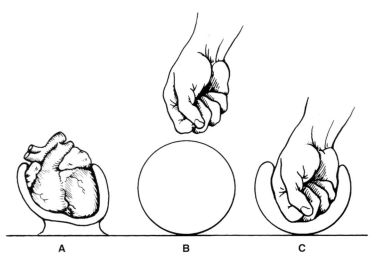

■ **FIGURE 1-14** Invagination of the serous membrane to form outer (parietal) and inner (visceral) layers (**A**). Development proceeded similar to a fist being pushed into a balloon (**B** and **C**). (From Frandson RD, Wilke WL, Fails AD. Anatomy and Physiology of Farm Animals. 6th Ed. Baltimore: Lippincott Williams & Wilkins, 2003.)

2. **Differentiate between visceral and parietal pleura.**
3. **What is the mediastinal space?**
4. **What structures occupy the mediastinal space?**
5. **Differentiate between the abdominal and pelvic cavities with regard to the structures contained in each.**
6. **What is the peritoneum?**
7. **Differentiate among omentum, mesentery, and ligaments.**

A median plane view would show two main body cavities, the dorsal and ventral, and each has its subdivisions. The **dorsal cavity** contains the brain in its **cranial cavity** and the spinal cord in its **vertebral cavity**. The **ventral cavity** is subdivided by the diaphragm into the **thoracic cavity** cranially and the **abdominal** and **pelvic cavities** (collectively known as **abdominopelvic cavity**) caudally.

Thoracic Cavity

The thoracic cavity is divided into two lateral chambers. Each chamber is lined by a serous membrane called the **pleura**, and is termed a pleural cavity. The right and left lungs occupy their respective cavity and are enveloped by **visceral pleura**, which is continuous with the **parietal pleura** (mediastinal and costal). The envelopment occurs during embryonic development. An analogy is that of pushing one's fist into a partially inflated balloon, as shown for the heart in *Figure 1-14*. The space between the two lungs is known as the **mediastinal space** or **mediastinum** (*Fig. 1-15*). It is a partition between the two pleural cavities. The heart, thoracic parts of the esophagus, trachea, vessels, and nerves are contained in the mediastinum, which is bounded laterally by mediastinal pleura. The **mediastinal pleurae** are the parietal pleurae that cover the sides of the partition between the two pleural cavities, and the **costal pleurae** line the walls of the thorax. The partition completely separates the right and left pleural cavities for all of the domestic animals except the dog and horse.

The Abdominopelvic Cavity

The abdominal cavity contains the kidneys, most of the digestive organs, and parts of the

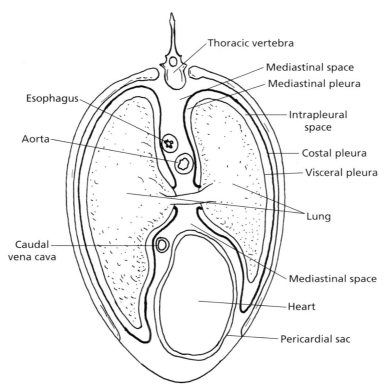

Esophagus

Aorta

Caudal
vena cava

Thoracic vertebra

Mediastinal space
Mediastinal pleura

Intrapleural
space

Costal pleura

Visceral pleura

Lung

Mediastinal space

Heart

Pericardial sac

■ **FIGURE 1-15** Schematic transverse plane of equine thorax. The thoracic portions of esophagus, aorta, caudal venae cavae, and the heart are shown in the mediastinal space.

internal reproductive organs in both sexes. The pelvic cavity contains the rectum (terminal part of the gastrointestinal tract) and the internal parts of the urogenital system not otherwise found in the abdominal cavity. A serous membrane similar to that surrounding the heart and lungs is also found in the abdominopelvic cavity and is known as peritoneum.

The Peritoneum

The peritoneum lines the abdominal cavity and extends into the pelvic cavity. The abdominal organs begin development in a subserous (outside of the peritoneum) location, near the body wall. During development the organs enlarge and migrate into the abdominal cavity.

They carry the peritoneum before them (introversion), and folds are formed that suspend them from the wall (*Fig. 1-16*). The connecting folds are termed omenta, mesenteries, and ligaments. They contain a varying amount of connective tissue, fat, and lymph glands, and provide a pathway for vessels and nerves of the organs. An **omentum** is a fold that passes from the stomach to other viscera (soft structures). A **mesentery** is a fold that attaches the intestine to the dorsal wall of the abdominal cavity. **Ligaments** are folds that pass between viscera, other than parts of the digestive tube, or connect them with the abdominal wall. The coronary ligament (*Fig. 1-16*) is a sheet of peritoneum that passes between the diaphragm and the liver around the caudal vena cava and hepatic veins.

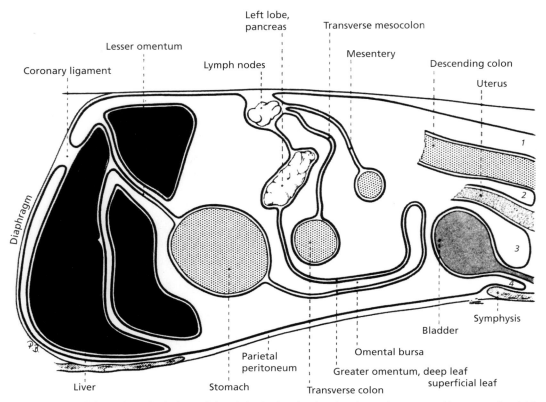

■ FIGURE 1-16 Schematic sagittal plane of the abdominal cavity showing the peritoneum and its connecting folds. (From Evans HE, deLahunta A. Guide to the Dissection of the Dog. 5th Ed. Philadelphia: WB Saunders Company, 2000.) 1. Pararectal fossa. 2. Rectogenital pouch. 3. Vesicogenital pouch. 4. Pubovesical pouch.

■ SUGGESTED READING

Cormack DH. Essential Histology. 2nd Ed. Baltimore: Lippincott Williams & Wilkins, 2001.
Evans HE, deLahunta A. Guide to the Dissection of the Dog. 5th Ed. Philadelphia: WB Saunders Company, 2000.

Frandson RD, Wilke WL, Fails AD. Anatomy and Physiology of Farm Animals. 6th Ed. Baltimore: Lippincott Williams & Wilkins, 2003.
Nelson DL, Cox MM. Lehninger Principles of Biochemistry. 3rd Ed. New York: Worth Publishers, 2000.

☑ SELF EVALUATION—CHAPTER 1

THE CELL, ITS STRUCTURE AND FUNCTIONS

1. The Golgi apparatus is associated with:
   a. cell reproduction.
   b. energy production.
   c. packaging materials for transport.
   d. protein synthesis.

2. The endoplasmic reticulum:
   a. is entirely separate from the nucleus.
   b. has agranular locations associated with protein synthesis.
   c. has granular locations with ribosome attachments and is associated with protein synthesis.

d. has an internal fluid with the same composition as that found in the cytoplasm.

3. Which one of the organelles is the site of the citric acid cycle?
   a. Mitochondria
   b. Lysosomes
   c. Centrioles
   d. Endoplasmic reticulum

ENERGY PRODUCTION

4. The aerobic stage of energy production from carbohydrate, lipid, and protein catabolism involves:
   a. acetyl-Co A.
   b. NAD and FAD.
   c. the citric acid cycle.
   d. all of the above.

5. The electron transfer chain is located in the:
   a. endoplasmic reticulum.
   b. mitochondria.
   c. nucleus.
   d. Golgi apparatus.

6. In the electron flow in the electron transfer chain:
   a. ATP is synthesized from ADP (oxidative phosphorylation).
   b. NADH and $FADH_2$ are oxidized.
   c. oxygen is consumed and metabolic water is produced.
   d. all of the above.

FUNCTIONS OF DNA AND RNA

7. A chromosome is:
   a. the same as a gene.
   b. a large molecule of DNA.
   c. a large molecule of RNA.
   d. the histone portion of DNA.

8. Chromatids:
   a. are paired, identical chromosomes formed from chromatin in early prophase.
   b. is another name for chromatin.

c. are the paired centrioles.
d. are formed during telophase.

9. Mitosis:
   a. is a phenomenon of cell division in which each cell after division has a haploid chromosome number.
   b. is the division of somatic cells in which nuclear division precedes cytoplasmic fission.
   c. is the division of reproductive cells (oocytes and spermatozoa) in which each cell after division has a diploid chromosome number.
   d. concludes with the anaphase stage.

10. The sequence of bases on one strand of DNA is TGCCAT. What would be the sequence of bases of its complementary strand within a DNA double helix?
    a. ACGGTA
    b. CATTGC
    c. GTAACG
    d. TGCCAT

11. During replication of DNA:
    a. the double helix is not split and a new double helix forms by its side.
    b. the double helix is split and each nucleotide chain is identified as the new chromosome.
    c. the double helix is split and each nucleotide chain becomes paired with a new complementary strand, forming two double-helix chromosomes.
    d. the duplicated attached chromosomes are called centromeres.

12. The synthesis of protein:
    a. occurs in the cytoplasm and is accomplished by RNA molecules.
    b. occurs in the nucleus and is accomplished by DNA molecules.
    c. occurs within the endoplasmic reticulum.
    d. has nothing to do with the DNA.

13. During the synthesis of protein:
    a. only one tRNA is involved in its synthesis.

b. tRNA is synthesized by the Golgi apparatus in the cytoplasm.

c. tRNA enters the nucleus with its attached amino acid for the nuclear synthesis.

d. tRNAs, specific for each of 20 amino acids, move to the cytoplasm to pick up respective amino acids and carry it to the mRNA, where it is fitted into the code for a specific protein molecule.

EMBRYOLOGY

14. Meiosis:
    a. is the same as mitosis except that it occurs in reproductive cells, the oocytes and spermatozoa.
    b. begins after fertilization of the oocyte by the spermatozoa.
    c. results in a reduction of chromosome numbers by one-half (haploid or n) while still in the reproductive systems of the male and female.
    d. happens beyond fertilization and during the formation of a new individual.

15. The nervous system develops from the germ layer known as:
    a. ectoderm.
    b. mesoderm.
    c. endoderm.
    d. hypoderm.

16. The celom is the forerunner of:
    a. skeletal, smooth, and cardiac muscle.
    b. the pericardial, pleural, and abdomino-pelvic cavities.
    c. the skin and all of its derivatives.
    d. the placenta.

TISSUES

17. Epithelial tissues are derived from:
    a. ectoderm.
    b. endoderm.
    c. mesoderm.
    d. both a and b.

18. Epithelium that appears to consist of many layers but actually only has one layer is known as:
    a. stratified squamous.
    b. transitional.
    c. simple columnar.
    d. pseudostratified columnar.

19. Glands with cells that accumulate secretory products in their cytoplasm and then die and disintegrate are known as:
    a. apocrine glands.
    b. merocrine glands.
    c. holocrine glands.
    d. pep glands.

20. Mucous membranes:
    a. line body cavities and cover the surfaces of related organs.
    b. line the hollow organs and cavities that open on the skin surface of the body.
    c. are represented by pleura, pericardium, and peritoneum.
    d. both a and c.

21. Tissues that produce intercellular substances (e.g., cartilage and bone), store fat, and produce various blood cells are known as:
    a. connective tissues.
    b. epithelial tissues.
    c. nervous tissues.
    d. muscle tissues.

22. Collagenous or white fibers, and elastic or yellow fibers:
    a. are intercellular substances produced by fibroblasts.
    b. are found in loose connective tissue.
    c. are found in dense connective tissue.
    d. a, b, and c.

DIRECTIONAL TERMS AND PLANES

23. Within the head, rostral means:
    a. toward the nose.
    b. the same as cranial.
    c. toward the tail.
    d. the same as caudal.

24. A sagittal plane is:
    a. one that divides the body into cranial and caudal parts.
    b. any plane parallel to the median plane.
    c. one that would divide the body into upper (dorsal) and lower (ventral) segments.
    d. equipped with jets.

25. The part of a limb, artery, or nerve that is nearest the center of the body or point of origin is referred to as:
    a. proximal.
    b. palmar.
    c. distal.
    d. superficial.

26. The position in which the dorsal aspect of the body or any extremity is uppermost is known as:
    a. supine.
    b. upside.
    c. prone.
    d. downer.

BODY CAVITIES

27. The mediastinum:
    a. is located in the abdominal cavity.
    b. contains the heart, thoracic parts of the esophagus, trachea, vessels, and nerves.
    c. is bounded by peritoneum.
    d. contains the lungs.

28. A mesentery is a connecting fold of the peritoneum that:
    a. attaches the intestine to the dorsal wall of the abdominal cavity.
    b. passes from the stomach to other soft structural viscera.
    c. passes between viscera other than parts of the digestive tube, or connects them with the abdominal wall.
    d. separates the abdominal cavity from the pelvic cavity.

29. The serous membrane that lines the wall of the thoracic cavity is:
    a. parietal pleura.
    b. parietal peritoneum.
    c. visceral pleura.
    d. visceral peritoneum.

30. Omentum refers to a peritoneal fold:
    a. passing from the stomach to other soft structure viscera.
    b. passing between viscera other than parts of the digestive tube.
    c. that attaches the intestine to the dorsal wall of the abdominal cavity.
    d. in the thoracic cavity.

ANSWERS TO SELF EVALUATION—CHAPTER 1

1. c	9. b	17. d	25. a
2. c	10. a	18. d	26. c
3. a	11. c	19. c	27. b
4. d	12. a	20. b	28. a
5. b	13. d	21. a	29. a
6. d	14. c	22. d	30. a
7. b	15. a	23. a	
8. a	16. b	24. b	

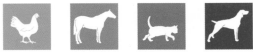

Body Water: Properties and Functions

CHAPTER OUTLINE

■ **PHYSICOCHEMICAL PROPERTIES OF SOLUTIONS**
Diffusion
Osmosis and Osmotic Pressure
Tone of a Solution
Interconversion of Units of Measurement
■ **DISTRIBUTION OF BODY WATER**
Total Body Water and Fluid Compartments
Intracellular and Extracellular Fluid
■ **WATER BALANCE**
Water Gain

Water Loss
Water Requirements
■ **DEHYDRATION, THIRST, AND WATER INTAKE**
Dehydration
Stimulus for Thirst
Relief of Thirst
■ **ADAPTATION TO WATER LACK**
Camels
Sheep and Donkeys

Water is the most abundant constituent of the body fluids, about 60% of the total body weight. It is the solvent for the many chemicals of the body, and the solutions thus formed provide the diffusion media for the body cells.

The physical properties of water make it ideal for this transport function. It has a relatively high specific heat, whereby heat from the cells is absorbed with a minimum of temperature increase. Water also provides the lubrication necessary for minimizing friction associated with fluid flow, cell movement, and movement of body parts.

■ PHYSICOCHEMICAL PROPERTIES OF SOLUTIONS

1. **How does facilitated diffusion differ from simple diffusion?**
2. **What parts of a cell membrane (protein or lipids) account for the diffusion of water-soluble substances? What parts are considered to be the pores?**
3. **How does active transport differ from facilitated diffusion?**
4. **Define osmosis.**
5. **Define a semipermeable membrane.**
6. **Define osmotic pressure and how it is determined.**
7. **How does a selectively permeable membrane differ from a semipermeable one?**
8. **As related to tone, how does effective osmotic pressure for a solution differ from a measured osmotic pressure?**
9. **What is the difference between hemoglobinemia and hemoglobinuria?**

An understanding of the physicochemical properties of solutions can be considered just as important to the study of physiology as knowledge of anatomy. These properties will be encountered when studying most of the systems that follow. Further, successful fluid replacement and correction of deficiencies in live animals require an understanding of solution composition and effects of their administration. Mark Twain said, "Education that consists in learning things and not the meaning of them is feeding upon the husks and not the corn." It is in this context that the basic principles of physicochemical properties of solutions are presented.

Diffusion

Simple diffusion refers to the random movement of molecules, ions, and suspended colloid particles under the influence of brownian (thermal) motion. If a concentration gradient (differential) exists, molecules, ions, and colloidal particles tend to move from the area of their higher concentration to the area of their lower concentration, "downhill." The movement is specific to each substance (i.e., Na^+ will diffuse from the area of its higher concentration to the area of its lower concentration, regardless of the presence and concentrations of other substances). If the molecules and ions are dispersed equally, the random motion continues but does not accomplish net movement or flow; this represents a state of equilibrium. Energy is not required for simple diffusion.

Barriers to diffusion are generally the membranes of cells. These consist of a lipid bilayer, which is a thin film of lipid only two molecules thick through which fat-soluble substances (especially carbon dioxide and oxygen) can readily diffuse (*Fig. 2-1*). There might be **facilitated diffusion** for other substances, in which a carrier is required (*Fig. 2-2*). Facilitated diffusion for any substance, however, still occurs from the area of its higher concentration to that of its lower concentration, and as in simple diffusion, energy is not required. Because cell membranes are predominantly lipid, they are relatively hydrophobic (water repelling), and the diffusion of water through the lipid bilayer proceeds with difficulty, but water can diffuse through protein channels. **Protein channels** (*Fig. 2-1*) consist of large protein molecules interspersed in the lipid film; they provide structural pathways ("pores") not only for water, but also for water-soluble substances. Some substances might be excluded from diffusion through the pores because of their large size; conversely, diffusion might be facilitated because of other factors, such as a substance's relatively smaller size, its electrical charge (e.g., negative pore charge assists Na^+ diffusion), or the protein channel's specificity (e.g., specific ion channels). Other protein channels act as carrier proteins for transport of substances in a direction opposite to their natural diffusion direction. This is known as **active**

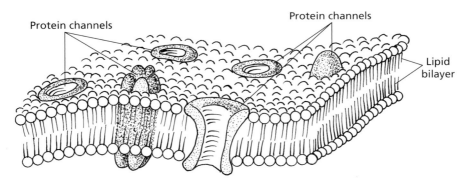

■ **FIGURE 2-1** Structure of a cell membrane. The lipid bilayer is represented by a thin film of lipid that is two molecules thick. The protein channels (pores) may be composed of a single protein or a cluster of proteins. The channels may have specificity for certain substances, or they may be restrictive because of size. Virtually all water diffuses through the protein channels.

Lipid Bilayer

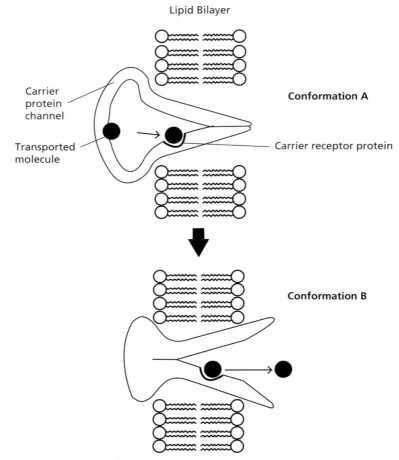

Conformation A

Carrier protein channel

Transported molecule

Carrier receptor protein

Conformation B

■ **FIGURE 2-2** A postulated mechanism for facilitated diffusion. **A**. The transported molecule enters the protein channel and binds with the receptor at the binding site. **B**. Subsequent to binding, the protein channel undergoes a conformational change to open the channel on the opposite side, and the transported molecule is released, causing return of the protein channel to its original conformation.

transport. Whereas the transport of glucose into most cells of the body is accomplished by facilitated diffusion, exceptions exist in the lumens of the kidney tubules and intestines, where active transport is involved. In these locations, glucose is continually transported into the blood even though its concentration in the lumen may be minute. Loss of glucose from the body is thereby prevented by active transport directed "uphill." Active transport not only requires a carrier, but also requires energy.

Osmosis and Osmotic Pressure

The most abundant substance in the body that diffuses is water. Diffusion of water occurs throughout the body relatively easily. The amount diffusing into cells is usually balanced by an equal amount diffusing out. **Osmosis** is the process of diffusion of water through a semipermeable membrane from a solution of higher water concentration to a solution of lower water concentration. A **semipermeable membrane** is one that is permeable (permits

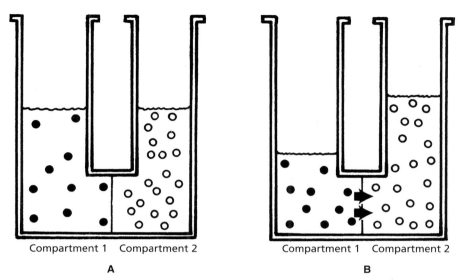

Compartment 1   Compartment 2

A

Compartment 1   Compartment 2

B

■ **FIGURE 2-3** Osmosis. **A**. Before osmosis. Equal volumes of aqueous solutions (solutes represented by black circles and open circles) are placed in compartments that are separated by a membrane permeable to water but not to the solutes (semipermeable membrane). The aqueous solution in compartment 1 has the highest concentration of water (lowest concentration of solute). **B**. During osmosis. Osmosis (diffusion of water) occurs from compartment 1 to compartment 2 (highest water concentration to lowest water concentration) and the water level rises in compartment 2.

passage) to water but not to solutes. When comparing water concentrations of solutions, it is implied that the solution with the highest water concentration has the lowest solute concentration. A situation in which osmosis could occur is illustrated in *Figure 2-3*. Net diffusion has occurred from the compartment with the highest water concentration to the one with the lowest water concentration.

The quantitative measure of the tendency for water to osmose is the **osmotic pressure**. This is the pressure that would have to be applied to the compartment with the lowest water concentration to prevent net diffusion of water from the compartment with the highest water concentration. This is really a potential pressure because it is the pressure that would have to be applied to prevent osmosis (i.e., in the body, osmosis is not prevented when water imbalances exist). The number of **particles in a solution** (i.e., ions, molecules) determines its osmotic pressure. The greater the number

of particles, the higher the osmotic pressure. For two aqueous solutions of NaCl separated by a membrane that permits diffusion of water, but not NaCl, the highest osmotic pressure is measured for the solution with the highest concentration of NaCl (lowest concentration of water). Water diffuses to the area of greatest osmotic pressure.

Osmolar concentrations are used to express the osmotic strength of solutions (e.g., urine, plasma, NaCl). One mole of an undissociated (not ionized) substance is equal to 1 **osmole (osm)**. If a substance dissociates into two ions ($NaCl \rightarrow Na^+$ and Cl^-), 0.5 mole of the substance equals 1 osmole. The number of particles, not the mass of the solute, determines osmotic pressure. One liter of a solution that contains 300 milliosmoles (mOsm) (0.3 osm) of 0.3 M glucose (undissociated) exerts the same osmotic pressure as one that contains 300 mOsm of 0.5 M NaCl. Similarly, the osmolality of a urine sample (many substances,

TABLE 2-1 OSMOLALITY OF SEVERAL SOLUTIONS AS DETERMINED BY VAPOR PRESSURE LOWERING OSMOMETRY*

SOLUTION IDENTIFICATION	OSMOLALITY (mOSM/kg H_2O)
Bovine plasma	302
Bovine urine	1,031
Bovine milk (skim)	272
Canine plasma	312
Canine urine	1,904
Tap H_2O	58

*Values obtained from student laboratory exercises.

ionized and undissociated) that is measured as 300 mOsm exerts the same osmotic pressure as the previous solutions of glucose and NaCl.

A comparison of osmotic pressure for several solutions is shown in *Table 2-1*. Values were determined using an osmometer and are given in **osmolality (mOsm/kg H_2O)**. An **osmometer** is an instrument for measuring osmolality by freezing point depression or vapor pressure lowering techniques (colligative properties). Values obtained are representative of diffusion through semipermeable membranes. Note that bovine urine has an osmotic pressure 3.3 times greater than bovine plasma (water concentration lower, solute concentration greater than bovine plasma). Canine urine has an osmotic pressure 6.1 times greater than canine plasma. Urine is formed from plasma, and canines have a greater potential for concentrating urine than bovines.

Tone of a Solution

The membranes of the body vary in their permeabilities and allow certain solutes (as well as water) to diffuse through them. They are **selectively permeable membranes**. The mea-

sured osmotic pressure for a solution containing solutes that could diffuse through membranes would then not be an index for its tendency to cause osmosis. Instead, the **tone of a solution** is defined, which is the **effective osmotic pressure**. Only those particles (molecules, ions) for which the membrane is not permeable contribute to the tone. The principles of osmosis continue to prevail, except that now water diffuses to the greatest effective osmotic pressure. *Figure 2-4* illustrates the tone of solutions. Two solutions of equal volumes and particle numbers are shown to be separated by a membrane that permits the passage of water and the particles in compartment 2. Each solution has the same measured osmotic pressure (same concentration of particles). Because compartment 1 has particles that cannot diffuse through the membrane, these particles are the ones that contribute to an effective osmotic pressure and, because the solution in compartment 2 has no effective osmotic pressure (because particles are diffusible), water diffuses to the greatest effective osmotic pressure, or from compartment 2 to compartment 1. In this example the net diffusion of water stops when the pressure resulting from the weight of the solution in compartment 2 opposes the diffusion resulting from the effective osmotic pressure in compartment 1.

From a practical standpoint, the tone of a solution that can be infused into the blood of animals is usually compared with the solution inside red blood cells (erythrocytes). The solution of erythrocytes is in osmotic equilibrium with plasma (the fluid part of blood). An infused solution is **hypotonic** if it has a lower effective osmotic pressure than the solution of erythrocytes, and it is **hypertonic** if it has a higher effective osmotic pressure than the solution of erythrocytes.

The effect of solutions with different tones on erythrocytes is illustrated in *Figure 2-5*. An erythrocyte placed into solution A enlarges. This solution must have a lower effective osmotic pressure than the erythrocyte solution

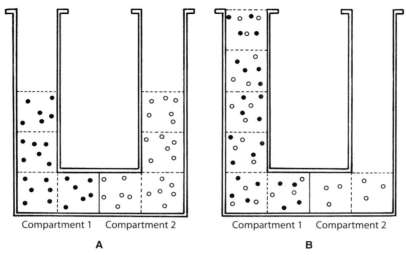

■ **FIGURE 2-4** Hypothetical example of tone of a solution. **A**. Before osmosis. Two aqueous solutions (solutes represented by black circles and open circles) of equal osmotic pressure are separated by a membrane permeable to water and open circle solutes (selectively permeable membrane). **B**. During osmosis. Effective osmotic pressure is exerted only by black circle solute, and water diffuses from compartment 2 to compartment 1. At equilibrium, open circle solute has a new, lower concentration that is equal throughout compartments 1 and 2. (Dashed lines represent divisions of equal volume.)

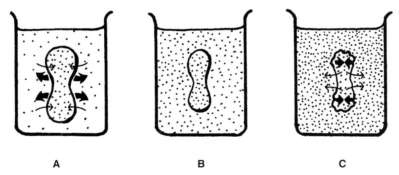

■ **FIGURE 2-5** Effect of the tone of a solution on erythrocytes (red blood cells). **A**. The solution is hypotonic, and the erythrocyte expands. **B**. The solution is isotonic, and no change occurs in erythrocyte size. **C**. The solution is hypertonic, and the erythrocyte decreases in size. The thick arrows indicate the direction of cell volume change. The thin arrows indicate the direction of water diffusion.

(water diffuses to the higher effective osmotic pressure) and is classified as hypotonic to plasma. In solution B there is no change in the size of the erythrocytes. The solution in the beaker and in the erythrocyte must have the same effective osmotic pressure, and the beaker solution is classified as **isotonic** to plasma. The erythrocyte in solution C decreases in size, indicating a loss of erythrocyte water to the beaker solution. In this case the higher effective osmotic pressure is found in solution C (water diffuses to the higher effective osmotic pressure). The loss of water from erythrocytes caused by hypertonic solutions makes the cells wrinkled in appearance, and they are said to be **crenated**.

TABLE 2-2 CHANGES IN VOLUME OF CANINE ERYTHROCYTES ATTRIBUTABLE TO TONE OF SUSPENDING NaCL SOLUTION*

SUSPENDING SOLUTION		VOLUME CHANGE
MOLARITY	PERCENT	PERCENT
0.3	1.76	−16.7
0.167	0.977	0.0
0.15	0.877	+2.0
0.10	0.585	+16.7

*Values obtained from student laboratory exercises.

TABLE 2-3 OSMOTIC FRAGILITY OF ERYTHROCYTES FROM NORMAL DOGS (CANINE) AND NORMAL GOATS (CAPRINE)*

SUSPENDING SOLUTION	NORMAL DOGS	NORMAL GOATS
PERCENT NaCl	PERCENT HEMOLYSIS	PERCENT HEMOLYSIS
0.85	0.0	0.0
0.75	0.6	2.1
0.65	0.7	88.0
0.60	1.7	93.6
0.55	14.0	97.7
0.50	67.4	97.7
0.45	94.4	97.7
0.40	95.7	100.0
0.35	100.0	100.0
0.30	100.0	100.0

*Values obtained from student laboratory exercises.

Table 2-2 presents the results of a laboratory exercise in which erythrocytes from a dog were placed in different concentrations of NaCl solutions. The 0.167-M NaCl solution (0.977%) was considered isotonic for the erythrocytes of this dog (no change in volume). Both of the 0.15-M (0.877%) and 0.10-M (0.585%) solutions were hypotonic (increased volume), and the 0.3-M (1.76%) solution was decidedly hypertonic (decreased volume).

Erythrocytes vary in their ability to withstand **hemolysis** (rupture of erythrocytes with release of hemoglobin). Older erythrocytes are more fragile and would be the first to hemolyze in solutions with reduced tone. Fragility of erythrocytes can also be increased by certain disease conditions or exposure to toxins and drugs. The degree of fragility can be determined by an **osmotic fragility test**. Blood from an animal is placed in NaCl solutions with decreasing concentration. The percent hemolysis is determined for each solution by its comparison with a solution in which hemolysis would be expected to be 100%. The results of an osmotic fragility test for a normal dog (canine) are presented in *Table 2-3*, and are compared with those of a normal goat (caprine). It is apparent that goat erythrocytes are less resistant to hemolysis than dogs when placed in solutions with increasing hypotonicity. Whereas dog erythrocytes are described as biconcave disks, goat erythrocytes are more spherical; therefore, expansion potential is minimal and hemolysis occurs earlier.

Solutions that cause erythrocytes to enlarge can be sufficiently hypotonic to cause hemolysis of the erythrocytes. Hemoglobin (red in color) in the erythrocyte imparts its color to the solution. Plasma from an animal in which hemolysis has occurred has some degree of redness, depending on the extent of the hemolysis (plasma is usually light yellow to colorless). When this occurs it is known as **hemoglobinemia**. Sometimes hemolysis occurs to such an extent that hemoglobin enters the kidney tubules and appears in the urine. In this condition, called **hemoglobinuria**, a red color is imparted to the urine.

Interconversion of Units of Measurement

Solution composition and strength is variably expressed in moles, osmoles, and equivalents, and each has a reference to the weight in grams from which they can be derived. These units are related, and interconversions can be made and must proceed according to the pathways shown in *Figure 2-6*.

The problems listed below are frequently encountered when preparing solutions for infusion or when interpreting contents shown on labels for solutions commercially prepared. These will enhance your understanding and skill related to physicochemical properties of solutions.

1. How many grams would be needed to prepare 1 L of a 5% glucose solution?
   Answer:
   Step 1: Percent solution = the concentration of solute in grams per 100 mL of aqueous solution. Accordingly, a 5% glucose solution would contain 5 g per 100 mL.
   Step 2: Because one liter (1,000 mL) is needed, the amount of glucose would be (5 g × 1,000) ÷ 100 = 50 g.
2. What is the molarity (M) of a NaCl solution that contains 8.775 g per L?
   Answer:
   Step 1: M = g per L ÷ MW (molecular weight)

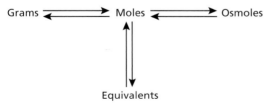

■ FIGURE 2-6 Pathways for the interconversion of grams, moles, osmoles, and equivalents. (From Reece WO. Physicochemical properties of solutions. In: Reece WO, ed. Dukes' Physiology of Domestic Animals. 12th Ed. Ithaca, NY: Cornell University Press, 2004.)

Step 2: Molecular weight of NaCl = 58.5; therefore, M = 8.775 ÷ 58.5 = 0.15 M.
3. What is the osmolarity (osm) of a 0.1 M $CaCl_2$ solution?
   Answer:
   Step 1: Osmolarity is a measure of osmotic pressure and is determined by numbers of particles.
   Step 2: One molecule of $CaCl_2$ when placed in solution would ionize and provide three particles (one Ca^{2+} and two Cl^-).
   Step 3: The osm (for molecules that ionize in solution) = number ions from molecule × M = 3 × 0.1 M = 0.3 osm = 300 mOsm (milliosmole).
4. How many grams would be required to make 1 L of a 300 mOsm NaCl solution?
   Answer:
   Step 1: 300 mOsm NaCl = 150 mM NaCl = 0.15 M NaCl
   Step 2: g/L = M × MW = 0.15 × 58.5 = 8.775 g
5. How many equivalents (mEq/L) of Na^+ and Cl^- are contained in a 0.15 M solution of NaCl?
   Answer:
   Step 1: NaCl is a monovalent molecule.
   Step 2: Eq for each ion = 1 (valence) × M = 0.15 Eq Na^+ and 0.15 Eq Cl^- = 150 mEq Na^+ + 150 mEq Cl^-.
6. How many equivalents (mEq/L) of Ca^{2+} and Cl^- are contained in a 0.1 M solution of $CaCl_2$?
   Answer:
   Step 1: $CaCl_2$ is a bivalent molecule.
   Step 2: Eq for each ion = 2 (valence) × M = 2 × 0.1 = 0.2 Eq Ca^{2+} and 0.2 Eq Cl^- = 200 mEq Ca^{2+} and 200 mEq Cl^-.
7. What is the osmolarity (mOsm/L) of a $CaCl_2$ solution labeled to contain 200 mEq Ca^{2+} and 200 mEq Cl^-?
   Answer:
   Step 1: Convert milliequivalents to millimoles (mEq ÷ valence) = 200 ÷ 2 = 100 mM $CaCl_2$.

Step 2: Convert mM to mOsm = 100 mM × number of atoms per molecule (particles) = 100 × 3 = 300 mOsm.

8. One liter of a solution contains the following: 155 mEq Na^+; 5 mEq K^+; 10 mEq Ca^{2+}; 145 mEq Cl^-; 25 mEq lactate. How many millimoles (mM) are there of NaCl, KCl, $CaCl_2$, and Na lactate? What is the milliosmolarity of the solution?

Answer:

Step 1: Determine electrolytes used to make the solution. These would be NaCl, KCl, $CaCl_2$, and Na lactate (all water soluble salts).

Step 2: Determine the milliequivalent contribution from each electrolyte.

	Na^+	K^+	Ca^{2+}	Cl^-	$Lactate^{-1}$
NaCl	130			130	
KCl		5		5	
$CaCl_2$			5	10	
Na lactate	25				25

Step 3: Convert milliequivalents determined for each electrolyte to millimoles.

NaCl = 130 mM; KCl = 5 mM; $CaCl_2$ = 5 mM; Na lactate = 25 mM

Step 4: Convert millimoles to milliosmoles for each electrolyte, and the total osmolarity of the solution is the sum of the individual values.

	mM	mOsm
NaCl	130	260
KCl	5	10
$CaCl_2$	5	15
Na lactate	25	50
Total		335

■ DISTRIBUTION OF BODY WATER

1. How do water and fluid differ from each other?
2. What percent of the body weight is water?
3. What are the two major body water compartments, and what percent of the body weight is represented by each?
4. Define interstitial fluid. What space does it occupy?
5. What substance gives interstitial water the characteristics of a gel?
6. Are intravascular fluid and plasma synonymous? Why would plasma volume have a greater value than plasma water?

The terms **water** and **fluid** are nearly the same but do differ inasmuch as a fluid, as found in the body, contains not only water but also solutes. The measurement of a compartment's volume usually includes the entire space occupied by the water and solutes. For example, blood plasma is a fluid, and the measurement of its volume is larger than the space occupied by the water it contains. For practical purposes, the compartments are referred to as **fluid compartments** because the fluid volume rather than water volume is that which is usually measured.

Total Body Water and Fluid Compartments

The **total body water (TBW)** is the sum of the water that is contained in arbitrary divisions of its distribution between the intracellular and extracellular compartments. The extracellular compartment can be further divided into interstitial, intravascular, and transcellular compartments.

TBW is variable and depends mostly on the amount of fat in the body. A lean animal might have water equivalent to 70% of its body weight, whereas an obese animal might only have 45% of its body weight as water because of the nature of fat cells (the cytoplasm is almost filled with fat). The fat and water are immiscible, and most of the cell mass is fat, rather than water. The average animal (neither fat nor lean) probably has water equivalent to 60% of its body weight.

Intracellular and Extracellular Fluid

About two-thirds of the body water is found within the cells; this is the **intracellular fluid (ICF)**. The amounts given for percentage of body weight are average values and can vary. All water that is not in cells is considered to be **extracellular fluid (ECF)**, or outside the cells. This includes the **interstitial fluid (ISF)**, **intravascular fluid (IVF)**, and **transcellular fluid (TCF)**. Intravascular fluid is the same as **plasma volume (PV)**. The divisions of TBW among the compartments are shown in *Figure 2-7*.

Interstitial fluid is fluid outside of capillaries that immediately surrounds the cells. It is the environment of the cells. It occupies the **intercellular space** (also called **interstitial space** and **interstitium**) along with a number of **intercellular substances** (e.g., collagen and elastic fibers, fibroblasts, and plasma cells and mast cells). It is important to visualize the location of the interstitial space (*Fig. 2-8*) because of references made to it throughout the text (e.g., edema, see Chapter 9). In addition to elastic and collagen fibers of the intercellular substance, an **amorphous** (without definite form or shape) **ground substance** is present; its principal component is **hyaluronic acid**. Hyaluronic acid is a highly hydrated gel that holds tissue fluid in its interstices. Because of the gel form, fluid is not observed to flow and accumulate in lower body parts, nor does fluid flow from a cut surface.

The IVF is the liquid part of blood known as **plasma**. About 92% of the plasma volume is water; the remaining 8% of PV is mostly protein, but also there are many ions and molecules found in plasma.

TCF is the fluid found in body cavities and is usually minimal. It includes intraocular fluid and cerebrospinal fluid. The most plentiful TCF is in the digestive tract. Its amount is greatest in ruminants, in which stomach compartments for fermentation are found.

■ WATER BALANCE

1. What is meant by water turnover?
2. What is the derivation of metabolic water? Why does 5 g of fat yield more metabolic water than 5 g of protein or carbohydrate?
3. What are examples of insensible water loss?
4. Why are excess water losses (e.g., diarrhea) more critical in young animals than in adults of the same species?

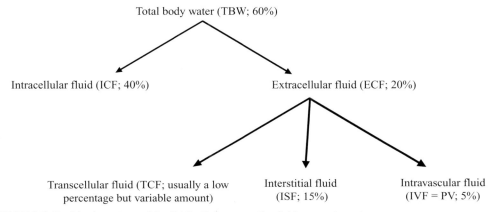

■ **FIGURE 2-7** Total body water and its distribution among the fluid compartments.

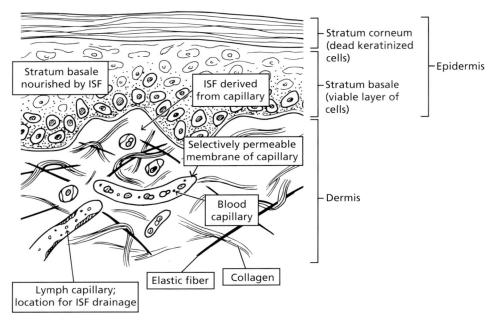

■ **FIGURE 2-8** Schematic representation of the outer part of skin from a pig with special emphasis on the interstitial space, the space outside of the capillaries and cells. The fluid of the interstitial space is interstitial fluid (ISF). Hyaluronic acid of the amorphous ground substance gives ISF the characteristics of a gel. An abnormal increase of ISF in this location is evident in a condition known as edema.

From day to day in any one animal the water content of the body remains relatively constant, with a balance between gains and losses. Water turnover is that amount of water gained by an animal to balance that which is lost. An example of daily water balance is shown in *Table 2-4*. The water turnover for the nonlactating cow is 29 L/day and is 56 L/day for the lactating cow. The water intake in both cases is equal to the output—there is **water balance**. The "pool" size is constant, but the water in the pool changes (water turnover). The output of the lactating cow has increased, not only because of the obvious milk production, but also because of the greater fecal output associated with eating nearly twice as much and because of greater urine and vapor losses associated with increased metabolism.

Water Gain

Water gains occur by ingestion of water in food and drink and from metabolic water. The food eaten by animals contains a variable amount of water; the usual drink is water or, in the very young, milk. **Metabolic water** is derived from the chemical reactions of metabolism in the cell mitochondria. At the end of the electron transfer chain, hydrogen is combined with oxygen to form water; this is metabolic water (see Chapter 1).

The metabolism of proteins, carbohydrates, or fats requires different amounts of cofactors, with the greatest amounts required for fats. Accordingly, the yield of metabolic water is greater for a certain amount of fat than for an equal amount of protein or carbohydrate. For example, the metabolic water yield from each

TABLE 2-4 DAILY WATER BALANCE OF HOLSTEIN COWS EATING LEGUME HAY (VALUES IN LITERS)

BALANCE	NONLACTATING	LACTATING
Intake		
Drinking water	26	51
Food water	1	2
Metabolic water	2	3
Total	29	56
Output		
Feces	12	19
Urine	7	11
Vaporized	10	14
Milk	0	12
Total	29	56

From Houpt TR. Water and electrolytes. In: Reece WO, ed. Dukes' Physiology of Domestic Animals. 12th Ed. Ithaca, NY: Cornell University Press, 2004.

of 100 g of protein, carbohydrate, and fat is 40, 60, and 110 mL, respectively. Energy in the form of adenosine triphosphate (ATP) is formed during the transfer of electrons. The amount of metabolic water formed varies but could be substantial under certain conditions. In domestic animals it is said to average about 5% to 10% of daily water gain, and it can approach 100% of the water gain for some small desert rodents.

Water Loss

Water loss from the body is classified as either an insensible loss or a sensible loss. **Insensible losses** are associated with vapor losses and occur constantly by evaporation from the skin and by loss of water vapor in exhaled air. Inhaled air becomes saturated with water vapor in the respiratory passages and lungs, but there is no body mechanism to remove moisture from the respiratory gases before exhalation. **Sensible losses** are the visible losses; they are part of the urine, feces, and body secretions that leave the body and are not subject to evaporation. Sensible losses can become excessive in certain conditions, such as diarrhea, and threaten body stores of water.

Water Requirements

No linear relationship exists between basal water needs and body weight. Accordingly, a 500-kg cow does not require 10 times more water than a 50-kg calf. The **basal daily needs** for water (that are needed to maintain water balance), however, are related to caloric expenditure. Under **basal metabolism conditions** (e.g., resting animal, thermally neutral environment, fasting state), **caloric expenditure** is related linearly to body surface area. The cow might require only three to four times more water than the calf because her body surface area is three to four times greater. If the ECF (20% of body weight) is considered to be that from which emergency water is drawn, the 500-kg cow has 100 kg of fluid and the 50-kg calf has only 10 kg. Therefore, the cow has considerably more reserve on which to draw to supply basal needs for water than does the calf. In other words, the cow has ten times more reserve water to supply her needs, and her needs are only three to four times greater than the calf's. It is because of the more limited reserves associated with their relatively higher needs that calves become distressed more quickly in conditions of uncontrolled water loss (such as diarrhea).

■ DEHYDRATION, THIRST, AND WATER INTAKE

1. In dehydration, what is the immediate source (compartment) of water lost from the body?
2. For most animals, what is considered to be a severe loss of body water?

3.   With a continuing loss of water (dehydration), is there a proportionate loss of electrolytes?
4.   Define thirst.
5.   Where is the thirst center located?
6.   How does dehydration stimulate thirst?
7.   How does hypovolemia stimulate thirst?
8.   How can thirst be temporarily relieved?

When water losses exceed water gains, a condition known as **dehydration** develops. The extent is variable, and when mild, physiologic mechanisms may be adequate to re-establish water balance via the thirst mechanism if water is available. Therapeutic measures (fluid replacement, treatment of underlying cause) may be necessary when water losses are moderate to severe and related to a disease condition.

Dehydration

In dehydration, the immediate source of water lost from the body is the extracellular fluid, followed by a shift from the intracellular to the extracellular fluid. A loss of water equal to 10% of the body weight is considered to be severe for most animals. The concentrations of electrolytes (ions) in the body fluids do not continue to increase during dehydration, but are excreted by the kidney in proportion to the water loss. With continuing dehydration, water and electrolytes are depleted. Therefore, rehydration requires not only water, but also appropriate electrolytes.

Stimulus for Thirst

When water losses exceed water gain, there is an effort on the part of the kidneys to conserve water. Also, animals are provided with a **thirst mechanism** to recognize the need for water intake greater than that provided by food and metabolic water. **Thirst** is the conscious desire for water. Central to the thirst mechanism is a thirst center located in the hypothalamus (see Chapter 4) of the brain and represented by thirst cells. The thirst cells are stimulated by an increase in their **osmoconcentration** (loss of water and increased salt concentration). Osmoconcentration of the thirst cells is a consequence of dehydration.

Another stimulus of thirst is the kidney hormone **angiotensin II** (see Chapter 11). This is formed in response to low blood pressure to bring about changes to increase blood pressure (e.g., salt retention, peripheral vasoconstriction, water ingestion). A loss of blood volume (**hypovolemia**), as in hemorrhage (an isotonic fluid loss), results in lowered blood pressure, and angiotensin II is formed. The thirst stimulation previously described causes an animal to drink water, which is subsequently absorbed, and blood volume and blood pressure are restored toward normal.

Relief of Thirst

An experiment can be performed with a dog to show the effect of dehydration on thirst stimulation. A hypertonic NaCl solution is slowly injected intravenously, which increases the osmoconcentration of plasma and subsequently that of the thirst cells in the hypothalamus. After a few minutes, water that was previously offered to the dog and ignored is now consumed. The amount consumed is approximately equal to the amount that would have been needed to make the hypertonic plasma isotonic. Even though there was insufficient time for the water ingested to be absorbed, the dog's thirst was relieved.

Thirst can be temporarily relieved by wetting the mouth and pharynx and by the distention of the stomach that accompanies water ingestion. The former method is used by many people seeking relief from thirst. The latter can be shown by distending a balloon placed into the stomach. Both of these temporary relief methods help to prevent overinges-

DISTRIBUTION OF BODY WATER

7. Which one of the following body fluid compartments would represent about 40% of the body weight?
   a. Transcellular
   b. Intravascular
   c. Intracellular
   d. Extracellular

8. Interstitial fluid is a component of the:
   a. intracellular fluid compartment.
   b. extracellular fluid compartment.
   c. transcellular fluid compartment.

9. Interstitial fluid is found:
   a. within the cells.
   b. between cells but outside of blood vessels.
   c. within the capillaries.
   d. in body cavities.

10. Hyaluronic acid (a component of the intercellular substance):
    a. maintains an optimal pH of the ISF.
    b. counteracts the effects of hyaluronidase.
    c. is a highly hydrated gel that holds ISF in its interstices.

11. Body fluid volumes were measured, and the values were reported as milliliters per kilogram of body weight but in a scrambled order with no body compartment identification. Total body water was reported as 610 ml/kg body weight, and the compartment volumes were reported as 170, 230, 380, and 60. Select the series below that corresponds with the values shown.
    a. ECF, ICF, ISF, PV
    b. PV, ISF, ECF, ICF
    c. ISF, ECF, ICF, PV
    d. ECF, ICF, ISF, PV

WATER BALANCE

12. Water lost from the body when air is exhaled or by evaporation from the skin is considered a vapor loss or insensible loss. It usually exceeds sensible losses, water lost in feces or urine.
    a. True
    b. False

13. The water requirement of a 1,000-lb cow is about 30 L each day. If a calf weighs 100 lb and has about 1/5 of the body surface area of the cow, what would be its approximate water requirement each day?
    a. 30 L
    b. 3 L
    c. 6 L

14. The basal daily needs for water are directly related to:
    a. body weight.
    b. caloric expenditure and body surface area.
    c. animal color.

15. More metabolic water is obtained from the metabolism of 100 g of fat than from 100 g of either protein or carbohydrate because:
    a. animals drink more when eating fat.
    b. more cofactors are reduced (and therefore need to be reoxidized) when fat is metabolized.
    c. 1 g of fat is heavier than 1 g of either protein or carbohydrate.

DEHYDRATION, THIRST, AND WATER INTAKE

16. If the effective osmotic pressure in the plasma becomes greater than the effective osmotic pressure within the thirst cells in the hypothalamus, which of the following would be predicted?
    a. The animal would seek water.
    b. The animal would not seek water.

17. Thirst can be stimulated by:
    a. osmoconcentration of the extracellular fluid.
    b. low blood pressure associated with blood loss.
    c. both a and b.

18. Which one of the following solutions would cause a dog to begin drinking water (become thirsty) if it were infused into the dog's blood?
    a. Hypertonic NaCl
    b. Isotonic NaCl
    c. Hypotonic NaCl

19. With continuing dehydration:
    a. only water is depleted.
    b. only electrolytes are depleted.
    c. both water and electrolytes are depleted.

ADAPTATION TO WATER LACK

20. Which one of the following statements is correct as it relates to tolerance to dehydration?

    a. Cattle have better tolerance than sheep.
    b. Sheep have better tolerance than cattle and pigs.
    c. Sheep, cattle, and pigs have the same tolerance.
    d. Pigs have better tolerance than sheep.

21. During the heat of the day, which one of the following is most productive in conserving body water?
    a. Elimination of body heat while it is being produced via evaporation
    b. Storing body heat during the day while it is being produced and eliminating the heat when ambient temperature is cooler
    c. Retention of urine

ANSWERS TO SELF EVALUATION—CHAPTER 2

1.	b	7.	c	13.	c	19.	c
2.	c	8.	b	14.	b	20.	b
3.	b	9.	b	15.	b	21.	b
4.	a	10.	c	16.	a		
5.	a	11.	c	17.	c		
6.	a	12.	b	18.	a		

CHAPTER 3

Blood and Its Functions

CHAPTER OUTLINE

- **GENERAL CHARACTERISTICS**
  Hematocrit
  Blood Color
  Blood Volume
  Blood pH
- **LEUKOCYTES**
  Classification and Appearance
  Life Span and Numbers
  Function
  Diagnostic Procedures
- **ERYTHROCYTES**
  Hemoglobin and Its Forms
  Erythropoiesis
  Numbers
  Shape
  Size
  Erythrocyte Indices
  Life Span

- **FATE OF ERYTHROCYTES**
- **IRON METABOLISM**
- **ANEMIA AND POLYCYTHEMIA**
- **HEMOSTASIS: PREVENTION OF BLOOD LOSS**
  Hemostatic Components
  Platelet Reactions
  Clot Formation (Blood Coagulation)
  Fibrin Degradation
- **PREVENTION OF BLOOD COAGULATION**
  Prevention in Normal Circulation
  Prevention in Withdrawn Blood
- **TESTS FOR BLOOD COAGULATION**
  Coagulation Defects
  Species Differences
- **PLASMA AND ITS COMPOSITION**
  Plasma Proteins
  Other Plasma Constituents

The blood vascular system evolved to provide for the transport of nutrients to the cells after they had become so numerous and so distant from the surface that diffusion was no longer adequate. The circulating medium came to be known as blood. The functions of blood are generally related to transport (e.g., nutrients, oxygen, carbon dioxide, waste products, hormones, heat, and immune bodies). There are additional functions of blood relating to its role of maintaining fluid balance and pH equilibrium in the body. Because blood must be maintained in a closed system for transport efficiency, it is provided with a mechanism for preventing blood loss if the normally closed system is opened.

■ GENERAL CHARACTERISTICS

1. **What are the components of the hematocrit?**

2. **What accounts for the color of blood and for the color of plasma?**

3. **A dog weighs 10 kg and has a packed cell volume of 42% and a plasma volume of 500 mL. What is its blood volume expressed as percent of body weight?**

4. **Why is venous blood more acidic than arterial blood?**

5. **If the blood pH is measured to be 7.1 and the H^+ concentration has doubled, what is an approximate pH of that blood before the H^+ increase? Has the blood become more alkaline or more acidic?**

Blood is composed of cells and plasma. The cells of blood are the: 1) **erythrocytes** (red blood cells [RBCs]), 2) **leukocytes** (white blood cells [WBCs]), and 3) **platelets**, also known as thrombocytes. **Plasma** is the liquid component of blood, within which the cells and colloids are suspended and other transported substances are dissolved.

Hematocrit

The relative proportion of cells to plasma is a clinically useful measure that can be determined by the hematocrit. **Hematocrit** means to centrifuge; by centrifugation, a column of blood can be divided into its component parts according to their relative specific gravity (*Fig. 3-1*). Accordingly, the erythrocyte mass occupies the lower portion and is known as the **packed cell volume (PCV)**, the leukocytes and platelets occupy the middle portion, known as the buffy coat, and the plasma occupies the top portion. The PCV is the most useful

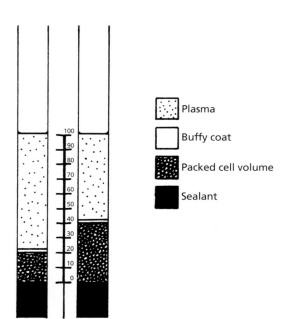

Plasma

Buffy coat

Packed cell volume

Sealant

A   **B**

■ **FIGURE 3-1** The microhematocrit as it might appear for an anemic **(A)** and a normal **(B)** animal. The buffy coat occupies an insignificant volume and is not accounted for. Accordingly, in the normal hematocrit, the plasma volume would be noted as 60%.

component for helping to distinguish abnormal conditions.

For greater precision of measurement and for uniformity, a standard procedure (microhematocrit method) is used in the determination of the hematocrit. A thin column of blood is allowed to fill about three-fourths of the length of the capillary tube. One end of the tube is closed with a sealant, and it is then centrifuged for 5 minutes at 11,000 rpm. The centrifuge used is a microhematocrit centrifuge. The proportion of the blood column length occupied by the RBCs can be obtained by measurement. PCV values are reported as percentages.

Blood Color

The red color of blood is imparted by the hemoglobin contained within the erythrocytes. Gradations of color from bright red to bluish-purple are seen, depending on the degree of saturation of hemoglobin with oxygen. The greater the saturation, the brighter the red color. Plasma is yellow to colorless, depending on the quantity and species examined. Plasma that is ordinarily light yellow when observed in a test tube might be almost colorless in a capillary tube. The color of plasma results principally from the presence of **bilirubin**, a degradation product of hemoglobin. It is a darker yellow in the cow and even darker in the horse, which has a relatively high bilirubin concentration.

Blood Volume

Blood volume (BV) is a function of the lean body weight and is generally 8% to 10% of the body weight. Blood volume cannot be measured directly because exsanguination (removal of blood) results in the loss of only about 50% of the blood; the remainder is trapped in capillaries, venous sinuses, and other vessels. Erythrocyte volume and **plasma volume (PV)** can be measured by various techniques. If one or the other is measured and the PCV is known, the BV can be calculated according to the hematocrit relationship. For example, if the PV is 600 mL and the PCV is 40%, the PV represents 60% of the BV. BV is then determined by the following relationship: BV = PV ÷ 1 − PCV (decimal equivalent) = 600 ÷ 0.60 = 1,000 mL. If these values were obtained from a 12.5-kg dog, the BV of 1,000 mL translates to 80 mL/kg. Further calculation shows that this is the same as 8% of the body weight if correction for specific gravity is not made and if 1 mL of blood is considered to weigh 1 g (80 mL = 80 g ÷ 1,000 g = 0.08 = 8%).

Blood pH

Blood has a pH of about 7.4. Venous blood is slightly more acidic than arterial blood. Thus, if the arterial blood pH is 7.4, one would expect the venous blood pH to be about 7.36. The higher acidity of venous blood is related to the transport of carbon dioxide; higher concentrations of CO_2 exist in venous blood. The hydration of carbon dioxide in venous blood (CO_2 + H_2O × H_2CO_3 × H^+ + HCO_3^-) forms hydrogen ions, thus resulting in its higher acidity and lower pH.

The **pH symbol** is the chemical notation for the logarithm of the reciprocal of the **hydrogen ion concentration** [H^+] in gram-atoms per liter of solution. For monovalent substances, equivalent measurements are the same as gram-atom measurements; when the pH is 7.4, the [H^+] is 0.00000040 g-atoms of H^+ in 1 L of solution, or 40 nEq (nanoequivalents). When the [H^+] doubles (80 nEg) or halves (20 nEq), the pH changes by 0.3 units as follows:

pH   [H^+]
7.4   Normal
7.1   Double normal
7.7   Half-normal
6.8   Four times normal

Even though the pH might seem to change very little, the [H^+] changes considerably. Therefore, the pH of the body fluids must be regulated precisely.

Data obtained from blood-gas analysis, which includes pH values, is presented in Appendix A for equine, bovine, canine, and feline species.

■ LEUKOCYTES

1. How are leukocytes classified? Where are the various cells produced? What do segmented and band cells refer to?
2. Which one of the leukocytes seems to have the longest life span?
3. How do the numbers of RBCs and WBCs compare?
4. Which WBC predominates in the horse, dog, and cat? In the pig, cow, sheep, and goat?
5. Describe the movement of neutrophils from the circulation to sites of inflammation.
6. What is a principal function for each of the leukocytes?
7. Which WBC is classified as a mononuclear phagocytic system cell? Which mononuclear phagocytic system cell is in a fixed position in the liver?
8. Which one of the WBCs becomes more numerous in certain types of parasitisms?
9. Differentiate between the functions of lymphocyte T cells and B cells.
10. What are plasma cells and mega karyocytes?
11. Differentiate among leukopenia, leukocytosis, and leukemia.
12. What is meant by absolute numbers of leukocytes?
13. Define phagocytosis, pinocytosis, and endocytosis.

Classification and Appearance

Leukocytes are classified either as **granulocytes**, containing granules in the cytoplasm, or as **agranulocytes**, containing few if any granules in the cytoplasm. There are three types of granulocytes, named according to which component of the hematoxylin and eosin (H&E) stain (hematoxylin, basic and colored blue; eosin, acidic and colored red) stains their granules. **Neutrophils** are neither markedly acidophilic nor basophilic and incorporate both basic and acidic components into their granules. **Basophils** only accept the basic (hematoxylin) component, and eosinophils only accept the acidic (eosin) component. There are two types of agranulocytes: **monocytes** and **lymphocytes**. Granulocytes and monocytes are produced in the bone marrow from myeloid stem cells known as myeloblasts and monoblasts, respectively. Lymphocytes originate from a lymphoid stem cell, known as a lymphoblast, in lymph tissue, such as lymph nodes, spleen, tonsils, and various lymphoid clusters in the intestine and elsewhere. The different types of leukocytes are shown in *Figure 3-2* for humans; there are many similarities for those in animals.

The nuclei of the granulocytes assume various shapes as they proceed to maturity (*Fig. 3-3*). The nuclei of the mature forms are generally divided into lobes or segments connected by filaments; these are sometimes called **segmented cells**. The younger forms have a nucleus that appears as a curved or coiled band without segmentation; these are known as **band cells**.

Life Span and Numbers

After their development, leukocytes are circulated in the blood until the (relatively short) time they leave the circulation to perform their extravascular function. Granulocytes can be present in the blood for 6 to 20 hours and are constantly leaving. Granulocyte time in the tissues varies considerably, but can be 2 or 3 days. Once granulocytes leave the blood, they do not normally return. They leave the body either from inflammatory sites or by way of the gastrointestinal, urinary, respiratory, or reproductive tracts. These organs are normally lined with neutrophils, which help prevent entry of organisms or foreign particles. Monocytes

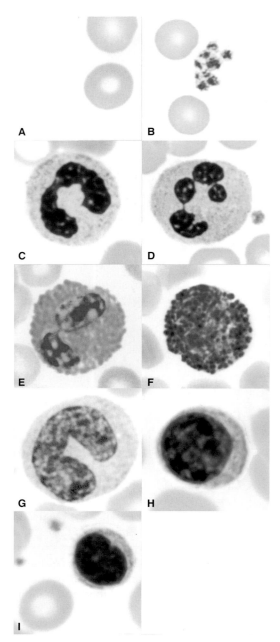

■ **FIGURE 3-2** Cell types found in smears of normal peripheral blood. **A.** Erythrocytes. **B.** Platelets (thrombocytes). **C.** Band neutrophil (granules stain various shades of pink and blue). **D.** Segmented neutrophil (granules stain various shades of pink and blue). **E.** Eosinophil (granules stain reddish-orange). **F.** Basophil (granules stain dark blue). **G.** Monocyte. **H.** Large lymphocyte. **I.** Small lymphocyte. (From Cormack DH. Essential Histology. 2nd Ed. Baltimore: Lippincott Williams & Wilkins, 2001.)

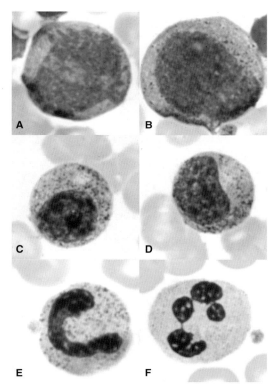

■ **FIGURE 3-3** Granulocytic (myelocytic) system. **A.** Myeloblast. **B.** Promyelocyte (progranulocyte). **C.** Neutrophilic myelocyte. **D.** Neutrophilic metamyelocyte. **E.** Neutrophilic band. **F.** Neutrophilic segmented. (From Cormack DH. Essential Histology. 2nd Ed. Baltimore: Lippincott Williams & Wilkins, 2001.)

have a circulation time of 24 hours or less, but can remain in the tissues for several months. Many monocytes become fixed macrophages in the sinusoids of the liver, spleen, bone marrow, and lymph nodes; in this way they continue to function in the blood and lymph.

Lymphocytes recirculate repeatedly from the blood to the tissues, to the lymph, and back to the blood. The **lymphocyte population** consists of **T cells** and **B cells**. Their life span varies, depending on classification. Generally T cells are long-lived (100 to 200 days), B cells are short-lived (2 to 4 days), and memory T and B cells are very long-lived (years).

The circulating leukocytes are considerably less numerous than erythrocytes. The numbers range from 7,000 to 15,000 per microliter (μL) among the domestic animals (*Table 3-1*). To appreciate the volume from which the number is obtained, recall that a microliter (μL) is one millionth of a liter, whereas a milliliter (mL) is one thousandth of a liter. Accordingly, there are 1,000 μL in 1 mL. The percentage distribution of the various types of leukocytes is not the same among the domestic species. There is a higher percentage of lymphocytes than neutrophils among the cloven-hoofed animals (pig, cow, sheep, goat). The reverse (higher percentage of neutrophils than lymphocytes) is true for the horse, dog, and cat. A more complete listing of blood variables is presented in Appendix A for each of these species.

Function

As a group, the WBCs serve as a defense mechanism against bacterial, viral, and parasitic infections and proteins foreign to the body. Each of the WBCs has a specific role in this broad function.

Neutrophils

The cell membranes of certain cells can engulf particulate matter (e.g., bacteria, cells, degenerating tissue) and extracellular fluid and bring them into their cytoplasm. The ingestion of particulate matter is known as phagocytosis, the ingestion of extracellular fluid is pinocytosis, and both are forms of endocytosis.

Neutrophils have two types of granules in their cytoplasm. Azurophilic granules are the lysosomes of the neutrophil and supply enzymes to digest the ingested bacteria, viruses, and cellular debris. Neutrophils produce hydrogen peroxide, a bactericidal substance, which is potentiated (made more active) by peroxidase, one of the lysosomal enzymes.

Substances within specific granules include collagenase and an iron-binding protein called lactoferrin. Lactoferrin has a very high affinity for ferric iron and can deprive phagocytized bacteria of the iron they need for further growth.

TABLE 3-1 TOTAL LEUKOCYTES PER MICROLITER OF BLOOD AND PERCENTAGE OF EACH LEUKOCYTE

SPECIES	TOTAL LEUKOCYTE COUNT OF EACH LEUKOCYTE (RANGE; NO./μL)	PERCENTAGE OF EACH LEUKOCYTE				
		NEUTROPHIL	LYMPHOCYTE	MONOCYTE	EOSINOPHIL	BASOPHIL
Pig						
1 day	10,000–12,000	70	20	5–6	2–5	<1
1 week	10,000–12,000	50	40	5–6	2–5	<1
2 weeks	10,000–12,000	40	50	5–6	2–5	<1
6 weeks and older	15,000–22,000	30–35	55–60	5–6	2–5	<1
Horse	8,000–11,000	50–60	30–40	5–6	2–5	<1
Cow	7,000–10,000	25–30	60–65	5	2–5	<1
Sheep	7,000–10,000	25–30	60–65	5	2–5	<1
Goat	8,000–12,000	35–40	50–55	5	2–5	<1
Dog	9,000–13,000	65–70	20–25	5	2–5	<1
Cat	10,000–15,000	55–60	30–35	5	2–5	<1
Chicken	20,000–30,000	25–30	55–60	10	3–8	1–4

From Reece WO, Swenson MJ. The composition and functions of blood. In: Reece WO, ed. Dukes' Physiology of Domestic Animals. 12th Ed. Ithaca, NY: Cornell University Press, 2004.

Neutrophils are highly phagocytic and this, coupled with their mobility, provides for an effective body defense mechanism. Their numbers increase rapidly during acute bacterial infections. The mechanism for their movement from the blood to an inflammatory site is described as follows (*Fig. 3-4*):

1. Degenerative products of inflamed tissue or bacterial cells can be **chemotactic** (chemically attracting) and diffuse through interstitial spaces to capillaries and venules.
2. Chemotactic substances increase porosity of these vessels and also provide for adhesion of neutrophils to endothelium (**margination**).
3. Neutrophils squeeze through endothelial openings (**diapedesis**).
4. Neutrophils proceed to inflammatory sites by **ameboid** movement.

This mechanism probably applies to the other leukocytes as well. When the neutrophils arrive at the inflamed site, they phagocytize bacteria and cell debris. The neutrophil life span is relatively short; dead neutrophils and their liquid is known as **pus**. The accumulation of pus within a connective tissue capsule is known as an **abscess**.

The comparable leukocyte in birds is known as the **heterophil**. Whereas the granules in mammals are neutrophilic, those in birds are acidophilic. Also, many of the granules are rod- or spindle-shaped instead of spherical. The nucleus is polymorphic with varying degrees of lobulation.

Monocytes

Monocytes are usually the largest leukocyte seen on a stained blood film. They occur in

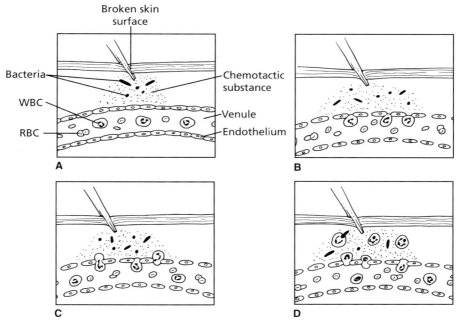

■ FIGURE 3-4 Mechanisms by which neutrophils are attracted to sites of injury. **A.** Tissue injury and introduction of bacteria causes diffusion of a chemotactic substance to capillaries and venules. **B.** Chemotactic substance increases endothelial porosity and adhesion of neutrophils to endothelium. **C.** By a process known as diapedesis, the adhered neutrophils squeeze through endothelial pores. **D.** Neutrophils proceed to injury site by amoeboid movement and phagocytize bacteria and other debris. WBC, white blood cell; RBC, red blood cell.

normal blood to only a limited extent. Compared with other leukocytes, they have a copious cytoplasm. Circulating monocytes phagocytize bacteria, viruses, and antigen-antibody complexes from the bloodstream. Their circulatory phagocytic function is not as pronounced, however, as that which occurs in the tissues. The movement of neutrophils from capillaries and venules is accompanied by similar margination and diapedesis of monocytes. On entering the tissues, monocytes are transformed into **macrophages (large phagocytic cells)** and initially participate in the phagocytosis of bacterial cells. Macrophages kill phagocytized microbes by their acidic pH, bacteriostatic proteins, and degradative enzymes. They also produce hydrogen peroxide in greater quantity than neutrophils. Macrophages eventually predominate at the inflammatory site because of their longer life span. Also, they are attracted

to some organisms that neutrophils ignore and they phagocytize the cellular debris that remains when inflammation subsides.

The enzyme systems of monocytes are designed to degrade engulfed tissue debris from chronic inflammatory reactions, and monocyte numbers increase in chronic infections. They are especially valuable in the defense against long-term inflammation be cause of their larger size and longer life span. Lysosomes within the cytoplasm of the neutrophils and monocytes help in the digestion of the phagocytized materials.

Monocytes are the cells that make up the **mononuclear phagocytic system (MPS)**. The MPS was formerly known as the reticuloendothelial system. Its cells either are monocytes (intravascular) or are derived from monocytes (extravascular). The cells are mobile (macro phages) or become fixed in position (e.g., the

Kupffer cells in the liver sinusoids and others in the spleen and lymph nodes). The fixed cells are also phagocytic.

Monocytes in birds are comparable in morphology to avian large lymphocytes, but in general they have relatively more cytoplasm than large lymphocytes.

Eosinophils

On a stained blood film, eosinophils can be seen to have cytoplasmic granules that are red or reddish-orange (eosinophilic). These are about the same size as neutrophils. The granules contain several enzymes (e.g., histaminase) that dampen and terminate local inflammatory reactions of allergic origin. Eosinophils become more numerous in certain types of parasitisms. The parasitic forms are **opsonized (attacked by antibodies)**, and the eosinophils discharge their granular contents onto the surface of the opsonized parasite, inflicting lethal damage.

In **Cushing's disease** there is an oversecretion of adrenocorticosteroid hormones (see Chapter 6). When **cortisol (an adrenocorticosteroid)** is injected, this condition is simulated and the number of circulating eosinophils decreases. Cortisol reduces the eosinophil count by enhancing eosinophil diapedesis and by diminishing the release of eosinophils from the bone marrow. Cortisol production increases during stress, and lowered eosinophil blood counts have been associated with stress.

Because of their eosinophilic granules and polymorphic nuclei, avian eosinophils have similarities to avian heterophils. However, the eosinophil granules are spherical and are dull red instead of the heterophil granule brilliant red. Also, the nucleus is most often bilobed and stains a richer blue than the heterophil.

Basophils

Basophils of the blood are somewhat similar to the **mast cells** that are present in the inter-

stitial spaces outside the capillaries (see Chapter 1). They seem to lack phagocytic power. Basophil granules contain histamine, bradykinin, serotonin, and lysosomal enzymes, substances that initiate an inflammatory response. Basophils and mast cells have receptors on their cell membranes for immuno globulin E (IgE) antibodies (those associated with allergies). When the antibody on the cell membrane contacts its antigen, the basophil ruptures, releasing its granular contents, and the local vascular and tissue reactions of allergies are manifested. Basophils are rare in normal blood, and their distribution in blood is usually considered to be less than 1%.

Basophils enhance allergic reactions, whereas eosinophils tend to dampen them. There is a balance between their functions in that inflammatory reactions proceed quickly (basophils) and then are modified (eosinophils) so that overreaction does not occur.

Avian basophils are about the same size and shape as heterophils. The nucleus is usually round or oval and weakly basophilic. Deeply basophilic granules are numerous in cytoplasm that is devoid of color.

Lymphocytes

Lymphocytes can be classified morphologically as small or **large lymphocytes**. It is believed that the large lymphocytes represent immature lymphocytes, whereas the **small lymphocytes** represent more mature forms. Lymphocytes are involved in immune responses, and on this basis are classified as T cells or B cells. Both T and B cells are derived from hematopoietic stem cells (lymphoblasts) that differentiate to form lymphocytes. For mammals, shortly before or after birth, the site of early processing and differentiation of the stem cells for T lymphocytes is the thymus gland; for B lymphocytes, the sites are the fetal liver, spleen, and bone marrow. T cells are involved in **cell-mediated immunity**, which involves the formation of large numbers of lymphocytes to destroy foreign substances

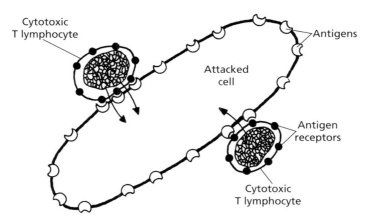

■ **FIGURE 3-5** Mechanism by which sensitized cytotoxic T lymphocytes destroy a foreign cell. The attacked cell is killed by the release of cytotoxic and digestive enzymes from the T lymphocytes directly into the cytoplasm of the attacked cell. The T lymphocytes can proceed to other cells after their attack on a cell.

(antigens). The three different types of T cells are: 1) **cytotoxic T cells**, 2) **helper T cells**, and 3) **memory T cells**. Cytotoxic T cells are sometimes called killer cells. T-cell receptors bind to specific antigens, and cytotoxic substances are released into the foreign cell (e.g., bacteria, virus, tissue cell; *Fig. 3-5*). Cytotoxic cells also attack cells of transplanted organs. Because cancer cells generate unique antigens when they become cancerous, cytotoxic T cells recognize the cancerous cells as foreign to the body and attack them. Helper T cells are the most numerous of the T cells. When helper T cells are activated, they assist in the activation of cytotoxic T cells and of B cells. Antigens ordinarily activate these cells, but activation is more intense when assisted by helper T cells. Memory T cells are long-lived and respond to the same antigen when exposed at a later date.

B lymphocytes were first discovered in birds, and early processing and differentiation were found to be in the bursa of Fabricius, from which the name was derived (B for bursa). After exposure to an antigen, **activated B cells** proliferate and transform into **plasma cells** and a smaller number of **memory cells**. The memory B cells have a function similar to memory T cells and are readily converted to effector cells by a later encounter with the same antigen. B cells do not attack foreign substances directly, but instead the plasma cells produce large quantities of **antibodies (globulin molecules called immunoglobulins)** that inactivate the foreign substance. This type of immunity is known as **humoral immunity**. Antibodies can produce inactivation by causing **agglutination**, **precipitation**, **neutralization** (antibodies cover toxic sites), or **lysis** (rupture of the cell). Agglutination and precipitation reactions are shown in *Figure 3-6*.

A more common humoral method of immunity is represented by the **complement system**, which is composed of a number of enzyme precursors that are activated successively. From a small beginning, a large reaction occurs. Examples of **complement reactions** are: 1) **opsonization**, in which foreign substances are covered by antibody and become vulnerable to phagocytosis by neutrophils and macrophages, and 2) **chemotaxis**, in which the complement product attracts neutrophils and macrophages into the local region of the antigenic agent. Several other complement products can be formed and result in lysis, agglutination, inflammation, and activation of mast cells and basophils, which produce a number of inflammatory effects in an effort to incapacitate the antigenic agent.

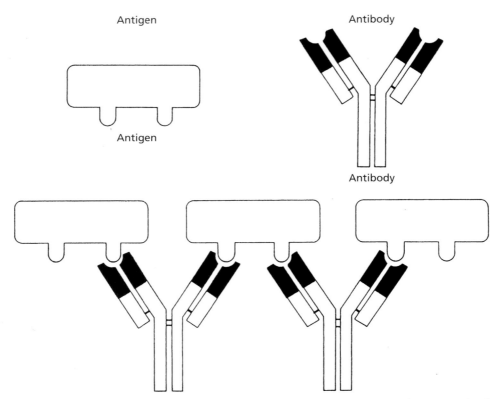

■ **FIGURE 3-6** Antigen–antibody agglutination and precipitation. Antigens (molecules or cells) are grouped with other antigens by bivalent (two binding sites) antibodies. This causes them to agglutinate or precipitate. (From Vander AJ, Sherman JH, Luciano DS. Human Physiology: The Mechanisms of Body Function. 4th Ed. New York: McGraw-Hill, 1985.)

Lymphocytes comprise about two-thirds of the leukocytes in birds and in this regard are similar to the cloven-hoofed animals. There are large and small lymphocytes as in mammals, with varying amounts of cytoplasm (meager in small lymphocytes and abundant in large) that is weakly basophilic.

Diagnostic Procedures

Diagnostic procedures related to white blood cells include determination of their total number and distribution of the leukocyte types. The total number can be determined by dilution and subsequent counting, either manually in a hemacytometer or with an electronic counter. An increase in leukocyte numbers is called

leukocytosis; this usually occurs in bacterial infections. A decrease in numbers is called **leukopenia**; this is usually associated with the early stages of viral infections. Leukemia is a cancer of white blood cells and is characterized by leukocytosis. The determination of the percentage distribution of WBCs is known as a **differential white blood cell count**. In this procedure a smear is made of a blood drop and is subsequently stained. The cells are observed under a microscope, and the different types are counted and classified until a total of 100 has been tallied. The number for each type is then estimated as the percentage distribution in the blood (see Table 3-1).

The **absolute number of leukocytes** is calculated after the total number and differential count have been determined. The absolute number refers to the number per microliter for each leukocyte type. Determination of the absolute number can prevent misinterpretation of the differential count. For example, the total WBC count for a normal cow might be 9,000/µL. This number could be 30% neutrophils and 60% lymphocytes, in which the absolute numbers would be 2,700/µL ($0.30 \times 9{,}000$) and 5,400/µL ($0.60 \times 9{,}000$), respectively. If traumatic reticuloperitonitis (hardware disease) is present, this same cow might have a total WBC count of 27,000/µL and a differential count of 70% neutrophils and 20% lymphocytes. A first interpretation might be that a lymphopenia exists (60% lymphocytes decreased to 20%). Further calculation shows, however, that the absolute number of lymphocytes remains the same ($27{,}000/\mu L \times 0.20 = 5{,}400/\mu L$), whereas the absolute number of neutrophils increases ($27{,}000/\mu L \times 0.70 = 18{,}900/\mu L$). The neutrophil increase would indicate inflammation. Refer to Appendix A, where normal absolute values (range and average) are presented for the domestic animal species.

■ ERYTHROCYTES

1. What chemical atom associated with hemoglobin binds loosely and reversibly with oxygen? How many molecules of O_2 can be transported by one molecule of hemoglobin?
2. What is the valence of iron before and after its binding with oxygen?
3. What are methemoglobin, myoglobin, and carbonmonoxyhemoglobin, and how do they differ from hemoglobin?
4. What is the average concentration of hemoglobin in the blood of domestic animals?
5. What is the physiologic name for the production of erythrocytes?
6. Where does RBC production occur during the postnatal, growth, and adult periods?

7. How does reticulocyte presence relate to life span of erythrocytes?
8. What substance controls the rate of erythropoiesis? Where is it produced?
9. How long does it take for new RBCs to enter the circulation after their formation begins?
10. If there are 7 million RBCs in each microliter of cow blood, how many would there be in one milliliter?
11. What are advantages of a discoid RBC shape? What is tolerance to RBC shape change known as?
12. Which domestic animal has the largest RBC? The smallest?
13. Which one of the erythrocyte indices relates to an erythrocyte's volume? What is the unit of expression? What is the unit of expression for the amount of hemoglobin in each RBC?

Hemoglobin and Its Forms

The principal component of erythrocytes is **hemoglobin (Hb)**, which makes up about one-third of the erythrocyte content, the remainder being water and stroma (structural components). The hemoglobin molecule (*Fig. 3-7*) has a molecular weight of about 67,000 and is composed of four heme groups combined with one molecule of globin (the protein component). Globin is composed of four polypeptide chains, each containing one of the heme groups. Each heme group contains an iron atom that combines loosely and reversibly with one oxygen molecule. Therefore, one molecule of hemoglobin contains four iron atoms and can carry four molecules of oxygen. The iron atom of heme has a valence of +2 (Fe^{2+}, ferrous) regardless of whether molecular oxygen is combined with it. Because of the presence of hemoglobin, blood can transport about 60 times more oxygen than would be possible by its simple solution. Certain conditions cause the ferrous iron of heme to be oxidized to its ferric state. In one such

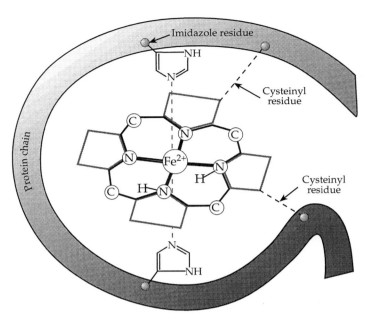

■ **FIGURE 3-7** Schematic representation of one heme group and its associated polypeptide chain. Four of these combinations, at different orientations to each other, make up hemoglobin. The heme is held to its specific polypeptide chain (one of four in the protein globin) by cysteine (an amino acid) bridges and by bonding of the iron to imidazole groups of histidine (an amino acid). Molecular oxygen binds with iron. (Modified from Conn EE, Stumpf PK. Outlines of Biochemistry. New York: John Wiley & Sons, 1963.)

condition, nitrate poisoning, the hemoglobin formed is known as methemoglobin, and it cannot transport oxygen. Another abnormal form of hemoglobin is carbonmonoxyhemoglobin (sometimes called carboxyhemoglobin). As the name implies, carbon monoxide occupies the site normally occupied by oxygen. Hemoglobin has an affinity for carbon monoxide that is about 200 times greater than its affinity for oxygen. Thus, small concentrations of carbon monoxide compete more favorably for sites on Hb than normal concentrations of oxygen.

The hemoglobin of muscle is known as **myoglobin**. It differs from hemoglobin in that it has only one polypeptide chain and one associated heme group, so it can only combine with one molecule of oxygen instead of four. The concentration of hemoglobin in the blood of domestic animals averages about 12 g/dL (*Table 3-2*).

Erythropoiesis

The production of erythrocytes is known as **erythropoiesis**. Before birth, erythrocyte formation occurs in the liver, spleen, and bone marrow. During the postnatal, growth, and adult periods, erythropoiesis is restricted almost exclusively to the bone marrow. It seems that most bones are involved in erythropoiesis, and the axial and appendicular skeletons account for about 35% and 65% of RBC production, respectively. This pattern has been observed in 1-year-old beagle dogs and can vary in other animals. The **axial skeleton** includes almost all bones except those of the limbs, which belong to the **appendicular skeleton** (see Chapter 7). The erythrocytes are continually formed and destroyed. Considering the large number of RBCs in the blood, one should appreciate the dynamic aspect of this phenomenon. For example, approximately

TABLE 3-2 AVERAGE VALUES FOR SEVERAL BLOOD VARIABLES[a]

VARIABLE	ANIMAL					
	HORSE[b]	COW	SHEEP	PIG	DOG	CHICKEN
Total RBC/µL blood ($\times 10^6$)	9.0	7.0	12.0	6.5	6.8	3.0
Diameter of RBC (µm)	5.5	5.9	4.8	6.0	7.0	elliptic 7×12
PCV (%)	41.0	35.0	35.0	42.0	45.0	30.0
Sedimentation rate (mm/min)	2–12/10	0/60	0/60	1–14/60	6–10/60	1.5–4/60
Hemoglobin (g/dL)	14.4	11.0	11.5	13.0	15.0	9.0
Coagulation time (capillary tube method; min)	2–5	2–5	2–5	2–5	2–5	[c]
Specific gravity (g/dL)	1.060	1.043	1.042	1.060	1.059	1.050
Plasma protein (g/dL)	6–8	7–8.5	6–8	6.5–8.5	6–7.8	4.5
Blood pH (arterial)	7.40	7.38	7.48	7.4	7.36	7.48
Blood volume (percent of body weight)	8–10	5–6	5–6	5–7	8–10	7–9
Mean corpuscular volume (MCV; fL)	45.5	52.0	34.0	63.0	70.0	115.0
Mean corpuscular hemoglobin (MCH; pg)	15.9	14.0	10.0	19.0	22.8	41.0
Mean corpuscular hemoglobin concentration (MCHC; %)	35.0	33.0	32.5	32.0	34.0	29.0

[a]Data compiled from Swenson MJ. Physiological properties and cellular and chemical constituents of blood. In: Swenson MJ, Reece WO, eds. Duke's Physiology of Domestic Animals, 11th Ed. Ithaca, NY: Cornell University Press, 1993, and Jain NC. Essentials of Veterinary Hematology. Philadelphia: Lea & Febiger, 1993.
[b]Hot blooded.
[c]See Species Differences.

35,000,000 erythrocytes are formed and destroyed in a 450-kg horse each second.

Erythrocytes are formed in the bone marrow from a beginning cell known as a **rubriblast**. Several intermediate forms are recognized in the genesis of the erythrocyte (*Fig. 3-8*). The distribution of these forms can be studied by preparation and examination of bone marrow smears. Just before the developing erythrocyte's entrance into the circulation, the nucleus is expelled. The polyribosomes and ribosomes are retained and might still be apparent on stained smears for a day or so after their arrival in the circulation. If they are present, they are identified as **reticulocytes** because of the netlike appearance of the polyribosomes and ribosomes. **Polyribosomes (polysomes)** consist of several ribosomes joined together by the same messenger RNA molecule. During periods of rapid RBC production, reticulocyte numbers can increase. Reticulocytes are usually present in the blood of animals when the life span of erythrocytes is less than 100 days. The dog is an exception. Adult ruminants, and especially horses, with longer RBC life spans, do not have reticulocytes in the circulating blood in health. The nuclei of avian erythrocytes are not expelled before

| Rubriblast | Basophilic rubricyte | Polychromatophilic rubricyte | Metarubricyte | Reticulo- cyte | Erythro- cyte |

■ FIGURE 3-8 The stages of erythrocyte development.

entry into the circulation, and they persist throughout the life of the erythrocytes.

The rate of erythropoiesis seems to be controlled by the tissue need for oxygen. The reduced oxygen concentration at the tissue level results in the secretion of a hormone by the kidneys known as **erythropoietin**. Erythropoietin stimulates the bone marrow to begin formation of new erythrocytes. The life span of erythropoietin is less than 1 day; this short life span helps provide greater flexibility in the adjustment of erythrocyte numbers to regulate the tissue need for oxygen more precisely. New erythrocytes do not appear in the circulation until about 5 days after their formation begins. Thus, additional erythropoietin can be formed to allow for continued production during the interim. When the new erythrocytes appear in the circulation, the tissue need for oxygen begins to be met, and erythropoietin is no longer secreted.

Numbers

The number of erythrocytes can be determined by making known dilutions and counting the number of RBCs in a known volume using the counting chamber of a hemacytometer with the aid of a microscope. The Unopette® microcollection system (Becton Dickinson and Company, Franklin Lakes, NJ) is widely used for this purpose. In addition to erythrocytes, leukocytes and platelets can also be enumerated with this system. Using various multiplication factors (which make allowance for dilution and for the limited volume that is

counted), the number of RBCs per microliter of blood can be determined. More accurate determinations can be made by using electronic counting equipment. A number of systems are available that are capable of counting erythrocytes, leukocytes, and platelets and of determining hemoglobin concentration. The cells are counted as they stream by a photoelectric cell in single file. A computer within provides printouts of means, ranges, and call-outs for highs and lows. The erythrocyte indices are also calculated for erythrocytes. Generally, there are about 7,000,000 RBCs/μL blood in the cow, pig, and dog (see Table 3-2). More RBCs are seen for hot-blooded horses (9,000,000/μL) and for sheep (11,000,000/μL). Values for the goat are not given in Table 3-2, but they average about 13,000,000/μL blood. See Appendix A for erythrocyte profiles (range and average) for each of the domestic animal species.

Shape

Erythrocytes are generally considered to be discocytes, with some degree of concavity. The dog's RBCs have typical biconcave disks, whereas the goat's RBCs are more spherical. The camel has elliptical RBCs, and the deer has RBCs that are somewhat sickle-shaped. The advantages of a discoid shape are: 1) the provision of a larger surface area–volume ratio, 2) minimal diffusion distance, and 3) greater osmotic swelling (water intake) possible without threatening the integrity of the membrane.

The characteristic shape of erythrocytes is maintained by the molecular constitution of hemoglobin and by certain contractile proteins of the cell membrane. An altered shape, because of a difference in hemoglobin constitution, can result in disease, such as sickle cell anemia in humans. A genetically induced substitution of the amino acid valine for the usual glutamic acid in the amino acid sequence of hemoglobin causes RBCs to assume a sickle shape, rather than the usual biconcave disk shape, when hemoglobin is deoxygenated. The altered shape makes the cells more vulnerable to destruction, and the anemia results.

Erythrocytes are tolerant of shape changes as they circulate. Many variations are noted as they pass through the small lumen (duct) of capillaries or rebound from a collision with a vessel bifurcation (branch). This property of tolerance for shape change is known as **plasticity**.

Size

Among the domestic animals, dogs have erythrocytes with the largest diameter (7 μm), and sheep and goats have those with the smallest (4 to 4.5 μm). It seems that this was an adaptive feature, because RBCs of the smallest size are greater in number. Because the sheep and goat were commonly found in regions of high altitudes with lower oxygen concentrations, the available hemoglobin was placed in a greater number of smaller packages so that a greater surface area would be available for diffusion.

Erythrocyte Indices

The **erythrocyte indices** are determinations that are calculated after the erythrocytes (RBCs) have been enumerated and PCV and Hb concentration ([Hb]) determined. There are three indices, and each relates to a value for a single RBC. Accordingly, the units are small and are shown for each as follows:

1. MCV = mean corpuscular volume in femtoliters (fL); femto = one quadrillionth (10^{-15})

2. MCH = mean corpuscular hemoglobin in picograms (pg); pico = one trillionth (10^{-12})
3. MCHC = mean corpuscular hemoglobin concentration in g/dL (deciliter) or g percent.

Derivations of values are as follows: (exponent manipulations completed but not included)

1. MCV = (PCV ÷ RBC) × 10
    Example: PCV = 42%; RBC = 7 million/μL
    42 ÷ 7 × 10 = 60 fL
2. MCH = ([Hb] ÷ RBC) × 10
    Example: [Hb] = 14 g/dL; RBC = 7 million/μL
    14 ÷ 7 × 10 = 20 pg
3. MCHC = ([Hb] ÷ PCV) × 100
    Example: [Hb] = 14 g/dL; PCV = 42%
    14 ÷ 42 × 100 = 33.3%

It is easier to visualize the above derivations by considering the following:

1. For MCV. The RBCs in 1 L of blood occupy a volume of 420 mL. Because there are 7 million RBCs/μL, one can determine the volume of each RBC by dividing the total volume (420 mL) by the number of RBCs contained in that volume.
2. For MCH. There are 140 g of Hb in 1 L of blood. The amount of Hb in each RBC can be determined by dividing the total amount of Hb in 1 L (140 g) by the number of RBCs in the liter.
3. For MCHC. Assume that the RBC mass (PCV) in 1 dL weighs 42 g, therefore, the percent of that mass attributed to Hb is obtained by division as shown and multiplying by 100.

The values for these indices are shown for each species in Table 3-2. The indices are valuable aids in the diagnosis of various anemias.

Life Span

The life span of erythrocytes varies with species. Reported values for horses are 140 to 150 days. In adult ruminants (cattle, sheep, and goats), erythrocyte life span varies from 125 to 160 days, in pigs from 75 to 95 days, in dogs from 100 to 120 days, and 70 to 80 days in cats. The life span of erythrocytes of chickens is 20 to 30 days.

■ FATE OF ERYTHROCYTES

1.   What cell accounts for removal of about 90% of aged RBCs? What are the organs where this occurs?
2.   How can icterus (jaundice) occur during the degradation of hemoglobin?
3.   How can hemoglobinemia and hemoglobinuria occur as a result of RBC destruction?

As erythrocytes age, several metabolic changes occur: the membrane becomes more rigid and fragile, and the discocyte converts to a poorly deformable spherocyte. Accordingly, some intravascular hemolysis of erythrocytes occurs (10%), and the remainder of the aged RBCs (about 90%) is selectively removed from the circulating pool by cells of the MPS, mostly by the fixed cells in the spleen, liver, and bone marrow.

When erythrocytes are phagocytized by MPS cells, they undergo hemolysis within the phagocytic cell (**extravascular or intracellular hemolysis**), and the Hb, other proteins, and membrane lipids of the phagocytized RBCs are catabolized. A summary of Hb degradation begun in this way is shown in *Figure 3-9*. The iron and globin are separated from heme, globin is degraded to its amino acids, and they are reutilized. Iron is stored in the MPS cells in the form of **ferritin** and **hemosiderin** or is transferred to plasma, where it combines with a plasma protein, apotransferrin, to become **transferrin**. Transferrin circulates to the bone marrow, where the iron is used for the synthesis of new hemoglobin. During Hb synthesis, iron released from decomposing RBCs is used in preference to storage iron.

Heme is converted to **biliverdin** (a green pigment) and then reduced to **bilirubin** (a

yellow pigment). **Free bilirubin** (water-insoluble) is released into the plasma, where it becomes bound to albumin (a plasma protein) and is transported to the liver and is "dumped." In the liver, the insoluble bilirubin conjugates with glucuronic acid to form **bilirubin glucuronide**, mainly diglucuronide, which is water-soluble. It is secreted into the bile in this form and enters the intestine. Bacteria within the large intestine reduce bilirubin glucuronide to **urobilinogen**. Most urobilinogen is excreted with the feces in the oxidized forms of **urobilin** or **stercobilin**, which are pigments that give feces its normal color. Part of the urobilinogen is reabsorbed into the enterohepatic circulation, from which most is re-excreted into the bile. Some of the absorbed urobilinogen bypasses the liver, enters the general circulation and is excreted in the urine to become a part of the normal pigment of the urine as urobilin. Carbon monoxide (CO) is formed when the porphyrin ring of heme is opened. This is the only reaction in the body in which CO is formed and is excreted by the lungs.

Because of liver disease, free bilirubin combined with albumin might not be "dumped" and would continue to circulate and appear in high concentration in the plasma and interstitial fluids. Also, if the bile duct becomes blocked, the bilirubin glucuronides (soluble bilirubin) could spill over into the plasma. Both of these conditions can produce a yellow color in the tissues known as **icterus**, or **jaundice**.

When erythrocytes are hemolyzed intravascularly, the Hb is first bound to **haptoglobin** (a plasma protein). This complex is rapidly removed by cells of the MPS, and the Hb is degraded as described above for extravascular hemolysis. Because the complex is a large molecule, it is not filtered through the kidney glomeruli. Excessive intravascular hemolysis (hemolytic disease) can occur, however, and sufficient haptoglobin might not be available. The plasma takes on a reddish appearance, and the condition is known as **hemoglobine-**

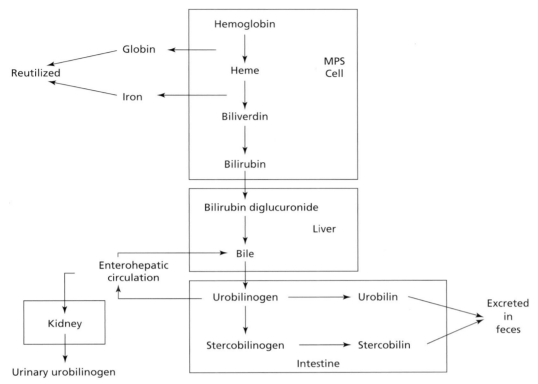

■ FIGURE 3-9 Degradation of hemoglobin that began within mononuclear phagocytic system (MPS) cells. Iron release as shown, used preferentially for synthesis of new hemoglobin. Protein (globin) degraded to amino acids and reutilized. Bilirubin released from MPS cells is insoluble and combines with a protein (known as free bilirubin) and is transported to the liver, where it is converted to bilirubin diglucuronide (soluble form of bilirubin). The soluble form enters the biliary system and is transported to the intestine. Bacterial reduction of bilirubin diglucuronide produces urobilinogen that may be recirculated via the enterohepatic circulation or further reduced to urobilin or stercobilinogen. Some of the recirculated urobilinogen bypasses the liver, enters the general circulation, and is excreted in the urine. (From Reece WO, Swenson MJ. The composition and functions of blood. In: Reece WO, ed. Dukes' Physiology of Domestic Animals. 12th Ed. Ithaca, NY: Cornell University Press, 2004.)

mia. The free Hb is then filtered at the glomeruli and enters the kidney tubules. Much of it is reabsorbed from the tubules, but can surpass the renal threshold for reabsorption and continue into the urine to give it a reddish color, a condition known as **hemoglobinuria**.

■ IRON METABOLISM

1. **What is the oxidation state of the storage form of iron?**
2. **What is the oxidation state of iron for transfer across cell membranes?**
3. **What is the name of the transport form of iron?**
4. **Would iron in its transport form be toxic? If not, why not?**
5. **What are the normal limitations to iron absorption? Can iron toxicity occur as a result of excess ingestion and subsequent absorption?**

Free iron (Fe^{2+}) catalyzes the separation of free radicals from molecular oxygen, and oxygen free radicals are toxic. To avoid toxicity, intracellular iron is either bound to or incorporated into various proteins. It is transported and stored in the protein-bound form in its **ferric (Fe^{3+}) oxidation state**. To be transported across membranes, iron must be in its **ferrous (Fe^{2+}) oxidation state**.

A large proportion of ingested iron is reduced to ferrous iron (Fe^{2+}) in the stomach.

Within the duodenum and jejunum, most of the ferrous iron is absorbed into the intestinal epithelial cells. Iron absorption, transport, storage, and usage are summarized in *Figure 3-10*. From the intestinal cell, it enters the blood or can combine with a cellular protein (apoferritin) to become ferritin, a storage form of iron. Within 2 or 3 days, the ferritin is either

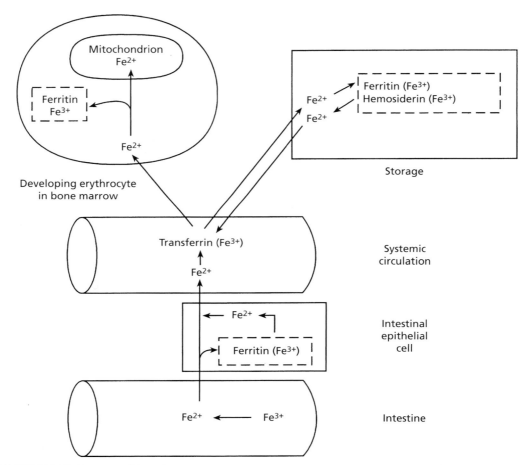

■ **FIGURE 3-10** Summary of iron absorption, storage, and use. Iron must be in the ferrous (Fe^{2+}) oxidation state to be transported across membranes. Intracellular iron is bound to or incorporated into various proteins or other chelates in its ferric (Fe^{3+}) oxidation state to reduce its toxicity because free iron can catalyze free radicals from molecular oxygen and hydrogen ions and can have disastrous consequences for biological materials. Transported iron is bound to the protein apotransferrin and is known as transferrin. Iron is stored in tissues as either a diffuse, soluble, mobile fraction (ferritin) or as insoluble, aggregated deposits (hemosiderin). Principal locations of iron storage are the liver and spleen, followed by the kidney, heart, skeletal muscle, and brain. In the bone marrow, all erythroid forms have surface membrane receptors for transferrin. When internalized, released iron is transported into the mitochondria of developing erythrocytes, where it is incorporated into the heme molecule or it combines with the protein apoferritin to be stored as ferritin. (From Reece WO, Swenson MJ. The composition and functions of blood. In: Reece WO, ed. Dukes' Physiology of Domestic Animals. 12th Ed. Ithaca, NY: Cornell University Press, 2004.)

converted back to its free form (Fe^{2+}) and absorbed into the blood or is cast into the intestinal lumen. The latter situation would be a result of the normal turnover of intestinal epithelial cells as they migrate from the crypts to the tips of the villi, from which they are exfoliated (passed off into the lumen) (see Chapter 12). The iron that enters the blood combines with apotransferrin (a plasma protein) to form transferrin. Combining with a protein prevents it from being excreted by the kidneys (the combination is poorly filtered at the glomerulus).

Within the bone marrow, all of the erythroid forms, including reticulocytes, have surface membrane receptors for transferrin. Plasma transferrin binds to these receptors, becomes internalized by endocytosis, and releases its iron, and the apotransferrin is returned to the plasma. The internalized iron is either transported into the mitochondria of the developing erythrocyte, where it is incorporated into the heme molecule, or it combines with apoferritin to be stored as ferritin in its ferric (Fe^{3+}) oxidation state.

Two factors generally affect the absorption of iron from the intestinal epithelium into the blood: 1) the extent of the iron stores in the body, and 2) the rate of erythropoiesis. If the requirement for iron increases and the iron stores are empty, absorption increases. If the requirement for iron decreases and the iron stores are adequate, absorption of iron from the intestine decreases. It seems that there is a self-limiting mechanism for iron absorption based on need. Excess iron can be ingested and subsequently absorbed, however, inducing iron toxicity. The excretion of iron is minimal so that the regulation is unidirectional—that is, controlled absorption. Iron with transferrin can be released to tissue cells anywhere so that excess iron can be deposited in all cells, especially those of the liver. **Ferritin** is a storage form of iron (see previous text). In addition, a more insoluble form, **hemosiderin**, accumulates in times of excess. The liver is the principal organ for iron storage. When liver stores are adequate, the production of apotransferrin decreases, and when they are depleted, the production of apotransferrin increases. Animals with iron deficiency anemia have high concentrations of apotransferrin.

■ ANEMIA AND POLYCYTHEMIA

1. Define anemia and polycythemia.
2. Without supplemental iron, why would anemia be common in baby pigs?
3. Differentiate between absolute and relative polycythemia.
4. What are some primary conditions that cause absolute polycythemia?

A reduction in the number of erythrocytes, the concentration of hemoglobin, or both is referred to as **anemia**, which can have several causes. It is considered **functional** if the tissues do not become hypoxic because of lack of exertion and because erythropoietin is not formed. **Blood loss** for any reason (e.g., trauma, parasitism) can also cause anemia. A common type of anemia in baby pigs is iron deficiency anemia. This type is common in baby pigs because of their rapid growth and consequent need for greater blood volume, and also because of the lack of iron in their normal diet, which is sow's milk. Because of iron deficiency, an insufficient quantity of hemoglobin is produced. Anemia can also occur from poor erythrocyte production, such as when certain nutritional factors are missing, or if the bone marrow has been poisoned. This latter type is known as aplastic anemia.

A condition opposite to that of anemia is **polycythemia**. In this condition, the erythrocyte mass is greatly increased. The condition may be relative or absolute. In **relative polycythemia**, there is an increase in red cell mass and a decrease in plasma volume. This is commonly encountered in conditions of shock and dehydration and in animals being treated with diuretic or cardiac medications. **Absolute polycythemia** is associated with an increased red cell mass without a decrease in plasma volume. It is secondary (not the primary condition) if associated with hypoxemia (decreased O_2 in arterial blood) or a tumor because either condition increases erythropoietin production. In the absence of hypoxemia or tumors, and when erythropoietin concentrations are normal or decreased, the condition is classified as a myeloproliferative disorder (increased bone marrow production) or **polycythemia vera**. Polycythemia vera is rare in animals, although it has been described in cats, dogs, and cattle.

■ HEMOSTASIS: PREVENTION OF BLOOD LOSS

1. What is the sequence of events from the time of vascular injury to a return to normal?
2. What is the principal chemical component of the clotting factors? Note the major sites of their synthesis.
3. What vitamin is required for the synthesis of several coagulation factors?
4. What chemical element is required for nearly all of the hemostatic reactions?
5. What is the substance contained in the basement membrane of capillaries and throughout the interstitial space that provides for platelet adhesion?
6. What are the properties of vascular endothelium that prevent activation of platelets and procoagulants?
7. What is another name for platelets?
8. Study the fine structure of the platelet and relate its structure to the release of the granular contents.
9. What is the first response of platelets to disrupted endothelium and contact with subendothelial tissues?
10. In addition to collagen, what substance is required for the initial adhesion of platelets?
11. What is the principal messenger that is formed after platelet stimulation that will release Ca^{21} from granule storage?

12. What is the role of aspirin in the blood coagulation scheme?
13. What is the platelet release reaction, and how is it initiated?
14. What is accomplished by platelet aggregation?
15. What are the four key reactions involved in the formation of a clot?
16. What are the relationships of the tenase and prothrombinase complexes to the formation of thrombin?
17. Know the difference between the extrinsic and intrinsic systems (tissue factor and contact activation pathways, respectively) and their relationship to each other.
18. In what way is the activation of factor X a focal point in the blood coagulation scheme?
19. What is the significance of factor XIII? What is its origin?
20. How is clot retraction accomplished? What is its function?
21. Once initiated, what prevents blood coagulation from spreading (clot growth)?
22. What is the role of plasmin? What is the principal plasminogen activator?

The effectiveness of blood function depends on its circulation within a closed system of vessels. The vessels might open because of disease or accident, and blood loss can be prevented or minimized by **hemostasis**.

When a blood vessel is damaged, endothelial cells are separated, the underlying collagen is exposed, and the surface loses its usual smoothness and nonwettability. Often the vessel is torn, cut, or separated, and the hemostatic crisis is exacerbated. Regardless of the severity, platelets begin to contact the damaged surface. This initiates the adhesion process because the platelets develop projections (pseudopods) and become sticky (*Fig. 3-11*). The adhered platelets undergo a reaction in which aggregating agents are released

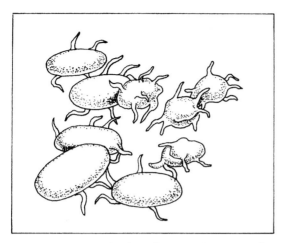

■ **FIGURE 3-11** Platelet adhesion. This is the first response to blood vessel injury. The platelets lose their discoid shape and form sticky projections (pseudopods) for their continued adherence to the injured vessel and entrapment of other platelets.

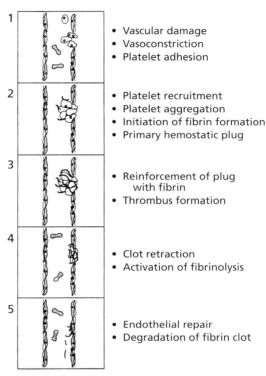

1
- Vascular damage
- Vasoconstriction
- Platelet adhesion

2
- Platelet recruitment
- Platelet aggregation
- Initiation of fibrin formation
- Primary hemostatic plug

3
- Reinforcement of plug with fibrin
- Thrombus formation

4
- Clot retraction
- Activation of fibrinolysis

5
- Endothelial repair
- Degradation of fibrin clot

■ **FIGURE 3-12** The five major stages in the formation and dissolution of a blood clot, or thrombus, around the site of vascular injury extending from the initiation of platelet activation after vascular damage through endothelial repair. (From Gentry PA. Blood coagulation and hemostasis. In: Reece WO, ed. Dukes' Physiology of Domestic Animals. 12th Ed. Ithaca, NY: Cornell University Press, 2004.)

and cause the accumulation of more platelets. If a vessel is separated, a loose platelet plug is formed that impedes blood loss. When this occurs, blood coagulation soon becomes evident at the damaged site, and the platelet plug is strengthened by the formation of a fibrin meshwork. Clot retraction (reduction in size) occurs, and fibrinolysis (dissolution of fibrin) begins. Finally, the damaged vessel is repaired by connective tissue and endothelial cell growth, and there is a return to normal when the platelet–fibrin complex and other cell debris is removed (Fig. 3-12).

Hemostatic Components

A complex series of biochemical reactions make up the hemostatic process. The major contributors to the process are proteins, vascular endothelium, and platelets.

Proteins

The protein components of the blood coagulation pathway, their synonyms or common abbreviations, and site of synthesis are pre-

sented in *Table 3-3*. The factor association with Roman numeral designation was described when first discovered and included factors I to XIII. As shown in Table 3-3, many still persist, but the identification of others was discontinued (e.g., VI was initially described but found later not to exist; IV identified Ca^{2+} and discontinued because it was not a protein). The major components now shown are proteins, and the list has grown because of continued discovery. These proteins are present in the blood or tissues and simply await an activation mechanism.

It is important to recognize that Ca^{2+} is required for nearly all of the reactions and that

TABLE 3-3 THE MAJOR COMPONENTS OF THE COAGULATION PATHWAY (ENZYMES, PROTEIN COFACTORS, AND SUBSTRATES) INVOLVED IN FIBRIN FORMATION AND FIBRIN DEGRADATION

COMPONENT	SYNONYM	SITE OF SYNTHESIS
Fibrinogen	Factor I	Liver
Prothrombin	Factor II	Liver[a]
Thrombin		Plasma
Tissue factor	Thromboplastin	Vascular endothelium
Factor V		Vascular endothelium
Factor VII		Liver[a]
Factor VIII	Antihemophilic factor	Vascular endothelium
Factor IX	Christmas factor	Liver[a]
Factor X	Stuart factor	Liver[a]
Factor XI	Plasma thromboplastin antecedent	Liver
Factor XII	Hageman factor	Liver
Factor XIII	Fibrin stabilizing factor	Liver
von Willebrand factor	vWF	Vascular endothelium
Prekallikrein	PK, Fletcher factor	Liver
High-molecular-weight kininogen	HK, HMWK	Liver
Protein C		Liver[a]
Protein S		Liver[a]
Thrombomodulin	TM	Vascular endothelium
Plasminogen		Liver
Tissue-type plasminogen activator	t-PA	Liver
Urokinase-type plasminogen activator	uPA, prourokinase	Unknown

[a]Vitamin K dependent protein.
From Gentry PA. Blood coagulation and hemostasis. In: Reece WO, ed. Dukes' Physiology of Domestic Animals. 12th Ed. Ithaca, NY: Cornell University Press, 2004.

vitamin K is required for production by the liver of prothrombin, protein C, protein S, and factors VII, IX, and X.

Vascular Endothelium

The entire cardiovascular system is lined by a single layer of flattened cells known as the endothelium (see Chapter 9). It not only lines the heart, but also the vessels. At the capillary level, all that remains is the endothelial layer. Regardless of its location, it is underlain with a basement membrane that contains collagen. Collagen fibers are also present throughout the interstitial space (see Chapter 1). Collagen in the subendothelial tissue, as well as

fibronectin released from endothelial cells, provide for the adhesion of platelets to the site of vascular injury.

As long as the endothelium is intact, the platelets and the proteins that are associated with blood coagulation (**procoagulants**) are not activated. The properties of the endothelium that prevent activation include: 1) the negative charge on the endothelial cell surface that repels the negatively charged platelets, 2) synthesis of inhibitors of platelet function (e.g., prostacyclin) and of fibrin formation (e.g., thrombomodulin), and 3) the generation of activators of fibrin degradation (e.g., tissue plasminogen activator [t-PA]).

Platelets

Platelets are also known as **thrombocytes**. An appreciation for the complexity of the platelet can be obtained from *Figure 3-13*. The band of microtubules that encircles the platelet contracts when platelets are activated and results in change of shape and extrusion of platelet granule contents into the open canalicular system and subsequent release from the plate-

let to its exterior. The granules (α granules and dense granules) contain many of the coagulation factors, other proteins, calcium, serotonin, adenosine diphosphate (ADP), and adenosine triphosphate (ATP), all of which assist or potentiate the coagulation process. Release of the granule contents requires energy from the mitochondria and glycogen particles and ionized calcium from the dense tubular system, a component of the membrane system of the platelet.

Platelet Reactions

Circulating platelets are recruited at the site of vascular injury, where they undergo structural changes. These changes are associated with platelet reactions and, coupled with release of granule components, provide for a highly reactive surface for the formation of thrombin and fibrin.

Platelet Adhesion

The first response of platelets to disrupted endothelium and contact with subendothelial

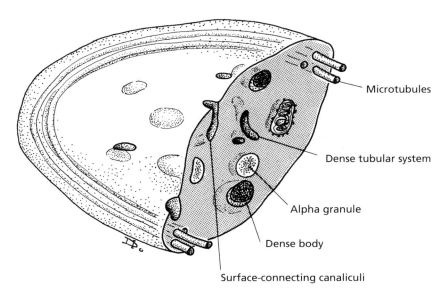

Microtubules

Dense tubular system

Alpha granule

Dense body

Surface-connecting canaliculi

■ **FIGURE 3-13** Internal details of a platelet discernible at the electron microscope level. Dense bodies are also known as dense granules. (From Cormack DH. Essential Histology. 2nd Ed. Baltimore: Lippincott Williams & Wilkins, 2001.)

tissues is their adhesion or attachment to these surfaces. When this happens, a monolayer of platelets adheres to the site and they lose their discoid shape and form **pseudopods** as shown in Figure 3-11. The pseudopods permit greater contact with other platelets flowing by the site of damage and also with those already adhering to the disrupted endothelium and exposed subendothelium. The initial adhesion requires collagen that is present in the subendothelium and fibronectin from the endothelial cells. Continued adhesion results from **von Willebrand factor (vWF)** and fibronectin presence in platelet granules that are extruded from activated platelets.

Platelet Activation

This is the means whereby platelets are stimulated to begin their further role in assisting hemostasis. The interaction of an **agonist** (e.g., collagen, thrombin, ADP) with its specific receptor on the platelet surface initiates the transmission of a signal through the cell membrane, which in turn activates **intracellular messengers**. Intracellular messenger activation results in the release of Ca^{2+} from storage pools into the platelet cytoplasm. The principal messenger, **thromboxane A_2 (TXA$_2$)**, is produced from platelet membrane phospholipids after agonist interaction with the membrane receptors. Aspirin blocks the formation of TXA$_2$, thus preventing the messenger from mobilizing Ca^2 from the granules to the cytoplasm.

Platelet Release Reaction

This event is initiated by the increase in intracellular calcium in response to the intracellular messenger, and granular contents are secreted. It involves clustering of **granular content** into the center of the platelet after **microtubular contraction** and, finally, granule content extrusion to the exterior from the **open canalicular system**. The mechanisms of release are illustrated in *Figure 3-14.*

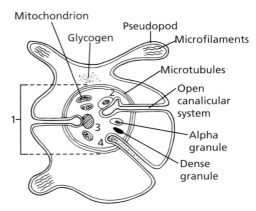

■ **FIGURE 3-14** Platelet cross-section showing how microtubular contraction results in extrusion of platelet granule contents into the open canalicular system and release from the platelet. 1) Clustering of granules into center of the platelet after microtubular contraction; 2) contact of granule membrane with open canalicular system membrane; 3) fusion of granule membrane with open canalicular system membrane; 4) granule content extruded from open canalicular system. (Modified from MacIntyre DE. The platelet release reaction: Association with adhesion and aggregation and comparison with secretory responses in other cells. In: Gordon JL, ed. Platelets in Biology and Pathology, Vol. 1. Amsterdam: Elsevier, 1976.)

Platelet Aggregation

The exterior presence of the granule contents provides high concentrations of fibrinogen (needed to form fibrin), fibronectin and vWF (both needed for adhesion), factor V, and other proteins that assist conversion of prothrombin to thrombin at the platelet surface which, by piling platelets on each other, can lead to the formation of the primary platelet plug. After the release reaction, the platelets lose their individual integrity, lipoprotein membranes are fused, receptors are exposed for coagulation proteins (factors), and thus a highly reactive surface (platelet aggregates) is exposed for the formation of thrombin and fibrin.

Clot Formation (Blood Coagulation)

Thrombin formation is the penultimate (next to last) stage in the formation of **fibrin**, which is insoluble and stabilizes the platelet plug. The stabilized platelet plug, formed by blood coagulation, is known as the secondary hemostatic plug or clot. Once the clot is formed, blood loss through the damaged endothelium is completely stopped. It was recognized previously that, after the platelet reactions, the stage was set for blood coagulation. Most of the proteins that participate in the hemostatic process circulate in plasma as inactive proenzymes, and each undergoes activation in sequence as coagulation proceeds. The sequence is referred to as a **cascade phenomenon**—each reaction represents an amplification point, whereby a small stimulus results in a larger response.

There are four key reactions involved in the formation of a clot: 1) activation of factor IX, 2) activation of factor X, 3) formation of thrombin, and 4) fibrin formation (*Fig. 3-15*). Activated factor IX (FIXa) is a component of the **tenase complex**, and activated factor X (FXa) is a component of the **prothrombinase complex**. These are key enzyme complexes assembled in close proximity on the surface of platelet aggregates. They accelerate the rate of the biochemical cascade reactions resulting in the **generation of thrombin** (see Fig. 3-15).

Pathways to Thrombin Formation

The conversion of prothrombin to thrombin (the key enzyme in hemostasis) is catalyzed by the prothrombinase complex (FXa, activated factors V [FVa], phospholipids [PL], and

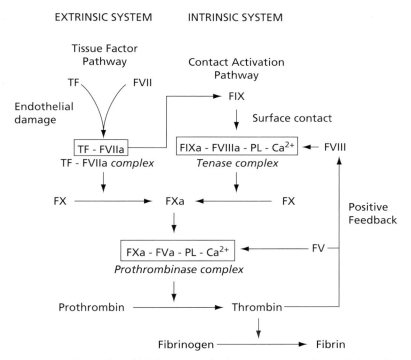

■ **FIGURE 3-15** The two pathways by which factor X activation can occur. In the extrinsic pathway (tissue factor pathway), activated factor X (FXa) is generated by the direct action of the tissue factor (TF)–factor VIIa complex, whereas in the intrinsic pathway (contact activation pathway), factor IXa must combine with factor VIII, phospholipids (PL), and calcium to form the tenase complex before factor X can be activated at a physiologically relevant rate. The final common steps in fibrin formation involve the formation of the prothrombinase complex, which activates prothrombin, allowing thrombin to convert fibrinogen to fibrin. (From Gentry PA. Blood coagulation and hemostasis. In: Reece WO, ed. Dukes' Physiology of Domestic Animals. 12th Ed. Ithaca, NY: Cornell University Press, 2004.)

Ca^{2+}). There are two separate activation mechanisms leading to the formation of the prothrombinase complex (see Fig. 3-15). The **tissue factor pathway (extrinsic system)** and the **contact activation pathway (intrinsic system)**. The tissue factor pathway begins with a traumatized vascular wall or traumatized extravascular tissues that come in contact with the blood. The contact activation pathway begins with trauma to the blood itself or exposure of the blood to collagen from a traumatized blood vessel wall. The pathways are not independent of each other, and after blood vessels rupture, clotting occurs by both pathways simultaneously. **Tissue factor (TF)**, also known as **thromboplastin**, initiates the tissue factor pathway, whereas contact of Factor XII and platelets with collagen in the vascular wall initiates the contact activation pathway (Fig. 3-16).

Following vascular damage, TF and binding sites for FVII, FIX, and FX are exposed on the surface of endothelial cells. In the presence of Ca^{2+}, the TF-VIIa complex forms first and then activates FIX and FX. Activated FIX (FIXa) can then become a part of the tenase complex without having FIX being activated via factor XII in the contact activation pathway as shown in Fig. 3-16. The rate of FXa formation by the proteolytic action of the tenase complex occurs at a much faster rate than that produced by the TF-VIIa complex acting alone and accordingly, provides an amplification step in thrombin generation. In addition, the initial formation of thrombin accelerates FXa production by a positive feedback response that activates factor VIII, a component of the tenase complex, and factor V, a component of the prothrombinase complex (see Fig. 3-15). The contact activation pathway is required to sustain thrombin formation at the site of severe trauma.

After activation of FX, there is a common pathway to the formation of thrombin, after which fibrin is formed from fibrinogen.

Fibrin Formation

The final step of blood coagulation is the conversion of **fibrinogen (a plasma protein)** to fibrin. This begins when thrombin has been

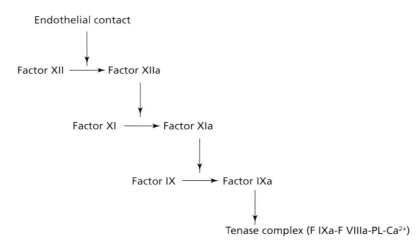

■ **FIGURE 3-16** The contact phase for the activation of factor IX, initiated when factor XII is activated by contact with damaged endothelium. Factor XIIa activates factor XI (accelerated by prekallikrein [PK] and high-molecular-weight kininogen [HK]). Activated factor XI, in the presence of Ca^{2+}, activates factor IX (FIXa). FIXa, in association with other components of the tenase complex, allows for the activation of factor X and Fxa's association with the prothrombinase complex. PL, phospholipid.

formed. The first reaction produces fibrin monomers that spontaneously polymerize, and a loosely knit mesh is formed, held together by covalent peptide bonds. This polymer structure is permeable to blood flow and is referred to as soluble fibrin. The stabilization (formation of isopeptide bonds) of soluble fibrin to an insoluble fibrin clot is catalyzed by activated factor XIII (FXIIIa). Factor XIII is released from entrapped platelets, and its conversion to the active form is induced by thrombin in the presence of calcium. Stabilization renders fibrin more elastic and less subject to lysis.

Clot Retraction

After stabilization, **clot retraction (shrinking of the clot)** occurs and is provided by the action of the platelet **contractile proteins, thrombosthenin, actin, and myosin.** These proteins are exposed when platelets are activated. The activation brings changes that activate thrombosthenin, actin, and myosin to react in a manner analogous to that which occurs during muscle contraction, and the clot retracts (serum is squeezed from the coagulum). Clot retraction permits greater blood flow in the damaged area while the tissue is being repaired. Failures of clot retraction can be associated with reduced platelet numbers.

Clot Growth

Once blood coagulation has been initiated, the process extends into the surrounding blood; this is known as **clot growth.** Clot growth stops when blood flows fast enough to remove the thrombin that has been generated; this thrombin has not been otherwise absorbed by the fibrin that is formed and by the other activated factors. The thrombin and activated factors washed away by the blood are not effective because they have been diluted and because natural anticoagulant substances in plasma (e.g., antithrombin III) are present.

These substances can prevent unwanted coagulation when procoagulants (substances favoring coagulation) are present in small quantities.

Fibrin Degradation

After hemostasis has been established, the damaged vascular area is repaired by new tissue growth assisted by growth factors released from activated platelets. The fibrin that was formed to assist in the hemostatic process undergoes degradation (**fibrinolysis**) by a proteolytic enzyme called **plasmin** (*Fig. 3-17*). **Plasminogen**, a protein that is present in plasma, becomes entrapped within the clot when it is formed. Plasminogen is activated to become plasmin by substances in blood and tissues known as plasminogen activators. The principal endogenous plasminogen activator is **tissue-type plasminogen activator (t-PA)**, which is released from endothelial cells when they are stimulated by the presence of thrombin or by stasis of blood. Plasmin degrades the fibrin molecule into protein fragments known as **fibrin degradation products (FDPs)**. When the outer surface of the fibrin clot is removed, fresh surfaces are exposed and degraded until clot removal is complete. The FDPs, platelets, and other cell debris are removed from the circulation by the MPS. Tissue-type plasminogen activator is produced commercially for human medical use to dissolve clots that are lodged in vessels and that block blood flow (e.g., coronary arteries).

■ PREVENTION OF BLOOD COAGULATION

1. **What are some preventatives against coagulation in the normal vascular system?**
2. **How does heparin prevent intravascular clotting?**
3. **What is the significance of mast cells? Why are there great numbers of them in the lung?**

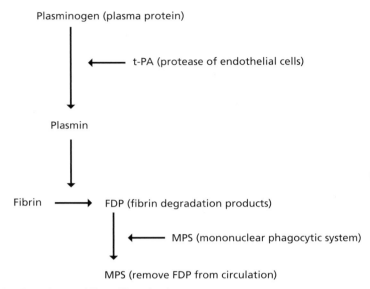

■ **FIGURE 3-17** The degradation of fibrin (fibrinolysis).

4. How do chelating agents prevent clotting in withdrawn blood?

In addition to procoagulants in the blood, there are also anticoagulants. Their presence balances and prevents coagulation that might otherwise occur because of small amounts of the procoagulants normally present. Also, when blood is withdrawn for analytical purposes or for storage, anticoagulants are added to the blood containers to prevent coagulation.

Prevention in Normal Circulation

The formation of thrombin occurs through a series of chemical reactions, so it is normal to have a small amount of thrombin in the circulation. The thrombin that is present could cause the conversion of fibrinogen (a normal plasma protein) to fibrin except that another protein, **antithrombin III**, blocks the action of thrombin on fibrinogen and also inactivates the thrombin that it binds.

In addition to antithrombin III action, coagulation in the normal vascular system is prevented by the **smoothness of the endothelium**. This prevents contact activation of factor XII, which is involved in the activation of factor IX in the intrinsic system (see Fig. 3-16). Also, **a monomolecular layer of protein (net-negative charge)** is adsorbed to the surface of the endothelium that repels clotting factors and platelets. When endothelial damage occurs, both the smoothness and the protein layer are lost at the damaged site.

Heparin, an anticoagulant, is produced by mast cells that reside in the pericapillary connective tissues. Mast cells are particularly abundant in the lungs because of the vulnerability of the lungs to emboli, which are clots that have broken loose from their original site and flow freely in the blood. The plasma concentration of heparin is normally low. The effectiveness of heparin in preventing normal intravascular clotting depends on its combining with antithrombin III to form a complex that removes not only thrombin but also factors IX, X, XI, and XII.

Because of the biological potency of thrombin, there are mechanisms that limit the rate and extent of thrombin generation around sites of vascular damage. One of these, the **anticoagulant protein C pathway**, involves the high-affinity binding of thrombin to thrombomodulin (TM), a membrane protein of endothelial and peripheral blood cells. When bound to TM, thrombin loses its ability to activate platelets and to clot fibrinogen and becomes an activator of protein C. Activated protein C destroys the activity of factors Va and VIIIa (thrombin modified FV and FVIII), which are cofactors in the prothrombinase and tenase complexes, respectively (see Fig. 3-15).

Prevention in Withdrawn Blood

It is often desirable to prevent blood coagulation when blood is withdrawn from an animal for later examination and analysis. Anticoagulants are used for this purpose. **Chelating agents** are used most frequently; they bind the calcium ions so that they are not available for the coagulation process. Either trisodium citrate, sodium oxalate, or ethylenediaminetetraacetic acid (sodium EDTA, disodium salt) is added in an appropriate quantity to the collection container and mixed with the withdrawn blood. Heparin is also available commercially and can be used to prevent coagulation of withdrawn blood. It is also used to prevent coagulation of blood in the body in certain disease conditions that predispose to clot formation.

■ TESTS FOR BLOOD COAGULATION

1.   What is the range in minutes for normal coagulation times among domestic animals by the capillary tube method?

2.   Why would low platelet counts be associated with delayed coagulation times?

3.   How is dicoumarol associated with coagulation defects?

4.   Why would liver disease be suspect as a cause of coagulation defects?

5.   How is vWF associated with coagulation defects?

6.   Why does blood withdrawn from birds, in which endothelial cell damage does not occur, coagulate with difficulty?

7.   In the absence of the contact activation system, why do birds not show hemorrhagic problems?

Tests for blood coagulation are used to determine the adequacy of coagulation in an animal. Several techniques are available. Blood is withdrawn and subjected to standard methods, and the time interval is observed from withdrawal to coagulation. One of these is the capillary tube method, in which the blood is collected directly into a nonheparinized capillary tube. The tube is manually broken at 1-minute intervals until the blood in the broken ends remains connected by a fibrin thread. The time in minutes for this to occur is the coagulation time (see Table 3-2 for normal values). A prolonged time interval indicates an inadequate mechanism in the body. Because platelets supply various factors to the coagulation mechanism, in addition to forming a platelet plug, an estimation of their number is also helpful in assessing coagulation adequacy.

A common laboratory screening test is the one-stage prothrombin time. In this test, plasma is activated with a mixture of TF and phospholipids. Calcium is added, and the time to coagulation is determined. If clotting time is prolonged, there may be abnormalities in plasma FV, FVII, FX, prothrombin activity, or fibrinogen concentration.

Coagulation Defects

Knowledge of the coagulation process is helpful in understanding coagulation defects when they occur. Vitamin K deficiency results in hemorrhage because of inadequate formation of prothrombin and factors VII, IX, and X. Also, dicoumarol interferes with the utilization of vitamin K and hence with prothrombin production.

Dicoumarol is a product of research on a hemorrhagic disease of livestock known as sweet clover poisoning. Both yellow and white sweet clover have high coumarin content susceptible to metabolism by several common molds, with resultant dimerization of coumarin when mold growth occurs. Sweet clover hay is thick-stemmed and subject to incomplete drying when harvested and stored (bales, stacks, haylofts). Mold growth is favored, and dicoumarol is produced. Because of its hemorrhagic properties, dicoumarol is commercially available in rodenticides, in which it is laced with rodent edibles, and a derivative is used as "blood thinners" in human medicine.

Other causes of coagulation defects are related to liver disease, platelet defects, a complex problem known as disseminated intravascular coagulation, and those that are inherited. The most common inherited defects identified in domestic animals are those associated with factor IX activation and formation of the tenase complex. In this category, factor VIII (antihemophilic factor) deficiency is the most widespread. Other common inherited defects are deficiencies of factor IX and vWF (von Willebrand factor). In the latter, platelet aggregates are poorly anchored to the damaged endothelium and are more susceptible to dislodgement by circulating blood. This deficiency is known as von Willebrand disease (vWD).

Species Differences

The interaction of activated platelets with damaged endothelium and coagulation proteins is a requirement among all animals for a normal hemostatic mechanism, even though platelet numbers and morphology may vary. The absence of factor XII (a factor of the intrinsic mechanism) from the blood of marine mammals and reptiles prolongs the clotting time of their withdrawn blood.

In birds, the entire contact activation pathway appears to be absent, whereby activation of factor IX by that pathway does not occur. This is noticeable if blood is withdrawn atraumatically whereby there is neither trauma to blood nor to endothelium. A coagulum will form, but serum is extracted with difficulty. For this reason, when chemical analysis is desired, one should use an appropriate anticoagulant and harvest plasma (assuming plasma compatibility with the analysis). The blood will clot extremely rapidly if trauma to the vessel wall occurs during collection. In this case, the tissue factor pathway is activated to form thrombin and associated enhancements to activate the tenase complex (see Fig. 3-15). This is the reason that avian species have an intact coagulation mechanism, even though they do not have a functional contact activation system.

■ PLASMA AND ITS COMPOSITION

1. **What differentiates plasma from serum?**
2. **What is the concentration of protein in plasma?**
3. **What are the three major classes of plasma proteins?**
4. **Which one of the immunoglobulins is most abundant in normal animals?**
5. **What is meant by a state of equilibrium among plasma proteins, amino acids, and tissue proteins?**
6. **What plasma protein represents the major contribution to intravascular effective osmotic pressure? Why is this?**
7. **Which cation is most abundant in plasma? Which anion?**

8.   What is the concentration of glucose in the pig and dog? Is it lower in the ruminants and horse?

Plasma, the noncellular, liquid part of the hematocrit, may be obtained from drawn blood in which coagulation has been prevented. When blood has been allowed to clot, the coagulation factors are effectively removed, and the liquid is known as **serum**. All of the coagulation factors are present in plasma. Plasma is a complex fluid (contains substances existing in chemical form in the body) that provides the medium of exchange between the blood vessels and the cells of the body. A number of these substances that are often referred to clinically are shown in *Table 3-4* for several species. The major constituent of plasma is water (about 92% to 94%), and the percentage will vary depending mostly on the concentration of protein. **Proteins** are the most abundant of the substances dissolved or suspended in the water, and their concentration varies from 6 to 8 g/dL.

Plasma Proteins

The three major classes of plasma proteins are **albumin**, **globulins** (α1, α2, β1, β2, and γ), and **fibrinogen**. In humans, sheep, goats, and dogs, albumin predominates over the globulins; in horses, pigs, cows, and cats, the relative proportions of albumin and globulins are nearly equal.

The γ **globulins** contain antibodies called **immunoglobulins** and are produced by lymphocytes and plasma cells. There are five major isotopes of immunoglobulins, which are classified as IgG, IgE, IgA, IgM, and IgD. IgG is the most abundant immunoglobulin of normal animals. It crosses the dam's placental barrier to provide immunity to newborns in some species (primates and rodents) but not others. In the latter, transfer depends on IgG presence in colostrum and early ingestion by the newborn (see Chapter 16). IgE, IgA, IgM, and IgD provide the immune response to allergic conditions or parasitisms (release of histamine), the microorganisms present in the mouth and gastrointestinal tract (via colostrum), activation of the complement system, and clone formation of lymphocytes, respectively.

The **alpha and beta globulins** serve as substrates for new substances and also perform transport functions (e.g., lactoferrin, a globulin, transports iron).

Origin

Plasma albumin, part of the globulins, and fibrinogen (and other coagulation factors) are formed in the liver. The balance of the globulins, including δ globulins, are formed in the lymph nodes and mucosal tissues.

The plasma proteins, amino acids, and tissue proteins are in a state of equilibrium (*Fig. 3-18*). When the amino acid concentration in tissue cells decreases below that of plasma, amino acids enter the cells and are used for synthesis of essential plasma and tissue proteins. The plasma proteins, formed mainly in the liver, may also be broken down into amino acids by MPS cells and made available for cellular protein synthesis. This occurs especially when the amino acid supply from digestive processes is not adequate. Plasma proteins do leak from capillaries into the interstitial fluid and are returned to the blood via the lymphatics. In this way, there is a 12- to 24-hour turnover (time within which all protein is leaked and returned).

Plasma Proteins and Colloidal Osmotic Pressure

The **plasma colloidal osmotic pressure** (also called **oncotic pressure**) is the **effective osmotic pressure of the plasma** (see Chapter 2). It is intimately associated with the balance of body fluids between the intravascular and interstitial fluid compartments. It occurs because of the presence of the protein molecules and cations retained by the net negative charge of protein. The proteins are colloidal

TABLE 3-4 VALUES OF SOME CONSTITUENTS OF BLOOD FROM MATURE DOMESTIC ANIMALS

VALUE (RANGE) CONSTITUENTS	HORSE	COW	SHEEP	PIG	DOG	CHICKEN
Glucose (mg/dL)	60–110	40–80 80–120 (calf)	40–80 80–120 (lamb)	80–120	70–120	130–270
Nonprotein nitrogen (mg/dL)	20–40	20–40	20–38	20–45	17–38	20–35
Urea nitrogen (BUN) (mg/dL)	10–24	10–30	8–20	8–24	10–30	0.1–1.0
Uric acid (mg/dL)	0.5–1	0.1–2	0.1–2	0.1–2	0.1–1.5	1–2 1–7 (laying hen)
Creatinine (mg/dL)	1–2	1–2	1–2	1–2.5	1–2	1–2
Amino acid nitrogen (mg/dL)	5–7	4–8	5–8	6–8	7–8	4–10
Lactic acid (mg/dL)	10–16	5–20	9–12		8–20	47–56 20–98 (laying hen)
Cholesterol (mg/dL)	75–150	80–180	60–150	60–200	120–250	125–200
Bilirubin						
Direct (mg/dL)	0–0.4	0–0.3	0–0.3	0–0.3	0.06–0.1	
Indirect (mg/dL)	0.2–5	0.1–0.5	0–0.1	0–0.3	0.01–0.5	
Total (mg/dL)	0.2–6	0.2–1.5	0.1–0.4	0–0.6	0.10–0.6	
Electrolytes (mEq/L)						
Sodium	132–152	132–152	139–152	135–150	141–155	151–161
Potassium	2.5–5.0	3.9–5.8	3.9–5.4	4.4–6.7	3.7–5.8	4.6–4.7
Calcium	4.5–6.5	4.5–6.0	4.5–6.0	4.5–6.5	4.5–6.0	4.5–6.0 8.5–19.5 (laying hen)
Phosphorus	2–6	2–7	2–7	3–6	2–6	3–6
Magnesium	1.5–2.5	1.5–2.5	1.8–2.3	2–3	1.5–2.0	
Chlorine	99–109	97–111	95–105	94–106	100–115	119–130

From Reece WO, Swenson MJ. The composition and functions of blood. In: Reece WO, ed. Dukes' Physiology of Domestic Animals. 12th Ed. Ithaca, NY: Cornell University Press, 2004.

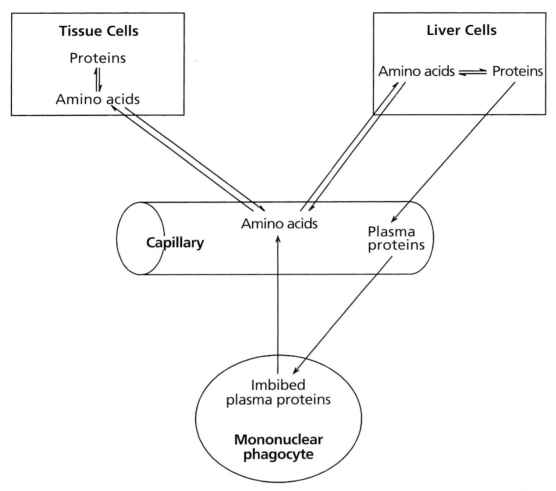

■ **FIGURE 3-18** Reversible equilibrium among the tissue proteins, plasma proteins, and plasma amino acids. (From Reece WO, Swenson MJ. The composition and functions of blood. In: Reece WO, ed. Dukes' Physiology of Domestic Animals. 12th Ed. Ithaca, NY: Cornell University Press, 2004.)

and nondiffusible. The effective osmotic pressure produced by them opposes the hydrostatic pressure of blood in the capillaries and is responsible for reabsorption of fluid at the venous end of capillaries (see Chapter 9). The albumins account for about 80% of the plasma colloidal osmotic pressure because of their abundance and smaller molecular weight. The osmotic pressure that each protein fraction contributes is inversely related to the molecular weight and directly related to its concentra-

tion in terms of number of particles in the plasma (recall that osmotic pressure relates to particle numbers rather than mass). The molecular weights of fibrinogen, albumin, and globulins are approximately 300,000; 70,000; and 180,000, respectively. The molecular weight of fibrinogen is high and its plasma concentration is low, therefore, its contribution to colloidal osmotic pressure is small. When the concentrations of globulins and albumin are nearly the same, albumin contributes two to three times as much osmotic pressure as globulins because there are two to three times more molecules (particles) in albumin than in an equal weight (concentration) of globulin.

Because of the many functions of plasma proteins, it is apparent that liver disease and resultant failure of adequate protein synthesis, or prolonged dietary protein deficiency, can lead to many body function problems.

Other Plasma Constituents

Oxygen, carbon dioxide, and nitrogen are the major gases of the atmosphere and are found in plasma. Their concentration in plasma depends on their concentration in the atmosphere and on their solubility in plasma. The major types of lipids in plasma are triglycerides, phospholipids, and cholesterol. The principal nonprotein nitrogen (NPN) compounds are amino acids, urea, uric acid, creatine, cre-

atinine, and ammonium salts. Inorganic substances in the plasma are presented mainly by the electrolytes, including cations (Na^+, K^+, Ca^{2+}, Mg^{2+}) and anions (Cl^-, HCO^-_3, HPO_4^{-2}). Values for many of these constituents are shown in Table 3-4.

■ SUGGESTED READING

Feldman BF, Zinkl JG, Jain NC. Schalm's Veterinary Hematology. 5th Ed. Baltimore: Lippincott Williams & Wilkins, 2000.

Gentry PA. Blood coagulation and hemostasis. In: Reece WO, ed. Dukes' Physiology of Domestic Animals. 12th Ed. Ithaca, NY: Cornell University Press, 2004.

Jackson ML. Platelet physiology and platelet function: Inhibition by aspirin. Compend Contin Educ Pract Vet 1987; 9:627.

Jain NC. Essentials of Veterinary Hematology. Philadelphia: Lea & Febiger, 1993.

Reece WO, Swenson MJ. The composition and functions of blood. In: Reece WO, ed. Dukes' Physiology of Domestic Animals. 12th Ed. Ithaca, NY: Cornell University Press, 2004.

 SELF EVALUATION—CHAPTER 3

GENERAL CHARACTERISTICS

1. The PCV of a hematocrit determination refers to the:
   a. white cells and thrombocyte layer between the erythrocyte mass and plasma.
   b. erythrocyte mass at the bottom.
   c. yellowish liquid layer at the top of the hematocrit.
   d. total length of the hematocrit tube content.

2. Which one of the following most accurately approximates the amount of blood in an animal?
   a. 2% of body weight
   b. 16% of body weight
   c. 8% of body weight
   d. 24% of body weight

3. Arterial blood changes from a bright red color to a darker purplish color when it becomes venous blood. Which one of the following causes this?
   a. Loss of oxygen
   b. Gain of carbon dioxide

4. A normal value for arterial blood pH would be closest to which one of the following values?
   a. 3.8
   b. 6.5
   c. 7.4
   d. 8.2

5. The blood volume of a 25-kg dog is 2,000 mL, of which the plasma volume is 1,200 mL. What is the PCV of this dog?
   a. 8%
   b. 60%

c. 40%

d. Mitzie

LEUKOCYTES

6. Which WBC is most numerous in pigs, cows, sheep, and goats?
   a. Eosinophil
   b. Neutrophil
   c. Lymphocyte
   d. Monocyte
   e. Basophil

7. The neutrophil is the most numerous leukocyte in all of the domestic species.
   a. True
   b. False

8. Which leukocyte will become a macrophage when it enters tissue spaces or becomes attached to certain blood channels?
   a. Neutrophil
   b. Basophil
   c. Eosinophil
   d. Monocyte

9. A differential WBC count and a total WBC count have been determined. Sixty of the 100 WBCs counted in the differential were determined to be neutrophils. The total WBC count was 10,000/µL. What is the absolute number of neutrophils?
   a. 6,000/µL
   b. 10,000/µL
   c. 60%
   d. 60/µL

10. Which one of the following leukocytes has as its function to provide immunity to antigens (foreign substances)?
    a. Monocytes
    b. Eosinophils
    c. Lymphocytes
    d. Basophils
    e. Neutrophils

11. A term that refers to a reduced number of leukocytes is:

    a. anemia.
    b. leukopenia.
    c. leukocytosis.
    d. polycythemia.

ERYTHROCYTES

12. Which one of the following time periods would approximate the life span of erythrocytes in most domestic mammals?
    a. 150 to 180 hours
    b. 70 to 80 days
    c. 80 to 150 days
    d. 35 to 60 seconds

13. Which one of the following best describes the hemoglobin molecule of blood?
    a. Has ferric iron (Fe^{3+}), combines with one molecule of oxygen
    b. Has one heme group and one globin molecule
    c. Has ferrous iron (Fe^{2+}), combines with four molecules of oxygen
    d. Has ferrous iron (Fe^{2+}) when unoxygenated and ferric iron (Fe^{3+}) when oxygenated

14. What is an approximate value for hemoglobin concentration in a normal healthy dog?
    a. 5 g/dL
    b. 20 g/dL
    c. 15 g/dL
    d. 10 g/dL

15. An erythrocyte just entering the bloodstream and having a net-like appearance because of polyribosomes and ribosomes is known as a/an:
    a. reticulocyte.
    b. rubriblast.
    c. polychromatophilic rubricyte.
    d. eosinophil.

16. Where is erythropoietin produced?
    a. Bone marrow
    b. Lungs
    c. Spleen
    d. Kidneys

17. Which one of the following represents the number of erythrocytes for most domestic species?
    a. 7,000,000
    b. 7,000,000 per microliter of blood
    c. 7,000,000 per milliliter of blood
    d. 7,000,000 per pound of body weight

18. What is the stimulus for the production of erythropoietin?
    a. Tissue need for oxygen
    b. Iron deficiency
    c. No stimulus, but constantly produced
    d. Sympathetic division of ANS

19. Erythropoiesis refers to:
    a. blood coagulation.
    b. the recycling of iron.
    c. the disintegration scheme for RBCs.
    d. RBC production.

FATE OF ERYTHROCYTES

20. A reddish color of plasma that may be coupled with a red color of urine is caused by:
    a. hemoglobin.
    b. bilirubin.
    c. iron.
    d. bilinogen.

21. Which body organ is the site at which insoluble bilirubin that is released from MPS cells is made soluble before its transport to the intestine?
    a. Kidney
    b. Liver
    c. Bone marrow
    d. Spleen

22. When an erythrocyte is disintegrated, the hemoglobin remains intact and is incorporated into new RBCs.
    a. True
    b. False

23. Icterus is present in a dog. Severe liver disease is apparent. Which form of bilirubin would be the most likely cause of the icterus?

a. Free bilirubin
b. Conjugated bilirubin
c. Biliboy

24. Free hemoglobin, from intravascular hemolysis:
    a. invariably results in hemoglobinuria.
    b. is too large a molecule to enter the kidney tubules.
    c. when combined with haptoglobin will not enter the kidney tubules.
    d. combines with haptoglobin in all circumstances.

IRON METABOLISM

25. What is the name of the transport form of iron?
    a. Hemosiderin
    b. Transferrin
    c. Ferritin
    d. Iron ore

26. To avoid toxicity, iron is transported in the blood and/or stored in cells bound with a protein in its:
    a. ferric (Fe^{3+}) oxidation state.
    b. ferrous (Fe^{2+}) oxidation state.

27. Because the absorption of iron is relatively controlled, based on need, it is impossible to observe conditions of iron toxicity from excess ingestion.
    a. True
    b. False

28. Which one of the iron forms would be most visible in the liver cells during times of excessive Hb degradation, e.g., hemolytic disease?
    a. Hemosiderin
    b. Ferritin
    c. Transferrin
    d. Ferrous iron (Fe^{2+})

ANEMIA AND POLYCYTHEMIA

29. Someone tells you that the hemoglobin concentration in a baby pig is 4 g/dL. What would you say is the status of that pig?

a. Normal
b. Anemic
c. Leukopenic
d. Polycythemic

30. A sheep presented with an RBC count of $6.0 \times 10^6/\mu L$ and a hemoglobin concentration of 5 g/dL:
    a. would not be considered anemic because the RBC numbers are approximately normal.
    b. would be considered anemic because both RBC and Hb are below the normal range.
    c. would be considered anemic because only the Hb is below the normal range.
    d. would not be considered anemic because both RBC and Hb are in the normal range.

31. Polycythemia vera is:
    a. rare in animals.
    b. a form of anemia.
    c. associated with a low PCV (red cell mass).
    d. associated with hypoxemia, tumors, and elevated erythropoietin production.

32. Without supplemental iron, anemia is common in baby pigs because of:
    a. rapid growth and increase in blood volume.
    b. sow's milk deficient in iron.
    c. lack of iron for ingestion in environment.
    d. all of the above.

HEMOSTASIS: PREVENTION OF BLOOD LOSS

33. Which one of the following cells assists in hemostasis (prevention of blood loss)?
    a. Basophil
    b. Platelet
    c. Erythrocyte
    d. Lymphocyte

34. The mesh of the blood clot is:
    a. thrombin.
    b. fibrin.
    c. fibrinogen.
    d. prothrombin.

35. Which one of the following cations plays an important role in blood coagulation?
    a. Na^+
    b. Mg^{2+}
    c. K^+
    d. Ca^{2+}

36. Which one of the following substances provides for the breakdown of fibrin to fibrin degradation products?
    a. Plasmin
    b. Thromboxane A_2
    c. Fibrinogen
    d. EDTA

37. Nearly all of the clotting factors are:
    a. carbohydrates.
    b. proteins.
    c. lipids.
    d. minerals.

38. Most, but not all, of the clotting factors are produced in the:
    a. kidney.
    b. lung.
    c. liver.
    d. intestinal epithelium.

39. Loss of individual integrity, fusion of lipoprotein membranes, and exposure of receptors for coagulation factors is characteristic for:
    a. platelet adhesion.
    b. platelet activation.
    c. platelet release reaction.
    d. platelet aggregation.

40. Tissue-type plasminogen activator (t-PA) is associated with:
    a. heparin production.
    b. initiation of the extrinsic mechanism of blood coagulation.
    c. erythrocyte production.
    d. fibrin degradation.

41. What substance is formed during the coagulation process that converts fibrinogen to fibrin?
    a. Thromboxane A_2
    b. Thromboplastin
    c. Thrombin
    d. Prothrombin

42. The prothrombinase complex (FXa, FVa, phospholipids, and Ca^{2+}):
    a. is the same as the tenase complex.
    b. activates factor IX.
    c. catalyzes the conversion of prothrombin to thrombin.
    d. is activated only via the TF-FVIIa complex.

43. Blood withdrawn from mammals, without endothelial damage, into glass tubes will clot via:
    a. the TF-FVIIa complex pathway (extrinsic system).
    b. the (FIXa-FVIIIa-PL-Ca^{2+}) tenase complex (intrinsic system).
    c. both a and b.
    d. it will not clot.

PREVENTION OF BLOOD COAGULATION

44. Protein C:
    a. promotes blood coagulation.
    b. is activated by the thrombomodulin-thrombin bond and limits the generation of thrombin.
    c. becomes a part of antithrombin III.
    d. is a vitamin that prevents scurvy.

45. Antithrombin III:
    a. is not a normal plasma protein.
    b. must combine with heparin to be effective.
    c. blocks the action of thrombin on fibrinogen.
    d. promotes fibrin formation by deactivating the prothrombinase complex.

46. Heparin:
    a. is produced by mast cells in pericapillary tissues.
    b. is an important anticoagulant in the lungs.
    c. combines with antithrombin III for its effectiveness.
    d. all of the above.

47. The use of chelating agents in tubes used for withdrawing blood:
    a. promotes blood coagulation.
    b. allows for the collection of serum.
    c. binds calcium and prevents blood coagulation.
    d. assists the analysis for calcium concentration.

TESTS FOR BLOOD COAGULATION

48. Which one of the following time frames would be considered a normal clotting time for domestic mammals (capillary tube method)?
    a. 20 to 30 seconds
    b. 20 to 30 minutes
    c. 2 to 5 seconds
    d. 2 to 5 minutes

49. The vitamin needed for the production of prothrombin and factors VII, IX, and X is:
    a. C.
    b. D.
    c. E.
    d. K.

50. A deficiency of von Willebrand factor (vWF) is associated with:
    a. activation of factor VIII.
    b. poorly anchored platelet aggregates.
    c. activation of factor IX.
    d. accelerated blood coagulation.

51. The avian species do not have the entire contact phase and its associated activation of factor IX. Accordingly,
    a. the tissue factor pathway cannot proceed.
    b. blood withdrawn without endothelial damage clots rapidly.
    c. hemorrhage in birds is always fatal.

d. the tissue factor pathway proceeds to form thrombin and activation of the tenase complex.

PLASMA AND ITS COMPOSITION

52. Which one of the following best describes plasma?
    a. About 40% of blood composition, contains no protein.
    b. The cellular part of blood, about 40% of blood composition.
    c. About 60% of blood composition, contains fibrinogen.
    d. About 60% of blood composition, clot removed.

53. The plasma protein concentration in the dog would be close to:
    a. 7 g/L.
    b. 7 mEq/L.
    c. 7 mg/dL.
    d. 7 g/dL.

54. Which one of the following series represents the approximate respective plasma concentration of Na^+, K^+, and Cl^- in mEq/L?

a. 110, 5, 145
b. 145, 110, 5
c. 5, 145, 110
d. 145, 5, 110

55. Which one of the three major classes of plasma proteins (albumins, globulins, and fibrinogen) is present in the least concentration?
    a. Albumins
    b. Globulins
    c. Fibrinogen

56. Which one of the immunoglobulins is important as a component of colostrums because it relates to absorption by the newborn?
    a. IgE
    b. IgG
    c. IgD
    d. IgA

57. Which one of the three major classes of plasma proteins accounts for about 80% of the plasma colloidal osmotic pressure?
    a. Albumins
    b. Globulins
    c. Fibrinogen

ANSWERS TO SELF EVALUATION—CHAPTER 3

1.	b	16.	d	31.	a	46.	d
2.	c	17.	b	32.	d	47.	c
3.	a	18.	a	33.	b	48.	d
4.	c	19.	d	34.	b	49.	d
5.	c	20.	a	35.	d	50.	b
6.	c	21.	b	36.	a	51.	d
7.	b	22.	b	37.	b	52.	c
8.	d	23.	a	38.	c	53.	d
9.	a	24.	c	39.	d	54.	d
10.	c	25.	b	40.	d	55.	c
11.	b	26.	a	41.	c	56.	b
12.	c	27.	b	42.	c	57.	a
13.	c	28.	a	43.	b		
14.	c	29.	b	44.	b		
15.	a	30.	b	45.	c		

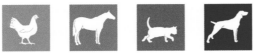

CHAPTER 4

Nervous System

CHAPTER OUTLINE

- **STRUCTURE OF THE NERVOUS SYSTEM**
  Neurons and Synapses
  Glial Cells
  Myelin Sheaths
- **ORGANIZATION OF THE NERVOUS SYSTEM**
  Central Nervous System
  Peripheral Nervous System
  Autonomic Nervous System
- **THE NERVE IMPULSE AND ITS TRANSMISSION**
  Mechanisms of Transmission
  Neurotransmitters
  Neuron Placement
- **REFLEXES**

Spinal Reflex
Somatic and Visceral Reflexes
Reflex Centers
Postural Reflexes and Reactions
- **THE MENINGES AND CEREBROSPINAL FLUID**
  Meninges of the Brain
  Meninges of the Spinal Cord
  Ventricles of the Brain
  Circulation and Function of
      Cerebrospinal Fluid
- **CENTRAL NERVOUS SYSTEM METABOLISM**
  Blood-Brain Barrier
  Blood Requirement

The nervous system is a communication network that enables an animal to adjust itself or its parts to changes in the external and internal environments. It has sensory components that detect the environmental changes, integrative components that process the sensory data coupled with the information stored in memory, and motor components that provide for a response to the processed information.

■ STRUCTURE OF THE NERVOUS SYSTEM

1. Differentiate between dendrites and axons.
2. Sketch a multipolar neuron.
3. What is a nerve fiber?
4. What is the difference between a neurilemma and the axolemma?
5. What is a nucleus?
6. What is a ganglion?
7. What is a tract?
8. What is a nerve?
9. What are the components of a synapse?
10. What are characteristics of a synapse?
11. Which one of the glial cells facilitates transport of blood constituents from capillaries to neurons?
12. Are myelin sheaths in the central nervous system and peripheral nervous system formed by the same cells?
13. How do myelin sheaths of the central nervous system and peripheral nervous system differ?
14. At what location does the axolemma have contact with extracellular fluid in myelinated nerve fibers?

The many complex functions of the nervous system are accomplished by two cell types:

neurons and glial cells, also called glia and neuroglia. Neurons transmit nerve impulses and join with others via synapses. Glial cells provide service to neurons and their environment. The human brain contains approximately 100 billion neurons and a 10-fold number more of glial cells.

Neurons and Synapses

The **neuron (nerve cell)** consists of the cell body and all its processes, the dendrites, and the axon (*Fig. 4-1*). A nerve cell process is a **dendrite** if it conducts impulses toward the cell body, and it is an **axon** if it conducts impulses away from the cell body. A neuron has only one axon but can have many dendrites. The dendrites provide the sites for receiving information from other neurons. They can be highly branched in order to provide a large surface area for communication with great numbers of axons.

The **polarity of a neuron** refers to the number of poles or processes that stem from its cell body. Mammalian neurons can be categorized as **bipolar** (one axon and one den-

drite extending from the cell body), **pseudounipolar** (in which the axon and dendrite of a bipolar neuron have fused near the cell body, giving the appearance of only one process), or **multipolar** (many branching dendrites and one axon extending from the cell body, see Fig. 4-1). Most primary afferent neurons are pseudounipolar and are further characterized under the heading Peripheral Nervous System. Bipolar neurons are found in the retina of the eye and the olfactory region (sense of smell) in the nose (see Chapter 5). Most neurons in the central nervous system (CNS) are multipolar, as shown in Figure 4-1.

The **axon** (and its myelin covering, if present) is called a **nerve fiber**. The part of the cell membrane that covers the axon is known as the **axolemma**. In a myelinated axon, the axolemma is surrounded by a **myelin sheath (neurilemma)** that is interrupted at regularly spaced intervals by myelin-free gaps, called **nodes of Ranvier**.

A group of nerve cell bodies within the brain or spinal cord is referred to as a **nucleus**, and a group of nerve cell bodies outside the

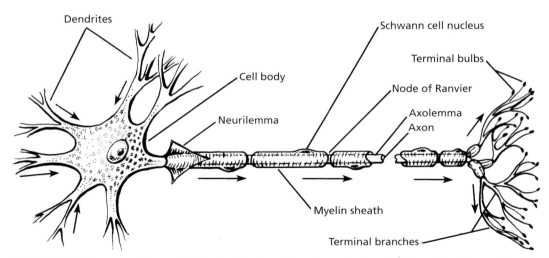

■ **FIGURE 4-1** The neuron. Arrows indicate the direction of impulse conduction. In this myelinated nerve fiber in a peripheral nerve are shown the neurilemma (sheath of Schwann), axolemma (plasma membrane of axon), and nodes of Ranvier. The terminal branches are also referred to as the telodendritic zone. The axon is shown as discontinuous to allow for variable length.

brain or spinal cord is called a **ganglion**. A bundle of parallel neuron fibers within the brain or spinal cord is known as either a **tract** or a **fasciculus**, and a bundle of neuron fibers outside the brain or spinal cord is called a **nerve**.

Continuity from one neuron to the next is provided by the **synapse** (*Fig. 4-2*). There is no physical contact of neurons at the synapse. A space exists between the neurons, the **synaptic gap**, and impulses from one neuron to the next are transmitted by chemical means through this space. This is **chemical synaptic transmission**, in contrast to electrical synaptic transmission. Because most synaptic transmission is chemical, our considerations will be limited to chemical transmission. Three notable characteristics of the synapse are: 1) one-way conduction (direction), 2) facilitation (repeated impulses provide for easier subsequent transmission), and 3) greater fatigability than the neuron (allows for repetitive impulses to fade).

Glial Cells

Glial cells are the nonneuronal cellular elements of the CNS. They outnumber neurons by about 10-fold and make up about half of its volume. The dense packing of neurons and the more numerous glial cells cause nervous tissue to have less interstitial space than other tissues. Glial cells are metabolically quite active.

Glial cells include oligodendrocytes, astrocytes, ependymal cells, and microglia. The most significant role of **oligodendrocytes** is their involvement in myelin sheath formation in the CNS. A similar function in the peripheral nervous system is performed by Schwann cells. **Astrocytes** are the most prominent glial cell, and their processes abut blood vessels, synaptic structures, and nerve cell bodies and processes. Because of their interposition between blood vessels and neurons, astrocytes not only provide support but also facilitate transport of blood constituents from capillaries to neurons. Also, astrocytes release excit-

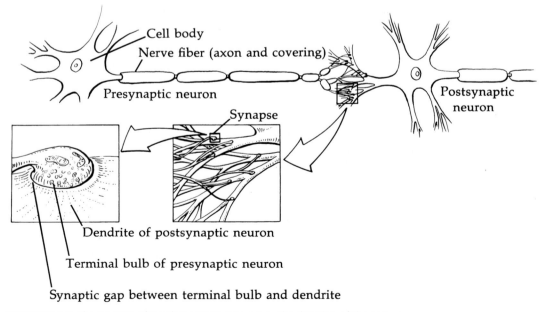

Cell body
Nerve fiber (axon and covering)
Presynaptic neuron
Postsynaptic neuron
Synapse
Dendrite of postsynaptic neuron
Terminal bulb of presynaptic neuron
Synaptic gap between terminal bulb and dendrite

■ **FIGURE 4-2** The synapse. The enlargements progress in the direction of the arrows.

atory neurotransmitter glutamate in response to stimulation. This permits a communication with the neurons by either stimulating or varying its response. Under some circumstances, too much glutamate may be released and lead to excitotoxicity, by which neurons can be killed. This could have implications with Alzheimer's or Parkinson's diseases in humans.

Ependymal cells line the ventricles of the brain and the central canal of the spinal cord. In these locations, the ependymal cells unite with the capillaries to form the choroid plexus, where cerebrospinal fluid is produced.

The **microglia** have a phagocytic function. They enter the CNS from blood vessels and increase in numbers during inflammatory processes or where neuron injury has occurred.

Myelin Sheaths

Myelin is a **white lipid (sphingomyelin)** substance that forms a sheath around nerve fibers and serves as an electrical insulator. It is formed by **oligodendrocytes** in the CNS and by **Schwann cells** in the peripheral nervous system (PNS).

Nerve fibers within the gray matter of the CNS are not myelinated; their white glistening appearance outside of the gray matter, as shown by the white matter and by peripheral nerves, is provided by the myelin that envelops the nerve fibers. Not all nerve fibers outside of the gray matter are myelinated, but because of the closeness of unmyelinated fibers to myelinated fibers, they tend to be invaginated (pressed) into the myelin substance. Even when this occurs, however, unmyelinated fibers are uninsulated because they maintain a direct association with extracellular fluid throughout their length.

The Schwann cell cytoplasm (which contains the myelin) is wrapped around a nerve fiber many times, and the nucleus lies within the Schwann cell just beneath the neurolemma external to the myelin sheath (see Fig. 4-1). The cytoplasm of the oligodendrocyte is dif-

ferent from that of the Schwann cell because several extensions exist, each of which forms a wrapping around a nerve fiber (*Fig. 4-3*). One cell, therefore, provides a sheath at several locations.

Interruptions of the myelin sheath that occur along the length of a fiber are called **nodes of Ranvier**. These nodes are the junctions of adjacent wrappings, either of the cytoplasmic extensions of oligodendrocytes or of Schwann cells. At these points, the nerve fiber plasma membrane (axolemma) is directly exposed to extracellular fluid. The exposure is more intimate in the CNS (*Fig. 4-4*). Whereas the sheathed portion of the nerve fiber is insulated, the nodes are uninsulated. Depolarization occurs at the nodes (see the following section), and the function of the myelin sheaths will become more apparent when nerve conduction is discussed.

■ ORGANIZATION OF THE NERVOUS SYSTEM

1. What are three major subdivisions of the nervous system?
2. What are the three gross divisions of the brain?
3. What are the subdivisions of the brain stem?
4. Is the hypothalamus a subdivision of the cerebrum, cerebellum, or brain stem?
5. List major characteristics of the cerebral hemispheres, cerebellum, and brain stem.
6. What are the five groups of vertebrae in order from their cranial location to their caudal location?
7. What is the vertebral formula for the dog?
8. How are the spinal nerves numbered in relation to the vertebrae?
9. What is the cauda equina?
10. Which root of a spinal nerve does an afferent fiber traverse? an efferent fiber?

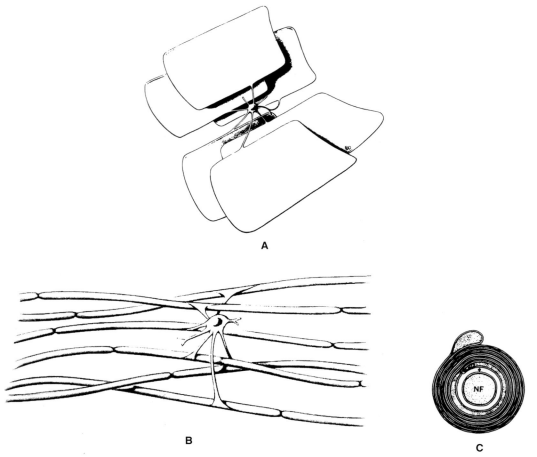

■ **FIGURE 4-3** An oligodendrocyte (myelin-forming cell) of the central nervous system. **A.** The cell with its cytoplasmic extensions unwrapped. **B.** Cytoplasmic extensions wrapped around several axons. **C.** Cross-section of a wrapped nerve fiber (NF). (From Bunge RP. Structure and function of neuroglia: Some recent observations. In: Schmitt FO, ed. The Neurosciences: Second Study Program. New York: Rockefeller University Press, 1970.)

11. What are the relative locations of nerve cell bodies and tracts within the spinal cord?
12. What is a spinal cord segment?
13. Are motor neurons located dorsally or ventrally in the gray matter of the spinal cord?
14. What is the general distribution of a spinal nerve?
15. What is a nerve plexus?
16. How many pairs of cranial nerves are there?

17. What is the general distribution of the cranial nerves?
18. Which one of the cranial nerves supplies parasympathetic fibers to visceral structures in the thorax and abdomen?
19. Are all spinal nerves mixed nerves?
20. Are all cranial nerves mixed nerves?
21. What tissues are innervated by autonomic nerves?
22. Which division of the autonomic nerves is associated with "fight, fright, and flight"?

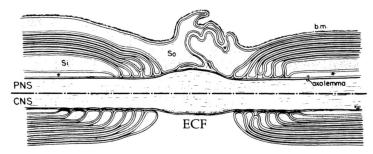

■ **FIGURE 4-4** The node of Ranvier as it would appear in the vertebrate central nervous system (CNS) and peripheral nervous system (PNS). Note the greater intimacy of the CNS node with extracellular fluid (ECF). b.m., basement membrane; Si, Schwann cell inside; So, Schwann cell outside. (From Bunge RP. Structure and function of neuroglia: Some recent observations. In: Schmitt FO, ed. The Neurosciences: Second Study Program. New York: Rockefeller University Press, 1970.)

23. **Where are the cells of origin for the sympathetic and parasympathetic neurons?**
24. **How do autonomic neurons get their structures innervated?**
25. **Study Table 4-2 (p. 102).**

All parts of the body are served by the nervous system. Based on the location of its components, it is subdivided as shown in the following schemes:

1. Central nervous system
   a. Brain
   b. Spinal cord
2. Peripheral nervous system
   a. Cranial nerves
   b. Spinal nerves

The autonomic nervous system (ANS) is another subdivision of the nervous system and is separate from the above scheme because it has both central and peripheral components with further subdivisions as follows:

1. Autonomic nervous system
   a. Sympathetic
   b. Parasympathetic
   c. Enteric

Central Nervous System

The CNS not only contains components of transmission, but the brain also provides for those functions that we associate with computers, such as memory, a central processing unit for problem-solving, and input-output capability (sensations resulting from sensory input).

The Brain

The gross divisions of the brain are the **cerebrum (paired cerebral hemispheres)**, **cerebellum**, and **brain stem**. An organizational scheme (*Fig. 4-5*) shows additional subdivisions. Another scheme (*Fig. 4-6*) is also commonly used; it has different names for the various parts. The relative locations of the various subdivisions to each other according to the first scheme are shown in *Figure 4-7*.

Cerebral Hemispheres. The right and left cerebral hemispheres are large structures that make up most of the cerebrum (*Fig. 4-8*). Each hemisphere is composed of a covering of gray matter, the **cerebral cortex**; a central mass of white matter, the **medullary substance** (made up of nerve fibers); and the **basal nuclei** (previously known as basal ganglia, but because they are in the CNS, they are now called basal nuclei).

The cerebral cortex has the following characteristics:

1. Acquired late in vertebrate evolution
2. Concerned with those nervous reactions that result in consciousness

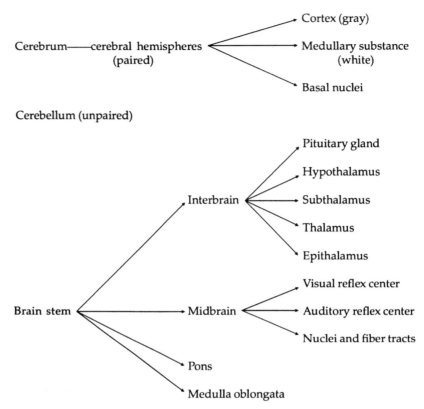

■ FIGURE 4-5 Subdivisions of the brain according to the major divisions, being the cerebrum, cerebellum, and brain stem.

3. Regarded as the seat of the highest type of nervous correlation (association)
4. Marked by a high degree of educability (especially in humans)
5. Possesses a motor area:
   a. Impulses from these areas in one hemisphere cause muscle movements on the opposite (contralateral) side of the body
   b. Size of motor area and number and complexity of skeletal muscle movements of which an animal is capable are directly related
6. Contains sensory areas, or centers, into which sensory fibers discharge

The sensory areas are: 1) the **somesthetic** or **body sense area**, which receives impulses from the skin concerned with touch, warmth, cold, and pain localization; impulses concerned with taste; and impulses from muscles, tendons, and joints; 2) the **visual area (sight)**; 3) the **auditory area (hearing)**; and 4) the **olfactory area (smell)**.

The **white matter** is composed of **myelinated nerve fibers** situated beneath the cerebral cortex. These include **association fibers**, which establish connection between the different parts of the cortex; commissural fibers, which connect the two hemispheres; and **projection fibers**, which connect the cerebral cortex with other parts of the brain and spinal cord.

The **basal nuclei** (see Fig. 4-7) lie deep within the cerebral hemispheres. They are composed of separate, large pools of neurons organized for the control of complex

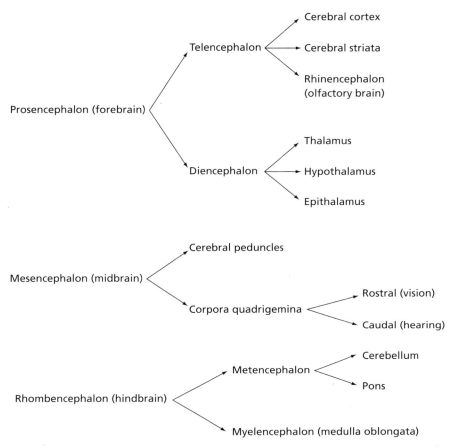

■ **FIGURE 4-6** Subdivisions of the brain according to its development from the primary embryonic vesicles, the prosencephalon, mesencephalon, and rhombencephalon.

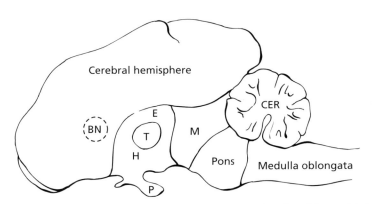

■ **FIGURE 4-7** Relative locations of brain subdivisions to each other. BN, basal nuclei; E, epithalamus; T, thalamus; H, hypothalamus; P, pituitary gland; M, midbrain; CER, cerebellum. Dotted line for boundaries of basal nuclei represents its location on the midline.

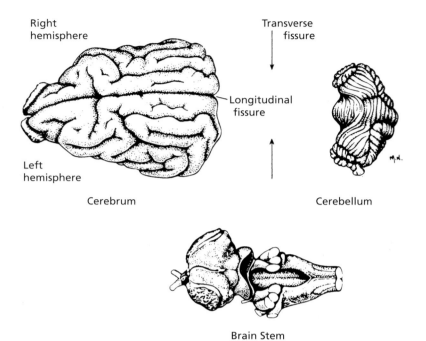

Right
hemisphere

Transverse
fissure

Longitudinal
fissure

Left
hemisphere

Cerebrum

Cerebellum

Brain Stem

■ **FIGURE 4-8** Gross subdivisions of the brain of the dog. (From Beitz AJ, Fletcher TF. The brain. In: Evans HE. Miller's Anatomy of the Dog. 3rd Ed. Philadelphia: WB Saunders Company, 1993.)

semivoluntary movements, such as walking and running. In birds the cerebral cortex is poorly developed, but the basal nuclei are highly developed. Because of this contrast, the basal nuclei perform nearly all of the motor functions, even the voluntary movements, in much the same manner as the motor area of the human cortex controls voluntary movement. In the cat, and to a lesser extent in the dog, removal of the cerebral cortex prevents many sophisticated motor functions. Because of the basal nuclei, however, this does not interfere with the ability to walk, eat, fight, and even participate in sexual activity.

Cerebellum. The **cerebellum** (see Figs. 4-7 and 4-8) is not concerned with consciousness or sensation, as is the cerebral cortex. Because of its motor function, the cerebral cortex can start a limb or body part in motion, but once in motion, inertial forces would tend to keep it in motion until opposing forces

stopped it. The cerebral cortex is not organized to mobilize the opposing force. The **cerebellum**, however, can make **automatic adjustments** to prevent the distortion of inertia and momentum. To accomplish this, the cerebellum receives impulses: 1) from the proprioceptive receptors (located in the internal mass of the body) found in all joints, muscles, and pressure areas (e.g., foot pads); 2) from the equilibrium apparatus of the inner ear; 3) from the visual cortex; and 4) directly from the motor cortex of all motor impulses being sent to muscles (*Fig. 4-9*). Whereas the motor area of a cerebral hemisphere exerts its effect on the opposite (**contralateral**) side of the body, the effect of one side of the cerebellum is exerted on the same (**ipsilateral**) side of the body. The cerebellum acts as a "collecting house" for all information regarding the instantaneous physical status of the body. Cerebellum malfunction is exemplified in feline cerebellar hypoplasia (arrested development) where the

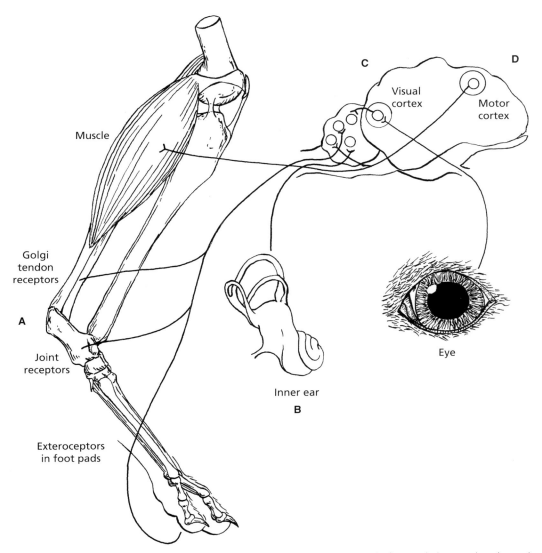

■ FIGURE 4-9 Sources of input to the cerebellum of the dog. **A.** Exteroceptors in foot pads (pressure) and proprioceptors in joints, muscles, and tendons (tension). **B.** Vestibular apparatus (equilibrium) of the inner ear. **C.** Visual cortex of the cerebrum. **D.** Cerebral motor cortex (simultaneous impulse to muscle).

mother cat acquires a virus infection while pregnant. Following birth, voluntary muscle movement of the kittens overreaches the intended goal (hypermetria); there is failure of muscle coordination (ataxia), and involuntary trembling or quivering (tremor). A very underdeveloped cerebellum is revealed when the kittens are necropsied.

Brain Stem.   The **brain stem** is composed of the **interbrain** rostrally followed caudally (in order) by the **midbrain**, **pons**, and **medulla oblongata** (see Figs. 4-7 and 4-8). The cerebral hemispheres and cerebellum arise from the brain stem. In addition to the many fiber tracts that ascend and descend between the spinal cord and the cerebrum and cerebellum, the brain stem is the origin of all the cranial nerves except for the optic, olfactory, and acoustic nerves (special senses). The cells of origin for the latter lie outside of the skull.

From below upward, the interbrain is composed of the **hypothalamus, thalamus**, and **epithalamus** (see Fig. 4-7). The **hypothalamus** contains the **hypophysis** or **pituitary gland**, which is an endocrine organ. Associated with the hypothalamus is a complex sensing and neurosecretory function. Also, the hypothalamus assumes a major role in the integration of functions carried out by the autonomic nervous system. For these functions, the anterior and middle portions contain parasympathetic components, and the posterior portion contains sympathetic components. The thalamus contains many nuclei and is truly a relay center. Impulses from all areas of the body are transmitted to the thalamus for transfer to the cerebral cortex. Other nuclei in the thalamus are associated with the relay of impulses within the brain. The **epithalamus** contains an olfactory (smell) correlation center and the pineal gland. The latter is a neurosecretory organ that regulates gonadal hormones and certain daily rhythms.

The **midbrain** (see Fig. 4-7) contains the auditory and visual reflex centers, the nuclei of two cranial nerves, and several descending tracts.

The **medulla oblongata** and **pons** (see Fig. 4-7) contain many ascending and descending pathways, the sensory and motor nuclei for all of the cranial nerves originating in the brain stem (except the two located in the midbrain), and a large part of the central mechanism of the postural reflexes (e.g., hopping, righting, placing). There are also several reflex centers associated with the regulation of important visceral functions such as heart rate, blood vessel muscle tone (vasomotor tone), respiration, and motor and secretory activities of the digestive tract.

Spinal Cord

The **spinal cord** is the caudal continuation of the medulla oblongata. **Segmentation** (asso-

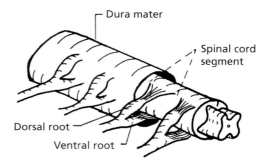

■ **FIGURE 4-10** Structure of the spinal cord of the dog, showing a spinal cord segment. (Redrawn from Breazile JE. Textbook of Veterinary Physiology. Philadelphia: Lea & Febiger, 1971.)

ciation with the vertebral segments) is noticeable, with each segment giving rise to a pair of spinal nerves. The spinal cord receives **sensory afferent (inflowing)** fibers by way of the dorsal roots of the spinal nerves and gives off **efferent (outflowing)** motor fibers to the ventral roots of the spinal nerves (*Fig. 4-10*).

The centrally located **gray matter** (which resembles a capital H and is sometimes called the gray H) consists primarily of nerve cell bodies and their processes. The peripherally arranged **white matter**, which has a white appearance because of its myelin sheath, is composed of many distinct tracts (*Fig. 4-11*). A **tract** is a bundle of nerve fibers having a common origin, termination, and function; and connects the brain stem and higher centers with the spinal nerves. Different sensory and motor tracts are segregated in the cord. **Proprioceptive** (referring to the sensing of position of limbs or other body parts without the use of vision) impulses from muscles, tendons, and joints have well-defined ascending tracts, as do sensory impulses for pain, temperature, and touch. Similarly, impulses associated with certain motor functions descend in definite tracts. Many of the tracts are named according to the structures they connect. For example, the ventral spinocerebellar tract carries impulses from the spinal cord to the cerebellum. The lateral spinothalamic tract carries

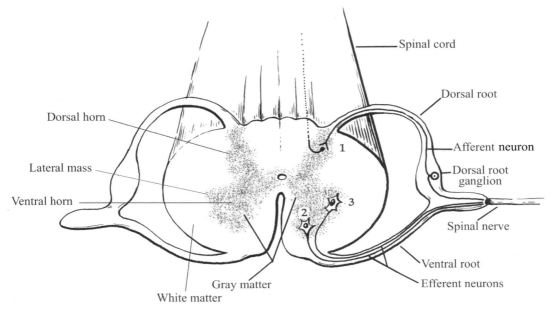

Dorsal horn

Lateral mass

Ventral horn

Spinal cord

Dorsal root

Afferent **neuron**

Dorsal root
ganglion

Spinal nerve

Ventral root

Efferent neurons

Gray matter

White matter

■ **FIGURE 4-11** Transverse section of the spinal cord of the dog. Located within the gray matter are: 1) nerve cell bodies for sensory neurons in dorsal horns; 2) somatic motor neurons in ventral horns; and 3) autonomic motor neurons in lateral masses of ventral horns.

impulses from the spinal cord to the thalamus. The cells of origin for sensory impulses to the brain or to other parts of the spinal cord are located in the **dorsal horns of the gray matter**, and the cells of origin of motor impulses to the spinal nerves are located in the **ventral horns of the gray matter**. The cells of origin of the autonomic motor impulses arising from the spinal cord are the **lateral masses** of the ventral horns (**intermediate location**) of the **gray matter** (see Fig. 4-11).

As the spinal cord descends and proceeds caudally, its cross-sectional area decreases. This is because the cranial parts not only have tracts with fibers from the caudal portions, but also contain fibers associated with the cranial aspects of the body. Finally, at the caudal extremity, the tracts terminate and the spinal nerves fan outward and backward, giving the appearance of a broom or horse's tail. Accordingly, the terminal part of the spinal cord, meninges, and nerves is called the **cauda equina** (*Fig. 4-12*).

Peripheral Nervous System

The peripheral nervous system consists of the spinal nerves and the cranial nerves.

Spinal Nerves

Spinal nerves, as well as **cranial nerves**, are referred to as **somatic** nerves because of their association with voluntary control of muscles. **Autonomic nerves** are referred to as **visceral** nerves because they are involved with involuntary functions such as control of smooth muscle, cardiac muscle, and glands. The spinal nerves are those that arise from the spinal cord and emerge from the vertebrae. In the dog, for example, there are 7 cervical, 13 thoracic, 7 lumbar, 3 sacral, and an average of 20 caudal vertebrae. With the exception of the cervical and caudal nerves, there is a pair of spinal nerves (one right and one left) that emerges behind the vertebrae of the same serial number and name. In this plan the first pair of thoracic nerves emerges through the intervertebral

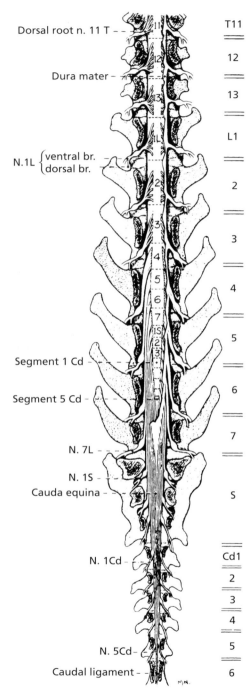

FIGURE 4-12 Caudal extremity of the spinal cord showing the cauda equina. (From Fletcher TF, Kitchell RL. Anatomical studies on the spinal cord segments of the dog. Am J Vet Res 1966; 27:1762.)

foramina located between the T1 and T2 vertebrae, and the last pair of thoracic nerves emerges through the intervertebral foramina between the T13 and L1 vertebrae (*Fig. 4-13B,C*). There are the same number of pairs of thoracic, lumbar, and sacral nerves as there are similar vertebrae. Instead of seven pairs of cervical nerves (corresponding with seven cervical vertebrae), however, there are eight pairs. The first pair of cervical nerves emerges through the foramina in the C1 vertebra, and the second pair emerges between the C1 and C2 vertebrae (*Fig. 4-13A*). Usually there are only six or seven pairs of caudal nerves.

A spinal nerve is composed of a dorsal and ventral root and its branches. The dorsal root enters the dorsal portion of the spinal cord. It carries afferent (sensory) impulses from the periphery toward the spinal cord (see Fig. 4-11). The nerve cell bodies of the neurons composing the dorsal root are located in the **dorsal root ganglion (DRG)**. This is visible as an enlarged part of the dorsal root close to the point where the dorsal and ventral roots join to form the spinal nerve proper. These neurons are embryologically bipolar, but the two processes later fuse near the cell body into one process so that it appears to be T-shaped. One branch of the process becomes a peripheral afferent nerve fiber, and the other branch passes into the CNS by way of the dorsal root. Both branches anatomically are axons and conduct action potentials. Nerve impulses apparently pass from the peripheral branch to the central branch without entering the cell body.

The ventral root emerges from the ventral horn of the spinal cord. It carries efferent (motor) impulses from the spinal cord to striated muscle fibers (see Fig. 4-11). Near the intervertebral foramen, the dorsal root joins with the ventral root to form the main part of the spinal nerve. The spinal nerve proper is classified as a **mixed nerve** because it contains both sensory and motor fibers. After the spinal nerve emerges from the intervertebral foramen, it divides into a **dorsal branch** and a **ventral branch**; these supply innervation to structures

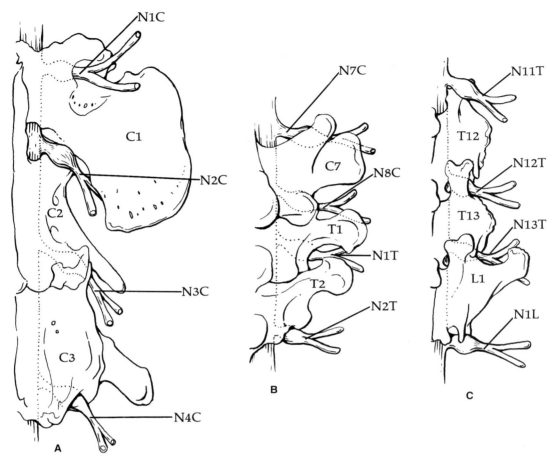

■ **FIGURE 4-13** A schematic representation of the association of spinal nerves with vertebrae in the dog. Only the right half of the spinal cord, vertebrae, and spinal nerve pair is shown. **A.** C1 to C3 vertebrae. **B.** C7, T1, and T2 vertebrae. **C.** T12, T13, and L1 vertebrae. Although not consistently shown, the dorsal root ganglions are medial to the emergence of spinal nerves through intervertebral foramina.

dorsal and ventral to the transverse processes of the vertebrae, respectively (*Fig. 4-14*). The spinal nerves generally supply sensory and motor fibers to the region of the body in the area where they emerge from the spinal cord, but this is not the case for the appendages. They are innervated by the ventral branches of several spinal nerves and, near the limb they supply, the nerves join together in braidlike arrangements known as plexuses. Each forelimb is supplied by nerves that arise from the **brachial plexus** (*Fig. 4-15*), and each hindlimb is supplied by nerves that arise from the **lumbosa cral plexus**.

Cranial Nerves

There are **12 pairs of cranial nerves,** with a right and left nerve making up each pair. The cranial nerves usually supply innervation to structures in the head and neck. The **vagus nerve** is an exception. In addition to its sensory and motor supply to the pharynx and larynx, it also supplies parasympathetic fibers to visceral structures in the thorax and abdomen (*Fig. 4-16*). These nerves have no dorsal or ventral roots and emerge through foramina in the skull. Some cranial nerves are strictly sensory (afferent), some are strictly motor

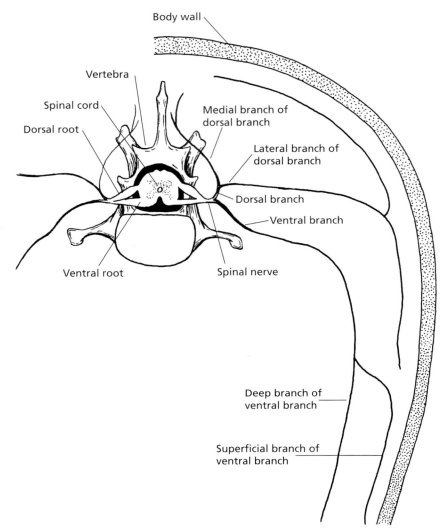

■ **FIGURE 4-14** A spinal nerve and its location relative to its branches, roots, spinal cord, and vertebra.

(efferent), and some are mixed (both sensory and motor). The cranial nerves are listed by number, name, type, and distribution in *Table 4-1.*

Autonomic Nervous System

The ANS, also known as the involuntary, vegetative, or visceral nervous system, is essential for maintaining normal organ function (homeostasis), adapting to environmental change (e.g.,

body temperature), and responding to stresses (e.g., excitement). These responses are accomplished by either simple or complex reflexes and with little, if any, conscious perception. The ANS has sympathetic, parasympathetic, and enteric subdivisions: 1) the **sympathetic nervous system (SNS)** is associated with the body's response to stress; 2) the **parasympathetic nervous system (PSNS)** is associated with homeostatic functions in the absence of stress;

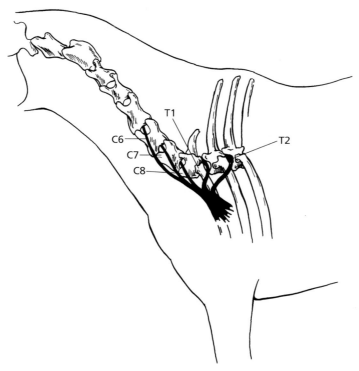

■ **FIGURE 4-15** Brachial plexus of the horse. It is formed by the contributions of the last three cervical and first two thoracic spinal nerves to supply the forelimbs. C, cervical; T, thoracic. The corresponding numbers refer to their respective spinal nerve.

and 3) the **enteric nervous system (ENS)** is associated with regulation of the gastrointestinal (digestive) system. The ENS functions mostly by itself but can be modulated by both the SNS and PSNS. The ENS will be described in more detail in Chapter 12. These subdivisions have mostly efferent activities, but not to be overlooked are the many sources of afferent information needed for its reflex functioning.

ANS innervation extends to smooth muscle, cardiac muscle, and glands. Most organs receive both sympathetic and parasympathetic innervation. Exceptions are sweat glands, most blood vessels, the uterus, and piloerector muscles of the skin, all of which receive only sympathetic innervation. The effect of sympathetic stimulation is generally opposite to that of parasympathetic stimulation. Accordingly, they can be considered as antagonistic to each other. To visualize their respective functions in regard to an organ, the so-called "**fight, fright, or flight**" concept can be considered. Those actions that would be considered favorable in a fighting, frightening, or retreating situation can be attributed to sympathetic activity, and those actions associated with restful or tranquil situations (**eat-or-sleep concept**) can be attributed to the parasympathetic activity. A comparison of their respective actions for various organs is presented in *Table 4-2.*

Central Components

The **central component** resides in the central processing that results from data received (e.g., blood pressure, organ distention) from afferent (inflowing) neurons. The central processing also relies on a number of blood signals

TABLE 4-1 CRANIAL NERVES

NO.	NAME	TYPE	DISTRIBUTION
I	Olfactory	Sensory	Nasal mucous membrane (sense of smell)
II	Optic	Sensory	Retina of eye (sight)
III	Oculomotor	Motor	Most muscles of eye
			Parasympathetic to ciliary muscle and circular muscle of iris
IV	Trochlear	Motor	Dorsal oblique muscle of eye
V	Trigeminal	Mixed	Sensory—to eye and face; motor—to muscles of mastication
VI	Abducens	Motor	Retractor and lateral muscles of eye
VII	Facial	Mixed	Sensory—region of ear and taste to cranial two-thirds of tongue; motor—to muscles of facial expression; parasympathetic—to mandibular and sublingual salivary glands
VIII	Vestibulocochlear	Sensory	Cochlea (hearing); semicircular canals (equilibrium)
IX	Glossopharyngeal	Mixed	Sensory—to pharynx and taste to caudal third of tongue; motor—muscle of pharynx; parasympathetic—to parotid salivary glands
X	Vagus	Mixed	Sensory—to pharynx and larynx; motor—to muscles of larynx; parasympathetic—to visceral structures in the thorax and abdomen
XI	Accessory	Motor	Motor—to muscles of shoulder and neck
XII	Hypoglossal	Motor	Motor—to muscles of tongue

Modified from Frandson RD, Wilke WL, Fails AD. Anatomy and Physiology of Farm Animals. 6th Ed. Baltimore: Lippincott Williams & Wilkins, 2003.

such as temperature, pH, glucose concentration, and others. The central processing for the reflex integration and modulation of body conditions by the ANS occurs in spinal cord sites and a number of brain locations. The latter is best represented by the hypothalamus. After central processing, reflex adjustments are made by the peripheral (efferent) components of the ANS.

Peripheral Components

The cells of origin for the sympathetic nerves are located in the lateral masses of the ventral horns of the thoracic and lumbar segments of the spinal cord, and the cells of origin of the parasympathetic nerves are located in the brain stem and sacral segments of the spinal cord, hence, the term for their origin is noted as **craniosacral** for the parasympathetics, as opposed to **thoracolumbar** for the sympathetics (*Fig. 4-17*). For both sympathetic and parasympathetic activity, two neurons (in series) are associated with the transmission of impulses from the cells of origin in the spinal cord or brain to the effector organ (glands or muscle). The cells of origin for the second neuron are located in ganglia. The first neuron

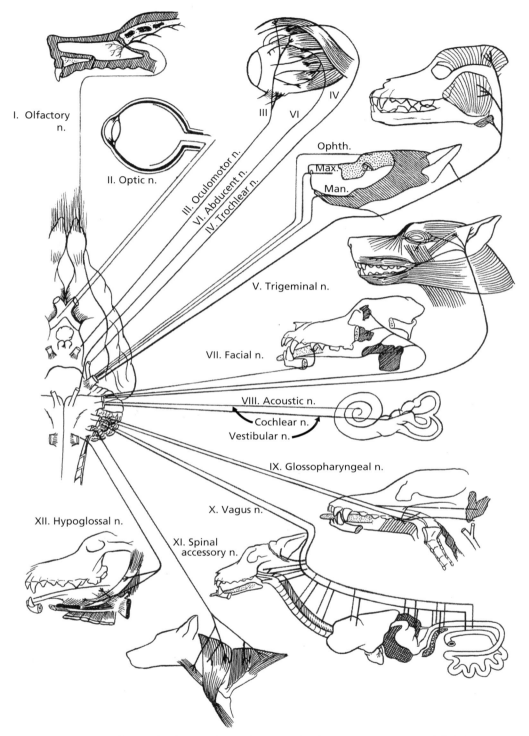

I. Olfactory n.

II. Optic n.

III. Oculomotor n.

VI. Abducent n.

IV. Trochlear n.

III   VI   IV

Ophth.
Max.
Man.

V. Trigeminal n.

VII. Facial n.

VIII. Acoustic n.
Cochlear n.
Vestibular n.

IX. Glossopharyngeal n.

X. Vagus n.

XII. Hypoglossal n.

XI. Spinal accessory n.

■ **FIGURE 4-16** Origin and major distribution of cranial nerves in the dog. N, nerve; OPHTH, ophthalmic nerve; MAX, maxillary nerve; MAN, mandibular nerve. Acoustic nerve (VIII) now called vestibulocochlear nerve and spinal accessory nerve (XI) now called accessory nerve. (From Hoerlein BF, Oliver JE, Mayhew JG. Neurologic examination and the diagnostic plan. In: Oliver JE, Mayhew IG. Veterinary Neurology. Philadelphia: WB Saunders Company, 1987.)

TABLE 4-2 ACTIONS OF AUTONOMIC STIMULATION

ORGAN/STRUCTURE	SYMPATHETIC ACTION	PARASYMPATHETIC ACTION
Eye		
Muscles of iris	Contraction of radial muscle (dilates pupil)	Contraction of circular muscle (contracts pupil)
Heart		
S-A node	Increase in heart rate	Decrease in heart rate
A-V node	Increase in conduction velocity	Decrease in conduction velocity
Muscle	Increase in force of contraction	Decrease in force of contraction
Intestines		
Muscle	Decreased	Increased
Secretions	Decreased	Increased
Lungs		
Bronchi	Dilation	Constriction
Kidney	Afferent arteriole constriction	None and renin secretion
Urinary bladder		
Bladder wall	None	Contraction
Sphincter	Contraction	Relaxation
Penis	Ejaculation	Erection
Piloerector muscles	Contraction	None
Salivary glands	Mucus secretion	Serous secretion

is called **preganglionic**, and the second neuron is called **postganglionic**.

Sympathetic Efferent Distribution. The preganglionic neuron for a sympathetic nerve traverses the ventral root of a thoracic or lumbar spinal nerve, enters the spinal nerve proper, and soon branches from it to enter a vertebral ganglion of the **sympathetic trunk**, a bilateral chain of ganglia ventral to the vertebrae (see Fig. 4-17) with a ganglion on each side of each vertebrae. It either synapses in a ganglion of the same vertebral segment, or it can continue over a considerable distance to another vertebral ganglion, where it synapses. The synapse might not occur in a vertebral ganglion at all, however, but might continue to some paired ganglia that are ventral to the sympathetic trunk; these are called **prevertebral ganglia**. The prevertebral ganglia are fewer in number and include the cranial cervical ganglion (with distribution to smooth muscle and glands of the head), middle cervical ganglion (heart and lungs), cervicothoracic ganglion (arteries in neck and thorax), celiac ganglion (stomach, liver, pancreas, kidney, adrenal), cranial mesenteric ganglion (small intestine and upper colon), and caudal mesenteric ganglion (lower colon and neck of the bladder). The postganglionic neuron leaves the vertebral or prevertebral ganglion and proceeds to the effector organ, usually by way of a blood vessel to that organ. It can also leave the vertebral ganglion, reenter a spinal nerve,

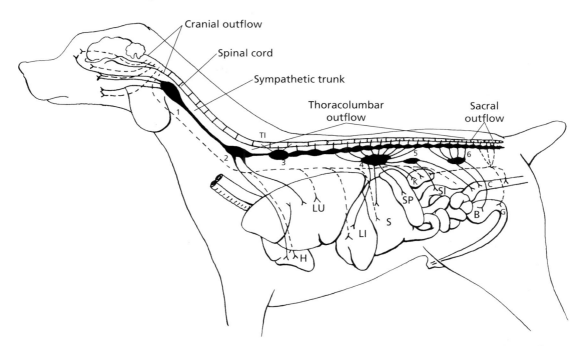

■ **FIGURE 4-17** Diagrammatic representation of the efferent autonomic nervous system of the dog. Only one chain of the bilateral sympathetic trunk is shown. The lines showing sympathetic outflow (thoracolumbar) are solid; lines for parasympathetic outflow (craniosacral) are broken. Numbers indicate sympathetic ganglia: 1) cranial cervical; 2) middle cervical; 3) cervicothoracic; 4) celiac; 5) cranial mesenteric; 6) caudal mesenteric. LU, lung; H, heart; LI, liver; S, stomach; SI, small intestine; SP, spleen; K, kidney; C, colon; B, urinary bladder; G, genitalia; T1, 1st thoracic vertebra.

and be distributed by the branchings of the spinal nerve.

Parasympathetic Efferent Distribution. The preganglionic neurons of the parasympathetic division are distributed to ganglia near the effector organs before they synapse with the postganglionic neuron. Accordingly, the preganglionic fibers are relatively longer and the postganglionic fibers are relatively shorter as compared with the preganglionic and postganglionic fibers of the sympathetic division. Most of the parasympathetic ganglia are microscopic and are an intimate component of the tissue they innervate. The parasympathetic preganglionic fibers that arise from nerve cell bodies in the brain are distributed to their respective organs in common with one of four cranial nerves (III, VII, IX, or X). The first

three supply regions of the head, and the last, cranial nerve X (the vagus nerve), supplies the heart and lungs in the thorax and nearly all of the abdominal viscera. The vagus nerve has sometimes been called the vagabond nerve because of its extensive wanderings. The parasympathetic preganglionic fibers that arise from nerve cell bodies in the sacral portion of the spinal cord supply the last part of the digestive tract and most of the urogenital system. These fibers emerge from the ventral branches of their respective segments and are distributed to the ganglia near the effector organs supplied by the pelvic nerve.

Autonomic Reflexes. Autonomic function is based on reflex activity, and these reflexes control such functions as blood pressure, heart rate, and the activity of the digestive and urogenital systems (see Table 4-2). Autonomic reflexes involve afferent transmission of sensory information from effector organs to the CNS, information processing, and return of a motor response to the effector organs. Autonomic afferents are not designated as sympathetic or parasympathetic (i.e., they transmit information regardless of which division of the ANS), and most travel to the CNS via SNS and PSNS nerves. Their cell bodies are in DRG and cranial nuclei. Some afferents (e.g., blood vessels in skeletal muscle) travel in spinal and cranial nerves. Most of the autonomic functions do not reach the conscious level. However, some afferent information carried by autonomic sensory neurons does reach conscious levels. This may be normal or pathologic. Normal would include feelings of fullness of the bladder or rectum, and pathologic might include gallbladder pain or angina pectoris as experienced by humans.

■ THE NERVE IMPULSE AND ITS TRANSMISSION

1. What is the function of the Na⁺-K⁺ ATPase pump in the axolemma?
2. What is the approximate value of the resting membrane potential?
3. What is the polarity of a resting neuron membrane?
4. What accomplishes depolarization?
5. What accomplishes repolarization?
6. Describe the sequence of events associated with neurotransmission in mammals.
7. What is an action potential?
8. What is threshold?
9. What is a refractory period?
10. What is meant by a nerve fiber being "fired"?
11. What is the "all-or-none" principle for nerve fibers?
12. How does neurotransmission differ in myelinated fibers?
13. What are two functions of saltatory conduction?

14. What kind of nerve fiber has the fastest impulse transmission?
15. What is the purpose of a neuro transmitter?
16. What are the neurotransmitters associated with the autonomic nervous system, and where are they located?
17. What is the nature of the central neurotransmitters?
18. Describe the final common pathway concept.
19. Differentiate between the different types of neuron circuits.
20. What is the minimum number of neurons required for the transmission of a nerve impulse from the periphery by way of a spinal nerve to the cerebral cortex?

Communication among neurons and with the cells of their control is accomplished by the transmission of a nerve impulse. A nerve impulse originates in response to a stimulus of an electrical, chemical, thermal, or mechanical nature that has been received by the cell membrane of a neuron. The stimulus elicits a wave of depolarization and repolarization that spreads along the axolemma, away from the site where the stimulus was received, which results in the transmission of the nerve impulse.

Mechanisms of Transmission

The word potential is used in regard to nerve cells as it is in the study of electricity, in which it refers to relative electrical charges between two points in a field or circuit. For the neuron, this is referred to as a transmembrane potential, and the two points are the inside and outside of the confines of the cell membrane. All cells of the body have a **transmembrane potential**, but the neurons are unique in being able to alter this potential to produce an impulse. The charged transmembrane potential is a local phenomenon close to the cell membrane and does not refer to a charge inside and outside the cell, which is electrically neutral. A measured potential is relatively small, however, and its units are in millivolts rather than volts.

Resting Membrane Potential

In a resting neuron, the potential between the two sides of the membrane is called the resting potential. The **resting membrane potential** results from the unequal distribution of sodium ions (Na^+) and potassium ions (K^+) on the outside and inside of the neuron. The active transport of Na^+ to the outside, coupled with the transport of K^+ into the neuron (the $Na^+ - K^+$ ATPase pump), keeps the concentration of Na^+ low on the inside of the membrane. If their rates of transport were equal to each other, electrical neutrality between the inside and outside of the membrane would be maintained. However, the outward active transport of Na^+ occurs at a faster rate than the inward active transport of K^+, and thus an electronegativity is maintained on the inside of the membrane and an electropositivity on the outside (*Fig. 4-18*). The membrane is therefore **polarized**. The resting membrane potential has been measured as about −70 millivolts (mV). It does not exceed −70 mV because, at this level, the electrical gradient is sufficient to cause Na^+ diffusion inward to balance the rate of outward active transport.

Depolarization, Repolarization, and the Nerve Impulse

Chemical or physical stimulation of a neuron increases the permeability of the membrane for Na^+ at the point of stimulation and, because there is a high concentration of Na^+ on the outside of the membrane in the extracellular fluid, Na^+ rushes inward. This reverses the membrane potential at the point of stimulation, so the membrane now becomes positive on the inside and negative on the outside; this is **depolarization**. The inflow of Na^+ soon stops and the permeability of the membrane

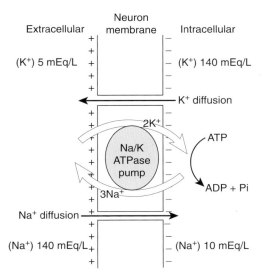

■ **FIGURE 4-18** Establishment of a resting membrane potential by active transport of three Na^+ outward coupled with the transport of two K^+ inward. The uneven distribution results in the electronegativity within the fiber. The large concentration gradients for sodium and potassium across the resting nerve membrane are caused by the sodium-potassium pump (Na/K ATPase pump). ATP, adenosine triphosphate; ADP, adenosine diphosphate; Pi, inorganic phosphate.

for K^+ increases; the K^+ then flows outward because it has a higher concentration inside the neuron than outside. The outflow of K^+ reestablishes the resting membrane potential at the point of stimulation; this is **repolarization**. Measurement of the membrane potential during membrane depolarization and repolarization and its continuous recording on a moving chart is shown in *Figure 4-19*.

When a microregion of a nerve fiber is stimulated and subsequently depolarized, a current flow occurs from the point of depolarization to the adjoining microregions. **Current flow** occurs because a positive charge now exists inside the membrane at the point of initial depolarization; because of the negative charge inside the membrane, beyond the point of stimulation, the positive charges (ions) flow toward the negatively charged portion. In addition, the outer aspect of the fiber membrane

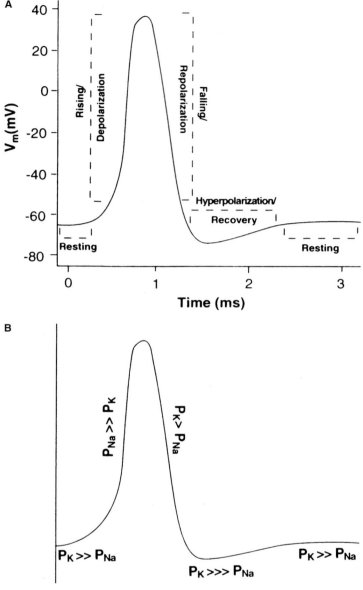

■ **FIGURE 4-19** Recording of a transmembrane potential during depolarization and repolarization of a nerve fiber microregion. A. The various phases of the action potential. B. The relative membrane permeability relationships between sodium and potassium ions associated with each of the phases (e.g., $P_{Na} \gg P_K$ refers to permeability for Na is greater than permeability for K, where >= greater and >>= much greater). V_m, transmembrane voltage; P_{Na}, membrane permeability to sodium; P_K, membrane permeability to potassium. (From Klein BG. Membrane potentials: The generation and conduction of electrical signals in neurons. In: Reece WO, ed. Dukes' Physiology of Domestic Animals. 12th Ed. Ithaca, NY: Cornell University Press, 2004:42.)

(which has become negatively charged at the point of depolarization) attracts positive ions to it from the charged membrane farther ahead. Because of these two events, the interior of the fiber just beyond the depolarized region becomes somewhat more positively charged and the exterior of the fiber just beyond the depolarized region becomes less positively charged. Accordingly, an electrical current flows outward through the fiber membrane from the interior (that gained positive charges)

to the exterior (where positive charges were drawn away). The passage of current out through the membrane, just beyond the site where depolarization has occurred, causes this region of the membrane to become depolarized in turn (because current flow increases permeability to Na$^+$), just as the membrane did at the site of the stimulus. The process of depolarization followed by current flow is repeated throughout the length of the nerve fiber and accounts for the nerve impulse (*Fig. 4-20*).

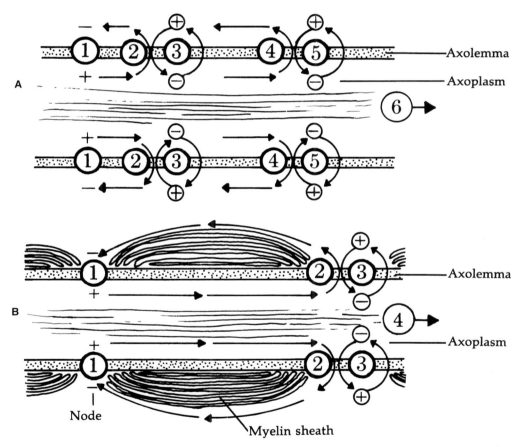

■ **FIGURE 4-20** Summary of neurotransmission in mammals. **A.** In unmyelinated nerve fiber, the sequence of events is as follows: 1) depolarization at point of stimulation has occurred (now negative outside and positive inside); 2) current flow; 3) depolarization of adjacent region begins (will become negative outside and positive inside); 4) current flow; 5) depolarization begins (will become negative outside and positive inside); 6) repetition of current flow and depolarization, and impulse travels to end of nerve fiber. **B.** In myelinated nerve fiber the sequence is: 1) depolarization; 2) current flow; 3) depolarization; 4) saltatory conduction to end of nerve fiber.

Action Potential

Action potentials are changes in the resting membrane potential that are actively propagated along the membrane of the cell. The application of a stimulus to a nerve cell membrane diminishes the resting membrane potential (zero direction). When the membrane potential reaches a critical value (usually 10 to 15 mV less than the resting level of −70 mV), an action potential occurs. The membrane potential at which an action potential is produced is referred to as **threshold**. Not all stimuli can depolarize the membrane to threshold.

During an action potential, depolarization can change the membrane potential from −70 mV to about +40 mV. During repolarization there is a return to the resting membrane potential of −70 mV. The recording shown in Figure 4-19 represents an action potential. The nerve fiber cannot be stimulated again until repolarization is nearly complete; this is known as the **refractory period**. When an action potential has been initiated, the nerve fiber is said to fire. If the stimulus is strong enough to initiate an action potential, the entire fiber will fire. This is known as the **all-or-none principle** for nerve fibers. There is no such thing as a weak impulse. If the stimulus is strong enough to initiate depolarization, the impulse will be conducted with action potentials of normal magnitude. Depolarization and repolarization proceed from one microregion to the adjoining microregion until the entire fiber has been traversed.

Saltatory Conduction

In myelinated fibers the depolarization and repolarization processes are the same, but the action potentials occur from one node of Ranvier to the next instead of over the entire area of the membrane. This process of impulse transmission is referred to as **saltatory conduction** (saltation refers to an abrupt movement, such as dancing or leaping). The axolemma is in intimate association with the extracellular fluid at the nodes of Ranvier, and the remainder of the membrane is relatively insulated from the extracellular fluid. Thus, current flow sufficient to increase membrane permeability leaps from one node of Ranvier to the next, rather than being dissipated at the adjoining microregion. Two functions are served by saltatory conduction. First, impulse transmission is accelerated; second, less membrane is depolarized and repolarized, hence reducing the energy requirement for "recharging" the membrane.

Transmission Velocity

The larger the diameter of the fiber and the thicker the myelin sheath, the faster the transmission of the impulse. The fastest transmission is about 100 m/s, and the slowest is about 0.5 m/s. Large myelinated fibers can transmit about 2,500 impulses/s, contrasted with about 250 impulses/s for small unmyelinated fibers.

Neurotransmitters

A nerve impulse causes an effect at a synapse or at the structure being innervated. Axons terminate by branching; the branches terminate with a structure known as a presynaptic terminal bulb at the synapse and with other similar, modified structures at the organs innervated (see Fig. 4-2). These terminations have vesicles containing chemical substances that are liberated when the impulse arrives. The chemical substance then diffuses to the membrane of the postsynaptic neuron or structure and influences the permeability of the membrane for sodium ions.

Peripheral Neurotransmitters

The neurotransmitters of the somatic peripheral nervous system are excitatory in nature—that is, they increase the permeability of the affected membrane for sodium ions. This substance is **acetylcholine (ACh)** for the somatic spinal and cranial nerves. ACh is also the preganglionic and postganglionic terminal

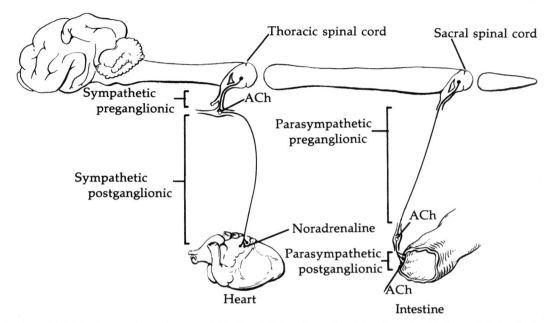

■ **FIGURE 4-21** The neurotransmitters acetylcholine (ACh) and norepinephrine (noradrenaline) associated with the autonomic nervous system of mammals.

neurotransmitter for the parasympathetic division of the autonomic nervous system (*Fig. 4-21*). This division of the autonomic nervous system is, therefore, sometimes referred to as the **cholinergic system**. The preganglionic terminal neurotransmitter of the sympathetic division is also ACh, but the postganglionic terminal secretion is usually **norepinephrine**. Another name for norepinephrine is **noradrenaline**, so the sympathetic division is often referred to as the **adrenergic system**.

Central Neurotransmitters

In the central nervous system there are not only excitatory but also inhibitory transmitters. In addition to ACh and norepinephrine, which are present in peripheral neurons, other excitatory transmitters are found in the central nervous system. At least two inhibitory transmitters are recognized within the brain and spinal cord, **gamma-aminobutyric acid**

(GABA) and **glycine**, which is a simple amino acid. A decrease in the permeability of the affected membrane for sodium ions is one mechanism of inhibition.

Final Common Pathway

Somatic **lower motor neurons (LMNs)** are motor neurons of the spinal cord and brain stem nuclei that innervate skeletal muscle effectors. **Upper motor neurons (UMNs)** are located in the brain and have fibers that descend to and modify the activity of LMNs. Usually, the branches of many axons (some UMNs), perhaps 2,000 or so, will impinge on the dendritic zone of an LMN, which then, depending on the algebraic sum of the inhibiting and facilitatory input, will either fire or not fire. Thus, the LMN serves as the **final common pathway** (and the last site for integration) for all output to striated skeletal muscle (*Fig. 4-22*).

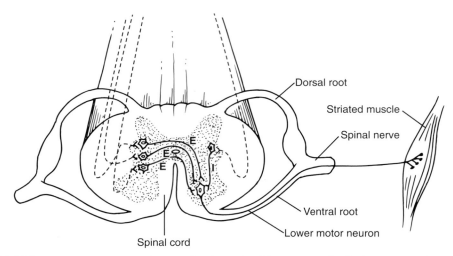

■ **FIGURE 4-22** Lower motor neuron going to striated muscle. This represents the final common pathway. To fire, a greater amount of excitatory (E) neurotransmitter must be released than inhibitory (I) neurotransmitter. Dashed lines represent axons of upper motor neurons.

Neuron Placement

Within the central nervous system are several schemes of neuron placement (circuits) that allow for different patterns of activity.

Converging Circuit

A circuit in which several neurons impinge on one neuron is known as a **converging circuit** (*Fig. 4-23A*). It allows impulses from many different sources to cause some response or provide a sensation.

Diverging Circuit

A **diverging circuit** is one in which the axon branches of one neuron impinge on two or more neurons, and each of these in turn impinge on two or more neurons (Fig. 4-23B). This type of circuit allows for amplification of impulses and is found in the control of skeletal muscles.

Reverberating Circuit

A **reverberating circuit** is one in which each neuron in a series sends a branch back to the beginning neuron so that a volley of impulses is received at the final neuron (Fig. 4-23C). This type is associated with rhythmic activities, and the volley continues until the synapse fatigues or some other mechanism of unknown type stops the reverberating circuit.

Parallel Circuit

A **parallel circuit** contains a number of neurons in a series, with each neuron supplying a branch to the final neuron (Fig. 4-23D). Because there is a delay of transmission at the synapse, a volley of stimuli reaches the final neuron. Unlike the reverberating circuit, the impulses then stop. This type provides reinforcement to a single stimulus.

Simple Circuits

Many complex neuron connections are possible, but neuron connections also can be direct and simple. In this regard, the neurons associated with the special senses might involve no more than two neurons for their projection to the cerebral cortex. A minimum of three neurons is required to transmit a nerve impulse from the periphery by way of a spinal nerve to the cerebral cortex (*Fig. 4-24*). The three-neuron circuit is the classic circuit for conscious sensations.

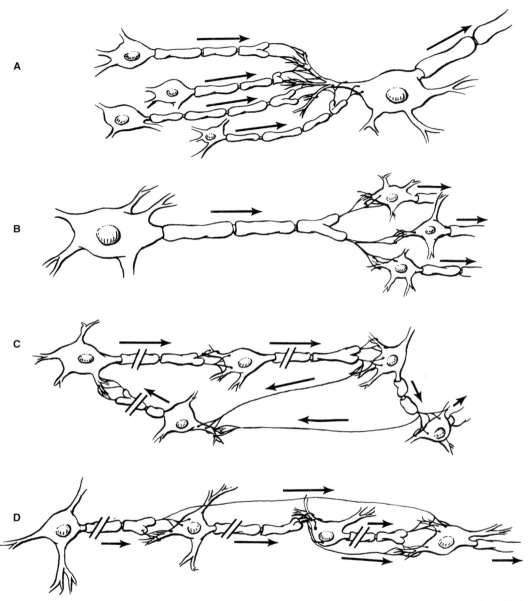

■ **FIGURE 4-23** Examples of neuron placement within the central nervous system of mammals. **A.** Converging circuit. **B.** Diverging circuit. **C.** Reverberating circuit. **D.** Parallel circuit.

■ Reflexes

1. What are the components of a reflex arc?
2. Describe the knee jerk reflex.
3. What is the purpose of the stretch reflex?
4. Why is the stretch reflex considered a postural reflex?
5. How does the crossed extensor reflex differ from the knee jerk reflex?
6. Differentiate between somatic and visceral reflexes.

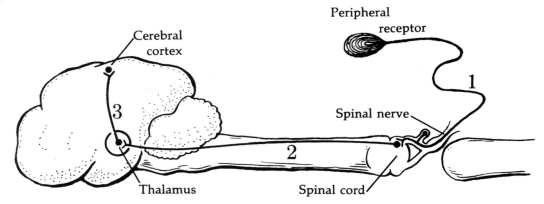

■ **FIGURE 4-24** A neuron circuit from periphery to cerebral cortex. A minimum of three neurons is required: 1) afferent neuron in a mixed spinal nerve; 2) neuron ascending in a spinal cord tract to the thalamus; 3) final neuron in the circuit that transmits the impulse to the cerebral cortex.

7. How are visceral reflexes transmitted?
8. List functions of reflex centers located in the: 1) medulla oblongata, 2) cerebellum, 3) hypothalamus, and 4) midbrain.
9. What is meant by muscle tone?
10. What is the basic element of muscle tone?
11. Describe standing, attitudinal, and righting reflexes.

A **reflex** is defined as an automatic or unconscious response of an effector organ (muscle or gland) to an appropriate stimulus. The components involved for a reflex to occur make up what is known as a **reflex arc** and consist of: 1) a receptor, 2) an afferent limb, 3) central connections, 4) an efferent limb, and 5) an effector organ.

Spinal Reflex

A reflex can involve parts of the brain and autonomic nervous system, but the simplest reflex is the **myotatic (stretch) spinal reflex**. An example of a spinal reflex is the knee jerk reflex (*Fig. 4-25*). The reflex is elicited by striking the middle patellar ligament. This

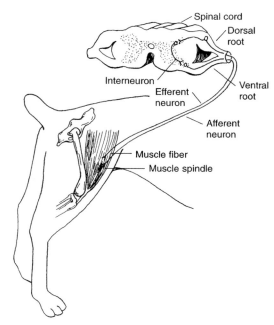

■ **FIGURE 4-25** The stretch reflex. Stretch of muscle stimulates the muscle spindle. The impulse travels to the spinal cord by way of an afferent neuron. Transmission of the impulse to an efferent neuron may be direct or by way of an interneuron as shown. Stimulation of an efferent neuron to striated muscle counteracts stretch by causing contraction. Muscle spindles, in addition to being involved in reflexes, also provide sensory input to cerebral and cortical levels as well as playing a role in voluntary control of muscular activity.

ligament, located at the knee, is the tendon of insertion for the quadriceps femoris and transmits its action to extend the tibia. Striking the middle patellar ligament stretches the quadriceps muscle, which in turn stimulates muscle spindles (receptors for muscle sense). An impulse is transmitted by way of the dorsal root of the appropriate spinal nerve to the applicable motor neuron in the ventral horn of the gray matter, and thence to muscle fibers of the quadriceps muscle, causing it to contract. The purpose of the reflex is to oppose stretch of the muscle. Because this reflex involves an intact and functioning spinal cord at a certain level of segmentation, the soundness of the cord at that level can be determined by this reflex action. Absence of the knee jerk reflex can help to confirm suspicion of damage or injury to the spinal cord or any of the five components of the reflex arc. This reflex is a postural reflex because it aids in maintaining a standing position.

Spinal reflexes can also be rather complex, in which the central connections of the reflex extend over several segments and also extend contralaterally as well as ipsilaterally. The crossed extensor response is an example of a complex spinal reflex. This is shown when there is painful stimulation of the skin or subcutaneous tissues and muscle. The response is flexor muscle contraction and inhibition of extensor muscles so that the part stimulated is flexed and withdrawn from the stimulus and at the same time there is extension of the opposite limb (assisting withdrawal).

Somatic and Visceral Reflexes

If the effector organs are composed of striated muscle, the reflex is somatic. If the effector organs are either smooth or cardiac muscle, or glands, the reflex is visceral. Visceral reflexes regulate visceral functions and are transmitted by the autonomic nervous system (by visceral afferent fibers and preganglionic and postganglionic efferent fibers of the sympathetic or parasympathetic division).

Reflex Centers

Reflex centers are located throughout the central nervous system. They are involved with the integration of more complex reflexes. The simplest reflexes are those associated with the spinal cord, and the more complex are carried out through reflex centers in the brain. Some of these centers are located in the pons and medulla oblongata and include reflex centers for the control of heart action, vessel diameter, respiration, swallowing, vomiting, coughing, and sneezing. The cerebellum contains most of the reflex centers associated with locomotion and posture. The hypothalamus is the main integration and regulation center for the autonomic nervous system, e.g., contains reflex centers associated with temperature regulation. The midbrain contains visual and auditory reflexes, which can bring about constriction or dilatation of the pupils and evoke a startle reaction to loud noises.

Postural Reflexes and Reactions

The **postural reflexes** and **reactions** aid in maintaining an upright position. Responses that involve the cerebral cortex are more properly called reactions than reflexes. **Muscle tonus (tone)** is that state of muscle tension that enables an animal to assume and remain in the erect attitude. The stretch reflex, previously described, is the fundamental element of muscle tone. The following are examples of postural reflexes and reactions:

1. Standing reflex—pushing down on the back of a dog causes muscle movements that compensate for and resist the displacement.
2. Attitudinal reflexes—displacement of one part of the body is followed by postural changes in other parts (e.g., lifting the head of a horse is followed by postural changes in the rear quarters so that a new attitude is assumed).
3. Righting reflex—dropping an inverted cat is followed by its landing in the upright position.

4. Hopping reaction—pushing a supported dog with three limbs elevated results in a placement correction of the intact leg to act as a rigid pillar.

The spinal cord of domestic animals constitutes a greater proportion of the CNS (brain and spinal cord) than in humans. This reflects the fact that more of the CNS activity in animals is accomplished by reflex than by cerebral activity. There is approximately 10 times more spinal cord activity in dogs than in humans.

■ THE MENINGES AND CEREBROSPINAL FLUID

1. Visualize the relative location of the meningeal layers to each other and to the skull and brain and to the vertebral canal and spinal cord.
2. What are the arachnoid villi extensions of, and what do they extend into?
3. What is an epidural injection?
4. Is cerebrospinal fluid circulated within the epidural space?
5. Which meningeal layer forms the lining of the perivascular spaces, and what is its extent?
6. What fluid fills the perivascular space?
7. Visualize the location of the brain ventricles.
8. What structures within the ventricles produce cerebrospinal fluid?
9. Describe the circulation of the cerebrospinal fluid.
10. What could cause the cerebrospinal fluid pressure to increase?
11. What are functions of cerebrospinal fluid?
12. Are blood cells normally not present in cerebrospinal fluid?

Within the bony cranium and vertebral column, the brain and spinal cord have three connective tissue wrappings known as the meninges. In addition, they are cushioned by

cerebrospinal fluid, which functions as a shock absorber. Cerebrospinal fluid is formed in the cavities of the brain, the ventricles.

Meninges of the Brain

The **meninges** are the coverings of the brain and spinal cord. From without inward they are the **dura mater**, **arachnoid**, and **pia mater**, respectively (*Fig. 4-26*). In the skull the outer aspect of the dura mater is intimately fused with the inner periosteum of the **calvaria** (**brain case**). Dorsally, between the cerebral hemispheres and between the cerebrum and cerebellum, there is a separation of the outer and inner aspects of the dura mater to form valveless venous sinuses into which drain the veins of the brain and its encasing bone. Venous sinuses are also located beneath the brain, and the paired cavernous sinus plays a big role in the ventral venation of the brain. These blood collection areas are continued as veins that return blood to the heart from the brain. The only space between the inner aspect

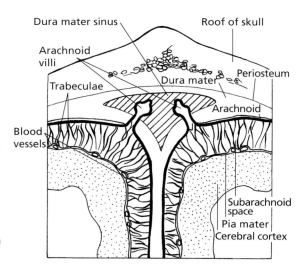

■ **FIGURE 4-26** Cerebral meninges and arachnoid villi. The meninges consist of the dura mater (thickness exaggerated to illustrate dura mater sinus), arachnoid (darkened line), and pia mater. The subarachnoid space contains cerebrospinal fluid. The arachnoid villi project into the dural sinus (blood sinus) and provide an outlet for cerebrospinal fluid.

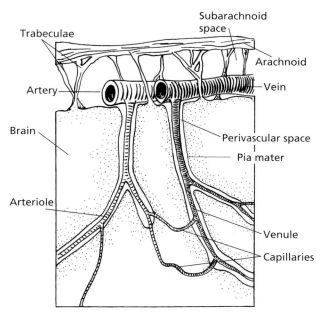

■ FIGURE 4-27 The perivascular space. The space is lined by pia mater that follows blood vessels into the brain substance. The space is filled with cerebrospinal fluid and communicates with the subarachnoid space. It extends only to the level of the capillaries, and serves a lymphatic function.

of the dura mater and the arachnoid is that which is sufficient for blood vessels. The **arachnoid** has projections (**trabeculae**) from its inner aspect to the most intimate covering of the brain, the pia mater. The trabeculae give the appearance of a spider's web—hence the name arachnoid (after the class name for spiders, Arachnida). The space between the arachnoid and the pia mater is significant and is known as the **subarachnoid space**. There are projections from the subarachnoid space into the dura mater sinuses, the microscopic **arachnoid villi**. Clusters of arachnoid villi, when there are enough to form a macroscopic structure, are called **arachnoid granulations**. The subarachnoid space contains cerebrospinal fluid, and the arachnoid villi allow for the resorption of this fluid back into the blood. The **pia mater** follows all of the grooves and fissures of the brain surface. It forms a sheath around blood vessels and follows them into the substance of the brain (*Fig. 4-27*). The perivascular spaces thus formed extend as far as the arterioles and venules, but not onto the

capillaries. The inner aspects of the brain, therefore, are in communication with cerebrospinal fluid (this might serve a "lymphatic" function because there are no lymph vessels in the brain). The meninges (and cerebrospinal fluid) continue for a short distance onto the cranial and spinal nerves. The vestibular (auditory) branch of the vestibulocochlear nerve (cranial nerve VIII), because of its closeness to the exterior of the body, subjects the meninges to some hazard if the inner ear becomes inflamed.

Meninges of the Spinal Cord

The meninges of the spinal cord are continuous with the meninges of the brain. The outer aspect of the dura mater is not fused with the vertebral canal (the hole through the vertebrae within which the spinal cord transcends), and an epidural (outside the dura mater) space exists, which contains fat (*Fig. 4-28*). Sites for entering the epidural space include those between L1-L2 (lumbar vertebrae), lumbosa-

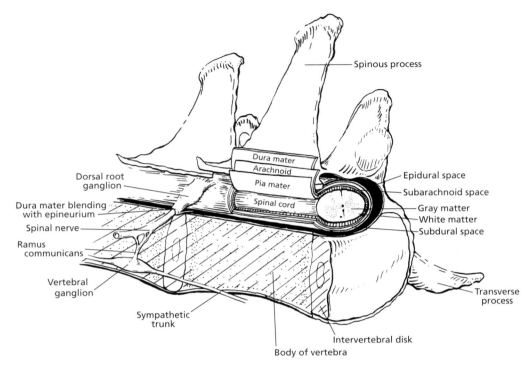

Spinous process

Dura mater
Arachnoid
Pia mater

Dorsal root
ganglion

Dura mater blending
with epineurium

Spinal nerve

Ramus
communicans

Vertebral
ganglion

Sympathetic
trunk

Spinal cord

Epidural space

Subarachnoid space

Gray matter
White matter
Subdural space

Transverse
process

Intervertebral disk
Body of vertebra

■ **FIGURE 4-28** The meninges of the spinal cord. Only half of the vertebra is shown to indicate the extension of dura mater onto the spinal nerves. Note the presence of an epidural space.

cral, and sacrocaudal for varying purposes and in varying species. The epidural space at the sacrocaudal location is used for the injection of local anesthetics in cattle. Spinal nerve projections are present in this location; when anesthetized, sensory and motor loss occurs in certain areas, which is advantageous for medical or surgical treatment. For example, a prolapsed uterus (uterus that has everted through the vagina) can be replaced in the cow without the straining that would otherwise occur.

Ventricles of the Brain

The four ventricles of the brain are cavities or hollowed-out spaces within the substance of the brain (*Figs. 4-29 and 4-30*). The **lateral ventricles** are paired cavities within each right and left cerebral hemisphere. Each is continuous with the single **third ventricle** through an interventricular foramen (foramen of Monro). The third ventricle is located within the interbrain and is continuous with the fourth ventricle through the **cerebral aqueduct** (mesencephalic aqueduct). The **fourth ventricle** is located beneath the cerebellum and above the medulla oblongata. It communicates in turn with the subarachnoid space by means of paired lateral recesses (see Fig. 4-29) and apertures (foramina of Luschka). In addition to the paired foramina of Luschka, primates have a single median aperture (foramen of Magendie). The fourth ventricle is continued caudad as the **central canal of the spinal cord**. Each of the four ventricles has a structure known as the **choroid plexus** projecting into it. The choroid plexus is a tuft of capillaries that secretes cerebrospinal fluid. The capillaries belong to the pia mater, but they are covered with ependymal cells (a glial cell) that unite with the capillaries to form the choroid plexus.

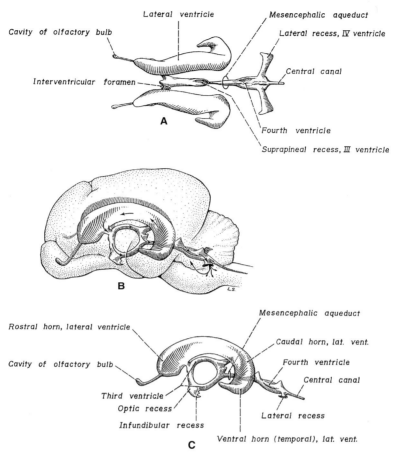

Lateral ventricle

Cavity of olfactory bulb

Mesencephalic aqueduct

Lateral recess, IV ventricle

Central canal

Interventricular foramen

A

Fourth ventricle

Suprapineal recess, III ventricle

B

L.S.

Rostral horn, lateral ventricle

Cavity of olfactory bulb

Mesencephalic aqueduct

Caudal horn, lat. vent.

Fourth ventricle

Central canal

Third ventricle

Optic recess

Infundibular recess

Lateral recess

Ventral horn (temporal), lat. vent.

C

■ **FIGURE 4-29** The canine brain ventricles. **A.** Dorsal view of ventricles without brain substance. **B.** Lateral view of ventricles, which shows their location within the brain. **C.** Lateral view of ventricles without brain substance. (From deLahunta A. Veterinary Neuroanatomy and Clinical Neurology. 2nd Ed. Philadelphia: WB Saunders Company, 1983.)

Circulation and Function of Cerebrospinal Fluid

Cerebrospinal fluid, formed by the choroid plexuses, flows through the cavities of the lateral and third ventricles, through the cerebral aqueduct and fourth ventricle, and finally through the foramina of Luschka to enter the subarachnoid space of the brain and spinal cord. Cerebrospinal fluid also enters the central canal of the spinal cord from the fourth ventricle. Cerebrospinal fluid then leaves the subarachnoid space of the brain through specialized structures (arachnoid granulations or villi) in which the subarachnoid space invaginates into the cerebral venous sinuses (the **dural sinuses**) (see Fig. 4-26). The relationship of the subarachnoid space with the venous sinuses is such that each villus functions as a valve regulating flow of cerebrospinal fluid into the venous sinus. The backward flow of blood into the subarachnoid space is prevented, but the forward flow of cerebrospinal fluid into the cerebral sinuses is allowed. Therefore, a higher pressure must exist within the subarachnoid space than within the venous system, and

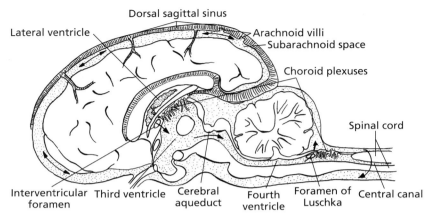

■ **FIGURE 4-30** Pathway of cerebrospinal fluid flow from choroid plexuses to the arachnoid villi that protrude into the dural sinuses. The interventricular foramina are openings from each of the two lateral ventricles (one in each cerebral hemisphere). The choroid plexuses produce the cerebrospinal fluid (stippled). The two foramina of Luschka (one shown) provide an exit from the sites of formation to the subarachnoid space of the brain and spinal cord. Note that cerebrospinal fluid circulates around the spinal cord. Cerebrospinal fluid circulates caudally through the central canal of the spinal cord as a continuation of the fourth ventricle. The central canal may not be patent all the way to caudal levels.

removal of cerebrospinal fluid is dependent on the venous pressure being at least 1 mm Hg less than the cerebrospinal fluid pressure. The normal pressure of cerebrospinal fluid ranges from 8 to 12 mm Hg, whereas the pressure within the dural sinuses ranges from 1 to 8 mm Hg.

Cerebrospinal fluid production is fairly constant regardless of pressures within the cranial cavity because it is an active process. Total amounts of cerebrospinal fluid vary with species and size of animal, with dogs producing at a rate around 0.05 mL/min and cats around 0.015 mL/min. In general, mammals produce about three to five times the total volume of their cerebrospinal fluid in a 24-hour period. If the pathway for flow from the choroid plexuses to the dural venous sinuses is occluded, the cerebrospinal fluid pressure increases and hydrocephalus can result. Cerebrospinal fluid that accompanies the meninges for a short distance onto the cranial and spinal nerves can enter lymphatics at that level and be returned to the blood. This is a particularly important outflow for cerebrospinal fluid that surrounds the spinal cord. In the

horse and in sheep, cerebrospinal fluid that enters the central canal has an exit at the caudal extremity via the terminal ventricle. The terminal ventricle then communicates with the subarachnoid space of the spinal cord. A similar arrangement is likely present in other animals.

The **cerebrospinal fluid** is thin and watery; it is derived from blood plasma by a secretion process. Except for a few lymphocytes, the normal cellular elements of the blood are absent. In cases of injury or inflammation of the meninges, the number of cellular elements of blood can increase.

The principal function of the cerebrospinal fluid is provision of a watery cushion for the brain and spinal cord. Displacement of the brain is therefore minimized when rapid directional changes occur in the head. The "lymphatic" function (see previous section) serves the brain and spinal cord for the return of protein that leaks from the capillaries. When blood volume in the brain increases, the volume of cerebrospinal fluid decreases, thereby keeping the volume of cranial contents constant. Determining the pressure of the cerebrospinal fluid can be helpful (e.g., in the neurologic examination of an animal), and is usually about 10 mm Hg.

■ CENTRAL NERVOUS SYSTEM METABOLISM

1. **What is the principal energy source for the CNS? How does it get into brain cells?**
2. **What percent of the body's oxygen requirement is used by the CNS?**
3. **What is meant by the blood-brain barrier?**
4. **What cells transport substances between the blood and brain tissue?**
5. **Is there a cerebrospinal fluid–brain barrier?**
6. **What are some maximum limits of oxygen deprivation to the CNS before injury occurs?**

The CNS receives its energy principally from carbohydrates, of which glucose is an important source. Unlike many tissues of the body, which require insulin for facilitated diffusion of glucose across cell membranes, the CNS receives glucose by simple diffusion, and insulin is not required. This is advantageous for the animal when insulin is lacking or in short supply because it enables CNS function to continue when other systems fail.

The relatively high rate of metabolism of the CNS compared with that of other tissues can be shown by noting its oxygen consumption. Although the CNS constitutes only 2% of body mass, it consumes approximately 20% of the total oxygen supplied to the body. Also, the metabolic rate of gray matter is three to four times higher than that of white matter.

Blood-Brain Barrier

Many substances in the blood do not readily enter the cells of the CNS, a limitation referred to as the **blood-brain barrier**. The capillaries of the CNS have tight junctions between their endothelial cells rather than slit pores, which limit the diffusion of substances from capillaries. Lipid-soluble substances, however, such as oxygen and carbon dioxide, readily diffuse. Transport for most substances is provided for by the CNS cells known as **astrocytes** (a glial cell), which are interposed between the capillaries and CNS cells. Astrocytes are selective regarding the materials they transport—hence, the blood-brain barrier. Some areas of the hypothalamus, as well as other portions of the brain that serve as chemoreceptor areas, lack a blood-brain barrier.

A barrier also exists between the cells of the choroid plexus and the cerebrospinal fluid that is provided for by the choroid plexus cells. A barrier probably exists between the cerebrospinal fluid and pia mater for certain substances, but most substances usually diffuse readily between the cerebrospinal fluid and the brain. Drugs in the blood might have no effect on the brain, but when placed directly into the cerebrospinal fluid, they can have a profound effect.

Blood Requirement

The CNS must have a continuous supply of blood for normal functioning. Other tissues can be deprived of a blood supply for extended periods and recover to normal function when blood supply resumes. Five to 10 minutes of little or no blood to the brain injures higher brain cells (in the cerebrum) so that no recovery occurs. Respiratory and cardiovascular centers (in the medulla oblongata) are more resistant to hypoxia (deficient oxygen), and revival has occurred after 10 minutes without blood. The tolerance of an adult brain to hypoxia is much lower than the tolerance of a newborn brain.

■ SUGGESTED READING

Behan M. Organization of the nervous system. In: Reece WO, ed. Dukes' Physiology of Domestic Animals. 12th Ed. Ithaca, NY: Cornell University Press, 2004:42.

Beitz AJ, Fletcher TF. The brain. In: Evans HE. Miller's Anatomy of the Dog. 3rd Ed. Philadelphia: WB Saunders Company, 1993:18.

Evans HE, deLahunta A. Guide to the Dissection of the Dog. 5th Ed. Philadelphia: WB Saunders Company, 2000.

Fletcher TF. Spinal cord and meninges. In: Evans HE. Miller's Anatomy of the Dog. 3rd Ed. Philadelphia: WB Saunders Company, 1993:16.

Frandson RD, Wilke WL, Fails AD. Anatomy and Physiology of Farm Animals. 6th Ed. Baltimore: Lippincott Williams & Wilkins, 2003.

Kitchell RL. Introduction to the nervous system. In: Evans HE. Miller's Anatomy of the Dog. 3rd Ed. Philadelphia: WB Saunders Company, 1993:14.

Klein BG. Membrane potentials: The generation and conduction of electrical signals in neurons. In: Reece WO, ed. Dukes' Physiology of Domestic Animals. 12th Ed. Ithaca, NY: Cornell University Press, 2004:43.

Oliver JE, Lorenz MD, Kornegay JN. Handbook of Veterinary Neurology. 3rd Ed. Philadelphia: WB Saunders Company, 1997.

Strain GM. Autonomic nervous system. In: Reece WO, ed. Dukes' Physiology of Domestic Animals. 12th Ed. Ithaca, NY: Cornell University Press, 2004:52.

 SELF EVALUATION—CHAPTER 4

STRUCTURE OF THE NERVOUS SYSTEM

1. The myelin sheaths of nerve fibers in the central nervous system are cytoplasmic extensions of:
   a. Schwann cells.
   b. oligodendrocytes.

2. Nerve fiber is another name for:
   a. nerve.
   b. neuron.
   c. axon.
   d. dendrite.

3. Which one of the following statements about the neuronal synapse is FALSE?
   a. One-way conduction (axon to dendrite or soma)
   b. Transmission by chemical means
   c. Physical contact of one neuron with the next
   d. Fatigue more readily than the neuron

4. Which one of the following statements about myelin sheaths is TRUE?
   a. The myelin sheath is formed by the cell body of the neuron of which it is a part.
   b. There is no chance for extracellular fluid to be in contact with the nerve fiber throughout its length when a nerve fiber is myelinated.
   c. Unmyelinated fibers may be nearly surrounded by myelin from adjacent myelinated fibers but maintain a direct association with extracellular fluid throughout their length.
   d. Nodes of Ranvier are the lymphatic structures of the nervous system.

ORGANIZATION OF THE NERVOUS SYSTEM

5. The autonomic divisions having cell origins in the cranial and sacral (craniosacral) regions of the spinal cord and the thoracic and lumbar (thoracolumbar) regions are the _____ and _____, respectively.
   a. sympathetic, parasympathetic
   b. parasympathetic, sympathetic

6. With the exception of the cervical and caudal vertebrae, spinal nerves:
   a. emerge in front of the vertebrae of the same serial number and name.
   b. emerge behind the vertebrae of the same serial number and name.

7. Afferent nerve fibers enter the spinal cord via the _____ root, and efferent nerve fibers leave via the _____ root.
   a. dorsal, ventral
   b. ventral, dorsal
   c. dorsal, dorsal
   d. ventral, ventral

8. Parasympathetic stimulation increases intestinal muscle and secretory activity.

a. True
b. False

9. Which one of the following best describes the function of the hypothalamus?
   a. Important in equilibrium
   b. Large pools of neurons for performing complex semivoluntary movement (walking and running)
   c. Central mechanism for most postural reflexes (hopping, righting, placing)
   d. Senses need for anterior pituitary hormones, forms posterior pituitary hormones, integration of autonomic nervous system functions

10. Which one of the following is an appropriate function for the cerebellum?
    a. Modulates (adjusts) motor activity
    b. Provides for consciousness
    c. Relay center to cerebral cortex
    d. Site of production of several hormones

11. Parasympathetic stimulation to the heart would decrease its activity.
    a. True
    b. False

12. Which division of the autonomic nervous system is referred to as the cholinergic system?
    a. Sympathetic
    b. Parasympathetic

13. Which one of the following brain structures is a subdivision of the brain stem, contains the pituitary gland, and assumes a major role in the integration of functions carried out by the autonomic nervous system?
    a. Basal nuclei
    b. Cerebral cortex
    c. Hypothalamus
    d. Thalamus

14. A myelin sheath on a peripheral nerve fiber:
    a. is uninterrupted throughout its length.
    b. is produced by the neuron of which it is a part.

c. prevents contact of the nerve fiber with extracellular fluid throughout its length.
d. increases the velocity of impulse conduction.

15. The vagus nerve (cranial nerve X) supplies autonomic fibers to visceral structures in the thorax and abdomen. Which division of the autonomics has fibers in this nerve?
    a. Sympathetic
    b. Parasympathetic

16. Sympathetic stimulation to the bronchi (air passages) of the lungs would result in:
    a. a decrease of their diameter.
    b. an increase of their diameter.

17. How many neurons are associated with the transmission of an autonomic impulse from its cell of origin (in brain or spinal cord) to its organ of influence?
    a. One
    b. Two
    c. Three
    d. Too numerous to count

18. Which division of the autonomic nervous system is known as the adrenergic nervous system (postganglionic neuron secretes norepinephrine)?
    a. Sympathetic
    b. Parasympathetic

THE NERVE IMPULSE AND ITS TRANSMISSION

19. A stimulus increases the permeability of the neuron for the sodium ion.
    a. True
    b. False

20. If a stimulus lowers the resting membrane potential of −80 mV to −70 mV and the threshold for an action potential is −65 mV, the nerve fiber will fire.
    a. True
    b. False

21. Which one of the following contains the respective neurotransmitters for postganglionic sympathetic and parasympathetic neurons?

    a. Acetylcholine, norepinephrine
    b. Acetylcholine, acetylcholine
    c. Norepinephrine, acetylcholine
    d. Norepinephrine, norepinephrine

22. The phenomenon of saltatory conduction is associated with:
    a. the flow of cerebrospinal fluid.
    b. unmyelinated nerve fibers.
    c. myelinated nerve fibers.
    d. nerve impulse transmission at a synapse.

23. When a resting membrane potential of -85 mV is being measured in a nerve fiber at a particular point and the threshold for firing is -70 mV, which one of the following is FALSE?
    a. There is a high concentration of Na^+ on the outside and a low concentration of Na^+ on the inside.
    b. There is a relative impermeability of the fiber for diffusion of Na^+.
    c. There is no current flow at that point.
    d. A stimulus that would decrease the resting membrane potential (from -85 to -80) would cause the nerve to fire.

24. Repolarization of a nerve fiber:
    a. is accomplished by Na^+ being actively transported from the inside to the outside.
    b. is accomplished by diffusion of K^+ from the inside of the fiber to the outside.

25. Which one of the following statements about impulse transmission velocity is FALSE?
    a. Fastest impulse transmission in the body would be a small-diameter, non-myelinated fiber.
    b. Where high velocity is required, greater space reduction would be achieved by myelination rather than by increased fiber size.

26. Acetylcholine is an excitatory neurotransmitter and accordingly increases the permeability of the nerve fiber membrane for Na^+.
    a. True
    b. False

27. A stimulus applied to a neuron causes depolarization of the membrane. This means that the membrane:
    a. becomes positive on the outside because of the outflow of Na^+.
    b. becomes positive on the inside and negative on the outside because Na^+ flows inward.
    c. will not be able to propagate a nerve impulse.

28. A stimulus of sufficient strength to cause an action potential means that the magnitude of depolarization was sufficient to:
    a. demyelinate the fiber.
    b. incite a riot.
    c. reach threshold.
    d. raise or lower the threshold.

29. The period of time when a nerve fiber cannot be caused to fire is known as:
    a. repolarization.
    b. saltatory conduction.
    c. leakage.
    d. the refractory period.

REFLEXES

30. Muscle tone:
    a. is a state of complete muscle relaxation.
    b. is a state of muscle tension (contraction) that enables an animal to assume and remain in an erect position.
    c. refers to the sound made by contracting muscle.
    d. is an autonomic nervous system function.

31. A muscle spindle is best described as:
    a. a reflex center located in the spinal cord for the purpose of muscle control.
    b. the point on a bone over which a muscle passes.
    c. a specialized receptor for maintaining muscle tone that, when stretched, causes contraction of the muscle in which it is located.
    d. a specialized receptor found in tendons that, when stimulated, causes the muscle of the tendon to be relaxed.

32. The ability of a cat to land on its feet when dropped from a position of its feet in a skyward direction is known as:
    a. an attitudinal reflex.
    b. hopscotch.
    c. a righting reflex.
    d. a placing reflex.

33. Lifting the head of a horse in a standing position permits greater activity of the hind legs (attitudinal reflex).
    a. True
    b. False

34. Which reflex is the fundamental element of muscle tone?
    a. Stretch
    b. Attitudinal
    c. Righting
    d. Crossed extensor

THE MENINGES AND CEREBROSPINAL FLUID

35. Cerebrospinal fluid pressure:
    a. would increase if there were resistance to venous blood flow from the head.
    b. would decrease if there were resistance to venous blood flow from the head.
    c. is independent of any change in venous blood pressure.

36. Cerebrospinal fluid is produced:
    a. by the choroid plexus in cavities (ventricles) within the brain.
    b. by the ciliary processes in the posterior chamber of the eye.
    c. as a neurosecretion by neurons in the hypothalamus.
    d. by the nerve cell bodies in the cerebrum and spinal cord.

37. Which one of the following does NOT apply to cerebrospinal fluid?
    a. Provides a watery cushion for the brain and spinal cord
    b. Assists in maintaining volume of cranial contents at a constant level
    c. Contains numerous blood cells
    d. Secreted by choroid plexus and returned to blood via arachnoid villi

CENTRAL NERVOUS SYSTEM METABOLISM

38. The blood-brain barrier:
    a. exists for all substances in the blood.
    b. applies to all areas of the brain.
    c. excludes transport of some substances from blood to brain and permits transport of others.

39. Brain injury occurs when it is deprived of blood for (select the most appropriate time interval):
    a. seconds.
    b. minutes.
    c. hours.
    d. days.

ANSWERS TO SELF EVALUATION—CHAPTER 4

1.	b	11.	a	21.	c	31.	c
2.	c	12.	b	22.	c	32.	c
3.	c	13.	c	23.	d	33.	b
4.	c	14.	d	24.	b	34.	a
5.	b	15.	b	25.	a	35.	a
6.	b	16.	b	26.	a	36.	a
7.	a	17.	b	27.	b	37.	c
8.	a	18.	a	28.	c	38.	c
9.	d	19.	a	29.	d	39.	b
10.	a	20.	b	30.	b		

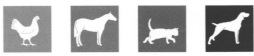

 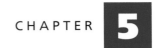

The Sensory Organs

CHAPTER OUTLINE

- **CLASSIFICATION OF SENSORY RECEPTORS**
- **SENSORY RECEPTOR RESPONSES**
  Graded Responses
  Adaptation
- **PAIN**
  Visceral Pain
  Referred Pain
- **TASTE**
  Taste Reception
  Taste Sensations
  Temperature and Taste
  Depraved Appetite
- **SMELL**
  Olfactory Region Structure
  Odor Perception
  Pheromones

- **HEARING AND EQUILIBRIUM**
  External Ear
  Middle Ear
  Inner Ear
  Vestibular Structure and Function
  Cochlear Structure and Function
  Summary of Sound Reception
- **VISION**
  Structure and Functions of the Eye
  Chemistry of Vision
  Adaptation to Varying Light
  Field of Vision
  Eyeball Movements and Accessory
    Structures

Sensations result from stimuli that initiate afferent impulses, which eventually reach a conscious level in the cerebral cortex. Sensations include the somatic senses—pain, cold, heat, touch, pressure, and a group known as the special senses—sight, hearing, taste, smell, and orientation in space. All sensations involve receptor organs; the simplest is a bare nerve ending, and the most complex are those associated with the special senses.

■ CLASSIFICATION OF SENSORY RECEPTORS

1. How do exteroceptors and interoceptors differ from each other?
2. What are proprioceptors?
3. Review muscle spindle function.
4. What is the relationship of myelination to speed of transmission of nerve impulses?

Sensory receptors are end organs of afferent nerves and belong to one of two main physiological groups: 1) **exteroceptors**, which detect stimuli that arise external to the body; and 2) **interoceptors**, which detect stimuli that originate within the body. The exteroceptors detect stimuli near the outer surface of the body and include those from the skin that respond to cold, warmth, touch, and pressure. The special receptor organs for hearing and vision are also classified as exteroceptors. The interoceptors detect stimuli from inside the body and include receptors for taste, smell, and those within the viscera that respond to pH, distention and spasm (as in the bowel), and flow (as in the urethra) and equilibrium sensors in the inner ear. The **proprioceptors** are a special class of interoceptors that signal conditions deep within the body to the central nervous system. Proprioceptors are located in skeletal muscles, tendons, ligaments, and joint capsules. Examples of proprioceptors are muscle spindles, Golgi tendon organs, and joint receptors. Just as muscle spindles prevent undue stretch of muscles (see Chapter 4), Golgi tendon organs in tendons and ligaments respond to stretch by countering muscle tension that caused the stretch. Muscle spindles and Golgi tendon organs are sensitive to stretching and reflexively prevent undue stretch of muscles, tendons, and ligaments. Muscle spindles also provide for muscle tone so that purposeful contraction is more effective and helps to prevent collapse of standing animals as a result of the force of gravity. Joint receptors are sensitive to the position or angle of joints and provide for a sense of body position. Because of the need for rapid transmission of proprioceptive impulses, the proprioceptive fibers have the heaviest myelination of all peripheral nerve fibers. Some examples of sensory receptors are shown in *Figure 5-1*.

■ SENSORY RECEPTOR RESPONSES

1. **Do sensory receptors respond to more than one energy type?**
2. **Does a sensory receptor have only one level of response?**
3. **Differentiate between a phasic and a tonic receptor. Are muscle spindles tonic or phasic receptors?**

A **sensory receptor** is the peripheral component of an afferent axon and the centrally located nerve cell body of that axon.

Sensory receptors convert different types of energy into action potentials; these include sound, light, chemical, thermal, and mechanical energy. Generally, the receptors are **specific** in that they respond more readily to one form of energy than another. For example, a Krause end-bulb receptor (sensitive to cold) would not generate an action potential if pressure were applied; in such a case, pacinian corpuscles would respond.

Graded Responses

Sensory receptors are subject to **graded responses**, depending on the intensity of the stimulus. The receptor can be regarded as a generator in which the amount of voltage produced is determined by the stimulus. If the voltage generation reaches threshold for the receptor, a nerve impulse (afferent) is created. As the intensity (amplitude) of the stimulus increases, the frequency of firing increases.

Adaptation

Receptors might not continue to fire at a rate consistent with the intensity of the stimulus, but they are subject to **adaptation**. The response to a prolonged stimulus might at first show a burst of action potentials at a high frequency, followed by a decrease in rate that quickly returns to zero. Receptors vary as to the degree of their adaptation. The previous response, in which the rate of discharge returns to zero, is characteristic of pacinian corpuscles (sensitive to pressure). This is an example of a **phasic receptor organ**—that is, one that quickly accommodates to prolonged stimulation. A rapidly adapting receptor is best suited for signaling sudden changes in the environment or vibratory fluctuations. The muscle spindle, which responds to stretch, is an example of a **tonic receptor organ** with regard to its adaptation. The application of a prolonged stimulus to the muscle spindle elicits a brief volley of action potentials at a high frequency, followed by an action potential rate that slows to a lower level and that is maintained throughout the duration of stimulus. This is known as a tonic receptor organ in the same sense that muscle tone (the result of muscle spindle stimulation) represents a continuous state of low-level muscle tension.

■ PAIN

1. **What is the name for receptors specific for pain?**

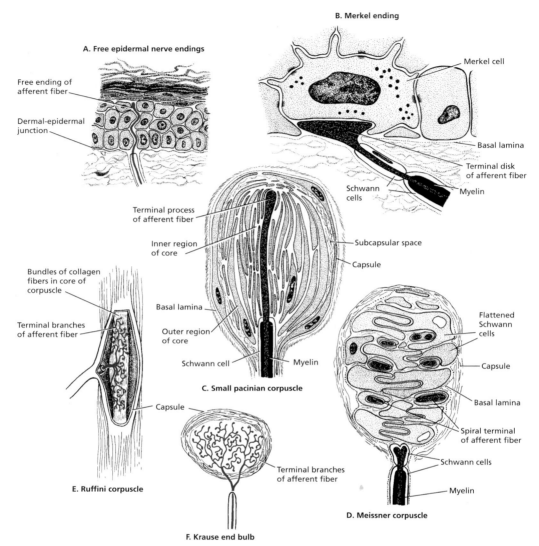

■ **FIGURE 5-1** Sensory receptors. Free nerve endings **(A)** act as thermoreceptors and nociceptors (pain). Merkel endings **(B)** are pressure-sensitive touch receptors. Pacinian corpuscles **(C)** respond to pressure and are widely distributed throughout the dermis and subcutaneous tissue, joint capsules, and other pressure sites. Meissner corpuscles **(D)** are highly sensitive to touch. Ruffini corpuscles **(E)** in subcutaneous connective tissue respond to tension. Krause end bulbs **(F)** are cold sensitive. (From Cormack DH. Essential Histology. 2nd Ed. Baltimore: Lippincott Williams & Wilkins, 2001:12.)

2. Can a receptor for cold or heat send an afferent impulse to the cerebral cortex to be recognized as pain?

3. What are the most sensitive visceral structures that produce pain?

4. How is pain that arises from the intestines produced?

5. What is a good example of referred pain in cattle?

Pain is a protective mechanism. Its sensation is aroused by damaging or noxious stimuli from almost all parts of the body, with the exception of the central nervous system (unless there is damage to the pain pathways). The specific receptors for pain are called **nociceptors**. Pain sensation does not arise from overstimulation of receptors that subserve a different sensation. The receptors are bare nerve endings of sensory neurons (pain neurons) that respond to all intense stimuli. The nerve endings are essentially chemoreceptors, and the pain stimulus (e.g., thermal, chemical, mechanical) produces cell injury, which produces a chemical reaction and causes the nerve to fire. **Pain fibers** are either **myelinated** or **unmyelinated**. The myelinated fibers have a short lag time between stimulus and reaction, and the pain has a so-called bright quality, whereas unmyelinated fibers have a longer lag time and the pain is more diffuse, with an aching, throbbing quality. Pain fibers, as are the fibers for other sensory modalities, are grouped in a specific tract of the spinal cord.

The **reaction threshold for pain** is highly variable among individuals. What is painful to one animal might not be so in another. Furthermore, the diversion of attention from a pained part or painful situation reduces pain perception. This can be demonstrated when a twitch (a handle with a rope loop at one end) is applied to the upper lip of a horse and tightened. The attention to discomfort of the twitch detracts from pain or manipulation of other body parts.

Visceral Pain

Pain does arise from the viscera (the organs within the abdominal, thoracic, and pelvic cavities); the most sensitive parts are the peritoneal and pleural linings of the abdominal and thoracic cavities, respectively. Peritonitis and pleuritis (inflammation of the peritoneum and pleura) evoke severe pain. Some of the thoracic viscera (the heart) might be a source of pain, whereas other viscera (the lungs) might not. Pain from hollow viscera (the intestines) within the abdomen is evoked by severe distention or powerful contractions (spasms). Normal distentions or contractions can be innocuous, but an inflammation can cause these to become painful.

Referred Pain

Referred pain is pain that is felt on the surface of the body. It usually has its source within the thoracic or abdominal viscera. It is caused by a convergence of cutaneous and visceral pain afferent fibers on the same neuron at some point in the sensory pathway (*Fig. 5-2*). The pain can be identified consciously as cutaneous (referring to the skin) because a previous cutaneous pain was actually seen and perceived as being cutaneous. When the pain source is of visceral origin, however, it is mistakenly perceived as coming from the site of the relevant cutaneous fibers (referred) because their common neuron has the same cerebral projection. Traumatic pericarditis (inflammation of the pericardium caused by perforation from the reticulum) in cattle is a form of referred pain. Pressure applied to the withers causes a painful response in cattle with traumatic pericarditis, whereas a minimal response would be noted in normal cattle. The cutaneous stimulation is additive to that coming from the inflamed heart sac because of the convergence of the nerve fibers.

■ TASTE

1. What is the physiological name for taste?
2. What is a function of taste in animals?
3. Where are most of the taste buds located?
4. Study the location of taste buds relative to papillae and the glands of von Ebner.
5. To stimulate taste hairs, what part of a taste bud must dissolved substances enter?

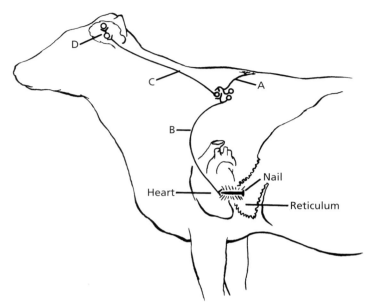

■ **FIGURE 5-2** The sensory pain pathway. A cutaneous pain afferent fiber **(A)** and a visceral pain afferent fiber **(B)** converge on a common neuron **(C)**. Neuron **(D)** conveys the pain impulse from the thalamus to the cerebral cortex.

6. How are taste substances classified in animals?
7. At what temperature does water rejection occur for poultry?
8. What is meant by depraved appetite in animals?

The sense of taste is referred to as **gustation**. The function of taste in animals seems to be one of discrimination; they seem to be able to discriminate between those substances that are healthful and harmful. Also, foods might be sought that contain nutrients that are lacking in the diet.

Taste Reception

The receptor organ for the sense of taste is the **taste bud**. Most of the taste buds are located on the tongue in association with the various papillae (*Fig. 5-3A*), and some are found on the palate, pharynx, and larynx. A collection of taste buds and their locations relative to a vallate papillus is shown in *Figure 5-3B*. A taste bud contains gustatory cells and supporting cells (*Fig. 5-3C*). The **gustatory cells** are the receptors for taste sensations. A tiny hair arises from each and extends into the **pit** of the taste bud. The pit communicates with the oral cavity by way of a **pore** (see Fig. 5-3C). Any substance to be tasted must get into solution and enter the pore of a taste bud. The hair of the gustatory cell that extends into the pit is affected in some way so that the gustatory cell is stimulated. The generated impulse is transmitted to the brain by branches of cranial nerves VII and IX (anterior two-thirds and posterior third of the tongue, respectively). The afferent ends of these cranial nerve branches originate at the deep ends of taste buds and are in intimate contact with the gustatory cells.

The **glands of von Ebner** (see Fig. 5-3B) are embedded deep within the underlying muscle tissue. Their watery secretion is conveyed to the moatlike furrow that surrounds the papillae by excretory ducts, and the substances to be tasted are dissolved in it.

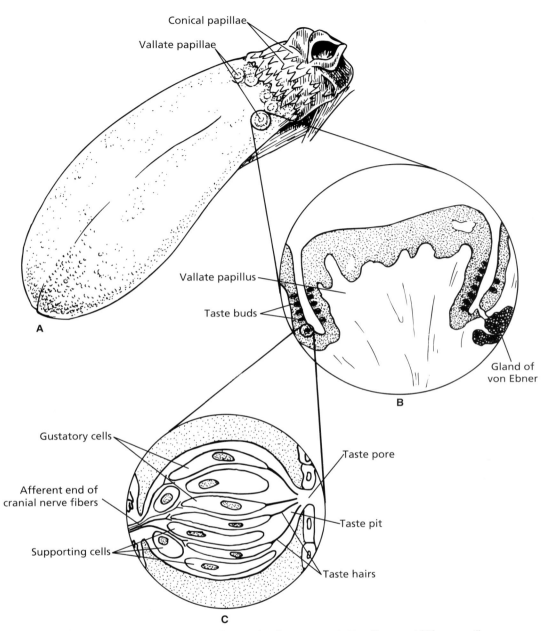

■ FIGURE 5-3 Taste buds associated with papillae on the dog tongue. **A.** Fungiform and filiform papillae are represented by the finer dots. Circumvallate and conical papillae are located at the base. **B.** A vallate papillus with taste buds lining its moatlike furrow. Glands of von Ebner provide a watery secretion for dissolving substances to be tasted. **C.** A taste bud with its gustatory (taste) cells and supporting cells.

Taste Sensations

Taste sensations in humans are classified according to verbal reports as being salty, sweet, bitter, or sour. Each taste sensation probably results from some combination of these basic tastes. Much of the current opinion about taste sensations that can be perceived by animals is based on casual observations and folklore.

A common method used to evaluate the sense of taste in animals is the **preference test**. Accordingly, responses are divided into **pleasant**, **unpleasant**, and **indifferent**. There is considerable individual variation within species. A substance considered to be pleasant by one dog might be regarded as unpleasant or indifferent by others. Similarly, variability of taste exists among pigs in the same litter for the same substances.

Temperature and Taste

In humans the temperature of a beverage or food markedly affects its taste. The effect of water temperature and its acceptance has been studied in domestic fowl. Acceptability of water decreases as its temperature increases above the ambient temperature. Water for domestic fowl that is placed in sunlight soon becomes warmer than the ambient temperature and is rejected. Chickens will suffer from acute thirst rather than drink water that is 5°C above their body temperature (41°C), but chickens readily accept water down to the level of freezing. Recognition of these preferences is important for maximum productivity and health in poultry production.

Depraved Appetite

A **depraved appetite** is recognized in animals when they are seen eating dirt, wood, and other materials not usually considered to be foodstuffs (this is different from similar habits that can develop in some animals). The depraved condition is termed **pica**. Its exact cause is difficult to determine, but it could be related to certain dietary deficiencies.

■ SMELL

1. **What is the physiological name for smell?**
2. **Where are the nerve cell bodies for smell located?**
3. **Why do dogs have a better sense of smell than humans?**
4. **Differentiate among anosmatic, microsmatic, and macrosmatic.**
5. **What is the function of the glands of Bowman secretion?**
6. **What is the function of olfactory epithelial basal cells?**
7. **Can more than one odor be perceived at one time?**
8. **What is meant by adaptation to smell?**
9. **What are pheromones?**
10. **What are some functions of animal pheromones?**

As development progressed from the simplest animal forms, nerve cell bodies migrated centrally so that only the nerve fibers remained in a peripheral position. Because nerve cell bodies are not regenerated, this central location provided for greater protection from destruction. If the neuron extensions are injured, regeneration can occur to some extent. Central migration did not occur for the nerve cell bodies of cranial nerve I (olfactory), however, and they are found in the mucous membrane of the nasal cavity. They are located in what is known as the **olfactory region**. The size of the olfactory region is directly related to the degree of development of the sense of smell, and its size varies among species. The individual olfactory receptor of the dog is probably no more sensitive than that of the human, but their larger olfactory region allows dogs to detect odorous substances at concentrations 1:1,000 of that detectable by humans.

The sensation of smell is known as **olfaction**. Animals with a greatly developed sense of smell (most domestic animals) are **macrosmatic**. A relatively lesser-developed sense of smell is known as **microsmatic**; humans, monkeys, and some aquatic mammals belong to this group. Animals with no sense of smell (e.g., many aquatic mammals) are **anosmatic**. Macrosmatic animals can become microsmatic or anosmatic, and microsmatic animals can become anosmatic because of disease loss of cells or temporary impairment. The peripheral location of the olfactory nerve cell bodies renders them more susceptible to destruction from inflammatory disease. Sensitivity to smell probably decreases with time.

Olfactory Region Structure

A microscopic view of a section taken from the olfactory region is shown in *Figure 5-4*. Each **olfactory receptor cell** has a cell body and a nerve fiber extending from each of its ends, one a dendrite and the other an axon (see Fig. 5-4). The dendritic process of the olfactory cell extends to the outside of the olfactory region membrane in crevices between the sustentacular cells. The **sustentacular cells** seem to provide major support to the dendritic processes and allow for the olfactory cell bodies to be shielded from the nasal cavity. At this location there might be several hairlike structures (olfactory cilia) extending into the nasal cavity from the olfactory vesicles (expanded part of a dendrite). Usually they are covered with a thin secretion from the **glands of Bowman** (subepithelial glands). The ducts of these glands lead through the epithelium to the surface. Their secretion constantly freshens the thin layer of fluid that continuously bathes the olfactory hairs on the surface of the olfactory region. Sniffing allows for the back-and-forth movement of air and provides a greater chance for the substance to be smelled to go into solution. This becomes the stimulus for the impulse to be transmitted to the brain.

The axons of the olfactory cells join with others and proceed with them as fibers and branches of the olfactory nerves. Basal cells divide and differentiate into either sustentacular cells or olfactory cells (replacement of a nerve cell). This is a safeguard against loss of smell that might otherwise occur as a result of nasal mucosal disease.

Odor Perception

Considering the great number of smell possibilities, it is unlikely that a specific type of olfactory cell exists for each smell. It is more probable that basic smells combine to provide the sensation for a particular odor.

Only one odor can be perceived at any one time. Some room deodorants are effective because they can stimulate olfactory cells more than the offensive odor. The offender is not eliminated; it is only masked. The olfactory cells become adapted to odors so that they do not persist for a particular individual. This is why the smell of fresh baked bread is so apparent when someone enters a bakery, whereas the baker might not even smell it anymore.

Pheromones

Animals use odors to communicate with each other. Black-tailed deer and Rocky Mountain mule deer have been found to use the tarsal glands on the insides of their hind legs as transmitters of odors to identify species as friendly or alien to their own kind. The scent is deposited on the skin and hair by the tarsal glands, and communication is established by sniffing other members of their group approximately once each hour. A chemical secreted by one animal that influences the behavior of other animals is known as a **pheromone**. The first chemical analysis of a mammalian pheromone was accomplished using the deer tarsal gland substance. Some animals have scent glands in the spaces between their hoof pads. Rabbits have a scent gland on the

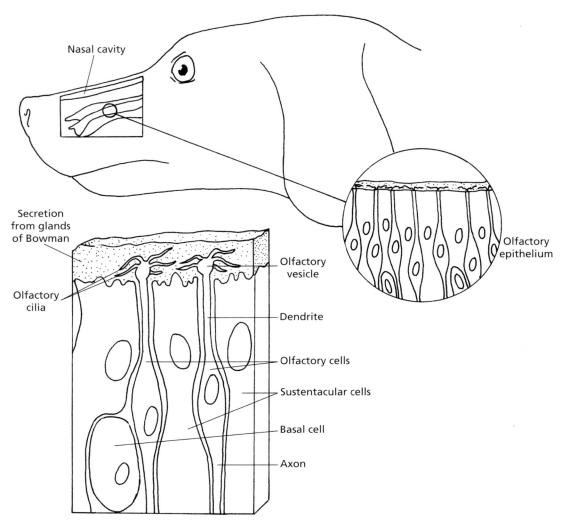

Nasal cavity

Secretion
from glands
of Bowman

Olfactory
cilia

Olfactory
vesicle

Dendrite

Olfactory cells

Sustentacular cells

Basal cell

Axon

Olfactory
epithelium

■ **FIGURE 5-4** The olfactory region of the dog and the cells associated with smell. **A.** Nasal cavity. **B.** Olfactory epithelium from nasal cavity mucous membrane. **C.** Olfactory cells, basal cells, and sustentacular (supporting) cells are associated with olfactory epithelium. Subepithelial glands of Bowman (not shown) provide secretion-covering olfactory cilia.

chest and around the anal opening. Cats have glands on the forehead and mark people or objects by rubbing their heads on them. Pheromones provide for a chemical language among animals for certain purposes, such as marking trails or boundaries, recognizing individuals from the same herd or nest, marking the location of food sources, and emitting alarms.

■ HEARING AND EQUILIBRIUM

1. Be able to follow the motion initiated by a sound wave from the tympanic membrane through the cochlear window (round window).
2. What is the function of the two striated muscles located in the middle ear?

3. What reflex is inherent to the function of the middle ear muscles?

4. What are the respective functions of the vestibular and cochlear portions of the inner ear?

5. Why is the cochlea coiled?

6. Differentiate between membranous labyrinth and osseous labyrinth and their respective fluids.

7. How are the cristae (located in the semicircular canals) stimulated?

8. How are the macula receptors stimulated?

9. What are the divisions of the cochlea brought about by extension of the membranous labyrinth into the cochlea?

10. Which cochlear division contains the organ of Corti?

11. What function is served by the organs of Corti?

12. Summarize sound reception (which relates to item 1).

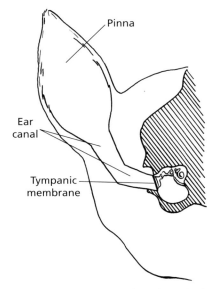

■ **FIGURE 5-5** Transverse section through the dog head. The external ear (pinna and ear canal) provide for transfer of sound waves to the tympanic membrane. The ear canal in the dog has a vertical and an oblique component.

The ear has components associated with the special sense of hearing and those involved with positional equilibrium. Sound waves are directed to the receptors for hearing in the inner ear via the external ear and middle ear. The inner ear has the receptors not only for hearing, but also for equilibrium.

External Ear

The external ear (*Fig. 5-5*) consists of the outer visible part (the **pinna**) and ear canal (**external acoustic meatus**) that extends from the pinna into the substance of the skull to the middle ear (tympanic cavity). The pinna in most animals consists of a funnel-shaped cartilage that is lined on the outside with skin having a generous amount of hair and on the inside with relatively hairless skin. Varying degrees of muscle attachment lend mobility to the pinna, which is helpful in localizing and picking up sounds. The funnel-shaped cartilage concentrates sound waves and directs them through the ear canal toward the tympanic membrane, which separates the middle ear from the external ear.

Middle Ear

The middle ear and inner ear are shown in *Figure 5-6*. The middle ear is separated from the inner ear by membranes that close the **vestibular (oval) window** and **cochlear (round) window**. The middle ear communicates with the pharynx by way of the **auditory tube** (often called the eustachian tube). The auditory tube allows for equalization of pressures between an otherwise closed cavity and the outside. Within the middle ear a mechanical linkage is provided between the tympanic membrane and the membrane closing the vestibular window by three **auditory ossicles (bones)**. From without inward they are the **malleus**, **incus**, and **stapes**, or more commonly, the

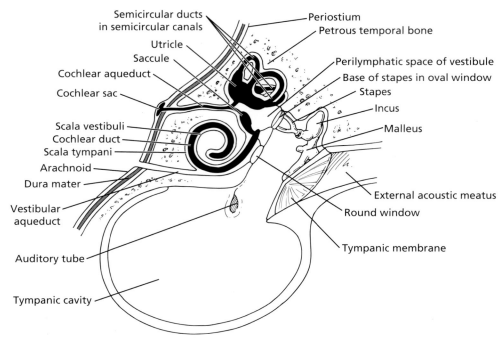

■ **FIGURE 5-6** A schematic of the middle ear and inner ear that features the membranous labyrinth (black), which contains endolymph within its ducts, within the osseous labyrinth, which contains perilymph within the semicircular canals and vestibule. The vestibular aqueduct communicates with the subarachnoid space and its cerebrospinal fluid. (Adapted from Getty R, Foust HL, Presley ET, Miller ME. Macroscopic anatomy of the ear of the dog. Am J Vet Res 1956; 17:366.)

hammer, anvil, and stirrup. Amplification of sound waves is provided by leverage of the ossicles and by the greater surface area of the tympanic membrane, which transmits sound waves to the smaller surface area of the vestibular window. Excessively loud noises are damped by two skeletal muscles in the middle ear, the **tensor tympani** and the **stapedius muscle** (*Fig. 5-7*). Muscle spindles within these muscles respond to muscle stretch by initiating a reflex that causes the muscles to contract. The tensor tympani muscle is attached to the malleus, and its contraction tenses the tympanic membrane, thus limiting its movement. The stapedius muscle (the smallest skeletal muscle in the body) is attached to the stapes. Its contraction tenses the stapes to reduce its movement. The degree of stretch is determined by the intensity (loudness) of the sound wave.

Loud noises are damped because of excessive muscle stretch and subsequent reflex muscle contraction, which prevents excessive movement of the ossicles.

Inner Ear

The inner ear can be divided into two parts according to function: 1) the **vestibular portion**, which is sensory for **position** and **equilibrium**; and 2) the **cochlear portion**, which is sensory for **sound** (*Fig. 5-8*). The cochlear portion receives the cochlear nerve, a branch of the vestibulocochlear nerve (cranial nerve VIII), and the vestibular portion receives the vestibular nerve branch of the same cranial nerve (VIII). The inner ear is contained within a bony excavation known as the **osseous labyrinth** (*Fig. 5-9*). Labyrinth refers to an intricate

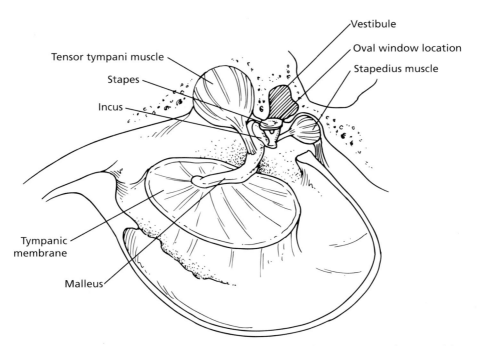

FIGURE 5-7 Inside view of the middle ear. The malleus is attached to the tympanic membrane, and the stapes is attached to the vestibular (oval) window. Muscle spindles in the tensor tympani and stapedius muscles initiate the stretch reflex in response to loud noises. Contraction of these muscles, respectively, tenses the tympanic membrane, limiting its movement, and reduces movement of the stapes.

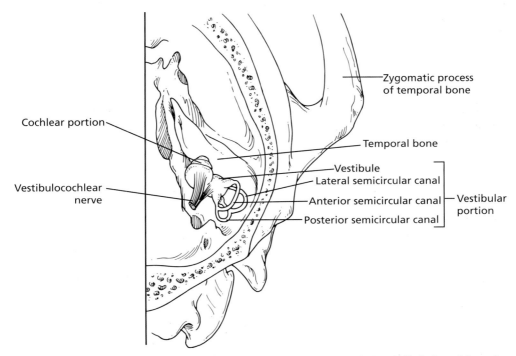

FIGURE 5-8 Right inner ear (viewed from above showing its orientation with the skull). (Adapted from Getty R, Foust HL, Presley ET, Miller ME. Macroscopic anatomy of the ear of the dog. Am J Vet Res 1956; 17:369.)

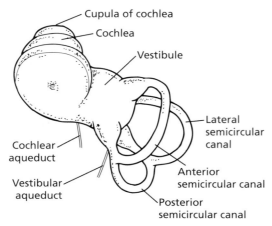

■ **FIGURE 5-9** Drawing of a latex cast of the inner ear of the dog, occupying the osseous labyrinth. The membranous labyrinth would occupy the space filled by the latex cast. (Adapted from Getty R, Foust HL, Presley ET, Miller ME. Macroscopic anatomy of the ear of the dog. Am J Vet Res 1956; 17:370.)

combination of passages. Because the cochlea is coiled, it can occupy limited space. An uncoiled cochlea would project into the brain.

Vestibular Structure and Function

The **vestibular portion** is housed in the parts of the osseous labyrinth known as the **vestibule** and **three semicircular canals** (anterior, lateral, and posterior). Each semicircular canal leaves and returns to the vestibule (see Fig. 5-9). In addition, each semicircular canal is arranged so that it is in a different geometric plane than the others (at right angles to each other). The cochlear portion is housed mostly in the cochlear portion of the osseous labyrinth that departs from the vestibule. Within the osseous labyrinth is a **membranous labyrinth**, which is a completely closed connective tissue structure (*Fig. 5-10*). It contains a fluid known as **endolymph** (a fluid high in potassium and low in sodium) that is secreted by the vascular tissue on the outer wall of the scala media. Outside the membranous labyrinth and within the osseous labyrinth is another fluid known as perilymph. By way of

the **vestibular aqueduct** (connection to the subarachnoid space), perilymph circulates freely with **cerebrospinal fluid** and shares similar composition (see Fig. 5-6). Because of the meningeal connection, a potential exists for inner ear infections to ascend to the meninges and produce meningitis (inflammation of the meninges). Within the vestibular portion, the membranous labyrinth also includes **three semicircular ducts** and two sacs within the vestibule known as the utricle and saccule. Both ends of each semicircular canal open into the utricle, and the **utricle** communicates with the **saccule** (see Fig. 5-10). The saccule has two other communications, a major one with the membranous labyrinth of the cochlea and another with the **cochlear aqueduct**, which leads to the **cochlear sac** that lies between the layers of the meninges (subdural) (see Fig. 5-6). The cochlear sac is a site for the active absorption of endolymph. Also, neutrophils and macrophages from the surrounding connective tissue can cross the epithelium to phagocytize cellular debris and other particulates that may accumulate in the lumen of the cochlear sac.

As each membranous labyrinth occupying the semicircular canals leaves the utricle, a dilated portion is noted—the **ampulla**. Each of the three ampullae contains sensory receptors for equilibrium known as a **crista** (*Fig. 5-11*). The utricle and saccule each contain a sensory receptor area known as a **macula** (*Fig. 5-12*). In both cases, the receptive regions are patches of epithelium containing hair cells, and the vestibular impulses that the hair cells generate contribute to an overall sense of orientation and balance.

The maculae in the utricle and saccule (see Fig. 5-12) have **receptor hair cells** that are embedded in an **otolithic membrane** consisting of a gelatinous material covered by a glycoprotein studded with calcium carbonate crystals called **otoliths (otoconia)**, which are relatively heavy. The utricle receptors lie in a horizontal plane, and those of the saccule lie in a vertical plane. Because of the pull of

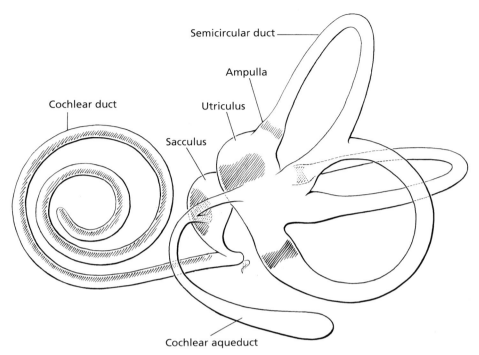

■ **FIGURE 5-10** Membranous labyrinth. Hatched regions indicate the sites of neuroepithelium, including the spiral organ of the cochlear duct, the maculae of the utriculus (utricle) and sacculus (saccule), and the crista ampullares of the semicircular ducts. (From Banks WJ. Applied Veterinary Histology. 2nd Ed. Baltimore: Lippincott Williams & Wilkins, 1986.)

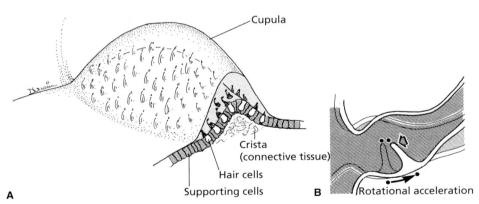

■ **FIGURE 5-11 A.** General structure of the ampullary crista in a semicircular duct. **B.** Ampullary hair cells responding to deflection of the cupula. (From Cormack DH. Essential Histology. 2nd Ed. Baltimore: Lippincott Williams & Wilkins, 2001.)

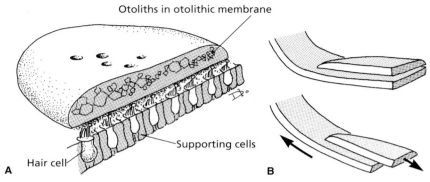

■ **FIGURE 5-12 A.** General structure of the utricular and saccular maculae. **B.** Macular hair cells respond to movement of otolithic membranes. From Cormack DH. Essential Histology. 2nd ed. Baltimore: Lippincott Williams & Wilkins, 2001.

gravity, and depending on the position of the head, the heavy otoliths on one or both of the maculae can apply shearing stresses to the hair cells. This force registers the position of the head. Because of the weight of the otoliths, sufficient inertia is provided to the otolithic membrane for the maculae to also sense linear acceleration or deceleration of the head.

Rotational acceleration or deceleration involving the head is detected in any given plane by the ampullary crista of the corresponding semicircular duct. Hair cells of the cristae are stimulated when the head is moved because the hair cells are mechanically moved through the endolymph, which does not move as a result of inertia. When the head stops, the endolymph is finally moved; this stimulates the hair cells in an opposite direction and further accommodation is inhibited.

Cochlear Structure and Function

The extension of the membranous labyrinth into the cochlea is known as the **cochlear duct** or, more commonly, the **scala media**. This occupies a central position within the cochlea extending from one side to the other and dividing the cochlea into a part above the scala media (**scala vestibuli**) and a part below (**scala tympani**) (*Fig. 5-13*). These latter divisions do not communicate with each other except for a

small opening at the apex or tip of the cochlea, known as the **helicotrema**. Along the length of the scala media are a large number of structures, each individually called an **organ of Corti** (see Fig. 5-13). These structures convert sound waves to nerve impulses, which in turn are transmitted to the cerebral cortex to provide the sensation of hearing. The nerve entries for these structures and for the larger basilar cells are arranged so that the thicker base is called the **basilar membrane**. The location of a particular organ of Corti within the scala media, from the base (near the middle ear) to the apex of the cochlea, with its individual innervation, determines the frequency of the sound wave perceived (*Fig. 5-14*).

Sound waves of different frequencies have different transmission patterns from the base to the apex. A weak sound wave (of any frequency) at the base strengthens when it reaches the portion of the basilar membrane that has a natural resonant frequency equal to its own. At this point, the basilar membrane can vibrate easily; the sound wave energy is dissipated and does not travel the remaining distance along the basilar membrane. Therefore, a **high-frequency sound wave** travels a short distance along the basilar membrane, where it reaches its resonant point and dies out. A **low-frequency sound wave** travels a longer distance, and a similar phenomenon occurs. All frequencies

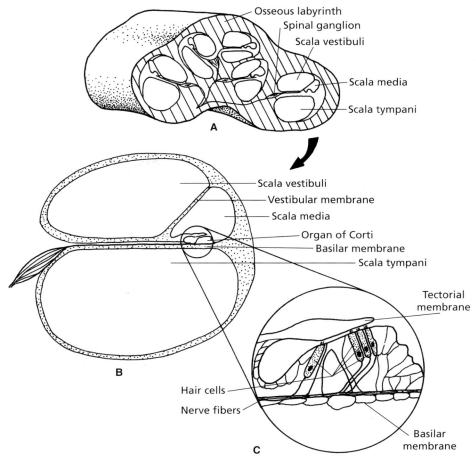

■ **FIGURE 5-13** The cochlear portion of the inner ear. **A.** Cross-section through the cochlea, illustrating its coiled nature. **B.** Schematic representation of a section through one of the turns of the cochlea. **C.** Details of an organ of Corti.

between high and low are represented at separate points on the basilar membrane between the base and apex of the cochlea.

An organ of Corti is composed primarily of sensory receptors called hair cells that have hairs projecting toward the **tectorial membrane** (see Fig. 5-13). Displacement of the hair cell cilia against the tectorial membrane caused by oscillations of the basilar membrane (resulting from dissipation of sound waves) causes the hair cells to depolarize and create a nerve impulse, which is transmitted to the auditory cerebral cortex by way of the **vestibulocochlear nerve**.

Summary of Sound Reception

The structures traversed and actions initiated for a sound wave to be heard may be summarized as follows (*Fig. 5-15*):

1. The sound wave is directed into the external auditory meatus by the pinna.
2. The sound wave strikes the tympanic membrane (eardrum) and sets it in motion.
3. The motion of the eardrum is transmitted through the middle ear by the auditory ossicles to the vestibular (oval) window.

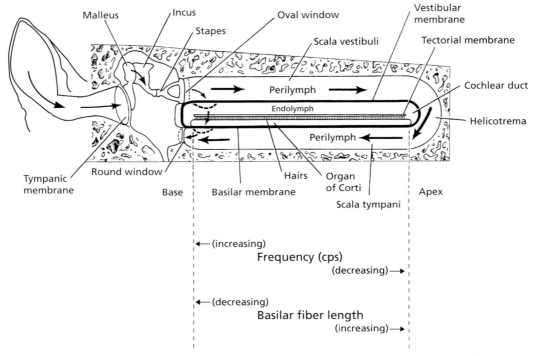

■ **FIGURE 5-14** Transmission of pressure waves in the cochlea. When the movement of the stapes is slow, pressure waves are transmitted through the perilymph with no movement of the basilar membrane. With greater movement of the stapes (higher frequency), pressure waves are directed through the endolymph with movement of the basilar membrane, hence sound is perceived. High and low frequency sounds are related to regions of the basilar membrane where different sound wave frequencies can cause displacement. Adapted from Spence AP, Mason EB. Human Anatomy and Physiology. 4th Ed. St. Paul, MN: West Publishing Co., 1992.

4. The vestibular window is set in motion and displaces perilymph in the vestibule of the inner ear.

5. The perilymph (a liquid) is incompressible and thus transmits the sound wave through the scala vestibuli of the cochlea.

6. An organ of Corti at a distance from the base characteristic of the approaching sound wave is stimulated when a sound wave is transmitted to the scala media and from there to the scala tympani.

7. The movement of the liquid in the scala tympani is finally compensated for by an outward movement of the cochlear (round) window into the cavity of the middle ear.

8. The stimulation of hair cells in an organ of Corti initiates a nerve impulse that is transmitted by the cochlear branch of the vestibulocochlear nerve to the brain.

The range of frequencies through which sound can be perceived varies among species. In humans, the limit seems to be between 20 and 20,000 cycles per second (cps). Dogs can perceive frequencies up to about 50,000 cps, which is the basis for dog whistles. These emit a high-frequency sound that is not perceived by humans, but the dog responds because its organ of Corti is stimulated.

■ VISION

1. **Identify the parts of the external eye.**
2. **Identify the basic structures of the eyeball.**

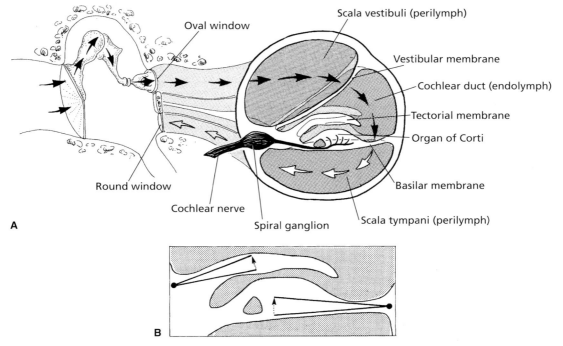

■ **FIGURE 5-15 A.** Schematic representation of the pathway of sound waves that enter the ear. **B.** Hair cells in the organ of Corti respond to shearing stresses generated by independent pivoting of the tectorial and basilar membranes on separate axes. (From Cormack DH. Essential Histology. 2nd Ed. Baltimore: Lippincott Williams & Wilkins, 2001.)

3. What is the normal arrangement of the corneal stroma?
4. Does the cornea have a blood supply?
5. Are there nerve fibers in the cornea?
6. How is accommodation accomplished by the lens of the eye?
7. What is the extent of accommodation among domestic animals?
8. How is the size of the pupil changed?
9. Are pupil shapes the same among all animals?
10. What would be the impact of a centrally located optic disk and a constricted circular pupil?
11. Review the production, location, circulation, function, and drainage of aqueous humor.
12. What visual chemical when excited by light begins to decompose and stimulates retinal rod cells?
13. What is the tapetum, and how does it provide for better vision in reduced light?
14. What is meant by field of vision? binocular vision? monocular vision?
15. Describe the conjunctiva.
16. If the nasolacrimal duct were plugged, explain the reason for a horse's wet face.
17. What is "cherry eye" in the dog?

The receptor organs for vision are the eyes. The receptor stimulus is light and, accordingly, many of the eye structures are adapted for transparency so that light rays can reach the receptors. The parts of the eye as seen from the front (the external eye) are shown in *Figure 5-16.* The basic structures of the eyeball are shown in *Figure 5-17.*

Structure and Functions of the Eye

The eye is composed of the eyeball (globe), the optic nerve, and the accessory structures, which comprise the eyelids, conjunctivae, lacrimal apparatus, and the muscles of the eyeball.

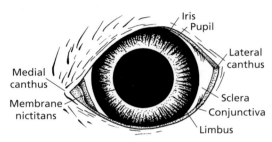

■ **FIGURE 5-16** The external eye. The medial canthus is on the nasal side. The nasolacrimal duct originates in the medial canthus. The limbus is the junction of the sclera with the iris.

Tunics of the Eyeball

The eyeball has three distinct layers or coats, known as **tunics**. The outermost external coat (**fibrous tunic**) is the supporting layer of the eyeball and is composed of the **anterior cornea** and **posterior sclera**. The sclera is the tough, white part of the fibrous tunic. The middle coat is the vascular tunic and is composed of the **choroid, ciliary body,** and **iris**. The innermost tunic is the **light-sensitive retina (nerve tunic)**. It consists of several layers; three of its layers are cells. The light-sensitive cell layer consists of the **rods (black-and-white vision)** and the **cones (color vision)**. These receptors convert light to a nerve impulse. The retina is black because of the presence of **melanin**. This black pigmentation not only assists in the absorption of light, but also prevents uncontrolled reflection to other parts of the eye.

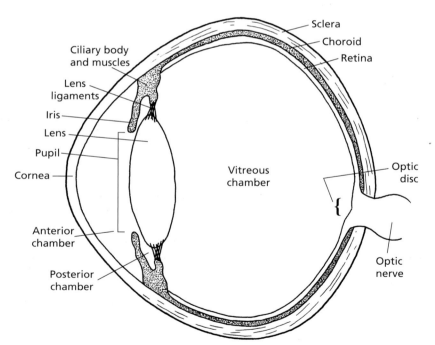

■ **FIGURE 5-17** Diagram of an eyeball showing its basic structure. The pupil is the opening between the central projection of the iris.

Cornea

The **cornea** is the transparent, forward continuation of the sclera. It is transparent to allow for the entrance of light. In a cross-sectional view of the cornea, five layers can be identified from the outside to the inside (*Fig. 5-18*): 1) the anterior epithelium (stratified squamous nonkeratinizing epithelium), 2) subepithelial basement membrane (Bowman membrane), 3) substantia propria, or stroma, 4) posterior limiting lamina (Descemet membrane), and 5) posterior endothelium (Descemet endothelium).

There is greater light transmission if the surface area ratio of cornea to sclera is increased. **Nocturnal animals** (nighttime) have relatively larger corneas than **diurnal animals** (daytime). About 17% of the eyeball in the dog is cornea (a diurnal animal), whereas about 30% of the eyeball in the cat is cornea (a nocturnal animal).

About 90% of the corneal thickness is a result of **collagen fibers** (called **stroma**). The collagen fibers have an orderly, laminated

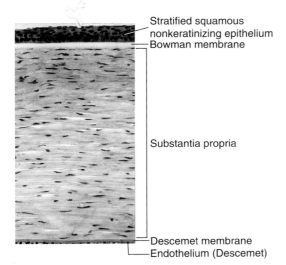

Stratified squamous nonkeratinizing epithelium
Bowman membrane

Substantia propria

Descemet membrane
Endothelium (Descemet)

■ **FIGURE 5-18** The histologic organization of the cornea (top, anterior surface; bottom, posterior surface). (From Cormack DH. Essential Histology. 2nd Ed. Baltimore: Lippincott Williams & Wilkins, 2001.)

arrangement, and this is related to the transparent nature of the cornea.

The **cornea is avascular** (without blood supply) so that blood vessels do not interfere with the inward transmission of light. The cornea is supplied abundantly with **nonmyelinated nerve fibers**, bare nerve endings that enter from the limbus and penetrate the outer epithelial layer. The cornea is one of the most sensitive tissues of the body.

Transparency of the cornea depends further on the degree of its hydration; the normal transparent cornea contains less water than it is able to imbibe. Increased uptake of water with a consequent reduction in transparency can occur as a result of damage to either the anterior epithelium or the posterior endothelium or to a reduction of oxygen. If this occurs, a rearrangement of the collagen fibers results, causing the cornea to become cloudy or white. Other causes of corneal cloudiness or whiteness are thinning from increased intraocular tension, disruption by trauma, or replacement by scar tissue.

The Lens and Accommodation

The **lens** is positioned between the cornea and retina. It is attached by suspensory ligaments (**zonular fibers**) to the ciliary body, which is a thickened forward ridge of the choroid that circumscribes the eyeball (*Fig. 5-19*). The ciliary body contains three sets of smooth muscle fibers (ciliary muscles), with each set oriented in a different direction. Normal ciliary muscle tone results in normal vision with a lens that is convex and that has a focal distance (distance from the lens to the retina) where the image is focused on the retina. Convex lenses converge light rays. A more convex lens would shorten the focal distance, and a less convex lens would lengthen the focal distance. Accordingly, when nearer objects are viewed, the focal distance is in back of the retina and the lens must become more convex to shorten the focal distance and bring it to focus on the retina. This is accomplished by increased ciliary

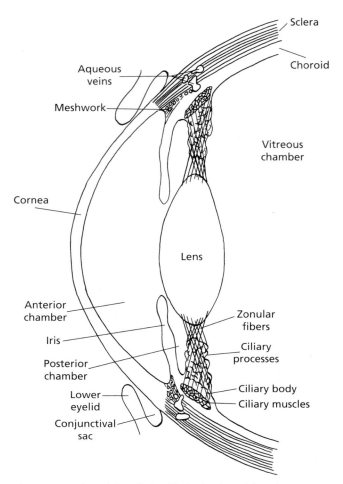

■ **FIGURE 5-19** Schematic representation of the relationship in the dog of the ciliary processes with the ciliary body, the zonular fibers (lens ligaments), and the posterior chamber. The ciliary muscles are a part of the ciliary body and are attached to the zonular fibers. The meshwork represents a collection location for aqueous humor that drains to scleral veins. The ciliary muscles encircle the eyeball. When contracted, tension on the lens ligaments is reduced and the lens becomes more convex.

muscle contraction. Because the ciliary muscles encircle the eyeball, contraction decreases the tension on the lens ligaments making them more slack (see Fig. 5-19). Because of its elastic capsule, the reduced tension on the ligaments allows the lens to assume a more convex configuration and the focal distance is shortened. When more distant objects are viewed, the focal distance is in front of the retina and the lens must become less convex (more divergent) in order to increase the focal distance to the retina. Greater relaxation of the ciliary muscles occurs and more tension is applied to the elastic lens capsule thereby making the lens less convex, and the focal distance is increased because of the greater divergence. The adjustments needed for near and far objects are known as **accommodation**. Accommodation among domestic animals seems limited. This is thought to be true because of the sparseness of ciliary muscles, except in the cat. In the cat, the convexity of the lens increases during accommodation for near objects to the extent that it may compress the iris anteriorly to the cornea.

Visual acuity is the extent to which details and forms of objects can be perceived accurately. A **foveal region** is an area of the retina where there is high visual acuity and is characterized by a pit (**fovea centralis**). In primates and birds it contains only **cone (color) cells**. Domestic mammals lack foveas but do have areas with high visual acuity called **visual streaks**.

Iris

The amount of light allowed to enter the eye is controlled by the **iris**, which is the colored part of the eye (see Fig. 5-19). The allowed opening, of varying size, is called the **pupil**. The pupil is horizontal in the domestic herbivores and pig, vertical and elliptic in the cat, and circular in the dog. The iris contains two sets of smooth muscles: 1) **circularly arranged fibers**, innervated by the **parasympathetic division** of the autonomic nervous system; and 2) **radially arranged fibers**, innervated by the **sympathetic division**. Contraction of the circularly arranged fibers decreases the size of the pupil and allows less light to enter the eye, whereas contraction of the radially arranged fibers increases the size of the pupil and allows more light to enter the eye.

Humors of the Eye

The spaces forward from the lens are divided by the iris into two parts. The space behind the iris and forward from the lens is called the **posterior chamber**, and the space behind the cornea but in front of the iris is called the **anterior chamber**. Projecting from the ciliary body and into the posterior chamber are structures known as **ciliary processes** (see Fig. 5-19). They present a considerable surface area because of their folded arrangement and are well vascularized. They actively secrete a liquid into the posterior chamber, the **aqueous humor** (*Fig. 5-20*). The aqueous humor has free communication with the anterior chamber and thus occupies all spaces anterior to the lens. The transparent material behind the lens that occupies most of the volume of the eyeball (the **vitreous chamber**) is called the **vitreous body**. It does not have the flow characteristics of a liquid, rather, it is more similar to a gelatinous mass—hence, the name vitreous body is more appropriate than vitreous humor.

Aqueous humor can diffuse through the mass of the vitreous body, but only slowly. The principal flow of aqueous humor after its formation is through the pupil into the anterior chamber and to where it is reabsorbed at the **iridocorneal angle**, which is the angle formed where the cornea meets the iris (*Fig. 5-21*). Inasmuch as there is a constant formation of aqueous humor, there must also be a constant removal. It enters the **corneoscleral meshwork** at the iridocorneal angle and is directed to **aqueous collecting veins** and the **scleral venous plexus** for its return to blood. A **canal of Schlemm** does not exist for domestic animals as described for humans. Aqueous humor functions to: 1) provide nutrition to the avascular lens and cornea, 2) remove waste products of metabolism from these structures, and 3) occupy space and maintain a constant distance for the refractive parts. The pressure maintained by the aqueous humor within the eyeball can be measured; it is about 20 mm Hg in the dog. This pressure maintains the normal shape and firmness of the eyeball. If the reabsorption of aqueous humor is impeded, the pressure increases. This situation is recognized clinically as glaucoma and can lead to blindness if left untreated.

Retina

The innermost tunic of the eye is the **nerve tunic**, or **neural retina** (*Fig. 5-22*). The **photoreceptors**, the **rods** and **cones**, are located near the outer aspect, immediately inward from the pigmented epithelium. Impulse transmission is directed inwardly toward the vitreous. Considerable convergence of impulses from the photoreceptors occurs on two interposed cell

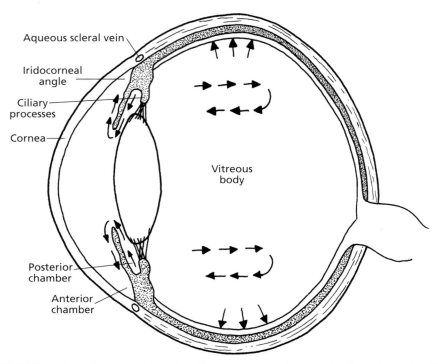

■ **FIGURE 5-20** Formation of aqueous humor by ciliary processes and its anterior flow. Arrows in vitreous body indicate flow by diffusion of aqueous humor through the vitreous body. Some absorption occurs from the vitreous into choroidal vessels.

layers, of which the innermost cell layer is that of ganglion cells. The unmyelinated axons of the ganglion cell layer arc toward the **optic disc**, also known as optic nerve head. Here they become myelinated and turn to form the **optic nerve**. The intraocular myelinated portion of the nerve forms the optic disc. There are no photoreceptors overlying the disc, hence the optic disc represents a blind spot. It is located ventrolateral to the posterior pole of the eyeball. The posterior pole is the posterior location of the **optical axis**, which is a line drawn from the center point of the cornea to the center point of the posterior sphere.

The retinas of **domestic mammals** contain mostly **rods** and the retinas of **domestic birds** contain **mostly cones**. The **rods** are the photoreceptors associated with **black-and-white vision**, and the **cones** are those associated with **color vision**. The rods are extremely sensitive

to light and are used for night vision, whereas cones function best in day vision.

The part of the retina and all associated structures that are visible with the ophthalmoscope are referred to clinically as the **ocular fundus**. The fundi of several domestic animals are shown in *Figure 5-23*.

Chemistry of Vision

Light that enters the eye stimulates biochemical reactions in the rods and cones. Chemicals in the rods and cones decompose on exposure to light. The chemical in the rods is called rhodopsin, and the light-sensitive chemicals in the cones are only slightly different from rhodopsin. The reaction scheme shown in *Figure 5-24* is characteristic of the visual cycle.

Rhodopsin (also known as **visual purple**) is a light-sensitive pigment in the outer part

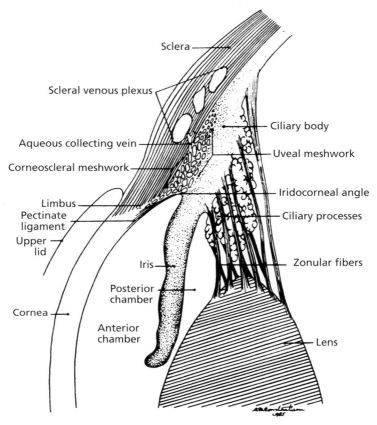

■ **FIGURE 5-21** Schematic drawing of the iridocorneal angle region of a dog. This is the location for drainage of aqueous humor. (From Dellmann HD. Textbook of Veterinary Histology. 4th Ed. Philadelphia: Lea & Febiger, 1993.)

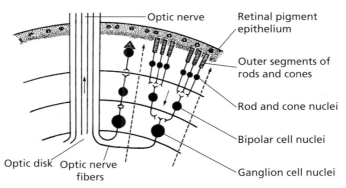

■ **FIGURE 5-22** A simplified version of the retina. The arrows indicate the direction of impulse transmission from rods and cones in the outer aspect to the ganglion cells in the inner aspect. Impulse transmission is opposite to the direction of light. Dashed lines represent direction of light from the lens. From Cormack DH. Essential Histology. 2nd Ed. Baltimore: Lippincott Williams & Wilkins, 2001.

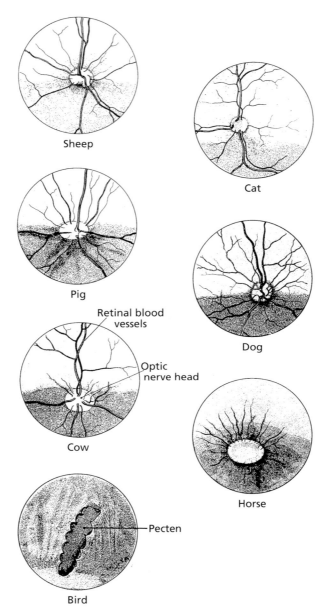

FIGURE 5-23 Drawings of fundi of seven domestic animals as seen by ophthalmoscopy. The disc-shaped structures are optic discs shown as optic nerve head. Pecten, as shown for birds, is responsible for nourishment of the inner eye and retina. (From Coulter DB, Schmidt GM. Special senses I: Vision. In: Swenson MJ, Reece WO, eds. Dukes' Physiology of Domestic Animals. 11th Ed. Ithaca, NY: Cornell University Press, 1993.)

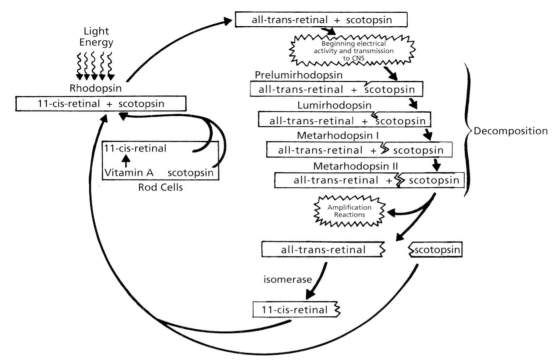

■ **FIGURE 5-24** Photochemistry of the visual cycle. Metarhodopsin II, called photoexcited rhodopsin, triggers highly amplified visual excitation. CNS, central nervous system.

of the rod that is located in the pigmented epithelium. It is composed of 11-cis-retinal (also known as retinene) and scotopsin. **Scotopsin** is a **rod protein**, and the similar opsin in cones is **photopsin**. Exposure of rhodopsin to light energy immediately begins its decomposition, in which a number of unstable, short-lived (nanoseconds for prelumirhodopsin and seconds for metarhodopsin II) intermediates are formed. The final one, metarhodopsin II, triggers highly amplified visual excitation and splits into scotopsin and all-*trans*-retinal. All-*trans*-retinal is chemically the same as 11-*cis*-retinal but has a different physical structure; it is a straight rather than a curved molecule. Its conversion to 11-*cis*-retinal requires the presence of the retinal enzyme isomerase. All-*trans*-retinal is converted to 11-*cis*-retinal, which then recombines with scotopsin to reform rhodopsin.

Rod stimulation is believed to occur at the instant that the rhodopsin molecule becomes excited by light. The stimulation resulting from an instantaneous flash of light can persist for about 0.05 to 0.5 s, depending on the intensity of the light. Rapidly successive flashes with alternating intensity become fused to give the appearance of being continuous. This effect is observed when watching motion pictures or television.

There is a relationship between vision and vitamin A. A lack of vitamin A results in inadequate formation of rhodopsin. Night vision requires optimum amounts of rhodopsin, and its shortage, because of vitamin A deficiency, is referred to as night blindness.

Adaptation to Varying Light

Dark adaptation refers to an adaptation to relatively dark environments. Because of less light, the concentration of rhodopsin increases, allowing for maximum reaction to the available light. When first entering a dark room, one might be almost unable to see anything, but after dark adaptation, objects can be perceived more readily.

Light adaptation refers to an adaptation to lighter environments. The higher concentration of rhodopsin decomposes because of the abundance of light. The images perceived seem to be overexposed. Normal vision returns when the rhodopsin concentration is balanced with the available light.

Concurrent with the adaptation processes are the **visual reflexes**, which increase or decrease the diameter of the pupil (see previous section). Consequently, not only does rhodopsin concentration increase in the dark, but the pupil diameter also increases to allow for maximum light entry. Conversely, rhodopsin concentration decreases in light, and pupil size decreases to minimize light entry.

The **tapetum** is a light-reflecting layer of cells of the inner choroid, located just outside the retinal-pigmented epithelium (*Fig. 5-25*). Melanin is absent from the pigmented epithelium of the retina where the tapetum is present. The tapetum is not present throughout the choroid and varies in size among those domestic species in which it is present (e.g., cats, dogs, horses, ruminants). The tapetum allows light that has just stimulated the receptor cells to be reflected back onto them so that they receive another stimulation. In this way greater vision is obtained, even with minimal light. The reflected light continues on a forward path through the pupil and out of the eye again. This reflected light is termed **eyeshine**, which is when eyes glow at night in the presence of light.

Field of Vision

The **field of vision** for an animal is the spatial area from which the complete image is formed. The more lateral the placement of the eyes, the larger the field of vision. In fact, some animals might even see everything around them with the exception of objects directly behind their body, which can still be seen with only a slight movement of the head. If the field of vision for each eye overlaps that of the other, a **binocular area of vision** is formed; conversely, a **monocular area of vision** is formed if there is no overlap. Binocular vision provides greater depth perception, and this is more pronounced in animals that prey on other animals for food. Greater accuracy of position is necessary before the leap. Such animals characteristically have more forward-placed eyes (*Fig. 5-26*). In contrast, herbivores (plant eaters) have more laterally placed eyes and have a wider field of vision; this gives greater protection while grazing as far as predator observation is concerned (*Fig. 5-27*). In all domestic animals, regardless of how far their eyes are situated laterally, there is some central area of overlap providing a zone of binocular vision.

The horse has little or no accommodation. When observing more distant objects, the horse increasingly raises its head and lifts up the nose. When observing much closer objects, the horse may arch the neck and rotate the head on one side. In the past, these behaviors were explained as an attempt to make up for the lack of accommodation by using a **ramp-shaped retina**. This was presumed to provide a longer focal distance for viewing downward than for viewing along the axis of the eye. It was assumed that this retinal feature accounted for the alterations in head position whereby the animal was finding a distance from lens to retina appropriate for focusing the image.

It is now known that the ramp-shaped retina does not exist. Measurements have been made indicating that the horse has a retina that is equidistant from the lens except in the far dorsal and far ventral retina. In these peripheral regions, the retina is nearer to the lens, not farther as proposed for the ramp-shaped retina.

Ganglion cell densities in the horse have been mapped throughout the retina and correlated with maximum visual acuity. Densities

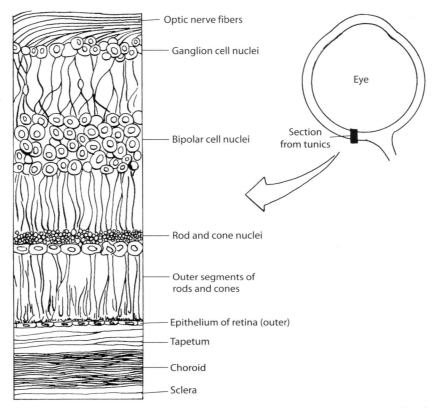

Optic nerve fibers

Ganglion cell nuclei

Bipolar cell nuclei

Rod and cone nuclei

Outer segments of
rods and cones

Epithelium of retina (outer)

Tapetum

Choroid

Sclera

Eye

Section
from tunics

■ **FIGURE 5-25** Location of the tapetum relative to the retina. The tapetum is shown as a broad band of cell layers between the choroid and the retina. Melanin is absent from the pigmented epithelium of the retina (outer layer of the retina), where tapetum is present. There is a pigmented layer in the choroid to aid light absorption.

of cells are low in the periphery and high in the ventrally placed visual streak, which is a strong narrow region visible in the ventral retina immediately above the optic nerve head. In retinal regions other than the visual streak, acuity in the horse is very low. Acuity is similar at any point along the narrow streak, and the horse can see a narrow, very circumscribed frontal and circular view. Because peripheral acuity is quite low, it would be of little benefit for a horse to use any part of the retina other than the visual streak for direct observation. When the horse lifts its head and points its nose forward to use its binocular field to scan the horizon, its monocular field is lessened and lateral vision becomes more limited (see

Fig. 5-27). When the animal lowers its head, such that the nose approaches the vertical, the binocular vision is directed toward the ground for grazing and the lateral monocular fields are again in position to scan the lateral horizon.

The horse can attend to either the frontal field with the head raised or the lateral field with the head lowered. The horse has a frontally placed blind field such that when the nose is drawn in and the face approaches the vertical, the animal is unable to see directly in front. This situation occurs when the horse is being ridden "on the bit" with the neck arched and the nose just in front of the vertical. If a show jumping horse is to see and judge the distance of a fence that it approaches,

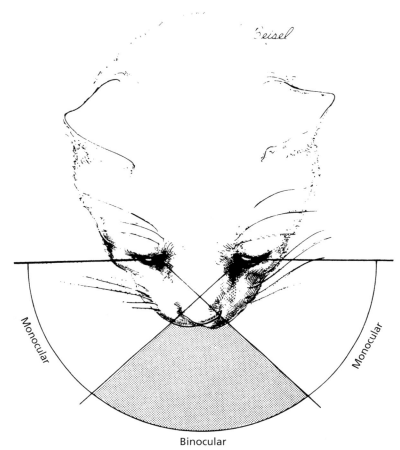

■ **FIGURE 5-26** Field of vision of the cat. The large central binocular area results from the forward position of the eyes. (From Coulter DB, Schmidt GM. Special senses I: Vision. In: Swenson MJ, Reece WO, eds. Dukes' Physiology of Domestic Animals. 11th Ed. Ithaca, NY: Cornell University Press, 1993.)

it must have the ability to raise its head and direct its binocular field forward.

Eyeball Movements and Accessory Structures

Movements of the eyeball are accomplished by skeletal muscles that are innervated by cranial nerves (*Fig. 5-28*). Up-and-down, side-to-side, rotational, and inward (retraction) movements are possible. These muscles also hold the eyeball within its orbit against a pad of fat. Side-to-side movements are made by contraction of a laterally placed muscle; up-and-down movements are made by contraction of a dorsally and ventrally placed muscle; and rotational movements are made by contraction of a dorsal or ventral obliquely placed muscle. The dorsal oblique muscle rotates the top of the eye medially, and the ventral oblique muscle rotates the ventral part of the eye medially. Retractor muscles are absent in humans; they seem to provide protection for animals in situations in which protruding eyeballs would be hazardous. Also, retraction of the eyeball causes the **third eyelid** (nictitating membrane) to slide over the eyeball and spread the tear film.

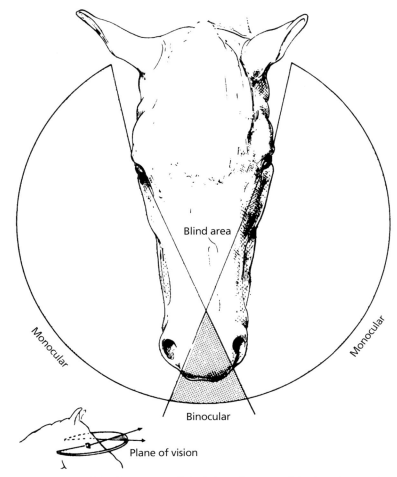

Plane of vision

■ **FIGURE 5-27** Field of vision of the horse. It is relatively large because of the horse's more laterally placed eyes. Note the small binocular area. (From Coulter DB, Schmidt GM. Special senses I: Vision. In: Swenson MJ, Reece WO, eds. Dukes' Physiology of Domestic Animals. 11th Ed. Ithaca, NY: Cornell University Press, 1993.)

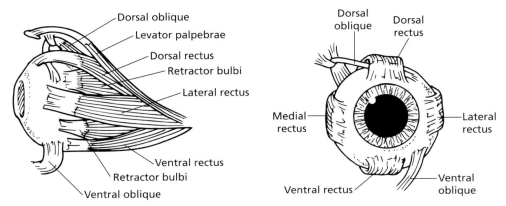

■ **FIGURE 5-28** Extrinsic muscles of the eye of the dog. (Adapted from Helper LC. Magrane's Canine Ophthalmology. 4th Ed. Philadelphia: Lea & Febiger, 1989.)

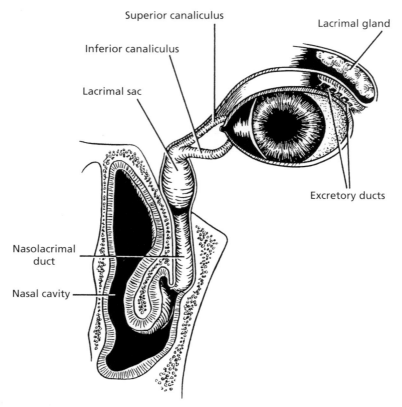

■ **FIGURE 5-29** The lacrimal production and drainage system of the eye of the dog. The accessory lacrimal glands are not shown. (From Helper LC. Magrane's Canine Ophthalmology. 4th Ed. Philadelphia: Lea & Febiger, 1989.)

Conjunctivae

The conjunctivae are the membranes that line the eyelids and that turn back onto the eyeball (see Fig. 5-19). The part lining the eyelid is the **palpebral conjunctiva**, and the part turned back onto the eyeball is the **bulbar or ocular conjunctiva**. The space between the palpebral conjunctiva and the eyeball forms the **conjunctival sac**. This is normally minimal and provides a reservoir for the accumulation of tears. It is also used for the application of eye drops and ointments. The conjunctival membrane, because of its superficial location, is useful for examining mucous membrane color. A pink color is considered normal, a blanched appearance indicates lack of blood or anemia, a blue color indicates lack of oxygen, and a yellow color is associated with icterus.

Lacrimal Apparatus

The lacrimal apparatus is associated with the formation of lacrimal secretions (tears), transport to the conjunctival sac, and drainage to the nasal cavity (*Fig. 5-29*). The **lacrimal gland** is located in the orbit, dorsal to the eyeball. Short ducts carry the secretion into the upper aspect of the dorsal conjunctival sac. The lacrimal secretion keeps the eyeball moist, provides lubrication, and keeps it clean and free of foreign materials. Ducts (nasolacrimal ducts) in the medial aspect of each eye conduct excess secretion to the nasal cavity, where it is dissipated. If these ducts become occluded, the lacrimal secretions accumulate in the conjunctival sac and overflow onto the face. Glands that secrete a waxy substance, known as **meibomian glands**, are located along the margin

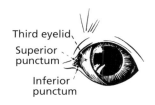 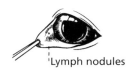 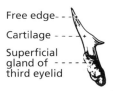

■ **FIGURE 5-30** Third eyelid in the dog. (From Evans HE, deLahunta A. Guide to the Dissection of the Dog. 5th Ed. Philadelphia: WB Saunders Company, 2000.)

of the eyelids. Their secretion helps to form a dam so that the lacrimal secretion does not ordinarily flow out onto the face.

Precorneal Film

The fluid layer on the cornea is known as the **precorneal film** (also called the **tear film**). It consists of an innermost layer of mucin, a middle layer of lacrimal secretions (tears), and an outer oil film.

The **outer oily layer** is formed by meibomian glands and accessory sebaceous glands. It reduces the rate of evaporation of the underlying tear layer and also helps to prevent overflow at the lid margin.

The **middle layer** of fluid is composed of **lacrimal secretions**, which wet the cornea and reduce evaporation from the eye. It is formed by the lacrimal glands and the accessory lacrimal glands (such as those associated with the third eyelid).

The **inner mucinoid layer** is formed by the **goblet cells** of the conjunctiva. In addition to mucin, it contains a high concentration of **lysozyme (an enzyme)**, which can digest bacterial cell walls. Lysozyme is present in most animal tissues and secretions, but it only is found in sufficiently high concentrations to be bactericidal in white blood cells, nasal secretions, and tears. In addition to lysozyme, a gamma globulin protein fraction also contributes to the antibacterial property of tears. Wettability (favorable surface tension between cornea and tears) is provided for by the mucin of the inner layer.

The tear film is reformed each time the eyelids close or when the third eyelid is swept across the eye by eyeball retraction.

Third Eyelid

The **third eyelid** arises as a fold from the ventromedial aspect of the conjunctiva (visible part shown as membrane nictitans in Fig. 5-16). It is well developed in the dog, is highly mobile, and is large enough to cover the entire anterior face of the cornea. The third eyelid is reinforced by a T-shaped cartilage surrounded at its base by a gland that contributes to the tear film (*Fig. 5-30*). Pigs and cattle also have a second, deeper gland. The third eyelid becomes prominent when all of the muscles of the eyeball are caused to contract, as in some clinical situations such as strychnine poisoning. The contraction retracts the eyeball and puts pressure on the cartilaginous plate, pushing it forward. Lymph nodules are also present on the underside of the third eyelid. When they become inflamed in the dog, they often protrude; the condition is referred to as "cherry eye."

■ SUGGESTED READING

Chibuzo GA. The tongue. In: Evans HE, ed. Miller's Anatomy of the Dog. 3rd Ed. Philadelphia: WB Saunders Company, 1993:396.

Cormack DH. Essential Histology. 2nd Ed. Baltimore: Lippincott Williams & Wilkins, 2001.

Dellman HD, Eurell JA. Textbook of Veterinary Histology. 5th Ed. Baltimore: Lippincott Williams & Wilkins, 1998.

Evans HE, deLahunta A. Guide to the Dissection of the Dog. 5th Ed. Philadelphia: WB Saunders Company, 2000.

Harman AM, Moore S, Hoskins R, Keller P. Horse vision and an explanation for the visual behaviour originally explained by the "ramp retina." Equine Vet J 1999;31:384–390.

Helper LC. Magrane's Canine Ophthalmology. 4th Ed. Philadelphia: Lea & Febiger, 1989.

Kare MR, Beauchamp GK, Marsh RR. Special senses II: Taste, smell, and hearing. In: Swenson MJ, Reece WO, eds. Dukes' Physiology of Domestic Animals. 11th Ed. Ithaca, NY: Cornell University Press, 1993:816.

 SELF EVALUATION—CHAPTER 5

CLASSIFICATION OF SENSORY RECEPTORS

1. Muscle spindles and Golgi tendon organs (proprioceptors) belong to the class of sensory receptors known as:
   a. interoceptors.
   b. nociceptors.
   c. exteroceptors.
   d. musculotendoceptors.

2. Stimulation of a Krause end-bulb (cold receptor) can result in the pain sensation.
   a. True
   b. False

PAIN

3. Pain that is felt on the surface of the body and is arising from the viscera is known as:
   a. heart pain.
   b. window pain.
   c. referred pain.
   d. pleuritis or peritonitis.

4. Which one of the following statements about pain is FALSE?
   a. Pain is a protective mechanism.
   b. The cornea of the eye is an insensitive structure.
   c. Diversion of attention reduces pain perception.
   d. Referred pain is that which is perceived as coming from an exterior part of the body but is actually coming from the viscera.

TASTE

5. The taste bud is a receptor organ for olfaction.
   a. True
   b. False

6. The greatest number of taste buds are associated with the:
   a. nasal cavity.
   b. tongue papillae.
   c. cheek.
   d. pharynx.

7. Water that is colder (even down to freezing) than environmental temperature is readily accepted by chickens and turkeys, whereas they may refuse water (that sitting in the sun) that is higher than their body temperature.
   a. True
   b. False

8. Which one of the following is NOT associated with gustation in animals?
   a. Papillae, taste buds, tongue
   b. Taste pore, pit, taste hairs
   c. Pleasant, unpleasant, indifferent
   d. Pheromone

SMELL

9. A chemical odorous signal secreted by one animal to influence the behavior of another animal is known as a:
   a. pheromone.
   b. scent.
   c. perfume.
   d. pheroscent.

10. Which one of the following cells from the olfactory region might provide for return of the smell sensation after olfactory receptor cell destruction?
    a. Sustentacular cells
    b. Olfactory receptor cells
    c. Basal cells

11. Pheromones are associated with which one of the following special senses?
    a. Taste
    b. Smell
    c. Hearing
    d. Vision

12. Which one of the following statements best explains why most domestic animals are macrosmatic?
    a. Individual receptors are more sensitive.
    b. Better able to sniff
    c. Have a more extensive epithelium containing the receptors

13. Which one of the following is NOT associated with olfaction in animals?
    a. Pica
    b. Sniffing
    c. Adaptation
    d. Macrosmatic, microsmatic, anosmatic

HEARING AND EQUILIBRIUM

14. High-frequency sounds are dissipated (and thus stimulate appropriate cells for the sense of hearing):
    a. near the base of the cochlea (closest to the vestibule).
    b. near the tip of the cochlea (farthest from the vestibule).
    c. near the base of the semicircular canals.
    d. in the curved portion of the semicircular canals.

15. Muscles in the middle ear that are attached to the auditory ossicles:
    a. amplify sound waves.
    b. protect the ear from excessive amplification.
    c. help direct sound waves into the ear canal.

16. The movement of fluid in the membranous semicircular canals moves hair cells of the ampullae therein. This apprises the brain about:
    a. equilibrium.
    b. hearing.
    c. smell.
    d. pain.

17. Which component of the ear relies on fluid conduction of sound waves for its function?
    a. External ear
    b. Middle ear
    c. Vestibular apparatus
    d. Cochlea

18. Equalization of pressure between the middle ear and the body exterior is accomplished by way of the:
    a. pinna.
    b. ear canal.
    c. auditory tube (eustachian tube).
    d. cochlear duct.

19. What proprioceptive sensory organ is present in the middle ear skeletal muscles that respond to stretch and dampen loud sounds?
    a. Bare nerve endings
    b. Muscle spindle
    c. Golgi tendon organ
    d. Vater-pacinian corpuscle

20. The observation of a pig with its head tilted and an awkward sense of body balance (equilibrium) would indicate malfunction within the:
    a. vestibular structure of the inner ear.
    b. cochlear structure of the inner ear.
    c. vestibular structure of the middle ear.
    d. cochlear structure of the middle ear.

21. The first fluid displaced by the inward movement of the stapes is:
    a. endolymph in the scala media (cochlear duct).
    b. endolymph in the vestibule.
    c. perilymph in the vestibule.
    d. perilymph in the scala media.

22. The sensory receptor of the inner ear that converts sound energy to a nerve impulse is known as the:
    a. organ of Corti.
    b. crista ampullaris.
    c. macula.
    d. harmonica.

VISION

23. A green dye placed into the conjunctival sac of a horse should later appear in the nasal cavity (near the nostrils) if the naso-lacrimal apparatus is functioning properly.
    a. True
    b. False

24. The fluid that provides nutrition to the avascular (without blood supply) cornea and lens is:
    a. vitreous humor.
    b. good humor.
    c. aqueous humor.
    d. endolymph.

25. The radially arranged muscles of the iris that dilate the pupil are innervated by the:
    a. sympathetic division of the autonomics.
    b. parasympathetic division of the autonomics.

26. The tear film:
    a. has little function.
    b. provides optical, mechanical, lubricating, and bactericidal functions.
    c. is a good movie.
    d. is secreted by glands in the nasal cavity.

27. Animals with eyes that are placed well forward on the head (such as the cat) have a more extensive field of vision than animals with eyes placed laterally, but have a more restricted binocular vision.
    a. True
    b. False

28. Which one of the following statements about the ciliary body is FALSE?

    a. It is a part of the vascular tunic.
    b. Contains ciliary muscles that when contracted decrease the tension on the lens ligaments, causing the lens to become more convex
    c. Has secretory processes known as choroid plexus
    d. Ciliary muscles within are poorly developed in most domestic animals.

29. The function of the tapetum is to:
    a. convert light to a nerve impulse.
    b. focus light on the retina.
    c. reflect light back to rod cells in the retina.
    d. secrete aqueous humor.

30. Which one of the following statements about the cornea is FALSE?
    a. The ratio of corneal area to eyeball area varies among animal species.
    b. Devoid of blood vessels
    c. Well supplied with bare nerve endings for pain reception
    d. Normally clear because of random arrangement of collagen fibers

31. Which one of the following statements about the retina is FALSE?
    a. The light-sensitive cells (rods and cones) are on the inside (nearest vitreous).
    b. Has highest metabolic rate per unit of weight of any tissue in the body
    c. May be damaged by deficiency or excess of oxygen
    d. Appears black because of outer pigment layer (in choroid if have tapetum)

32. Dark adaptation (greater vision in the dark) implies a depletion of rhodopsin.
    a. True
    b. False

33. The cornea is normally clear and transparent because the collagen fibers (stroma):
    a. have a lamellar (parallel) arrangement.
    b. are randomly arranged.
    c. have a good blood supply.
    d. have a poor oxygen supply.

34. For the lens to become more convex and to increase convergence of incoming light, the ciliary muscles must:
    a. relax.
    b. contract.

35. It seems that accommodation in domestic animals (as judged by ciliary muscle development) is:
    a. limited, and some may have auxiliary features.
    b. well developed in all species.

36. What are the two avascular structures of the eye that receive nutrition and have waste products removed by the aqueous humor?
    a. Retina and choroid
    b. Iris and ciliary muscles
    c. Lens and cornea
    d. Aqueous collecting veins and sclera

37. An expanded field of vision with more limited binocular vision would be noted in animals that have:
    a. more laterally placed eyes.
    b. more forward-placed eyes.
    c. a centrally placed eye.

38. When someone asks you what causes eye-shine in animals, you are now able to say that it is due to reflective cells in the inner choroid known as the:
    a. cone.
    b. vitreous body.
    c. ramp retina.
    d. tapetum.

ANSWERS TO SELF EVALUATION—CHAPTER 5

1. a	11. b	21. c	31. a
2. b	12. c	22. a	32. b
3. c	13. a	23. a	33. a
4. b	14. a	24. c	34. b
5. b	15. b	25. a	35. a
6. b	16. a	26. b	36. c
7. a	17. d	27. b	37. a
8. d	18. c	28. c	38. d
9. a	19. b	29. c	
10. c	20. a	30. d	

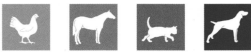

Endocrine System

CHAPTER OUTLINE

- **HORMONES**
  Modes of Transmission
  Biochemistry
- **PITUITARY GLAND**
  Anterior Pituitary
  Anterior Pituitary Hormones
  Posterior Pituitary and Its Hormones
- **THYROID GLAND**
  Thyroid Hormones
- **PARATHYROID GLANDS**
  Parathyroid Hormone and Calcium Ion
    Regulation
- **ADRENAL GLANDS**
  Hormones of the Adrenal Cortex

Glucocorticoid Functions and
  Regulations
Mineralocorticoid Functions and
  Regulation
Hormones of the Adrenal Medulla
- **PANCREATIC GLAND**
  Hormones of the Pancreas
  Control of Insulin and Glucagon
    Secretion
- **PROSTAGLANDINS AND THEIR
  FUNCTIONS**

The endocrine system is considered to be one of the animal body's communication systems, and its products (the hormones) help send messages to other cells. The other communication system is the nervous system, in which nerve networks conduct messages from cells in one part of the body to cells in another part. The nervous system uses physical structures (neurons) to transmit messages (impulses), but the endocrine system uses the body fluids (humors) as its medium to transmit messages (hormones). Because of this, control by the latter system is referred to as humoral control, in contrast to neural control.

The principal function of neural and humoral communication is control or regulation of various body functions. Nerve impulses traveling from the brain to the heart by way of the vagus nerve assist in the control of heart activities. Similarly, thyroid hormones are released from thyroid gland cells and circulated by the blood and interstitial fluids to all cells of the body to assist in the regulation of metabolic rate.

■ HORMONES

1. Are all hormones transported by blood? How does endocrine transmission differ from exocrine transmission?
2. What is an amine hormone? What is a peptide hormone? What is a steroid hormone? Finally, what is the biochemical derivation of the prostaglandins?
3. What is the common precursor of the steroid hormones?

Hormones have been classically defined as chemical substances produced by specialized ductless glands that are released into the blood and carried to other parts of the body to produce specific regulatory effects. Because of this, many substances that seem to have hormone-like activity are considered to be hormones, but are done so with apprehension, because they do not conform to one or more of the criteria in this definition. For example, the prostaglandins are not produced in any one gland of the body, but are produced by most cells of the body. Furthermore, prostaglandins can be transmitted by diffusion in the interstitial fluid rather than by circulation in the blood.

Therefore, it seems best to consider the hormones as chemical regulators and to recognize that they can be produced by cells with a specific location in a particular gland or by cells diffusely located in many parts of the body.

Modes of Transmission

The concept of the restriction of hormone transmission to blood circulation only must be abandoned and recognition given to other means of transmission. These are classified as epicrine, neurocrine, paracrine, endocrine, and exocrine transmission.

Epicrine Transmission

In **epicrine transmission**, hormones pass through gap junctions of adjacent cells without entering extracellular fluid.

Neurocrine Transmission

In **neurocrine transmission**, hormones diffuse through synaptic clefts between neurons, as do neurotransmitters. Also, the hormone (such as oxytocin) can be synthesized in the neuron cell body, stored in axons (like neurotransmitters), but can be secreted into the blood.

Paracrine Transmission

In **paracrine transmission**, hormones diffuse through interstitial fluid, as do prostaglandins.

Endocrine Transmission

In **endocrine transmission**, hormones are transported through the blood circulation. This is typical of most hormones.

Exocrine Transmission

In **exocrine transmission**, the regulatory agent (hormone) is secreted to the exterior of the body. The lumen of the intestine is considered to be exterior to the body, so that hormones secreted into it can affect cell activity more distal to the point of secretion. Some hormones, such as somatostatin, can have exocrine transmission (secretion to intestinal lumen), and subsequently act as inhibitors of many gastrointestinal functions, including intestinal motility and intestinal absorption. Inasmuch as pheromones are chemical communicators, they might be considered to have exocrine transmission because they are received by other animals of the same species (through olfaction) after they have been excreted to the exterior of the body.

Biochemistry

Under the classic definition, hormones are biochemically categorized as amines, peptides, or steroids. The **amine hormones** include thyroid hormone and the adrenal catecholamines, epinephrine and norepinephrine. All of the amine hormones are derived from the amino acid **tyrosine**. The **peptide hormones** include peptides, polypeptides, and proteins. All of the hormones of the hypothalamus and pituitary, as well as insulin and glucagon from the pancreas, are included in the peptide class. The **steroid hormones** include the adrenocortical and reproductive gland hormones and the active metabolites of vitamin D. Cholesterol is the common precursor of steroid hormones. The **prostaglandins** (not classic hormones) are derived from arachidonic acid (a fatty acid). More structural detail is provided in this chapter when some hormones of specific endocrine glands or other tissues are discussed.

■ PITUITARY GLAND

1. What is the hypophysioportal circulation? What is its function?
2. What are the abbreviated names of the anterior pituitary hormones?
3. Briefly list the functions of each of the anterior pituitary hormones. Is STH

needed throughout life or only during the growth phase?

4. What is meant by posterior pituitary hormones being known as neuro secretions?

5. Briefly list the functions for the posterior pituitary hormones.

The **pituitary gland** (hypophysis cerebri) has two distinct parts, the **anterior lobe** (anterior pituitary; **adenohypophysis**) and the posterior lobe (posterior pituitary; **neurohypophysis**). It is located in a bony recess (sella turcica) at the base of the brain. The divisions, blood supply, and neural connections to the hypothalamus are shown in *Figure 6-1*. Its location just below the hypothalamus provides for direct delivery of releasing and inhibiting hormones from the hypothalamus to the anterior lobe and for direct entry of secretory neurons from the hypothalamus to the posterior lobe. Assisting the delivery of hormones to the anterior lobe is a unique arrangement of blood vessels, the **hypophysioportal circulation** (see Fig. 6-1). Similar to other blood

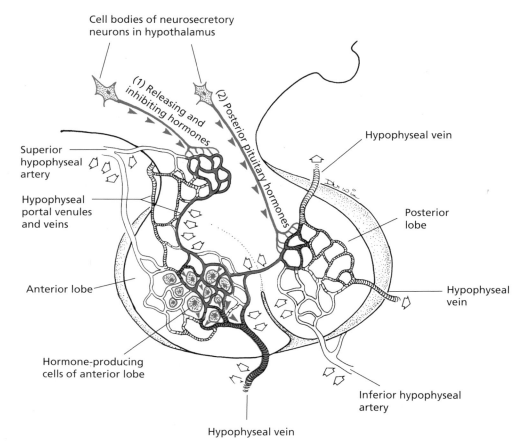

■ **FIGURE 6-1** Schematic representation of the pituitary gland and its hypophysioportal circulation. Hypothalamic releasing and inhibiting hormones **(1)** reach anterior pituitary cells by way of this circulation (left). Posterior pituitary hormones **(2)** enter capillaries of the posterior pituitary (right). Open arrows indicate direction of blood flow; arrowheads indicate direction of hormone transport toward axon terminals. (From Cormack DH. Essential Histology. 2nd Ed. Baltimore: Lippincott Williams & Wilkins, 2001.)

portal systems, the venous blood drained from the hypothalamus is redistributed by another capillary system within the anterior lobe. Shortages of hormones in arterial blood are detected by specific cells within the hypothalamus, which are stimulated to secrete releasing hormones. The hormones produced are distributed by the second capillary bed to their appropriate cells in the anterior lobe.

Anterior Pituitary

The anterior pituitary lies forward from the posterior pituitary and has five different cell types that secrete the seven hormones of the anterior pituitary: 1) **somatotrope cells**, which secrete growth hormone; 2) **corticotrope cells**, which secrete adrenocorticotropic hormone and beta-lipotropin hormone; 3) **mammotrope cells**, which secrete prolactin; 4) **thyrotrope cells**, which secrete thyroid stimulating hormone; and 5) **gonadotrope cells**, which secrete follicle-stimulating hormone and luteinizing hormone.

Because of the relatively large number of important hormones associated with the pituitary gland, it is sometimes called the master gland. Pharmaceutical companies obtain animal pituitary glands from slaughter houses and extract several hormones for commercial and experimental uses. Recovery of the pituitary gland at slaughter is laborious because of its protected location, and yields are low (340 g/100 cattle; 30 g/100 pigs) because of its small size.

Anterior Pituitary Hormones

The hormones of the anterior pituitary belong to the **peptide class**, ranging from polypeptides to large proteins. Differences in structure are noted among species, and replacement therapy from one species to another is not uniformly successful. Sometimes an active core of a hormone is identified that permits its subsequent use after the noncore portion is removed.

Growth Hormone

Growth hormone is also known as **somatotropic hormone (STH)** because of its stimulating effect on the somatic cells (body cells). It has invariably been referred to as growth hormone because of its stimulation of increase in body size. It causes growth of all tissues of the body that are capable of growth, and it promotes both increased cell size and increased mitosis with development of increased cell numbers. The epiphyseal plates of long bones are particularly sensitive to growth hormone; it stimulates mitotic activity, which results in lengthening. Growth hormone stimulates the liver to form several small proteins called **somatomedins**, which then act on cartilage and bone to promote their growth. Bone and cartilage are therefore not stimulated directly by growth hormone, but indirectly by this intermediate compound.

In addition to its general effect of causing growth, STH has several specific metabolic effects. Because of these, it is apparent that STH is needed throughout life and not only during the growth phase. These metabolic effects include: 1) increased rate of protein synthesis in all body cells, 2) increased mobilization of fatty acids from fat and increased use of fatty acids for energy, and 3) decreased rate of glucose uptake throughout the body. The preferential use of fats for energy conserves glucose and promotes glycogen storage. Because of glycogen storage, the heart can endure emergency contraction more effectively, whereby glycogen stored in the heart is converted to glucose. Probably most metabolic functions of growth hormone are caused not by its direct effects on the tissues, but by indirect effects through the somatomedins.

An effect of growth hormone in increasing milk yields in the lactating cow has received considerable research interest. Growth hormone does not produce its effects by stimulation of the mammary gland, but rather, it seems that the increased milk yield caused by continuous injections of exogenous STH is caused by the partitioning of available nutrients from body tissues toward milk synthesis.

Adrenocorticotropic Hormone

Adrenocorticotropic hormone (ACTH) causes increased activity of the adrenal cortex. It was formerly thought that ACTH only stimulated the secretion of glucocorticoids by the adrenal cortex, but it is now recognized that mineralo-corticoid (aldosterone) secretion is also enhanced. In addition, it has become apparent that ACTH has metabolic effects somewhat similar to those of STH, in which protein synthesis and fatty acid uptake are enhanced and glucose uptake is decreased.

Thyroid-Stimulating Hormone

Thyroid-stimulating hormone (TSH) stimulates the synthesis of colloid by thyroid gland cells and stimulates the release of thyroid hormone. Associated with these functions are the accumulation of iodine, organic binding of iodine, and formation of thyroxine within the thyroid gland. No extrathyroid activity is apparent for TSH, as for STH and ACTH.

Gonadotropic Hormones and Prolactin

The **gonadotropic hormones**, follicle-stimulating hormone (**FSH**) and luteinizing hormone (**LH**), have specific roles in male and female reproduction, and detailed accounts are provided in Chapter 14 (Male Reproduction) and Chapter 15 (Female Reproduction). Specifically, FSH stimulates oogenesis and spermatogenesis in the female and male, respectively. In the female, LH assists ovulation and development of a functioning corpus luteum, and in the male it stimulates the secretion of testosterone. Prolactin helps to initiate and maintain lactation after pregnancy. Also, in the ewe, it is associated with maintenance of the corpus luteum.

Beta-Lipoprotein Hormone

Beta-lipoprotein hormone (β-LPH) is secreted by the same cells (corticotrope) that secrete ACTH (see previous text). The physiologic role of β-LPH is still unknown. Products providing pain relief (e.g., endogenous opiates, which are the endorphins and enkephalins) might be derived from β-LPH. Inasmuch as they are associated with ACTH (same secreting cells), the response to stress might include β-LPH secretion and pain relief as a neural response.

Posterior Pituitary and Its Hormones

The posterior lobe is an outgrowth of the hypothalamus (see Fig. 6-1) and contains the terminal axons from two pairs of nuclei (supraoptic nucleus and paraventricular nucleus) located in the hypothalamus. The **supraoptic** and **paraventricular nuclei** synthesize antidiuretic hormone and oxytocin (neurosecretions), respectively, which are transported to the axon terminals in the posterior pituitary, where they are stored in secretory granules until released. An action potential, generated by the need for each of the stored hormones, causes the release of the hormone and subsequent absorption into the blood, where it is distributed to the receptor cells. The hormones of the posterior pituitary are of the peptide class, specifically **nonapeptides** (they contain nine amino acids).

Antidiuretic Hormone

When an animal is given an overload of water, a period of **diuresis** (increased output of dilute urine) occurs. Diuresis can be prevented by the administration of **antidiuretic hormone (ADH)**, also known as **vasopressin**. If dehydration occurs (osmoconcentration), osmoreceptors respond to the increased concentration by stimulating greater output of ADH by the axon terminals in the posterior pituitary. The target cells of the secreted ADH are the collecting tubules and the collecting ducts of the kidney. The presence of ADH renders the cells of the collecting tubules and collecting ducts more permeable to water, and more water is absorbed from the tubular fluid so that the plasma osmolality decreases (Na^+ concentration returns to normal) and the urine volume decreases (becomes more concentrated). ADH is therefore important for water conservation by animals. Other stimulators of ADH secretion include reduced blood volume, trauma, pain, and anxiety.

Oxytocin

The functional activity of **oxytocin** is related to the reproductive processes, which include lactation (see Chapter 16). Oxytocin is released from the posterior pituitary as a result of neuroendocrine reflexes. The act of suckling or similar teat stimulation causes release of oxytocin and subsequent milk letdown. Similarly, an estrogen-dominated myometrium, such as is found at ovulation and at parturition, is more responsive to oxytocin, and greater contraction of the uterus results. Oxytocin release at these times is associated with appropriate stimuli and subsequent myometrial contraction, which assists in the transport of sperm to the oviduct at copulation and in the expulsion of the fetus at parturition.

■ THYROID GLAND

1. What is the substance that fills the thyroid follicles?
2. Sketch the thyroxine molecule, and note the presence of iodine. How does T_3 differ from T_4?
3. What is thyroglobulin? How are T_3 and T_4 stored in the thyroid gland after their formation? Describe the release and absorption of T_3 and T_4 from the thyroid follicles.
4. What fraction of thyroid hormone release from the thyroid gland is T_4?
5. Describe the plasma transport, release, and cell use characteristics of T_3 and T_4.
6. What is the most well-known function of the thyroid hormones?
7. Note how low levels of thyroid hormones cause the secretion of the thyroid hormones.

8. What is calcitonin? Where is it secreted? Is it secreted in response to hypercalcemia or hypocalcemia? What, then, is its function?

In most mammals the thyroid gland is located on the trachea, just caudal to the larynx. In cattle it consists of two laterally placed, somewhat flattened lobes joined by an isthmus (*Fig. 6-2*). The lateral lobes have a less substantial isthmus in the horse and no isthmus in the dog and cat. Pigs have a compact thyroid form with a large median lobe (instead of an isthmus) in addition to the lateral lobes. The **thyroid gland** is composed of numerous **follicles** (*Fig. 6-3*) lined by simple cuboidal epithelial cells and filled with a fluid known as colloid. The surface area of the lining epithelium is increased by villi that project into the follicle.

Thyroid Hormones

The **thyroid hormones** belong to the **amine classification** of hormones—they are derived from the amino acid **tyrosine**. A further characteristic of the thyroid hormones is that they contain iodine. **Iodine** is bound organically in the thyroid gland in four forms. The thyroid hormones, 3,5,3′,5′-tetraiodothyronine (thyroxine [T_4]), and 3,5,3′-triiodothyronine (T_3) (*Fig. 6-4*), are combinations of two molecules of 3,5-diiodotyrosine, as in T_4, or one molecule of 3-monoiodotyrosine with one molecule of 3,5-diiodotyrosine, as in T_3. In both cases the combination results in the loss of one water molecule and an amino acid residue, glycine. Iodine trapping and iodination are unique features of the thyroid gland that are assisted by TSH.

Biochemistry of T_3 and T_4 Formation

Thyroglobulin is a large glycoprotein molecule secreted into the follicle by the lining cells. Thyroglobulin has a molecular weight of about 680,000. It contains many tyrosine molecules; when iodinated, they consist of both 3-monoiodotyrosine and 3,5-diiodotyrosine.

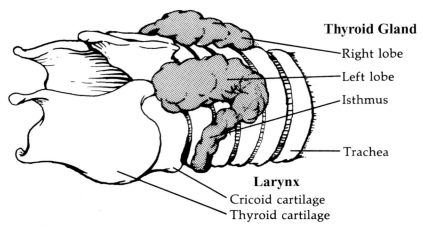

Thyroid Gland
Right lobe
Left lobe
Isthmus

Trachea

Larynx
Cricoid cartilage
Thyroid cartilage

■ **FIGURE 6-2** Thyroid gland (bovine).

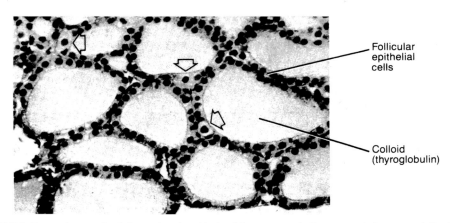

Follicular
epithelial
cells

Colloid
(thyroglobulin)

■ **FIGURE 6-3** Photomicrograph of the canine thyroid gland (lower power). The arrows indicate parafollicular cells (C cells that secrete calcitonin); the remainder are follicular cells. (From Cormack DH. Ham's Histology. 9th Ed. Philadelphia: JB Lippincott, 1987.

Tyrosine coupling occurs while the tyrosine residues are still attached to the thyroglobulin molecule. The lining cells of the follicles provide the enzymes required for coupling to form T_3 and T_4. The coupled tyrosines, still attached to the thyroglobulin molecule, are stored after synthesis within the follicle.

Release and Transport of T_3 and T_4

The thyroglobulin molecule, with enclosed T_3 and T_4, is not released into the blood from the thyroid follicles. Extensions from the follicle cells enclose parts of colloid so that colloid becomes a vesicle within the cell (endocytosis). Lysosomes release proteolytic enzymes that separate T_3 and T_4 from thyroglobulin and permit their absorption from the base of the cells. The 3-monoiodotyrosine and 3,5-diiodotyrosine freed similarly by digestion are not absorbed, but are deiodinated, and both the iodine and the tyrosine are recycled into new thyroglobulin. About 90% of thyroid hormone released is T_4.

A low plasma Ca^{2+} concentration stimulates secretion of PTH from the parathyroid gland, whereas hypercalcemia inhibits PTH secretion. A less effective stimulator of PTH secretion is hypomagnesemia.

Calcium and phosphorus are absorbed from bone under the influence of PTH by two processes. The most rapid means by which PTH increases the plasma Ca^{2+} concentration is called **osteolysis**; it involves osteoblasts and osteocytes (see Chapter 7). These cells are normally involved in calcium and phosphorus deposition, but in osteolysis they are involved in absorption. PTH inhibits osteoblast synthesis of new bone but increases osteoblast-initiated recruitment of osteocytes to transport calcium and phosphorus from the bone fluid to the extracellular fluid. In this instance absorption of Ca^{2+} and phosphorus occurs without loss of bone matrix. However, PTH also increases osteoblast-initiated recruitment of **osteoclasts (bone dissolvers)**. In contrast to osteolysis, osteoclastic activity causes loss of bone matrix and, over a period of time, excavations are visible. Osteolysis is considered to be the rapid phase of calcium and phosphate absorption, and activation of osteoclasts is considered to be the slow phase of bone absorption and calcium phosphate release.

Action of PTH on the Kidneys

PTH increases plasma Ca^{2+} concentration, but its action would be ineffective if a change did not occur in the kidneys to increase Ca^{2+} absorption from tubular fluid. This change is brought about by PTH. At the same time, phosphate reabsorption by the kidney diminishes. This change is also affected by PTH, and the calcium to phosphorus ratio of approximately $2:1$ in plasma is maintained.

PTH and 1,25-dihydroxycholecalciferol Formation

Parathyroid hormone greatly enhances both calcium and phosphate absorption from the intestines by increasing the rate of formation of 1,25-dihydroxycholecalciferol, known as **calcitriol**, the active form of vitamin D. The original forms of vitamin D, whether from the diet or by action of ultraviolet light on skin precursors, are converted through a succession of reactions in the liver and kidney. The first conversions occur in the liver and the final conversion to calcitriol occurs in the kidney under the influence of PTH. In the intestinal epithelium, calcitriol causes the formation of a calcium-binding protein that functions at the brush border to transport calcium into the cell cytoplasm. Calcium-binding protein remains in the cells for several weeks, providing a prolonged effect on calcium absorption.

Enhancement of intestinal phosphate absorption might result from the direct effect of calcitriol, but it could be a secondary result of the hormone's action on calcium absorption, in which calcium acts as a transport mediator for phosphate.

■ ADRENAL GLANDS

1. Where are the adrenal glands located?
2. What are the two principal hormones of the adrenal cortex? What is their biochemical classification?
3. What is the role of the glucocorticoids in carbohydrate metabolism? What is the main noncarbohydrate source of new glucose formation?
4. Do glucocorticoids have some mineralocorticoid activity?
5. What is the principal function of the mineralocorticoids? Do they possess some glucocorticoid activity?
6. What regulates the secretion of the glucocorticoids?
7. What are the processes by which aldosterone secretion increases?
8. What are the hormones of the adrenal medulla?
9. What is the biochemical classification for epinephrine and norepinephrine? Are they also considered catecholamines?

10. What division of the autonomic nervous system secretes norepinephrine? Is it a postganglionic or preganglionic secretion?

The **adrenal glands** are small, paired structures that lie immediately cranial to the kidneys and are close to the junction of the renal vein with the posterior vena cava (*Fig. 6-5*). A sagittal section of the adrenal gland (*Fig. 6-6*) shows an outer cortex and an inner medulla. The **adrenal cortex** has three distinct cell types: arranged in zones from the outside to the inside, the zona glomerulosa, zona fasciculata, and zona reticularis. The **adrenal medulla** is homogeneous in structure and contains secretory granules. Its nerve supply is by way of preganglionic sympathetic neurons. The cells of the medulla are thought to be modified postganglionic sympathetic nerve cell bodies.

Hormones of the Adrenal Cortex

The hormones of the adrenal cortex are steroids formed mainly from cholesterol. The membrane of the adrenal cortex has receptors for low-density lipoproteins (rich in cholesterol) and, after their attachment, these are absorbed by endocytosis. Seven adrenocortical hormones (corticosteroids) are recognized as secretions of the adrenal cortex. Four of these—corticosterone, cortisol, cortisone, and 11-dehydrocorticosterone—are termed **glucocorticoids**. The other three—11-deoxycorticosterone, 17-hydroxy-11-deoxycorticosterone, and aldosterone—are called mineralocorticoids. The structural formulas of the two principal adrenocortical steroids (**aldosterone** and **cortisol**) are presented in *Figure 6-7*.

Glucocorticoid Functions and Regulations

The **glucocorticoids** have a principal role in carbohydrate metabolism in that they enhance **gluconeogenesis**. The noncarbohydrate source from which new glucose is synthesized is mostly protein, but a definite affect on fat metabolism is also recognized. Two other hormones, **glucagon** and **epinephrine**, increase blood glucose levels by glycolysis of liver

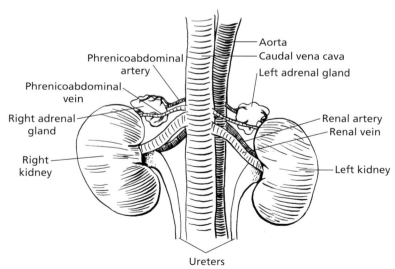

■ FIGURE 6-5 The canine adrenal glands (ventral view). Their blood supply and venous drainage is by way of branches from the phrenicoabdominal arteries and veins.

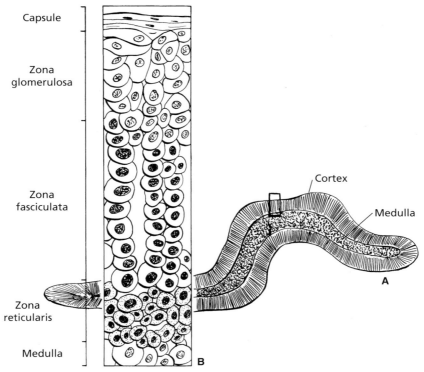

■ **FIGURE 6-6** Diagrammatic representation of the adrenal gland. **A)** Cross-section of the adrenal gland showing the contrasting appearance of the cortex and medulla. **B)** Magnification of boxed-in area in A that shows the different cell types associated with the three zones of the cortex.

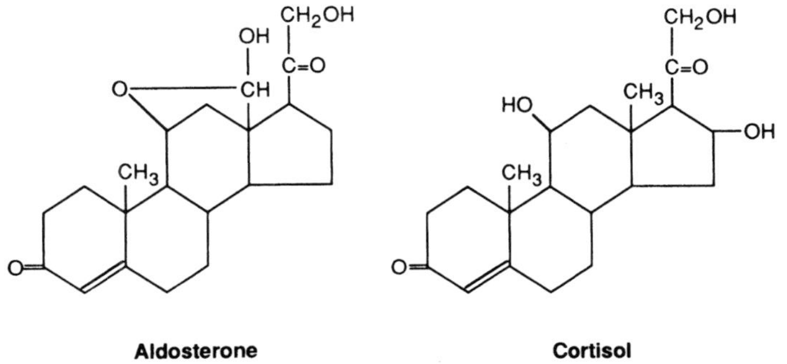

Aldosterone

Cortisol

■ **FIGURE 6-7** Structural formulas of the principal adrenocortical hormones.

glycogen. The glucocorticoids, however, seem to be necessary for glycolysis affected by glucagon and epinephrine. The gluconeogenic effect of the glucocorticoids is the basis for their use in the treatment of bovine ketosis (see Chapter 12).

A common therapeutic use of the glucocorticoids is related to their anti-inflammatory activity, and they are included in ophthalmic preparations, otic (ear) drops, and skin ointments. Injection of glucocorticoids into inflamed articulations or bursae provides temporary relief, and their systemic use is sometimes useful in the alleviation of some allergic responses. Prolonged systemic use is often associated with exaggeration of other physiologic functions of the glucocorticoids, such as sodium retention related to their having some mineralocorticoid activity (retention of Na^+ and H_2O). More potent pharmacologic preparations (which require smaller doses) can minimize these side effects, but do not eliminate them altogether.

The glucocorticoids are secreted by the zona fasciculata of the adrenal cortex. Their secretion is regulated by ACTH from the anterior pituitary. Free plasma cortisol (not protein-bound) concentrations influence ACTH secretion—low levels stimulate ACTH release and subsequent secretion of glucocorticoids from the zona fascicularis. Stimuli such as stress can also cause ACTH secretion that increases glucocorticoid concentrations above normal levels. An example of an adrenal response to adaptation can be seen with the overcrowding of domestic chickens whereby excess ACTH secretion results in adrenal hypertrophy because of greater output of glucocorticoids. The same phenomenon is observed in wild mammals whose population density increases.

Mineralocorticoid Functions and Regulation

The principal function of the **mineralocorticoids** can be illustrated by **aldosterone** and its action on the kidney to enhance sodium reabsorption and potassium excretion (see Chapter 11). The mineralocorticoids are also effective in promoting membrane transport in sweat glands, salivary glands, and intestinal mucosa, and between the intracellular and extracellular fluid compartments. Just as glucocorticoids

have some mineralocorticoid activity, the mineralocorticoids have some glucocorticoid activity. These secondary activities are most apparent when therapeutic uses are made of these compounds and the amounts used are in excess of normal endogenous amounts.

Three processes are usually considered to be the means by which aldosterone secretion from the zona glomerulosa increases: 1) renin–angiotensin system; 2) increased plasma concentration of potassium (hyperkalemia); and 3) ACTH stimulation. In the renin–angiotensin system (see Chapter 11), renin is secreted by juxtaglomerular cells in the kidney in response to their decreased perfusion by blood. Renin acts on a circulating blood globulin, angiotensinogen, to form angiotensin I. Angiotensin I is converted by the vascular endothelium to angiotensin II, which is the stimulus for the secretion of aldosterone from the zona glomerulosa. The result of this stimulation is promotion of Na^+ reabsorption and consequent retention of water, which expands blood volume and thus reestablishes normal blood pressure (low blood pressure was the cause for renin secretion). Systemically, angiotensin II causes arteriolar vasoconstriction, which increases vascular resistance and elevates systemic blood pressure.

The secretion of aldosterone in response to hyperkalemia provides a means for controlling the critical plasma concentration of potassium (see Chapter 11). Aldosterone secretion promotes Na^+ reabsorption with simultaneous K^+ excretion. This action of aldosterone occurs in the distal tubule, collecting tubule, and collecting duct. At other places in the nephron, K^+ is reabsorbed. Although Na^+ is reabsorbed in the process of K^+ excretion, the Na^+ concentration in the plasma is not regulated by aldosterone. Plasma Na^+ concentration decreases can cause aldosterone secretion, but the decreases necessary for stimulation are of greater magnitude than the effective increases of K^+ that cause aldosterone secretion.

The role of ACTH in promoting aldosterone secretion is of lesser significance. The increase in ACTH associated with stress causes some increased output of aldosterone and might augment the output produced by other means, such as angiotensin II.

Hormones of the Adrenal Medulla

The hormones of the adrenal medulla belong to the **amine chemical class** and are known as **epinephrine (adrenaline)** and **norepinephrine (noradrenaline)**. They are referred to as **catecholamines** and are derived from the amino acid tyrosine. The catecholamine hormones (including epinephrine and norepinephrine) are shown in *Figure 6-8*. Epinephrine is secreted only by the adrenal medulla, but nor-

epinephrine is also secreted by postganglionic sympathetic neurons. More epinephrine is secreted by the adrenal medulla than norepinephrine. The inactivation of the catecholamines is rapid—the half-life of epinephrine is about 20 to 40 seconds.

It seems that the adrenal medullary secretion is a continuous process, and it increases dramatically during an emergency. The continuous secretion enables the maintenance of a state of readiness or tone, and the larger outpouring provides for an immediate response to emergencies.

The actions of epinephrine and norepinephrine are similar and differences are expressed depending on the receptors, which

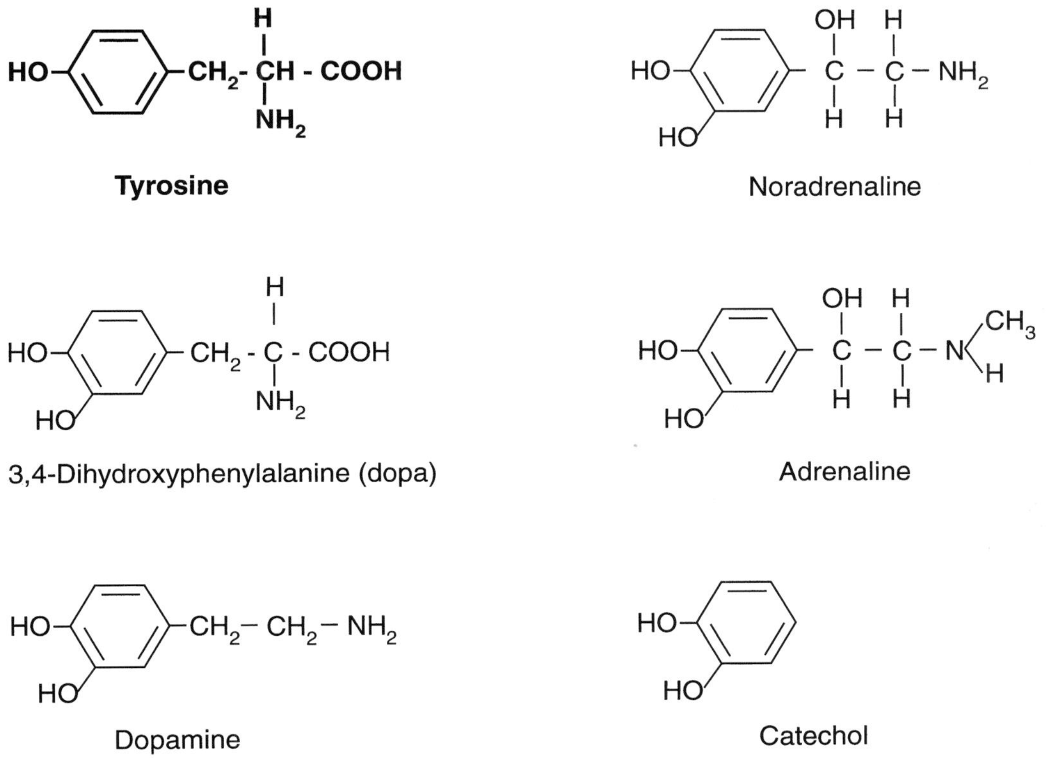

■ **FIGURE 6-8** Structural formulas of catecholamine hormones. They are formed from the amino acid tyrosine and are derivatives of catechol. The abbreviation "dopa" is derived from the German name of this compound, dioxyphenylalanine.

can have a preference for epinephrine or norepinephrine (see Chapter 4). The two adrenergic receptors are alpha and beta receptors. **Alpha receptors** are stimulatory (except in intestinal smooth muscle, where they are inhibitory), and **beta receptors** are inhibitory (except those in cardiac muscle, where they are stimulatory). Epinephrine and norepinephrine stimulate both receptors, but the alpha effect of norepinephrine is more potent than that of epinephrine, and epinephrine has a more potent action than norepinephrine on the beta receptors.

In addition to the "fight-fright-flight" reactions associated with the catecholamines, they have pronounced metabolic effects. These are associated with the increased activity caused by catecholamines and include hyperglycemia, increased calorigenesis, lipolysis, and an elevated blood lactate concentration. The hyperglycemia results from enhanced liver glycogenolysis, and the increased blood lactate level is caused by stimulation of muscle glycogenolysis. The calorigenic effect results from the increased muscle activity and an increase in lactic acid oxidation in the liver.

■ PANCREATIC GLAND

1. **Delineate the endocrine and exocrine functions of the pancreas.**
2. **What are the four pancreatic hormones? Briefly describe the functions of each (providing that they are known).**
3. **What are the pancreatic islets?**
4. **Does insulin activity increase or decrease blood glucose concentration?**
5. **How does glucagon increase blood glucose?**

The pancreas has both exocrine and endocrine functions. The exocrine functions are those associated with digestion and include digestive enzyme and bicarbonate secretion.

Hormones of the Pancreas

The hormones of the pancreas are **insulin**, **glucagon**, **somatostatin**, and **pancreatic polypeptide**. They are secreted by specific cells located in islets scattered throughout the pancreas. Four major types of cells are found in the islets, each responsible for the secretion of one hormone. The cells are identified as alpha cells (glucagon), beta cells (insulin), delta cells (somatostatin), and F cells (pancreatic polypeptide). The pancreatic hormones are polypeptides.

Insulin

The tissues differ in regard to their sensitivity to insulin. Whereas the liver, muscle, adipose tissue, and leukocytes respond readily to insulin, the brain, kidney, intestines, and erythrocytes show little response. The principal effect of insulin on carbohydrate metabolism in those tissues sensitive to insulin (except the liver) is to allow the transport of glucose across the cell membrane (see Chapter 11). In these tissues, insulin enhances facilitated diffusion. In the liver, insulin enhances glucose uptake by stimulating enzymes in the liver cells that assist in the production of glycogen and lipogenesis and by inhibiting enzymes that catalyze glycogenolysis. Generally, insulin promotes fat deposition and protein synthesis. The result of **insulin activity** is **lowering of the blood glucose concentration**.

Glucagon

The result of **glucagon activity** is **elevation of the blood glucose concentration**. This is achieved by the activation of adenylcyclase in liver cells, which in turn stimulates phosphorylase and results in the breakdown of glycogen. In addition, glucagon increases gluconeogenesis, increases metabolic rate, and stimulates lipolysis. Another action of glucagon is stimulation of the secretion of insulin (so that the new glucose can diffuse into cells) and of somatostatin.

Somatostatin

Somatostatin usually seems to act as an **inhibitory agent** to slow the output of nutrients into the circulation and to moderate the metabolic effects of insulin, glucagon, and growth hormone. In this regard, somatostatin inhibits the secretion of insulin and glucagon. Also, as a moderator, it inhibits the secretion of gastrin, secretin, cholecystokinin, pancreatic exocrine secretion, and gastric acid. Somatostatin also moderates gastrointestinal motility and the absorption of glucose.

Pancreatic Polypeptide

Pancreatic polypeptide secretion is stimulated by the ingestion of protein, by exercise, and by fasting. No definite function has been established for pancreatic polypeptide.

Control of Insulin and Glucagon Secretion

The secretion of insulin and glucagon is controlled directly by the blood glucose concentration. Because of the dual control (insulin decreases, glucagon increases) of glucose concentration, blood levels show little variation.

Important stimulatory effects on insulin secretion are caused by the gastrointestinal hormones, gastrin, secretin, cholecystokinin, and other hormones. The gastrointestinal hormones are secreted in response to food ingestion and actually cause insulin to be secreted before glucose absorption. Insulin secretion is also stimulated by pancreatic glucagon (see previous text).

Glucagon secretion is stimulated by hypoglycemia, gastrin, cholecystokinin, and stress and is inhibited by glucose, secretin, insulin, and somatostatin.

Somatostatin release is enhanced by almost every factor that increases insulin secretion.

■ PROSTAGLANDINS AND THEIR FUNCTIONS

1. How did the prostaglandins get their name?
2. What is the range of tissues associated with prostaglandin production?
3. Do prostaglandins promote or inhibit inflammation?
4. Do prostaglandins promote or inhibit blood coagulation?
5. Could aspirin use interfere with inflammation and blood coagulation?

The prostaglandins were first isolated from accessory sex gland fluids and were termed prostaglandins because of their association with the prostate gland. It is now recognized that they are secreted by almost all body tissues and, indeed, the prostate gland association is too narrow a definition.

The **prostaglandins** are derived from **arachidonic acid**. Their structure and synthesis are shown in *Figure 6-9*. The prostaglandins are usually short acting. Some forms never appear in the blood (so some have not been classified as hormones), and others are degraded after they circulate throughout the liver and lungs.

The functions of prostaglandins have been studied most in regard to their role in the reproductive process. Prostaglandin $F_{2\alpha}$ ($PGF_{2\alpha}$) is the natural luteolytic agent that terminates the luteal phase of the estrous cycle and allows for the initiation of a new estrous cycle in the absence of fertilization (see Chapter 15). $PGF_{2\alpha}$ is also particularly potent in terminating early pregnancy.

The prostaglandins promote inflammation. The antiinflammatory activity of aspirin (and perhaps of other drugs) is a result of its ability to inhibit the synthesis of prostaglandin G_2 (PGG_2) from arachidonic acid. The anti-inflammatory action of the glucocorticoids might also be caused by interference with prostaglandin synthesis. Other

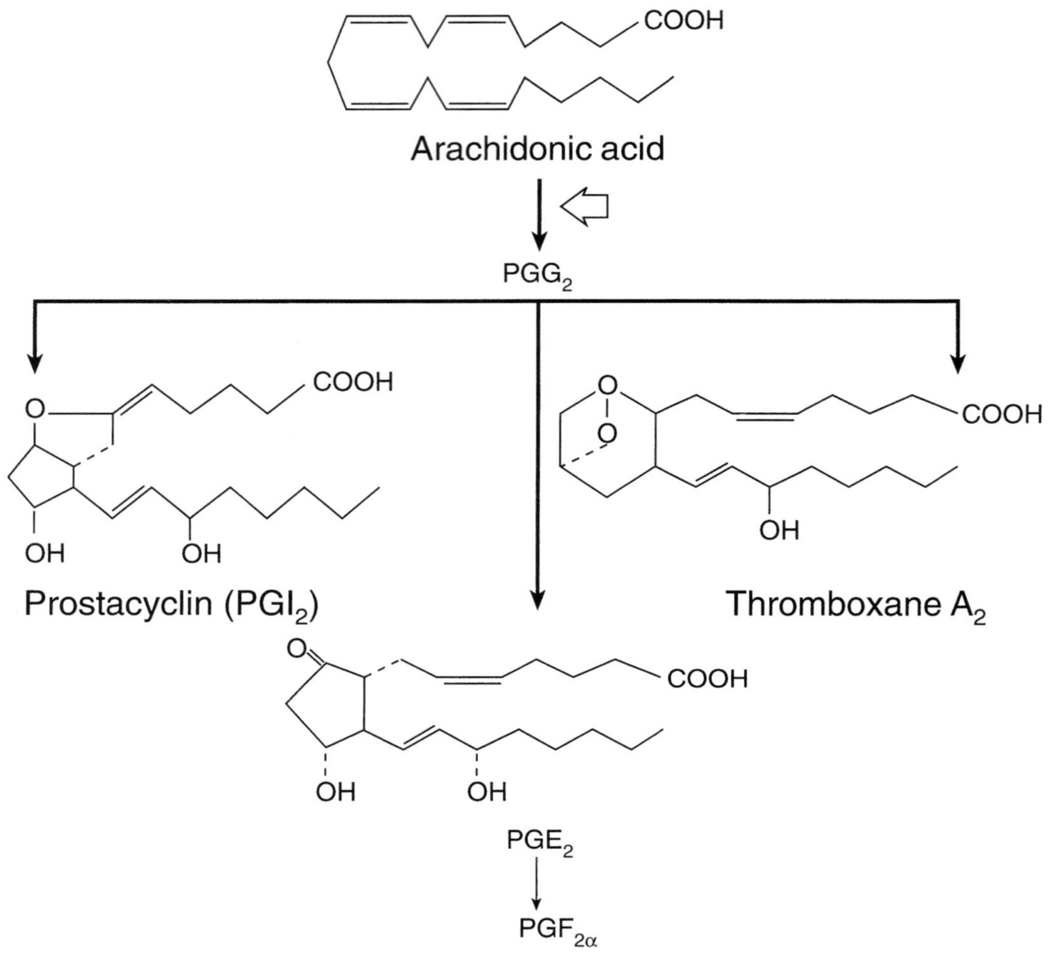

FIGURE 6-9 Three major pathways of prostaglandin synthesis. The open arrow indicates the site of aspirin inhibition. Thromboxane A_2 is biochemically related to the prostaglandins and is formed from them as shown. Thromboxane A_2 promotes the platelet release reaction associated with blood coagulation. Therefore, aspirin retards blood coagulation.

functions of some prostaglandins include inhibition of gastric secretion and relaxation of bronchial smooth muscle. One prostaglandin (prostacyclin, PGI_2) that is produced in the endothelium of blood vessels inhibits platelet aggregation (essential for blood coagulation), and a prostaglandin derivative (thromboxane A_2) favors platelet aggregation (see Chapter 3).

■ SUGGESTED READING

Cormack DH. Essential Histology. 2nd Ed. Baltimore: Lippincott Williams & Wilkins, 2001.

Eiler H. Endocrine glands. In: Reece WO, ed. Dukes' Physiology of Domestic Animals. 12th Ed. Ithaca, NY: Cornell University Press, 2004.

Frandson RD, Wilke WL, Fails AD. Anatomy and Physiology of Domestic Animals. 6th Ed. Baltimore: Lippincott Williams & Wilkins, 2003.

SELF EVALUATION—CHAPTER 6

HORMONES

1. Cholesterol and arachidonic acid are the respective precursors of:
   a. amino and peptide hormones.
   b. steroid and prostaglandin hormones.
   c. prostaglandin and steroid hormones.
   d. peptide and amine hormones.

2. What is the transmission classification for pheromones?
   a. Epicrine
   b. Endocrine
   c. Paracrine
   d. Exocrine

PITUITARY GLAND

3. The anterior pituitary hormone that causes growth of all body tissues that can grow and that also has several metabolic effects is:
   a. somatotropic hormone.
   b. adrenocorticotropic hormone.
   c. thyroid-stimulating hormone.
   d. gonadotropic hormone.

4. Which one of the following hormones is a neurosecretion of the posterior pituitary?
   a. Adrenocorticotropic hormone
   b. Antidiuretic hormone
   c. Epinephrine
   d. Somatotropic hormone

THYROID GLAND

5. Thyroxine (T_4) and T_3 are produced in the:
   a. thyroid follicle.
   b. epithelial cells, which line the thyroid follicles.
   c. anterior pituitary.
   d. blood after the components have been secreted by the thyroid epithelial cells.

6. Iodine is a part of which one of the following hormones?
   a. Growth hormone
   b. Hydrocortisone
   c. Parathyroid hormone
   d. Thyroxine

7. Which one of the following hormones is released in response to cooling of the anterior hypothalamus?
   a. Antidiuretic hormone
   b. Insulin
   c. T_4 and T_3 (thyroid hormones)
   d. Aldosterone

PARATHYROID GLANDS

8. Parathyroid hormone increases the absorption of calcium from the intestinal tract by its action on:
   a. intestinal epithelial cells.
   b. bone cells.
   c. the kidney to activate Vitamin D.
   d. cholesterol to form Vitamin D.

9. Plasma [Ca^{2+}] is decreased by:
   a. calcitonin.
   b. parathyroid hormone.
   c. 1,25-dihydroxycholecalciferol.
   d. cortisol.

ADRENAL GLANDS

10. The action of which one of the following would provide for gluconeogenesis (production of new glucose)?
    a. Growth hormone
    b. Norepinephrine
    c. Aldosterone
    d. Adrenocorticotropic hormone

11. The hormone that indirectly influences water reabsorption by the kidneys is:
    a. oxytocin.
    b. aldosterone.

    c. antidiuretic hormone.

    d. insulin.

12. The mineralocorticoids influence the plasma concentrations of:

    a. calcium and phosphorus.

    b. sodium and potassium.

    c. calcium and sodium.

    d. potassium and calcium.

13. Epinephrine and norepinephrine seem to be continuous secretions of the adrenal medulla with dramatic increases during an emergency.

    a. True

    b. False

PANCREATIC GLAND

14. What pancreatic function is associated with the secretion of insulin, glucagon, somatostatin, and pancreatic polypeptide?

    a. Endocrine

    b. Exocrine

15. Blood glucose concentration is decreased by the secretion of:

    a. glucagon.

    b. pancreatic polypeptide.

    c. insulin.

    d. glucocorticoids.

PROSTAGLANDINS AND THEIR FUNCTIONS

16. Aspirin use is associated with its ability to be anti-inflammatory and also to inhibit platelet aggregation that enhances blood coagulation. These characteristics are mediated through:

    a. specific prostaglandins.

    b. glucocorticoids.

    c. a thyroid hormone.

    d. beta-lipoprotein hormone.

ANSWERS TO SELF EVALUATION—CHAPTER 6

1. b	5. a	9. a	13. a
2. d	6. d	10. d	14. a
3. a	7. c	11. b	15. c
4. b	8. c	12. b	16. a

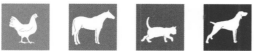

CHAPTER 7

Bones, Joints, and Synovial Fluid

CHAPTER OUTLINE

- **GENERAL FEATURES OF THE SKELETON**
  The Axial Skeleton
  The Appendicular Skeleton
- **BONE STRUCTURE**
  Composition of Bone
  Haversian Systems
  Cells of Bone
- **BONE FORMATION**
  Growth of Long Bones
  Bone Remodeling
- **BONE REPAIR**
- **JOINTS AND SYNOVIAL FLUID**
  Blood, Lymph, and Nerve Supply of
    Joints
  Synovial Membrane
  Articular Cartilage
  Lubrication of Synovial Joints

Bones are cellular structures in which the extracellular fluid environment of the cell is surrounded by a rigid, calcified frame. The framework of one bone, when combined with all of the other bones of the body, makes up what is commonly known as the **skeleton**. The skeleton gives an identifiable form to the body of an animal and provides protection to the cranial, thoracic, abdominal, and pelvic viscera. Also, the **medullary cavity** of the bones is the principal location of blood formation, and the calcified regions act as a sink and a source for many of the needed minerals (cations and anions). Movement of the body parts is enabled by the attachment of muscles to bones. Bones are dynamic structures that are capable of accommodating to different loads and stress by remodeling their shape. Also, function can be restored to broken bones (fractures) by the process of bone repair after appropriate fixation (alignment) of the bone parts.

An important aspect of bone study is the movable union between two bones known as a **joint**. This union is enclosed by a joint capsule. The inner aspect of the **joint capsule** is lined with a **synovial membrane**, which pro-

duces synovial fluid that provides for lubrication and nutrition of the joint surface.

The physiology of bones, joints, and synovial fluid is important not only because of the association of bones with other body systems, but also because bone and joint diseases are frequently encountered in animals.

■ GENERAL FEATURES OF THE SKELETON

1. Differentiate between the axial and the appendicular skeleton.
2. What are the components of the axial skeleton?
3. What is a collective term for the bones of the head?
4. What are the group names for the vertebrae, named in order, beginning with those most cranial?
5. What is an intervertebral disk?
6. What constitutes a prolapsed intervertebral disk?
7. What is the prominent bone in the pectoral girdle of domestic mammals?

8. What bones comprise the os coxae? Know the orientation of these bones to each other.
9. Note the location of the obturator foramen.
10. Name the bones in the hindlimb of the horse that are distal to the hock.
11. What are sesamoid bones?
12. What is the coffin joint

The bones of the body are generally similar among the animals but vary according to size, shape, and number. The skeletons of the horse (*Fig. 7-1*), the ox (*Fig. 7-2*), and the fowl (*Fig. 7-3*) are shown as examples that feature the general arrangement of the bones, and their similarities. The bones of the skeleton are clas-

sified as belonging to either the axial skeleton or the appendicular skeleton.

The Axial Skeleton

The components of the **axial skeleton** lie on the long axis (midline) of the body and include the skull, vertebrae, and those bones attached to the vertebrae, the ribs, and the ventral connections of the ribs, the sternum.

The skull comprises the **neurocranium (brain case)** and the **viscerocranium (bones of the face)**. Cranium is a collective term for the bones of the head. The brain case provides protection for the brain and openings for cranial nerve connections. The bones of the face provide a location and protection for the organs of the special senses and openings for

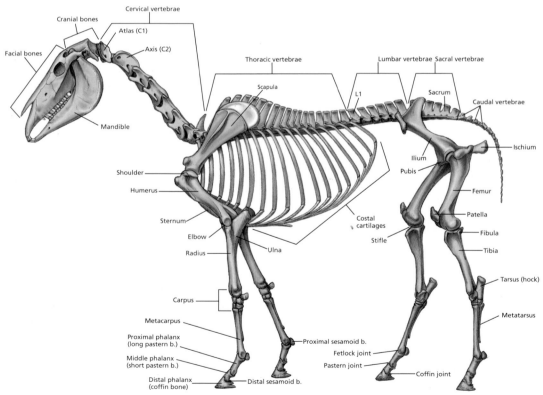

■ **FIGURE 7-1** Skeleton of the horse. (Adapted from McCracken TO, Kainer RA, Spurgeon TL. Spurgeon's Color Atlas of Large Animal Anatomy: The Essentials. Baltimore: Lippincott Williams & Wilkins, 1999.)

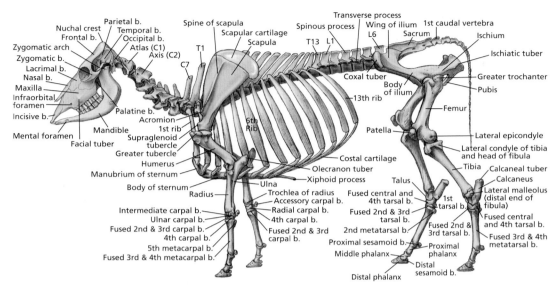

■ **FIGURE 7-2** Skeleton of the ox. (From McCracken TO, Kainer RA, Spurgeon TL. Spurgeon's Color Atlas of Large Animal Anatomy: The Essentials. Baltimore: Lippincott Williams & Wilkins, 1999.)

the digestive and respiratory systems. Special features are considered in respective chapters.

The ribs and sternum give limits and provide protection for the thoracic viscera (heart and lungs) and, because of their movement potential, assist respiration and blood flow.

General features of vertebrae are shown in *Figure. 7-4*. More specific information for the dog was presented when describing the relationship of vertebrae to spinal nerves (see Chapter 4). The numbers associated with the regions of their location, cervical (C), thoracic (T), lumbar (L), sacral (S), and caudal (Cd), are represented by a **vertebral formula** for each species. The vertebral formula for the horse is C7,T18,L6,S5,Cd15-20. The numbers of vertebrae for each region for the domestic animal species and human are presented in *Table 7-1*.

The bodies of contiguous vertebrae are held together by a **modified symphysis**, which is a slightly movable joint where bones are held together by a combination of hyaline cartilage and fibrocartilage. A **true symphysis** consists only of fibrocartilage. For the vertebrae, the modified symphysis is known as an **intervertebral disk** (*Fig. 7-5*). The cranial and caudal surfaces of contiguous vertebrae have a covering of hyaline cartilage, and the interconnection of these coverings is the intervertebral disc. The soft gelatinous interior of the disk is termed the **nucleus pulposus**. The fibrocartilaginous collar that supports the periphery of the disk is termed the **annulus fibrosus**. The intervertebral disk (nucleus pulposus and annulus fibrosus) provides for a compression-resisting cushion that permits limited movement between contiguous vertebrae. A **prolapsed** or **herniated intervertebral disk** occurs when the nucleus pulposus herniates (ruptures) through the annulus fibrosus. When inflammation proceeds at the site of herniation, there may be spinal nerve root compression at that level and peripheral nerve involvement with loss of function for the region served.

The Appendicular Skeleton

The **appendicular skeleton** is made up of the bones of the front (thoracic) and hind (pelvic)

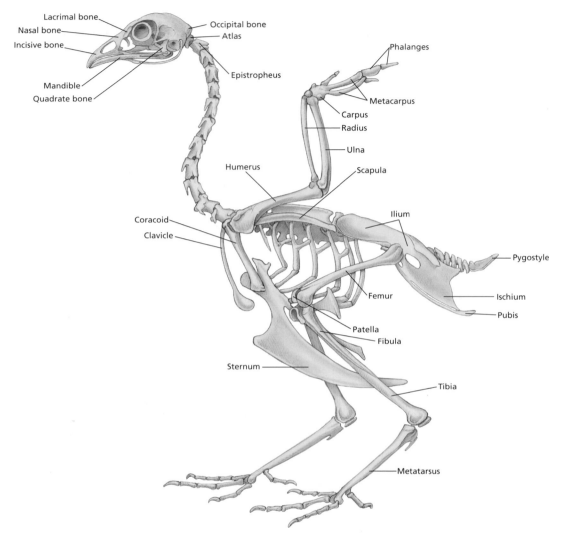

■ **FIGURE 7-3** Skeleton of the chicken. (Adapted from McCracken TO, Kainer RA, Spurgeon TL. Spurgeon's Color Atlas of Large Animal Anatomy: The Essentials. Baltimore: Lippincott Williams & Wilkins, 1999.)

limbs and their respective **pectoral girdle (shoulder)** and **pelvic girdle (pelvis)**. The pectoral girdle is composed of the scapula, clavicle, and coracoid, and the pelvic girdle is composed of the ilium, ischium, and pubis.

Whereas the pectoral girdle of birds has a visibly discernible **scapula**, **coracoid**, and **clavicle**, the only bone of prominence in the pectoral girdle of domestic mammals is the scapula

(shoulder blade). The coracoid is reduced to a small coracoid process projecting medially from the tuber scapulae (supraglenoid tubercle), from which the coracobrachialis muscle arises. This muscle stabilizes the shoulder. The clavicle is represented only by a fibrous identity in the brachiocephalicus muscle (a muscle of the forelimb) except in the cat, in which a very small clavicular bone is

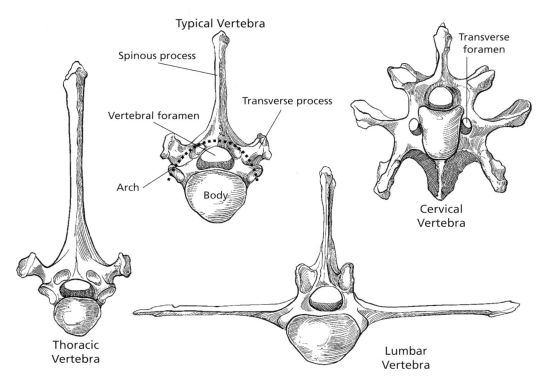

■ FIGURE 7-4 General features of typical vertebrae. (From Frandson RD, Wilke WL, Fails AD. Anatomy and Physiology of Farm Animals. 6th Ed. Baltimore: Lippincott Williams & Wilkins, 2003.)

TABLE 7-1 VERTEBRAL FORMULAS OF COMMON DOMESTIC ANIMALS AND HUMANS

SPECIES	CERVICAL	THORACIC	LUMBAR	SACRAL	CAUDAL
Horse	7	18	6	5	15–20
Ox	7	13	6	5	18–20
Sheep	7	13	6–7	4	16–18
Goat	7	13	7	4	12
Hog	7	14–15	6–7	4	20–23
Dog	7	13	7	3	20–23
Chicken	14	7	14 (lumbosacral)		6
Human	7	12	5	5	4

From Frandson RD, Wilke WL, Fails AD. Anatomy and Physiology of Farm Animals. 6th Ed. Baltimore: Lippincott Williams & Wilkins, 2003.

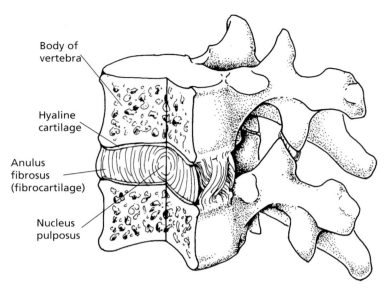

Body of
vertebra

Hyaline
cartilage

Anulus
fibrosus
(fibrocartilage)

Nucleus
pulposus

■ **FIGURE 7-5** Intervertebral disk, which is composed of hyaline cartilage and fibrocartilage and serves to interconnect the bodies of contiguous vertebrae. (From Cormack DH. Essential Histology. 2nd Ed. Baltimore: Lippincott Williams & Wilkins, 2001.)

embedded in this muscle. It has no function but will appear on radiographs, where it may be erroneously interpreted as a bone lodged in the esophagus. Medial and lateral views of the horse scapula are shown in *Figure. 7-6*.

The pelvic girdle consists of the os coxae (hip bone), which unites ventrally with the opposite bone at the symphysis pelvis and articulates with the sacrum dorsally (*Fig. 7-7*). The **os coxae** consists of the **ileum, ischium,** and **pubis,** which meet to form the **acetabulum,** the cavity that articulates with the head of the femur. The ilium is the largest of the three components and projects craniodorsally from the acetabulum to articulate with the sacrum at the tuber sacrale. The ischium projects caudally and ventrally from the acetabulum and forms much of the caudal floor of the pelvic cavity. The pubis is the smallest of the three pelvic bones and forms the cranial part of the floor of the pelvic cavity. The **obturator foramen** is bounded by the pubis cranially and the ischium caudally. The tuber coxae and tuber ischiadicum vary in prominence among domestic animals, and in cattle are referred to

as hook bones and pin bones, respectively. The obturator nerve passes through the obturator foramen to supply the adductor muscles of the pelvic limbs. Injury to the nerve during parturition (*Fig. 7-8*) can cause failure to bring the pelvic limbs together. Also, because of the support given to the pelvic limbs by the pelvis (via the acetabulum), a fracture to the pelvis can result in an inability to stand.

In general, among the domestic animals, the bones of the thoracic and pelvic limbs have like names but differ in size and shape and, for certain parts, differ in numbers. A comparison of the names for the bones between the thoracic and pelvic limbs is presented in *Table 7-2*. The relationship of these bones to each other is shown in *Figure. 7-9* and *Figure. 7-10* for the thoracic limb and pelvic limb, respectively, for comparison among the horse, ox, and pig. Because of lameness problems, more attention is given to the anatomy of the limbs of horses, and the further description that follows will relate to that species. Whereas humans, cats, and dogs have five metacarpal bones (corresponding to the hand), horses

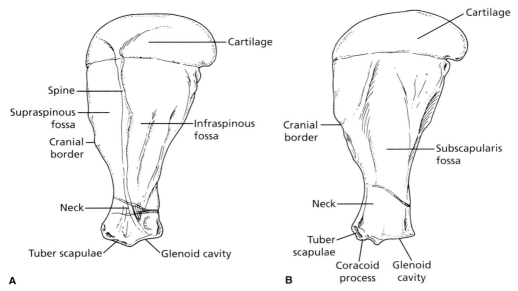

■ **FIGURE 7-6** Scapula of the horse. **A)** Lateral view. **B)** Medial view. The supraspinatus and infraspinatus muscles occupy the respective fossas noted on the lateral surface. The suprascapular nerve that innervates these muscles is a branch of the brachial plexus and arises from the medial surface at the neck of the scapula. Nerve injury is a cause for atrophy (reduction in size and loss of function) of the associated muscles.

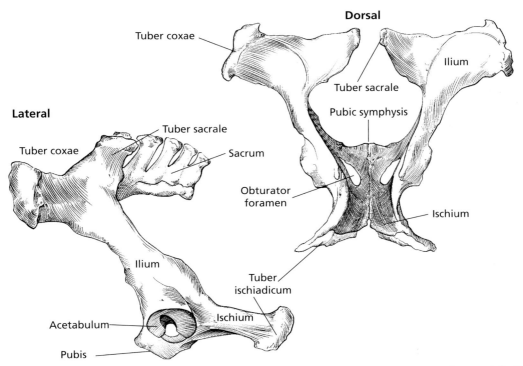

■ **FIGURE 7-7** Pelvis of the ox. Lateral view (left) and dorsal view (right). (From Frandson RD, Wilke WL, Fails AD. Anatomy and Physiology of Farm Animals. 6th Ed. Baltimore: Lippincott Williams & Wilkins, 2003.)

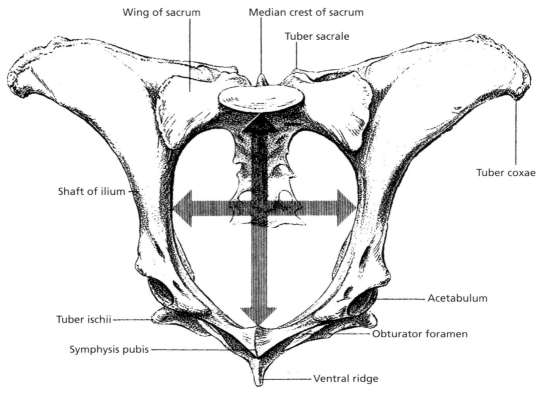

■ **FIGURE 7-8** The pelvic bones of the cow (viewed from in front and somewhat below) through which the calf must pass at birth. The caudal aspect of the sacrum erroneously appears as an obstruction because of the view. The arrows indicate the greatest transverse and dorsoventral diameters of the pelvic girdle. (From Salisbury GW, VanDemark NL, Lodge JR. Physiology of Reproduction and Artificial Insemination of Cattle. 2nd Ed. San Francisco: WH Freeman and Company, 1978.)

have one major **metacarpal (cannon bone)**, which is the third. The second and fourth exist as small bones alongside of the third and are referred to as **splint bones** (*Fig. 7-11A*). Fusion of these to the cannon bone along with excess bone formation may cause a lameness condition in horses that is known as splints. Distal to the cannon bone, the horse has a single digit (corresponds to the middle finger of humans) with three phalanges (*Fig. 7-11B*). The names for the joints (articulations) between the cannon bone and the first phalanx (long pastern bone), between the first and second phalanx (short pastern bone), and between the second and third phalanx (coffin bone) are

known as **fetlock**, **pastern**, and **coffin joints**, respectively. There are two proximal sesamoid bones and one distal sesamoid bone. Only the lateral proximal sesamoid is shown in Fig. 7-11B. These **sesamoid bones** serve for the attachment of ligaments directed for more distal parts, and because of the articulation with adjoining bones, friction is reduced that would otherwise occur without their placement. The distal sesamoid is known as the **navicular bone** and is situated behind the junction of the second and third phalanges. Inflammation in the region of the coffin joint (location of **distal sesamoid bone**) is called navicular disease. Because of the small size of

TABLE 7-2 COMPARISON OF BONES OF THORACIC AND PELVIC LIMBS

THORACIC LIMB		PELVIC LIMB	
PART OF LIMB	BONES	PART OF LIMB	BONES
Thoracic (shoulder) girdle	Scapula, clavicle, coracoid	Pelvic girdle	Sacrum
			Pelvis: ilium, ischium, pubis
Brachium (arm)	Humerus	Thigh	Femur
Antebrachium (forearm)	Radius, ulna	Crus (true leg)	Tibia, fibula
Carpus (knee)	Carpal bones	Tarsus (hock)	Tarsal bones
Metacarpus (cannon and splint bones)	Metacarpal bones	Metatarsus (cannon and splint bones)	Metatarsal bones
Phalanges (digit)	Proximal, middle, and distal phalanges	Phalanges (digit)	Proximal, middle, and distal phalanges
	Proximal and distal sesamoid bones		Proximal and distal sesamoid bones

From Frandson RD, Wilke WL, Fails AD. Anatomy and Physiology of Farm Animals. 6th Ed. Baltimore: Lippincott Williams & Wilkins, 2003.

the sesamoid bones, their name is derived from the small sesame seed. Not all sesamoid bones are small, however, and the **patella** (a **sesamoid bone**), which articulates with the femur, is an example.

The metatarsus and digits of the hindlimb are similar to the metacarpus and digits of the forelimb. The chief differences are in the form and size of the bones.

■ BONE STRUCTURE

1. What is another name for spongy bone?
2. Are the trabeculae (spicules) associated with compact or spongy bone?
3. How do trabeculae contribute to the strength of long bones?
4. Differentiate between epiphysis, metaphysis, and diaphysis.
5. How are bones associated with blood cell formation?
6. What is the epiphyseal plate? What parts of the bone does it separate?
7. What are periosteum and endosteum?
8. What percent of adult bone is water?
9. On a dry weight basis, what percent of adult bone is mineral content?
10. What part of bone is converted to gelatin when heated in aqueous solution?
11. What two elements are the major constituents of the mineral phase of bone?
12. What is the unit of structure of compact bone? Describe it.
13. What are lacunae and canaliculi? Where is bone interstitial fluid located?
14. What are interstitial and circumferential lamellae?

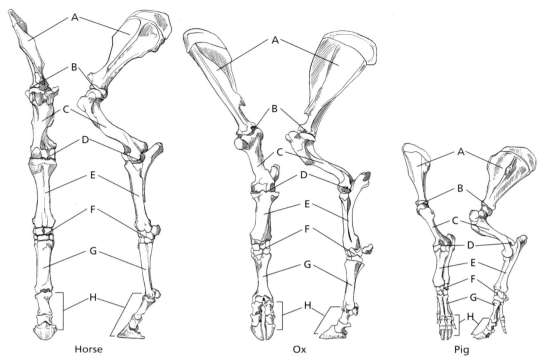

Horse   Ox   Pig

■ **FIGURE 7-9** Comparison of anatomy of bones of the thoracic limb. **A)** Scapula, **B)** scapulohumeral (shoulder) joint, **C)** humerus, **D)** elbow joint, **E)** antebrachium (radius and ulna), **F)** carpus, **G)** metacarpus, **H)** digit (phalanges). (From Frandson RD, Wilke WL, Fails AD. Anatomy and Physiology of Farm Animals. 6th Ed. Baltimore: Lippincott Williams & Wilkins, 2003.)

---

15. How are osteoprogenitor cells, osteoblasts, and osteocytes related?

16. Is the osteocyte more mature than the osteoblast?

17. How do osteocytes maintain communication with each other?

18. What is the name of the bone-resorbing cells? What is their origin?

The structure of a long bone (e.g., the femur) is shown in *Figure. 7-12*. A longitudinal section is shown to reveal its inner structure. Compact and spongy characteristics are noted. **Compact bone** appears to be solid, whereas **spongy bone** (also called cancellous bone) has the appearance of a sponge. In spongy bone there are **trabeculae (spicules)** of mineralized tissue, and the empty spaces between the trabeculae occupy a considerable volume. In living animals, the regions between the trabeculae are filled with **bone marrow**. The rigidity and strength of long bones is attributable not only to the hardness of its compact bone but also to the scaffolding arrangement of the trabeculae, which are generally parallel to lines of maximum stress and, therefore, act as pillars for stress points (see Fig. 7-12). The **epiphysis** refers to either extremity of a long bone, and the **diaphysis** is the cylindrical shaft situated between the two epiphyses. The **metaphysis** is the expanded or flared part of the bone at the ends of the diaphysis. The diaphysis contains the **marrow (medullary) cavity** that is surrounded by a thick-walled tube of compact bone. The

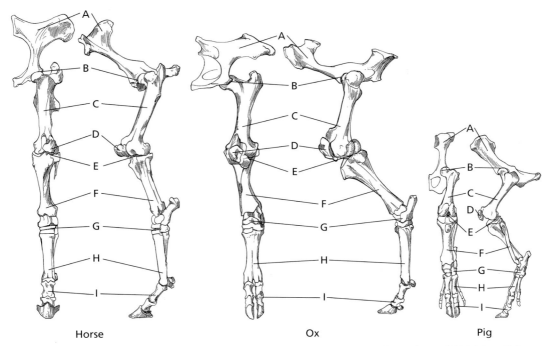

■ **FIGURE 7-10** Comparison of anatomy of bones of the pelvic limb. **A)** Pelvis, **B)** coxofemoral (hip) joint, **C)** femur, **D)** patella, **E)** stifle (knee) joint, **F)** crus (tibia and fibula), **G)** rarsus (hock), **H)** metatarsus, **I)** digit (phalanges). (From Frandson RD, Wilke WL, Fails AD. Anatomy and Physiology of Farm Animals. 6th Ed. Baltimore: Lippincott Williams & Wilkins, 2003.)

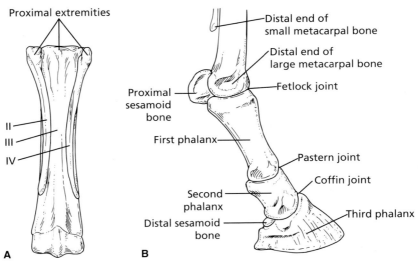

■ **FIGURE 7-11** Metacarpal and phalangeal bones of the thoracic limb of the horse. **A)** Right metacarpal bones (palmar view). The third (III) or large metacarpal bone (cannon bone) is fully developed; the second (II) and fourth (IV) are much reduced and are commonly called the small metacarpal or splint bones. **B)** The phalanges and distal part of right metacarpal bones (lateral view).

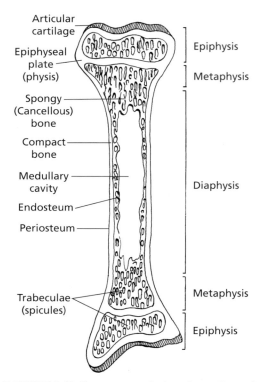

Articular cartilage

Epiphyseal plate (physis)

Spongy (Cancellous) bone

Compact bone

Medullary cavity

Endosteum

Periosteum

Trabeculae (spicules)

Epiphysis

Metaphysis

Diaphysis

Metaphysis

Epiphysis

■ **FIGURE 7-12** The structure of a long bone. The endosteum and periosteum designations refer only to their locations and do not reflect their cellular nature and extent. Note the parallel arrangement of the trabeculae to form scaffolding for maximum strength in response to its assumed load.

medullary cavity or bone marrow is the site of blood cell production. A small amount of spongy bone may line the inner surface of the compact bone. The epiphyses consist chiefly of spongy bone with a thin outer shell of compact bone. The **epiphyseal plate** (also called **physis**) is composed of hyaline cartilage and represents the point of growth in a longitudinal direction. **Hyaline cartilage** is the ordinary type and is so named because its matrix (intercellular substance) is a glassy bluish-white (hyalos is the Greek word for glass) and is somewhat translucent. In mature bones, the cartilage has been replaced by bone and epiphyseal lines remain where the plate last existed. The contact area of the bone that articulates

with its neighboring bone at a movable joint is covered with articular cartilage (described later in this chapter).

With the exception of the joint surfaces, all other outer surfaces of the bone are covered with periosteum. The **periosteum** is composed of an outer fibrous layer and an inner cell-rich layer containing **osteoblasts** (if bone formation is in progress) or other cells that can become osteoblasts in response to an appropriate stimulus (**osteoprogenitor cells**). Osteoblasts synthesize and secrete the organic substance of bone and participate in the mineralization of the organic matrix. The periosteum is responsible for the increase in diameter of bones and also functions in the healing of fractures. The endosteum is the lining tissue of all surfaces of the bone that face the medullary cavity and also of the trabeculae of the spongy bone. It is only one cell thick, and the cells can become osteoblasts when stimulated.

Composition of Bone

On a wet-weight basis, adult bone is approximately 25% water, 45% mineral, and 30% organic matter. Calcium constitutes about 37% of the mineral content and phosphorus about 18.5%. On a dry-weight basis, the mineral content is between 65% and 70%, whereas the organic fraction is 30% to 35%. The organic fraction is about 90% collagen, which is converted to gelatin when heated in aqueous solution. Several different elements are incorporated in the mineral phase of bone, but the major constituents are calcium and phosphorus.

Haversian Systems

Figure 7-13 is a three-dimensional illustration showing the appearance of both a cross section and a longitudinal section of the shaft of a mature long bone. The channels that run parallel to the long axis of the bone are the **haversian canals**, which contain blood vessels that

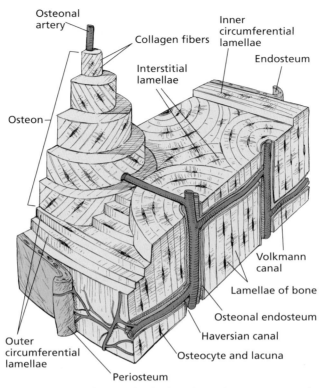

FIGURE 7-13 Three-dimensional view of the shaft of a long bone. (From Ross MH. Histology, A Text and Atlas. 4th Ed. Baltimore: Lippincott Williams & Wilkins, 2003.)

communicate with blood vessels serving the external surfaces and marrow cavity. The latter blood vessels are perpendicular to the long axis of the bone and are contained within **Volkmann canals**. The unit of structure of compact bone is the **haversian system** (also known as an **osteon**), which consists of a central haversian canal surrounded by concentric layers of bone, the **lamellae** (*Fig. 7-14*). Bone cells, the **osteocytes**, are contained within small cavities known as **lacunae (little lakes)**. The osteocytes communicate with each other and with the haversian canal through a branching network of canals, the **canaliculi**. The interstitial fluid for the osteocytes is contained within the lacunae and canaliculi. It diffuses through the canalicular network from the blood vessels in the canals for maintenance of the osteocytes. Facilitation of fluid transport

may be caused by periodic contraction of the osteocytes. Haversian systems are absent in spongy bone, but concentric lamellae with enclosed lacunae and osteocytes with intercommunicating canaliculi are present. In addition to the concentric lamellae that make up the haversian system, other lamellar patterns occur in the form of **interstitial lamellae** and outer and inner **circumferential lamellae** (see Fig. 7-13). The outer and inner circumferential lamellae are produced by the osteoblasts that cover the outer and inner surfaces of the bone while it is in the process of attaining its full width. During this time, haversian systems develop, and this gives the inner aspect of the outer circumferential lamellae and the outer aspect of the inner circumferential lamellae an interrupted appearance. Their uninterrupted aspects, however, give the outer and inner

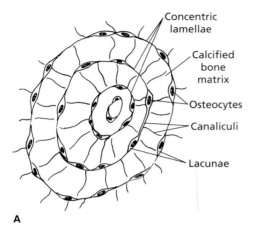

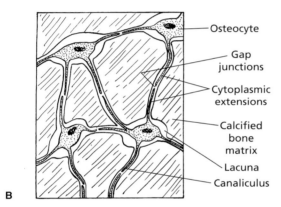

■ **FIGURE 7-14** An osteon (haversian system). **A)** Concentric lamellae, showing osteocytes within their lacunae and their communicating canaliculi. **B)** Cytoplasmic extensions of osteocytes into canaliculi for communication with other osteocytes.

lamellar surfaces a smooth look. The interstitial lamellae are remnants of older haversian systems or of circumferential lamellae.

Cells of Bone

Four different types of cells are associated with bone: osteoprogenitor cells, osteoblasts, osteocytes, and osteoclasts. The first of these, **osteoprogenitor cells**, comprise the population of cells in the innermost layer of the periosteum, the endosteal lining cells of the marrow cavities, and the lining cells of the haversian canals

and Volkmann canals. Their stimulation leads to the more active secretory cell, the osteoblast. Where active bone formation is not occurring, the surfaces are covered by bone-lining cells, which are analogous to osteoprogenitor cells except that they represent a more quiescent state.

The **osteoblast** is the differentiated bone-forming cell responsible for the production of bone matrix. Its secretion of collagen and ground substance makes up the initial unmineralized bone or osteoid. The osteoblast is also associated with calcification of the matrix.

The **osteocyte** is the mature bone cell and represents a transformed osteoblast. It is enclosed by the bone matrix that it had previously laid down as osteoid when it was an osteoblast. Osteocytes maintain the bone matrix and are able to synthesize and resorb matrix to a limited extent. They extend their cytoplasmic processes through the canaliculi to contact, by means of **gap junctions**, similar processes of neighboring cells. The gap junctions have a low electrical resistance that permit ionic and small molecule flow between cells. Communication among the osteocytes is thus possible such that the outermost cells, as well as those closest to blood vessels, can respond to stimuli (e.g., hormones). The osteocyte is smaller than in its previous state as an osteoblast because of reduced perinuclear cytoplasm. The appearance of osteocytes within their calcified bone matrix lacunae and their cytoplasmic extensions into the canaliculi is shown in Fig. 7-14B.

Osteoclasts are large, motile, often multinucleated bone-resorbing cells. Their precursors are stem cells in blood-producing tissue of bone marrow and spleen. These stem cells differentiate into bone-resorbing monocytes and then fuse with others to form the large multinucleated osteoclasts. Osteoclasts are considered to be members of the diffuse mononuclear phagocytic system (MPS) (see Chapter 3).

Although osteoprogenitor cells, osteoblasts, and osteocytes are featured as distinct cell types, they should be regarded as different functional states of the same cell type.

■ BONE FORMATION

1. What method of bone formation is represented by the os penis of some animals and the os cordis of the bovine heart?
2. What is endochondral ossification?
3. What method of bone formation forms the flat bones of the skull and face?
4. What is the name of the oldest zone within the epiphyseal plate?
5. Visualize the elongation of a bone by virtue of cells dividing, secreting matrix, and thus pushing the zone of reserve cartilage away from the diaphysis.
6. Does cartilage have a blood supply?
7. Are cartilage lacunae connected by canaliculi?
8. What causes chondrocytes to die?
9. What previously occupied the tunnels that exist in the zone of calcified matrix?
10. Note the invasion of the tunnels by capillaries as a prerequisite for new bone formation.
11. Visualize the development of lamellae (layers) around the capillary such that the tunnel is reduced to a narrow canal (a haversian system).
12. As a bone grows in width, why do the walls not become unduly thick? What is the appositional mechanism of bone growth?
13. What osteogenic layer accounts for the outer circumferential lamellae? The inner circumferential lamellae?
14. What cell provides for the erosion needed to form new channels during the process of bone remodeling?
15. After the erosion, what sequence of events forms new haversian systems?
16. How is bone mass correlated with increased muscle mass and exercise?

Bone formation (ossification) is identified according to the environment in which it is formed as either heteroplastic, endochondral, or intramembranous. Ossification is **heteroplastic** if it is formed in tissue other than the skeleton. This type occurs with the os penis of some animals and the os cordis of the bovine heart, but mostly it is pathologic. **Endochondral ossification** is that which develops from cartilage and is mostly preformed in the fetus but continues after birth from cartilage plates located between the metaphysis and epiphysis, and from the periosteum that surrounds the cortex. Most long bones are developed by this method. **Intramembranous** bone formation is that which is formed without the intervention of cartilage. These bones are preformed in a fibroid membrane that is then infiltrated with osteoid tissue that later becomes calcified. Bones formed by this method are the flat bones of the skull and face, the mandible, and the clavicle (cat). The previously mentioned mechanisms refer only to the manner in which existing bone was originally formed. Remodeling of bone is established on the preexisting bone, and the mechanism of remodeling is identical whether the original bone was formed by endochondral or intramembranous ossification. The sequence of actual bone formation during remodeling consists of osteoblasts laying down osteoid tissue that is subsequently calcified.

Growth of Long Bones

Increase in length of a bone depends on the presence of a cartilage plate (epiphyseal plate), wherein four zones are recognized that extend from the epiphysis to the diaphysis (*Fig. 7-15*). These are termed **zones of reserve cartilage** (the youngest), **proliferation, hypertrophy,** and **calcified matrix** (the oldest). Beyond the zone of calcified matrix are the developing trabeculae that make up the spongy bone of the metaphyses.

Cartilage does not have a blood supply, and nutrition of the **cartilage cells (chondrocytes)**

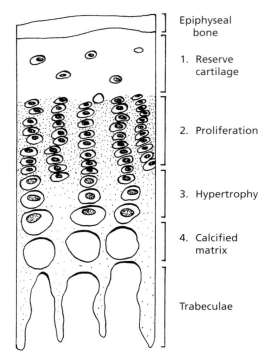

■ **FIGURE 7-15** The four zones of a cartilage (epiphyseal) plate.

Labels (top to bottom):
Epiphyseal bone
1. Reserve cartilage
2. Proliferation
3. Hypertrophy
4. Calcified matrix
Trabeculae

depends on diffusion of extracellular fluid from its source to the chondrocytes that lie within their lacunae. Also, unlike osteocytes, chondrocytes are still able to divide after they have become embedded in cartilage matrix. When the chondrocytes from the zone of reserve cartilage undergo division, the chondrocytes become organized into distinct columns, and a zone of proliferation that is directed toward the diaphysis is recognized. The columns are formed because of chondrocyte capture within lacunae. Each daughter cell within a lacunae produces matrix, and this causes the cartilage matrix to expand from within. This has the effect of pushing the epiphysis away from the diaphysis, thus, elongation of the bone.

Each division of chondrocytes brings about larger cells, hence the zone of hypertrophy (see Fig. 7-15). This has the effect of compressing the matrix into linear bands between the columns of hypertrophied cells. After several divisions, the hypertrophied cells become further removed from the epiphyseal plate and become active in bringing about calcification of the cartilage matrix. Calcification, coupled with increasing distance from the nutritional source, causes the chondrocytes to die, and the matrix becomes the zone of calcified matrix. The appearance of longitudinal and cross sections of different areas of the epiphyseal plate and metaphysis at the periphery of a growing shaft are presented in *Figure. 7-16*. A cross section at the level of calcified matrix (Fig. 7-16C2) would show that tunnels exist where nests of hypertrophied cells previously occupied the space between the linear bands of compressed cartilage matrix (now calcified). What are seen as trabeculae (columns) in longitudinal sections actually constitute a honeycombed structure in cross sections, and the spaces seen between the trabeculae in longitudinal sections are seen as tunnels in cross sections.

The tunnels are now invaded from the diaphysis by capillaries, and osteoblasts line up along the sides of the tunnels and deposit bone on their inner surfaces. The osteoblasts continue to divide, and each division of osteoblasts pushes the original osteoblast layer closer to the capillary in the center. Concentric lamellae of bone substance are thus established, with osteocytes occupying lacunae and canaliculi. After several layers of bone (concentric lamellae) have been deposited, the tunnel is reduced to a narrow canal, which contains a blood vessel, some osteoblasts or osteogenic cells, and perhaps a lymphatic vessel (Fig. 7-16C3). This arrangement is known as a haversian system, the unit of structure of compact bone.

While a long bone is growing in length, it is also growing in width. New layers of bone are being added to the outside of the shaft at the same time that bone is dissolved away from the inside of the shaft. Although the shaft of the bone becomes wider, its walls do not become unduly thick, and the width of the

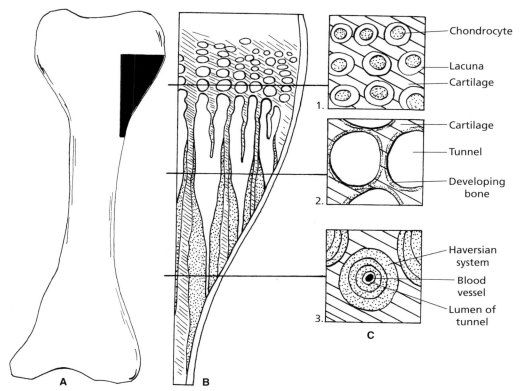

- Chondrocyte
- Lacuna
- Cartilage

1.

- Cartilage
- Tunnel
- Developing bone

2.

- Haversian system
- Blood vessel
- Lumen of tunnel

3.

C

A   B

■ **FIGURE 7-16** The appearance presented by both longitudinal and cross sections of different areas of the epiphyseal plate and metaphysis at the periphery of a growing shaft. **A)** The blackened area is the location on the long bone for parts B and C. **B)** Horizontal lines extend to their respective cross sections. White areas are tunnels or openings to tunnels. The oblique lines represent cartilage, and the stippled structures represent calcified matrix. **C1)** Chondrocytes in their lacunae in the zone of hypertrophy. **C2)** Tunnels formed in the zone of calcified matrix. Trabeculae are composed of both cartilage and bone. **C3)** Haversian system transforming tunnels into compact bone.

marrow cavity gradually increases. The shaft of a bone grows in width by the **appositional mechanism** (*Fig. 7-17*). The periosteum provides the osteogenic layer, and by repeated proliferation, new bone is formed to fill in the grooves between the longitudinal ridges of haversian systems that were formed while the bone was elongating. The same process of appositional growth occurs on the inner aspect of the bone shaft from endosteum. The bone formed from the periosteum and endosteum accounts for the outer and inner circumferential lamellae, respectively (see Fig. 7-13).

Bone Remodeling

As described previously, the growth of bones does not simply involve an increase in their thickness. Rather, there is a coordinated formation of new bone at the outer surfaces and resorption of bone at the inner surfaces (*Fig. 7-18*). This also occurs to the bones of the neurocranium to accommodate the growing brain during its maturation. In each instance, the two processes of appositional growth and bone resorption are the only ways that the shape and size of a bone can change during

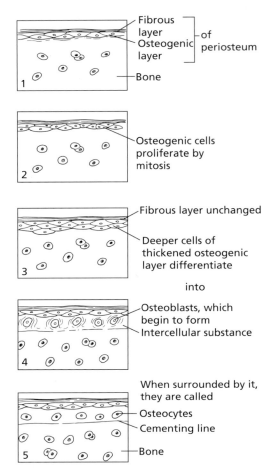

1 — Fibrous layer / Osteogenic layer —of periosteum / Bone

2 — Osteogenic cells proliferate by mitosis

3 — Fibrous layer unchanged / Deeper cells of thickened osteogenic layer differentiate / into

4 — Osteoblasts, which begin to form / Intercellular substance

5 — When surrounded by it, they are called / Osteocytes / Cementing line / Bone

■ **FIGURE 7-17** Bone growth by apposition. (Adapted from Ham AW. Histology. 1st Ed. Philadelphia: JB Lippincott, 1950.)

prenatal and postnatal life. Because this applies to long bones of the body, the shape of the bone does not grossly change during growth, and its marrow cavity is enlarged to ensure a sufficient area for blood cell requirements. During growth, haversian systems are being formed, resorbed, and remodeled. The general process for new haversian systems is generally initiated by osteoclasts concurrent with the invasion of blood vessels (*Fig. 7-19*). The osteoclasts are on the leading edge of the invading blood vessels. New tunnels are thus formed by erosion through the end osteal

surface that are oriented with the long axis of the shaft. A layer of osteoblasts forms on the surface of the eroded tunnel (that has a central blood vessel), and concentric lamellae are formed as previously described for haversian systems. The blood vessels grow and branch, with accompanying osteoclast and osteoblast activity, whereby new channels are made and new haversian systems form to fill them.

In addition to the remodeling that occurs to accommodate growth, remodeling also occurs in response to stress placed on bones. Reduction in bone mass accompanies loss of muscle mass and decreased mobility, whereas an increase in muscle mass and exercise is accompanied by an increase in bone mass. Therefore, the organization of bone changes to meet mechanical and other stresses placed on the skeleton, and it represents a balance between bone formation and bone resorption.

■ BONE REPAIR

1. What happens to osteocytes, the periosteum, and bone marrow when the blood supply is disrupted after bone fracture?
2. Will bone repair occur if a blood supply is not restored to a fracture site?
3. As related to bone repair, what is a callus?
4. What is the source of the osteogenic cells for the external and internal callus?
5. What determines whether a callus will be composed of spongy bone or cartilage?
6. What eventually happens to a cartilage callus?
7. Will spongy bone be replaced by compact bone at the fracture site?
8. What determines when remodeling of initial bone repair will occur?

Bone fractures are the most common consequences of bone injury. Fractures can result

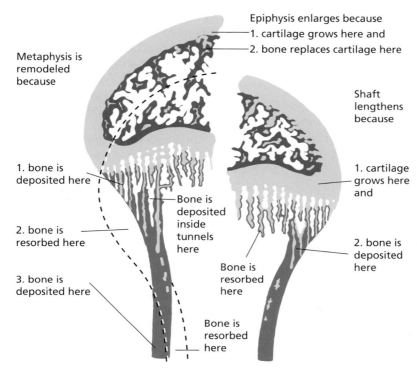

Epiphysis enlarges because
1. cartilage grows here and
2. bone replaces cartilage here

Metaphysis is remodeled because

Shaft lengthens because

1. bone is deposited here

Bone is deposited inside tunnels here

1. cartilage grows here and

2. bone is resorbed here

2. bone is deposited here

3. bone is deposited here

Bone is resorbed here

Bone is resorbed here

■ **FIGURE 7-18** Sites of bone deposition and resorption in the process of lengthening and remodeling of long bones. Bone is shown in black, cartilage in grey. (From Cormack DH. Essential Histology. 2nd Ed. Baltimore: Lippincott Williams & Wilkins, 2001.)

in separation of bone parts with loss of alignment, separation of periosteum and endosteum, and severe bleeding followed by clot formation. The torn blood vessels can be those that supply Volkmann canals, haversian systems, and the periosteum and endosteum at the fracture site. In the vicinity of the disrupted blood supply, the osteocytes begin to die and the periosteum and bone marrow become necrotic. The acute inflammatory condition that follows brings phagocytic cells into the area for clearance of blood clot components and necrotic tissue. New blood vessels enter the damaged area, and new bone formation begins. Bone formation does not occur until a blood supply has been established.

The most common type of bone repair involves the formation of a **callus**. This type takes place when the broken ends are not perfectly realigned and stabilized. A collar of repair tissue forms around the external surface of each broken end, and when a bridge is formed across the break, it is known as the **external callus**. The healthy intact periosteum is the source of the osteogenic cells for the external callus, whereas endosteum is the source for the **internal callus**. Depending on the richness of the periosteal capillaries, the callus will be composed of either spongy bone or cartilage. Inadequate blood supply predisposes to cartilage formation. When cartilage is formed, it is subsequently replaced by bone. The transformation from cartilage to bone is similar to that previously described for growth of long bones from the epiphyseal plate. The chondrocytes hypertrophy, and the cartilage matrix becomes calcified. The calcified cartilage is removed and replaced with spongy bone after the entrance of blood vessels. Any dead bone that was incorporated into the

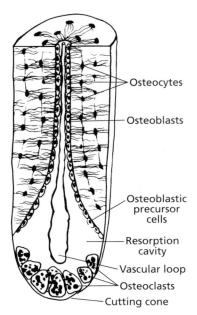

- Osteocytes
- Osteoblasts
- Osteoblastic precursor cells
- Resorption cavity
- Vascular loop
- Osteoclasts
- Cutting cone

■ **FIGURE 7-19** Osteoclastic activity that precedes bone remodeling. Osteoclasts advance a resorption cavity into the bone and are immediately followed by a vascular loop accompanied by precursor cells that multiply and differentiate into osteoblasts. Osteoblasts lay down new layers of osteoid. Canaliculi are formed, and osteoblasts become osteocytes. Successive layers of new bone are deposited to give the concentric lamellar rings of haversian bone. (From Whittick WG. Canine Orthopedics. 2nd Ed. Philadelphia, Lea & Febiger, 1990.)

callus is removed by the action of osteoclasts and is replaced by bone formed by osteoblasts that move into the spaces created by osteoclastic activity. As compact bone is formed at the fracture site, the spongy bone in the periphery of the callus is no longer needed to provide strength, and therefore it is resorbed. Final remodeling occurs when stresses associated with normal use return. A summary of fracture healing is shown in *Figure. 7-20*.

■ JOINTS AND SYNOVIAL FLUID

1. What is another name for the connection between component parts of the skeleton that is otherwise known as a joint?

2. What is the term used to describe inflammation of a joint?
3. What facilitates the gliding of two surfaces of a synovial joint over each other?
4. What is a joint capsule?
5. What part of the joint capsule secretes synovial fluid?
6. Do joints have a lymph drainage?
7. What functions are served by nerves that supply joints?
8. Are there pain nerve fibers in articular cartilage? What is the distribution of pain nerve fibers that are associated with a joint?
9. Does the synovial membrane cover the articular cartilage?
10. What are synoviocytes?
11. What are the chief functions of synovial fluid?
12. What component of synovial fluid provides for its viscosity?
13. What is the difference in viscosity of synovial fluid among joints of different sizes?
14. Are normal plasma constituents common to synovial fluid?
15. Describe adult articular cartilage. Does it have cells, blood vessels, and a nerve supply?
16. What provides the growth zone for endochondral ossification of the epiphysis?
17. How does intermittent pressure on articular cartilage relate to its nutrition?
18. What substances in synovial fluid contribute to its lubricating properties?
19. How does compression on articular cartilages contribute to lubrication?
20. What is weeping lubrication?

The connection between any of the skeleton's rigid component parts is known as a joint. These connections are also described as articulations. The study of joints is termed arthrology, and inflammation of joints is

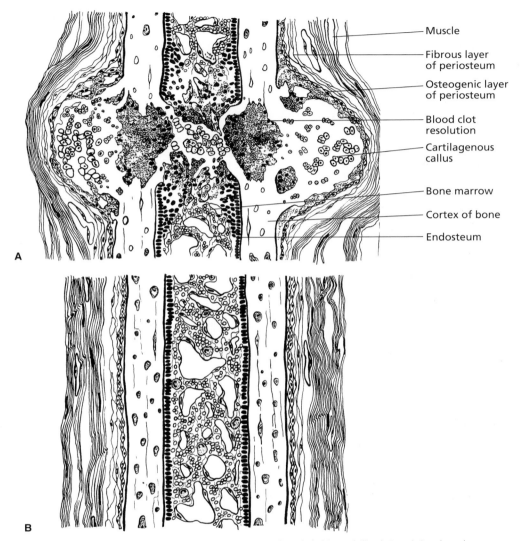

Muscle

Fibrous layer
of periosteum

Osteogenic layer
of periosteum

Blood clot
resolution

Cartilagenous
callus

Bone marrow

Cortex of bone

Endosteum

■ **FIGURE 7-20** Bone fracture repair. **A)** Fracture has been reduced and immobilized. Repair involves the appearance of a palpable callus. A cartilaginous callus precedes the mineralized callus. **B)** Fracture completely healed. The bone has been remodeled to conform to lines of stress. Original fracture site is obliterated. (From Whittick WG. Canine orthopedics. 2nd Ed. Philadelphia, Lea & Febiger, 1990.)

referred to as arthritis. Arthritis is a common malady among domestic animals; therefore, this brief study of the anatomy and physiology of joints is intended to assist students' understanding of joint diseases. A slightly movable joint was described for the connection of contiguous vertebrae (see Fig. 7-5).

Synovial joints are those that allow one surface to glide over another (*Figure 7-21*). This motion is facilitated by the presence of articular cartilage on each bone surface of the articulation and also by the presence of **synovial fluid**. The synovial joint is enclosed by a **joint capsule**. Synovial fluid is contained

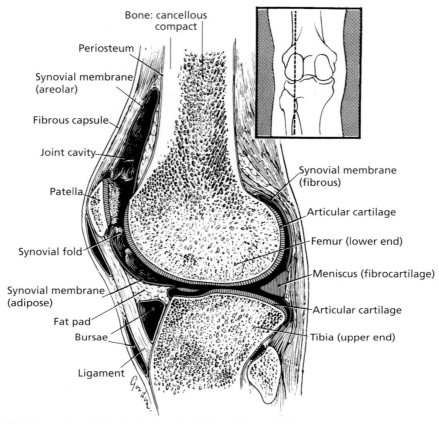

■ **FIGURE 7-21** Human knee joint (sagittal section indicated by inset). This is an example of a synovial joint. (From Cormack DH. Essential Histology. 2nd Ed. Baltimore: Lippincott Williams & Wilkins, 2001.)

within the cavity of the joint capsule and is secreted by its inner membrane, the **synovial membrane**. The outer layer of the joint capsule is a fibrous layer that extends from the periosteum of each bone and contributes to the stability of the joint. A **meniscus** within the joint capsule serves a cushioning function.

Blood, Lymph, and Nerve Supply of Joints

The blood and nerve supply of a synovial joint is shown in *Fig. 7-22*. The arteries that supply a joint and adjacent bone generally have a common origin. These arteries usually enter the bone near the line of capsule attachment and form a network around the joint. Capil-

laries from this network are one of the sources of nutrition to articular cartilage that was noted in the previous section. Lymph vessels are present with blood vessels, and the lymph vessels that leave a joint drain into regional lymph nodes. Diffusion between the joint cavity and the blood and lymph capillaries takes place readily.

Nerve supply to a joint has two principal functions. The first function has to do with pain and reflex responses that may accompany joint disease. The second function is associated with their role in posture, locomotion, and kinesthesia, which is a sense mediated by stimulation of end organs in muscles, tendons, and joints in response to body movements and tension (see Chapters 4 and 5). The pain fibers

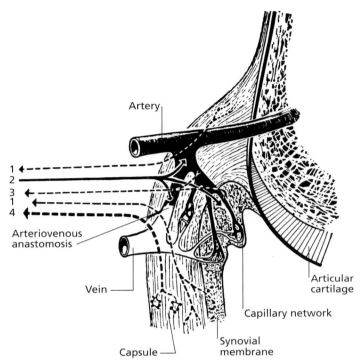

■ FIGURE 7-22 Blood and nerve supply of a synovial joint. An artery is shown supplying the epiphysis, joint capsule, and synovial membrane. Note the arteriovenous anastomosis. The articular nerve contains the following: **1)** sensory fibers (mostly pain) from the capsule and synovial membrane, **2)** autonomic fibers (postganglionic, sympathetic to blood vessels), **3)** sensory fibers (pain, and others with unknown functions) from the adventitia of blood vessels, and **4)** proprioceptive fibers from Ruffini endings and from small lamellated corpuscles (not shown). Arrows indicate direction of conduction. (From Gardner E, Gray DJ, O'Rahilley R. Anatomy. 4th Ed. Philadelphia: WB Saunders, 1975.)

are distributed within the fibrous layer and synovial membrane of the joint capsule.

Synovial Membrane

The synovial membrane is a vascular connective tissue that lines the inner surface of the joint capsule but does not cover the bearing surfaces (the **articular cartilage**). **Synoviocytes** within the synovial membrane synthesize synovial fluid by an active, energy-requiring process.

The chief functions of synovial fluid are joint lubrication and nourishment of the articular cartilage. Synovial fluid is a sticky, viscous fluid, often like egg white in consistency. It is usually slightly alkaline and ranges from colorless to deep yellow. The color and viscosity vary with species and type of joint. Fluid from large joints is usually less viscous than that from small joints. The viscosity of synovial fluid is attributable almost entirely to **hyaluronic acid**. Other chemical constituents of synovial fluid are those that are normally present in blood plasma. Synovial fluid normally contains a few cells that are mostly mononuclear. Examination of the cellular and chemical content and physical characteristics can be a valuable diagnostic aid when evaluating joint disease.

Articular Cartilage

Adult articular cartilage is usually hyaline in nature, avascular, and aneural, and has an acellular matrix that surrounds a relatively small number of cells called chondrocytes. It is a highly specialized connective tissue with biochemical and biophysical characteristics that enable it to play a dual role as a shock absorber and as a bearing surface. During the growth period, articular cartilage provides the growth zone for endochondral ossification in the epiphysis. During growth, articular cartilage is capable of regeneration and thus repairs defects that may arise. However, when growth ceases, it loses much of its power of repair. Cartilage is a resilient and elastic tissue that becomes thinner when compressed and slowly regains its original thickness when the pressure is released. Intermittent pressure associated with compression and release of compression causes cartilage to thicken by taking up fluid. Synovial fluid is absorbed by this spongelike property and diffuses through the cartilage matrix to provide for its nutrition. Other possible sources of nourishment for articular cartilage include diffusion from epiphyseal vessels that loop through subchondral bone and diffusion of fluid from capillaries associated with the arterial circle around the joint at the line of capsular attachment.

Lubrication of Synovial Joints

The fluids that lubricate a synovial joint are the synovial fluid and fluid pressed from artic-ular cartilage during compression. Substances within synovial fluid that contribute to its lubricating properties are **hyaluronic acid** and a glycoprotein known as **lubricin**. Both of these substances are secreted by the synovial membrane and lubricate the articular surface during light loads associated with minimal articular cartilage compression. During heavy loads, the synovial membrane fluids are displaced from the articular cartilages, and the compression causes fluid from the cartilage to be expressed and form a layer between the opposing surfaces. The lubrication provided by the cartilage fluid is known as **weeping lubrication**. Articular cartilage has been compared with a stiff sponge; it resists tensile stresses, shows elastic deformation under load, contains a high proportion of extracellular fluid (hyperhydrated), and exudes fluid under pressure (which is of major importance in lubrication).

■ SUGGESTED READING

Cormack DH. Essential Histology. 2nd Ed. Baltimore: Lippincott Williams & Wilkins, 2001.

Frandson RD, Wilke WL, Fails AD. Anatomy and Physiology of Farm Animals. 6th Ed. Baltimore: Lippincott Williams & Wilkins, 2003.

Goff JP. Cartilage, bone, and joints. In: Reece WO, ed. Dukes' Physiology of Domestic Animals. 12th Ed. Ithaca, NY: Cornell University Press, 2004.

 SELF EVALUATION—CHAPTER 7

GENERAL FEATURES OF THE SKELETON

1. The front- and hindlimbs and their respective shoulder and pelvic girdles are parts of the:
   a. axial skeleton.
   b. appendicular skeleton.

2. Intervertebral disks between contiguous vertebrae:
   a. are solid hyaline cartilage.
   b. are present only between lumbar vertebrae.
   c. provide compression-resisting cushions and permit limited movement.
   d. do not allow for movement.

3. The axial skeleton is composed of the:
   a. skull and vertebrae.
   b. skull, vertebrae, ribs, and sternum.
   c. skull, vertebrae, and pectoral and pelvic girdles.
   d. ribs, sternum, and pectoral and pelvic girdles.

4. Beginning cranially and extending caudally, the vertebral groups are:
   a. cervical, sacral, thoracic, lumbar, caudal.
   b. thoracic, cervical, lumbar, sacral, caudal.
   c. thoracic, lumbar, sacral, cervical, caudal.
   d. cervical, thoracic, lumbar, sacral, caudal.

5. The os coxae:
   a. is a part of the pectoral girdle.
   b. unites dorsally with its opposite bone, forming a symphysis without articulation.
   c. unites ventrally with its opposite bone at the symphysis pelvis.
   d. is another name for the bovine species.

6. In cattle, a prominent protuberance known as the hook bone is the:
   a. tuber sacrale.
   b. tuber ischiadicum.
   c. tuber coxae.
   d. simply tuber.

7. Proceeding distally from the cannon bone in the horse, the phalangeal articulations are referred to as:
   a. pastern, fetlock, coffin.
   b. fetlock, pastern, coffin.
   c. coffin, pastern, fetlock.
   d. pastern, coffin, fetlock.

8. Sesamoid bones:
   a. articulate with other bones, and thereby reduce friction by their attachment with ligaments directed for more distal locations.
   b. are firmly attached to other bones without visible movement.
   c. are the same as splint bones.
   d. got their name from Sesame Street.

BONE STRUCTURE

9. The cylindrical shaft of a long bone is known as the:
   a. epiphysis.
   b. metaphysis.
   c. diaphysis.

10. The principal location of hematopoiesis (blood cell production) is the:
    a. joint capsule.
    b. medullary cavity of the diaphysis.
    c. epiphyseal plate.
    d. lacunae.

11. The outer surface of bones (with the exception of joint surfaces) is covered by:
    a. endosteum.
    b. hyaline cartilage.
    c. periosteum.
    d. osteoblasts.

12. Osteoblasts:
    a. are the hematopoietic cells of bone.
    b. synthesize and secrete the organic substance of bone.
    c. are bone-dissolving cells.
    d. are the mature cells of bone.

13. The interstitial fluid of osteocytes:
    a. is contained within lacunae and canaliculae.
    b. diffuses from blood vessels within haversian canals.
    c. serves osteocytes in all concentric lamellae, even the outermost.
    d. is described in a, b, and c, above.

14. Stimulation of osteoprogenitor cells leads directly to:
    a. osteoclasts.
    b. osteocytes.
    c. osteoblasts.
    d. chondrocytes.

15. Production of osteoid and its subsequent calcification is accomplished by:
    a. osteoclasts.
    b. osteocytes.
    c. osteoblasts.
    d. chondrocytes.

16. Bone cells that represent transformed osteoblasts, communicate with each other by gap junctions in canaliculae, and maintain bone matrix are:
    a. osteoprogenitor cells.
    b. osteoblasts.
    c. osteoclasts.
    d. osteocytes.

17. Osteoclasts:
    a. are transformed osteocytes.
    b. are large bone-resorbing cells considered to be members of the diffuse mononuclear phagocytic system.
    c. are active in producing bone matrix.

18. Calcium and phosphorus:
    a. are the major constituents of the mineral phase of bone and exist in a ratio of $2:1$ (calcium:phosphorus).
    b. represent the organic matter of bone.
    c. are never recovered from bone once they are deposited in the mineral phase.

19. Haversian systems:
    a. are the units of structure of compact bone.
    b. develop within tunnels formed in the zone of calcified matrix.
    c. develop when capillaries invade the tunnels formed by nests of dead chondrocytes.
    d. are represented by a, b, and c.

BONE FORMATION

20. The os penis, os cordis, and pathologic bone deposits represent:
    a. endochondral bone formation.
    b. intramembranous bone formation.
    c. heteroplastic bone formation.

21. Most long bones are developed:
    a. without the intervention of cartilage.
    b. by endochondral ossification.
    c. by heteroplastic ossification.

22. The epiphyseal plate:
    a. is a cartilage plate between the epiphysis and diaphysis.
    b. has a profuse blood supply.
    c. has no distinguishable zones.
    d. is located on only one end of a long bone.

23. Bone forms:
    a. in both directions from the epiphyseal plate.
    b. toward the diaphysis, with a lifting effect on the epiphyseal plate.
    c. because the chondrocytes never die.
    d. because the zone of reserve cartilage dies.

24. Remodeling of bone:
    a. occurs during growth and in response to stress placed on bone.
    b. does not occur (once formed, not removed).
    c. does not involve osteoclastic activity.

BONE REPAIR

25. A prerequisite for fracture repair is:
    a. the alleviation of pain.
    b. perfect realignment.
    c. reestablishment of a blood supply.
    d. splinting.

26. Callus formation after bone fracture:
    a. is the most common type of bone repair.
    b. is located on the external surface only.
    c. whether on the internal or external surface, comes from the osteoblasts that originate from the periosteum.
    d. does not revert to compact bone and subsequent remodeling.

JOINTS AND SYNOVIAL FLUID

27. The synovial membrane:
    a. covers the bearing surface (articular cartilage) of a joint.
    b. is the outer fibrous layer of a joint capsule that contributes to the stability of the joint.
    c. is the lining inner surface of a joint capsule that contains synoviocytes, which secrete synovial fluid.

28. The chief function(s) of synovial fluid is (are):
    a. to serve as an adhesive to hold bones together at a joint.
    b. to provide for a popping noise when bones are pulled apart.
    c. to provide for joint lubrication and nourishment of the articular cartilage.

29. Synovial fluid:
    a. viscosity is almost entirely attributable to hyaluronic acid.
    b. color is always yellow.
    c. viscosity is the same in all joints.
    d. contains numerous cells.

30. Adult articular cartilage is:
    a. supplied with nerves and blood vessels.
    b. smooth but very rigid.
    c. a resilient and elastic tissue that becomes thinner when compressed and regains original thickness when pressure is released.

31. Nutrition of adult articular cartilage:
    a. is not needed.
    b. is provided by synovial fluid and fluid that diffuses from capillaries in the joint capsule.
    c. is provided from capillaries that infiltrate its substance.

32. Which one of the following items best describes lubrication of synovial joints?
    a. They do not need it because they are smooth.
    b. Aqueous humor
    c. Hyaluronic acid and lubricin, which are secreted by the synovial membrane
    d. Secretions of the choroid plexus

33. Nerve fibers for pain:
    a. are located in articular cartilage.
    b. are located in the joint capsule.
    c. do not exist in association with synovial joints.

ANSWERS TO SELF EVALUATION—CHAPTER 7

1. b	10. b	19. d	28. c
2. c	11. c	20. c	29. a
3. b	12. b	21. b	30. c
4. d	13. d	22. a	31. b
5. c	14. c	23. b	32. c
6. c	15. c	24. a	33. b
7. b	16. d	25. c	
8. a	17. b	26. a	
9. c	18. a	27. c	

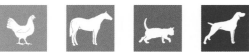

Muscle

- **CLASSIFICATION**
  Smooth Muscle
  Cardiac Muscle
  Skeletal Muscle
- **ARRANGEMENT**
- **SKELETAL-MUSCLE HARNESSING**
- **MICROSTRUCTURE OF SKELETAL MUSCLE**
  Muscle-Fiber Division
  Sarcotubular System
  Neuromuscular Junction

- **SKELETAL-MUSCLE CONTRACTION**
  Depolarization of Muscle Fibers
  Contraction Process
  Contraction versus Contracture
  Contraction Strength
- **COMPARISON OF CONTRACTION AMONG MUSCLE TYPES**
- **CHANGES IN MUSCLE SIZE**
  Hypertrophy and Hyperplasia
  Atrophy

Movements of the skeleton, changes in the amount of blood supplied to body parts, transport of ingesta through the intestinal tract, generation of body heat, and circulation of blood are examples of muscle function. Because of these diverse functions throughout the body, and because considerable work is required to perform them, it is not surprising that 45% to 50% of body weight is represented by components of the muscular system.

■ CLASSIFICATION

1. What kinds of nerves are associated with the activity of smooth, cardiac, and skeletal muscle?
2. What is the principal distinguishing characteristic between smooth muscle and cardiac and skeletal muscle?
3. What is the function of an intercalated disk in cardiac muscle?
4. What is the functional difference between red and white skeletal muscle fibers?

There are three types of muscle cells of the animal body: smooth, cardiac, and skeletal.

Each is characterized not only by microscopic structural differences, but also by location, function, and innervation.

Smooth Muscle

Smooth muscle is so named because it has no visible striations. The individual cells are spindle shaped and have a centrally located nucleus (*Fig. 8-1*). Smooth muscles are regulated by the autonomic nervous system and are located in visceral structures that require movements of an automatic nature. Aggregates of myofilaments in smooth muscle are composed of the contractile proteins actin and myosin. The filaments are not arranged in order (as in skeletal muscle), which accounts for the lack of visible striations.

Cardiac Muscle

Cardiac muscle is found only in the heart. It is regulated by the autonomic nervous system, like smooth muscle. In contrast to smooth muscle, however, on microscopic examination, cardiac muscle shows striations characterized by alternating light and dark bands. Cardiac muscle is composed of elongated,

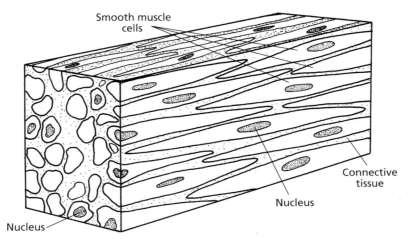

■ **FIGURE 8-1** Smooth muscle cells exposed in their longitudinal and cross-sectional planes. The cells are characteristically spindle-shaped and have a centrally located nucleus.

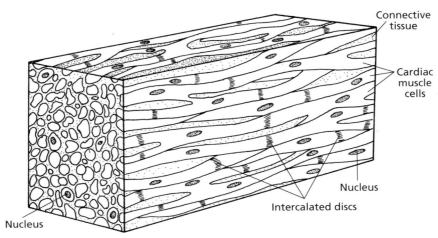

■ **FIGURE 8-2** Cardiac muscle cells exposed in their longitudinal and cross-sectional planes. Note elongated, branching cells with irregular contours at their junctions with other cells.

branching cells with irregular contours at their junctions with other cells (*Fig. 8-2*). The boundary area where the end of a cell anastomoses (joins) with the next cell is known as an **intercalated disc**. This highly specialized cell membrane structure facilitates the transmission of nerve impulses from one cell to the next because of its low electrical resistance. Each cell has one nucleus (sometimes two) that is centrally located.

Skeletal Muscle

Skeletal muscle cells (fibers) of many animals can be one of three types: 1) **red** or dark, 2) **white** or pale, or 3) **intermediate**, with characteristics between those of red and white fibers (*Fig. 8-3*). Red muscle fibers are characterized by having more myoglobin and more mitochondria than white fibers. All muscles are probably a mixture of these three types, but in some animals the red and in others the white predominates. A striking example of this is the crimson red pectoralis muscle (breast muscle) of pigeons, which contrasts sharply with the stark white color of the chicken pectoralis muscle. Red muscle fibers usually contract more slowly and fatigue less readily than white muscle fibers. In birds, the amount of red pigmentation in the pectoralis muscle can be correlated directly with the ability to sustain flight. Geese and ducks, as well as pigeons, are known for their sustained flight, and they have a predominance of red pectoralis muscle fibers.

Skeletal muscle makes up the major portion of the muscle mass of the animal body. An individual skeletal muscle fiber can extend the length of the muscle of which it is a part. As is characteristic of cardiac muscles, skeletal muscles are striated when viewed microscopically. They are not branched and do not anastomose (thus, no intercalated disc). Skeletal muscle is innervated by cranial and spinal nerves, and a nerve impulse to each muscle fiber is required for its stimulation. Multiple, peripherally arranged nuclei are present in each cell (*Fig. 8-4*), in contrast to both smooth and cardiac muscle cells.

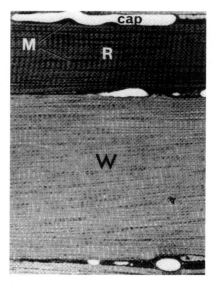

■ FIGURE 8-3 Photomicrograph of skeletal muscle showing red fibers (R) and white fibers (W). Red fibers have more mitochondria (M) packed between their myofibrils, especially in association with capillaries (cap). (From Cormack DC. Ham's Histology. 9th Ed. Philadelphia: JB Lippincott, 1987.)

■ ARRANGEMENT

1. **What is the difference between the origin and the insertion of a skeletal muscle?**
2. **What is the difference between a flexor and an extensor skeletal muscle?**
3. **What is the difference between an adductor and an abductor skeletal muscle?**

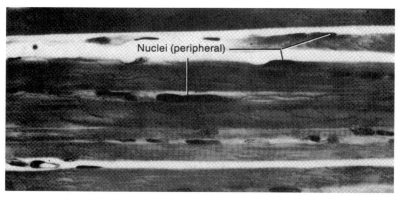

■ FIGURE 8-4 Photomicrograph of a longitudinal section of skeletal muscle fibers. Note the striations and the multiple, peripherally located nuclei. (From Cormack DC. Ham's Histology. 9th Ed. Philadelphia: JB Lippincott, 1987.)

The function of muscles is to contract or shorten. In doing this, they move a body part or body contents, or they provide resistance to some movement. A primary consideration in determining what muscles accomplish is their cell arrangement. Accordingly, the muscle cells might be arranged in sheets, sheets rolled into tubes, bundles, rings (sphincters), or cones, or they might remain as discrete cells or clusters for more precise or less forceful action. The emptying of visceral structures (e.g., urinary bladder, stomach, heart) or the conveyance of intestinal contents or organ secretions, as provided by smooth and cardiac muscle, is accomplished because of their intimate association with the affected part. Apart from the skeletal muscle sphincters, the effects of skeletal muscle may be noted at a point some distance from their location. This means that their contraction must be transmitted somehow to the affected part. For this to happen, one end of the muscle must be relatively fixed or anchored and the other end must be attached directly or by a tendon to the movable part. Accordingly, the anatomic description of a skeletal muscle sometimes refers to its origin and insertion, the **origin** being the least movable end and the **insertion** the most movable end. Contraction of skeletal muscle brings the origin and insertion closer together and, when attachments involve two bones, one or both of the bones will move.

Skeletal muscles are often described according to the type of movement performed. They are **flexors** if they are located on the side of the limb toward which the joint bends when decreasing the joint angle. They are **extensors** if they are located on the side of the limb toward which the joint bends when increasing the joint angle. **Adductors** are muscles that pull a limb toward the median plane, and **abductors** pull a limb away from the median plane. **Sphincters** are arranged circularly to constrict body openings. Muscles are strategically located to best serve the structure they affect. Lack of adduction occasionally occurs in the hindlimbs of cows after parturition or

calving. The adductor muscles are supplied by the obturator nerves (one to each leg), each of which passes through an opening (obturator foramen) in the birth canal (see Chapter 7). Its injury during the calving process can be followed by the inability to adduct one or both of the hind legs (obturator paralysis).

■ SKELETAL-MUSCLE HARNESSING

1.   **Differentiate between epimysium, perimysium, and endomysium. Which of these is most intimately associated with individual muscle fibers?**

The harness for skeletal muscle fibers is composed of connective tissue elements (**epimysium**, **perimysium**, **endomysium**) that are continuous from the individual muscle fibers to the connective tissue of the structure to which the muscle attaches and on which it exerts its pull when it contracts. Often the connective tissue of the structure to which it is attached is a **tendon** (*Fig. 8-5*). A broad connective tissue sheet that fulfills a similar function is an **aponeurosis**. The connective tissue elements of skeletal muscle are as follows:

1.   Muscle fibers that compose a muscle bundle (also called fascicles) are attached by their cell covering (sarcolemma) to a connective tissue division, the endomysium.
2.   The endomysium is continuous with connective tissue that envelops muscle bundles, the perimysium.
3.   The perimysium is continuous with connective tissue that envelops the muscle (collection of muscle bundles), the epimysium.
4.   The epimysium is continuous with the tendon or aponeurosis, which can travel some distance for its attachment.

Some muscles seem to arise directly from a bone, and their attachment could be considered a **fleshy attachment**. These muscle cells, however, do have a short tendinous attachment to the periosteum of the bone.

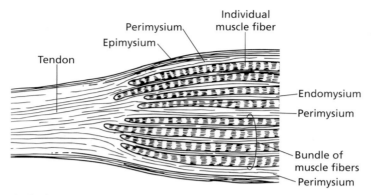

■ **FIGURE 8-5** Longitudinal section of a muscle. The connective tissue elements of muscle are continuous with a tendon. (Adapted from Ham AW. Histology. 7th Ed. Philadelphia: JB Lippincott, 1974.)

■ MICROSTRUCTURE OF SKELETAL MUSCLE

1. Is a muscle fiber the same as a muscle cell?
2. Understand the division of a muscle fiber into myofibrils, myofibrils into sarcomeres, sarcomeres into myofilaments, and myofilaments into actin and myosin.
3. Be able to sketch a sarcomere and the spatial arrangement of the myofilaments.
4. Relate the striations (banding) of skeletal muscle to the myofilaments.
5. Which tubule set of the sarcotubular system opens to the outside of the muscle fiber and contains extracellular fluid?
6. What is the location of the sarcoplasmic reticulum relative to T tubules and myofibrils?
7. What is the function of the sarcotubular system?
8. What is a neuromuscular junction, and how many are there for each muscle fiber?
9. What is a motor unit?

To understand how muscles contract, the microstructure of skeletal muscle fibers must be understood. Muscle fibers vary considerably in length, and they can be as long as the muscle of which they are a part.

Muscle-Fiber Division

The division of muscles into smaller parts, down to myofibrils, is shown in *Figure 8-6*. Depending on the diameter of the muscle fiber, there might be several hundred to several thousand **myofibrils** within one muscle fiber. Each myofibril has striations or banding. The further division of myofibrils into repetitive units (**sarcomeres**) and their components is shown in *Figure 8-7*. Sarcomeres contain the protein **myofilaments**, **actin** and **myosin**, which by their arrangement give rise to striations (Fig. 8-7B). Inasmuch as the striations are characteristic of the muscle fiber, it is apparent that the sarcomeres of a myofibril are in alignment with the sarcomeres of all the other myofibrils of the muscle fiber. The **Z line** is located at each end of a sarcomere and is common to both sarcomeres that it separates. Actin filaments project from the Z line into the sarcomeres that it separates (Fig. 8-7B). Thus, each sarcomere has actin filaments projected toward its center from each end. The actin of two sarcomeres common to the same Z line compose an **I band**. The myosin filaments are centrally located within a sarcomere and, coupled with the overlap of actin filaments, provide for the dark

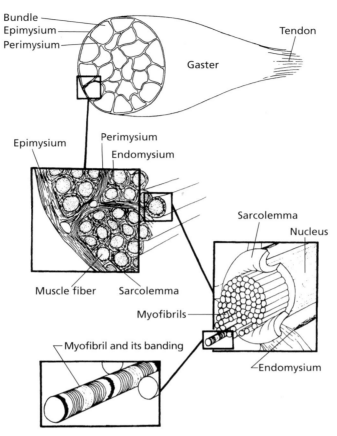

■ FIGURE 8-6 The division of muscles into smaller parts, down to myofibrils. (From Feduccia A, McCrady E. Torrey's Morphogenesis of the Vertebrates. 5th. Ed. New York: John Wiley & Sons, 1991.)

banding (**A band**) of the characteristic striations (*Fig. 8-8*). The actin and myosin filaments have a regular, spatial arrangement to each other, as shown in the cross section of a myofibril (Fig. 8-7C), which has a 2:1 ratio of actin to myosin. A longitudinal section of the spatially arranged myofilaments shows cross linkages extending from the myosin filaments toward the actin filaments (Fig. 8-7D). During muscle-fiber shortening, the actin filaments appear to slide deeper into the myosin filaments.

Sarcotubular System

Skeletal muscle fibers contain a network of tubules known as the **sarcotubular system**.

These tubules are located within the muscle fiber, but are outside the myofibrils. The sarcotubular system is composed of two separate tubule sets, with each set having a different arrangement among the myofibrils (*Fig. 8-9*). The tubules that are arranged parallel to the myofibrils and encircle them are known as the sarcoplasmic reticulum. The tubules that are arranged transversely (right angles) to the myofibrils are known as the **T tubules**. T tubules extend transversely from one side of the fiber to the other. They open to the outside of the fiber (surface of the sarcolemma), and therefore their lumens contain extracellular fluid. The T tubule openings are regularly spaced throughout the length of the muscle

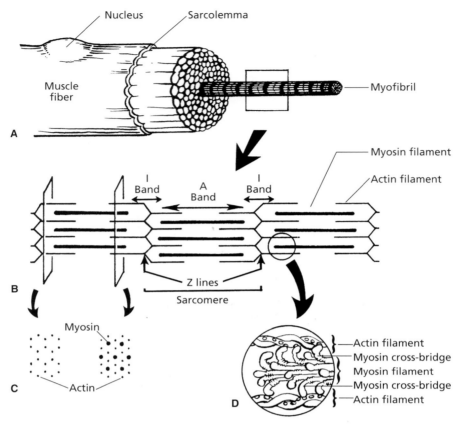

■ **FIGURE 8-7** The division of myofibrils into sarcomeres. **A)** Cross section of a muscle fiber. **B)** Longitudinal arrangement of myofilaments within sarcomeres. **C)** Spatial arrangement of the myofilaments within a sarcomere. **D)** Further details of the relationship between actin and myosin molecules.

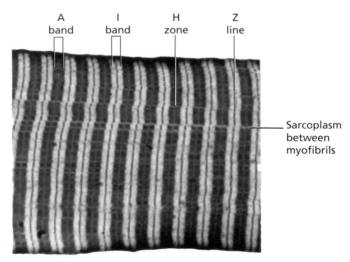

■ **FIGURE 8-8** Photomicrograph of a longitudinal section of a skeletal muscle fiber. Shown is the characteristic banding. (From Cormack DC. Essential Histology. 2nd Ed. Baltimore: Lippincott Williams & Wilkins, 2001.)

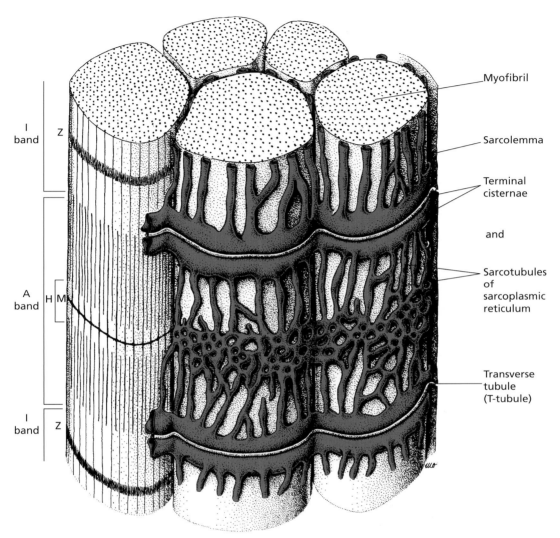

■ FIGURE 8-9 Cross section of part of a mammalian skeletal muscle fiber, showing the sarcoplasmic reticulum that surrounds myofibrils. Two transverse (T) tubules supply a sarcomere and are in close association with the sarcoplasmic reticulum. The T tubules open to the surface of the sarcolemma. (From Cormack DC. Essential Histology. 2nd Ed. Baltimore: Lippincott Williams & Wilkins, 2001.)

fiber because of their orientation to each sarcomere. Similarly, their openings are regularly spaced around the circumference of the fiber so that all myofibrils are intimately served by the sarcotubular system.

In reference to a sarcomere, the T tubules are located near the junction of the actin fila-ments with the myosin filaments. Therefore, each sarcomere is close to two T tubules (see Fig. 8-9). The individual tubules (sarcotubules) of the sarcoplasmic reticulum are located regularly throughout the length of the muscle fiber between the T tubules, and they in turn contain intracellular fluid. The T

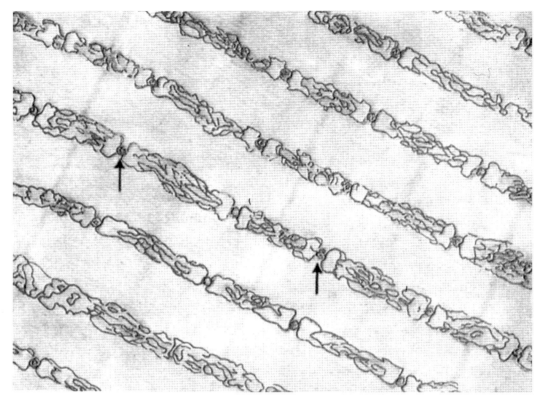

■ **FIGURE 8-10** Sarcoplasmic reticulum in the extracellular spaces between the myofibrils, showing a longitudinal system paralleling the myofibrils. Also shown in cross section are T tubules (arrows) that lead to the exterior of the fiber membrane and are important for conducting the electrical signal into the center of the muscle fiber. (From Fawcett DW: The Cell. Philadelphia: WB Saunders, 1981.)

tubules do not open into the sarcoplasmic reticulum; instead, the bulbous ends of the sarcoplasmic reticulum are closely associated with the T tubules (*Fig. 8-10*). The point of closeness of a T tubule with the bulbous ends of two adjoining sarcoplasmic reticula is known as a **triad**. The principal function of the sarcotubular system is to provide a means for conduction of an impulse from the surface of the muscle fiber to its innermost aspects.

Neuromuscular Junction

Each skeletal muscle fiber is provided with one specialized area, the **neuromuscular junction**. This junction is the intimate association of the terminal branch of a nerve fiber with the muscle fiber (*Fig. 8-11*). The nerve fiber ending is not continuous with the muscle fiber; there is a space between the neuromuscular junction and the muscle fiber. This space is centrally located on the surface of the muscle fiber. A nerve fiber can have a number of terminal branches, with each one going to a separate muscle fiber (*Fig. 8-12*). A **motor unit** consists of a nerve fiber and the muscle fibers that it innervates. A motor unit ratio of 1:150 means that one nerve fiber is innervating 150 muscle fibers, whereas a ratio of 1:4 means that one nerve fiber is innervating four muscle fibers. Hypothetically, a smaller ratio is helpful if greater precision is required for muscle contraction.

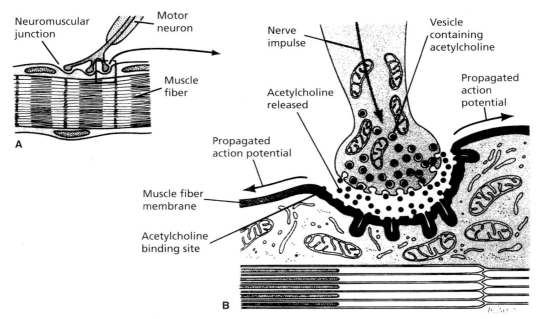

■ **FIGURE 8-11** A neuromuscular junction. **A)** General structure. **B)** Magnification of junctional area showing the events that occur after nerve impulse transmission. (From Spence A, Mason EB. Human Anatomy and Physiology. 4th Ed. St. Paul, MN: West Publishing Co, 1992.)

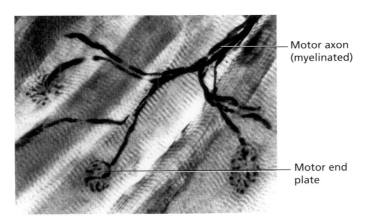

■ **FIGURE 8-12** Photomicrograph showing the distribution of terminal branches from a nerve fiber to individual muscle fibers to compose a motor unit. A motor end plate is a small, flattened mound on the muscle-fiber surface formed by the axon terminal branch and its myelin covering. (From Cormack DC. Essential Histology. 2nd Ed. Baltimore: Lippincott William & Wilkins, 2001.)

■ SKELETAL-MUSCLE CONTRACTION

1. Describe the chain of events that initiates muscle-fiber membrane depolarization.
2. What is the association of Ca^{2+} to acetylcholine release? How is this related to milk fever in dairy cows?
3. What is the trigger for release of Ca^{2+} from the sarcoplasmic reticulum? Where does Ca^{2+} go after release?
4. Study the molecular basis of muscle contraction with emphasis on sequence, and relate it to shortening and relaxation of muscle fibers.
5. What molecule seems to be necessary for relaxation?
6. What causes rigor mortis?
7. What is muscle tetany? Is this a reflection of motor unit summation or wave summation?
8. How is the bacterial disease, tetanus, related to central nervous system neurotransmitters?

Muscle tissue has basic physiologic properties other than contractility or the ability to shorten. These include excitability, extensibility, and elasticity. **Excitability** (also called irritability) is the capacity to receive and respond to a stimulus. **Extensibility** is the ability to be stretched. **Elasticity** is the ability to return to the original shape after contraction or after being stretched. All four of these properties are related to the ability of muscle to produce movement.

Depolarization of Muscle Fibers

The neuromuscular junction functions as an amplifier for a nerve impulse. The arrival of a spinal or cranial nerve impulse at the neuromuscular junction results in the release of **acetylcholine (ACh)** into the space between the nerve-fiber terminal branch and the muscle fiber (synaptic gap). The release of ACh is accelerated because **calcium ions** from the extracellular fluid enter the prejunctional membrane when the nerve impulse arrives. ACh is the stimulus that increases the permeability of the muscle-fiber membrane for sodium ions, after which membrane depolarization begins. Depolarization proceeds in all directions from the neuromuscular junction, and an impulse is generated. The impulse is conducted into all parts of the muscle fiber by the sarcotubular system (see previous text). Because the impulse initiates muscle contraction, a more synchronized contraction results when all parts of the fiber are depolarized nearly simultaneously as a result of sarcotubular transmission.

A low concentration of calcium in the extracellular fluid is recognized clinically in dairy cows after calving (parturient paresis, or milk fever) as a state of semiparalysis caused by partial neuromuscular block. When the calcium ion concentration is low, the amount of ACh released is lowered; this might not be sufficient to cause neuromuscular transmission, and thus neuromuscular block results.

Almost immediately after its release, ACh is hydrolyzed by the enzyme acetylcholinesterase into acetic acid and choline. Therefore, the next depolarization must await the arrival of the next nerve impulse.

The tubules of the sarcoplasmic reticulum have a relatively high concentration of calcium ions. Depolarization of these tubules results in a simultaneous release of calcium ions into the sarcoplasm, which in turn diffuse rapidly into the myofibrils (*Fig. 8-13*). The presence of calcium ions within the myofibrils initiates the contraction process. The calcium ions are returned rapidly by active transport to the sarcoplasmic reticulum after contraction is initiated and are released again when the next nerve impulse arrives.

Contraction Process

The shortening, or contraction, process involves an interaction between the actin and myosin filaments. There is a natural attraction

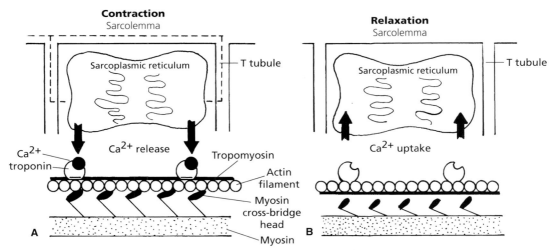

■ **FIGURE 8-13** A cycle of contraction followed by relaxation. **A)** The dashed line indicates transfer of depolarization from the sarcolemma and T tubules to the sarcoplasmic reticulum. Depolarization is followed by Ca^{2+} release from the sarcoplasmic reticulum with diffusion to the myofibrils. Ca^{2+} binds to troponin, removing blocking action of tropomyosin. Myosin cross-bridge heads attach to active sites on actin and bend toward center of myosin molecule. **B)** ATP binds to cross-bridge heads, causing their detachment from actin. Ca^{2+} is returned to the sarcoplasmic reticulum using energy supplied by ATP. Removal of Ca^{2+} from troponin restores blocking action of tropomyosin.

for actin and myosin molecules involving active sites on the actin molecule. Attraction is inhibited during relaxation because the active sites are covered, but when calcium ions enter the myofibril, the active sites are uncovered. The projecting portions of the myosin molecules (**cross bridges**) attach to the active sites and bend toward the center, causing the actin to slide toward the myosin molecule center (*Fig. 8-14*).

The actin filament has three major components (all protein): **actin**, **tropomyosin**, and **troponin** (*Fig. 8-15*). Actin and tropomyosin are arranged in helical strands interwoven with each other. Troponin is located at regular intervals along the strands and contains three proteins, two of which bind actin and tropomyosin together and the third of which has an affinity for calcium ions. Active sites (places where myosin cross bridges attach) are located on the actin strands and are normally covered by the tropomyosin strands. When calcium ions bind to the troponin complex, however, a conformational change occurs between the

actin and tropomyosin strands and causes the active sites to be uncovered. The uncovered sites favor activation of the natural attraction that exists between actin and myosin. A number of changes occur in the heads of the myosin cross bridges that cause muscle contraction, and these are summarized as follows (*Fig. 8-16*) (assume that cross-bridge heads have just bound with adenosine triphosphate [ATP] and have detached from the active sites of the actin filaments):

1. **Adenosine triphosphatase (ATPase)** of the myosin cross-bridge heads hydrolyze ATP to adenosine diphosphate (ADP) + inorganic phosphorus (Pi), leaving the ADP + Pi bound to the heads. Energy from the hydrolysis of ATP "cocks" the heads so that they increase their angle of attachment to the cross-bridge arm and become perpendicular to the active sites of the actin filaments.

2. After depolarization of the sarcotubular system, calcium ions diffuse from the

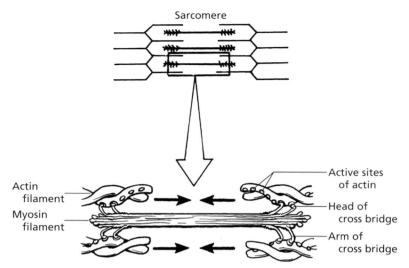

■ FIGURE 8-14 The components of the actin and myosin myofilaments associated with contraction of the sarcomere. Arrows indicate the direction of actin movement during contraction (shortening of myofibrils).

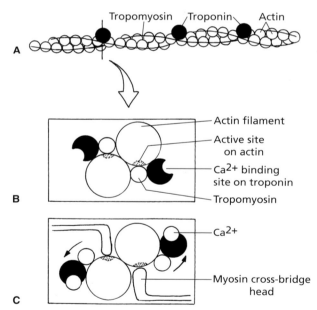

■ FIGURE 8-15 Conformational changes of the actin filament after calcium binding. **A)** The actin filament with its three proteins, actin, troponin, and tropomyosin. The vertical line indicates the cross-section location for B and C. **B)** The active sites on actin are covered by tropomyosin. **C)** Ca^{2+} binds to troponin, resulting in a conformational change that exposes the active sites on actin. Myosin cross-bridge heads attach to actin active sites, and myofibril contraction begins.

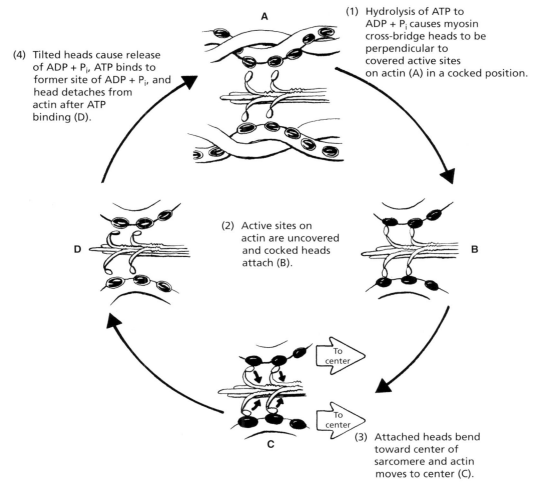

(4) Tilted heads cause release of ADP + P$_i$, ATP binds to former site of ADP + P$_i$, and head detaches from actin after ATP binding (D).

(1) Hydrolysis of ATP to ADP + P$_i$ causes myosin cross-bridge heads to be perpendicular to covered active sites on actin (A) in a cocked position.

(2) Active sites on actin are uncovered and cocked heads attach (B).

(3) Attached heads bend toward center of sarcomere and actin moves to center (C).

A

B

C

D

To center

To center

■ **FIGURE 8-16** The sequence of actin and myosin interaction. This results in muscle shortening. ATP, adenosine triphosphate; ADP, adenosine diphosphate; Pi, inorganic phosphorus.

sarcoplasmic reticulum into myofibrils and bind to the troponin complexes, whereby actin filament active sites are uncovered; calcium ions are returned rapidly to the sarcoplasmic reticulum once the shortening process begins (ATP is required for return). Natural attraction of myosin to actin is now permitted, and the "cocked" heads bind with active sites.

3. Bonding with actin causes conformational change in the heads ("uncocking"), causing them to bend (tilt) toward the cross-bridge arms (toward the center of the sarcomere), pulling actin with it (energy is derived from previous ATP hydrolysis).

4. The tilted heads cause release of ADP + Pi and expose sites on the heads for binding of new ATP.

The binding of new ATP causes detachment of myosin cross-bridge heads from actin filaments. The ATPase of heads hydrolyzes ATP as before, cocking the heads; the process is repeated when the next neuromuscular transmission causes depolarization of the sarcotubular system. Repetition of the process causes the actin filaments to be pulled farther into the center, thus shortening the sarcomere.

The immediate energy for muscle contraction is thus derived from ATP, forming ADP + Pi. The amount of ATP in muscle fibers is limited, and rephosphorylation of ADP must occur so that contraction can continue. This is accomplished by transfer from **creatine phosphate (CP)**, which is about five times more plentiful than ATP, according to the following reaction:

$$CP + ADP \xrightarrow{\text{kinase}} C + ATP$$

Because the amount of CP is also limited, the necessary rephosphorylation of creatine (C) and ADP is ultimately derived from intermediary metabolism within the muscle cell and from the associated reoxidation of reduced cofactors that occurs in the electron transfer chain of the mitochondria. The presence of ATP is required for relaxation, or detachment of the myosin from the actin, and also for the return of calcium ions to the sarcoplasmic reticulum.

Muscle contraction is 50% to 70% efficient in regard to the accomplishment of work. The nonwork portion is dissipated as heat. This heat source is important to the body for the maintenance of body heat. Body cooling results in shivering, which is an attempt by the body to generate heat by muscle contraction.

Contraction versus Contracture

Muscle shortening can occur in the absence of action potentials. This type of shortening is referred to as **rigor** or **physiologic contracture**, as opposed to contraction. The actin and myosin filaments remain in a continuous contracted state because sufficient ATP is not available to bring about relaxation (see previous text). Contracture that occurs after death is referred to as **rigor mortis**. Lack of ATP for relaxation in this case endures, however, and relaxation only occurs as a result of postmortem autolysis caused by enzymes released from the lysosomes 12 to 24 hours after death. Those muscles that were most active just before death are those that develop rigor mortis first (i.e., greater exhaustion of ATP and CP associated with greater muscle activity).

Contraction Strength

Contraction strength varies and is achieved by motor unit summation or by wave summation. The stimulation of one motor unit causes a weak contraction, whereas the stimulation of a large number of motor units develops a strong contraction. This is known as **motor unit summation**. All gradations of contraction strength are possible, depending on the number of motor units stimulated. Increasing the strength of contraction by **wave summation** occurs when the frequency of contraction is increased. When a muscle is stimulated to contract before the muscle has relaxed, the strength of the subsequent contraction, as measured by the height of a lifted load, is increased. When the frequency is sufficient such that the individual muscle twitches become fused into a single prolonged contraction, the strength is at a maximum; this condition is known as **tetany** (*Fig. 8-17*).

Tetanus

Tetanus is a bacterial disease caused by a potent neurotoxin elaborated by the organism Clostridium tetani. The neurotoxin reaches the central nervous system and prevents release of an inhibitory transmitter (glycine). The resulting sensitivity to excitatory impulses, unchecked by inhibitory impulses, produces generalized muscular spasms (tetany). Tetanus has been called lockjaw because the masseter muscles that close the mouth are stronger than the muscles that open the mouth and the jaws remain in a closed (locked) position.

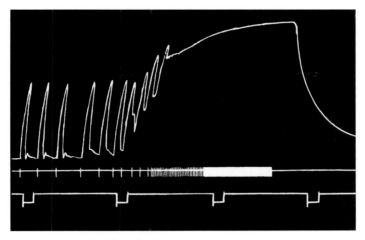

■ **FIGURE 8-17** Increasing muscle strength by increasing the frequency of contraction. This is known as wave summation. Tetany occurs when individual contractions are fused and cannot be distinguished from each other. (From Carlson AJ, Johnson V. The Machinery of the Body. 4th Ed. Chicago: University of Chicago Press, 1953.)

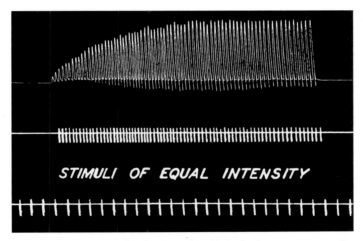

■ **FIGURE 8-18** The staircase phenomenon of skeletal muscle. This is also known as treppe. Successive stimuli of the same intensity produce contractions of increasing strength. (From Carlson AJ, Johnson V. The Machinery of the Body. 4th Ed. Chicago: University of Chicago Press, 1953.)

Treppe

Muscles seem to "warm up" to a maximum contraction state. This can be shown by applying stimuli of equal intensity a few seconds apart to a muscle. Each successive muscle twitch has slightly more strength than the previous one, until optimal contraction strength is reached (*Fig. 8-18*). This phenomenon is referred to as **treppe**, or the **staircase phenomenon**. Successive stimulations are believed to provide for an increasing concentration of calcium ions in the sarcoplasm during the beginning contractions of rested muscles.

■ COMPARISON OF CONTRACTION AMONG MUSCLE TYPES

1. What characteristic of muscle contraction is generally similar among smooth, cardiac, and skeletal muscle fibers?
2. Differentiate harnessing, innervation, and stimulus conduction between cardiac and skeletal muscle.
3. Do smooth muscle fibers have actin and myosin, a neuromuscular junction, a harnessing system, and a sarcotubular system?
4. How does the slower cycle of attachment and detachment of cross-bridge heads of smooth muscle relate to its function?

Brief structural differences among the three muscle classifications were noted earlier. The contraction process for all three is generally similar in that actin filaments slide between myosin filaments and cause a shortening of the cell. There is a greater similarity in arrangement of these filaments between cardiac and skeletal muscle (hence, their common description as striated muscle). The myofibrils of cardiac muscle constitute most of the muscle fiber, but instead of being discrete and cylindric, as in skeletal muscle, they join together and are of variable diameter. This might be related to the more circular contraction of the heart (cardiac muscle) as compared with the more linear contraction of skeletal muscle.

Whereas the work of skeletal-muscle fibers is harnessed to connective-tissue elements, cardiac-muscle fibers anastomose with each other. Thus, the contraction of each joins with others to decrease the diameters of their respective heart chambers. Also, each skeletal-muscle fiber receives separate stimulation through a spinal or cranial nerve and neuromuscular junction, but cardiac muscle receives its stimulus from rhythmic, contractile, specialized cardiac-muscle cells known as **pacemakers**. The autonomic nervous system regulates the pacemakers. Conduction of stimulation is from cell to cell (through the intercalated disc) and special conduction fibers (Purkinje fibers in the ventricular walls). The sarcotubular system of cardiac muscle is not as well developed as that of skeletal muscle.

Smooth-muscle myofilaments are not aligned into myofibrils, as in cardiac and skeletal muscles. Furthermore, a higher ratio of actin to myosin exists ($15:1$ instead of $2:1$). The actin filaments are attached to dense bodies that are dispersed inside the cell, and also some are attached to the cell membrane. The dense bodies correspond to the Z lines of skeletal muscle and are held in place by a framework of structural proteins that link one dense body to another. The actin filaments from two separate dense bodies extend toward each other and surround a myosin filament, thereby providing a contractile unit that is similar to a contractile unit of skeletal muscle (*Fig. 8-19*).

There also are differences between the contraction of smooth muscle and striated muscle. The cycle of attachment and detachment of cross-bridge heads that extend from myosin to actin is much slower in smooth muscle. This provides for prolonged tonic contraction, in contrast to rapid contractions of skeletal muscle. The slower cycles are a result of the much lower ATPase activity on the myosin cross-bridge heads than in skeletal muscle, and the heads remain in an "uncocked" position for a longer time. Coupled with the slower frequency of attachment-detachment cycling is the lower energy requirement for sustaining the same tension of contraction in smooth muscle as in skeletal muscle. This is important from the standpoint of energy conservation, wherein smooth-muscle organs (e.g., urinary bladder, intestines) must maintain tone throughout the day and night.

Smooth-muscle cells are able to shorten a much greater percentage of their total length than skeletal muscle. This feature enables a smooth-muscle organ, such as the urinary

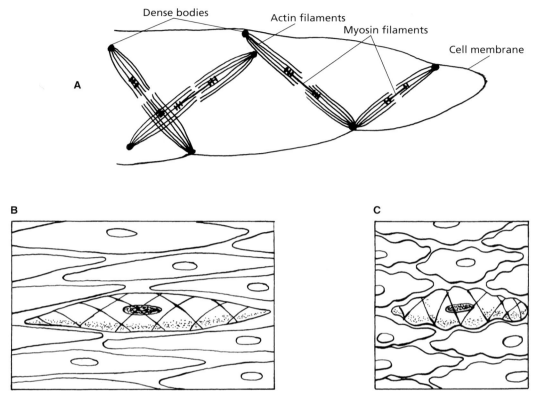

■ **FIGURE 8-19** Contraction of smooth muscle. **A)** Physical structure of smooth muscle. Dense bodies attach either to the cell membrane or to an intracellular structural protein that links several dense bodies together. The dense bodies are functionally similar to Z lines. **B)** A translucent view of a relaxed smooth-muscle cell. **C)** A translucent view of a contracted smooth-muscle cell. Dense bodies not shown in B and C.

bladder, to reduce its lumen diameter from its expanded state to virtually zero.

The neuromuscular junctions associated with smooth muscle are **diffuse junctions**. The autonomic nerve fibers that innervate smooth muscle do not make direct contact with the muscle fibers but form diffuse junctions that secrete their transmitter substance into the interstitial fluid, whereupon it diffuses to the smooth-muscle cells. The vesicles of the terminal axons contain either ACh or nor-epinephrine, depending on whether the post-ganglionic terminal fiber is parasympathetic or sympathetic, respectively. The vesicle secretion may be excitatory or inhibitory depending on the receptors that are located on the smooth muscle membrane. The receptors determine whether the smooth muscle will be excited or inhibited and which one of the two transmit-ters will be effective in causing the excitatory or inhibitory response. The sarcotubular system of smooth muscle fibers is poorly developed. Counterparts to the T tubules are **vesicles** (called **calveolae**) that open onto the surface of the fiber just under the cell membrane.

■ CHANGES IN MUSCLE SIZE

1. **What is the difference between hyperplasia and hypertrophy?**
2. **How do skeletal muscle fibers hyper-trophy (grow in size) after birth?**

3. Is regeneration of skeletal, cardiac, and smooth-muscle fibers possible?
4. What is muscle atrophy?

Muscle is the most adaptable tissue in the body of an animal. Individual muscle cells of skeletal, cardiac, and smooth muscle increase in size as a normal response to chronic mechanical stress, as with regular exercise. Similar stress in skeletal and smooth muscle causes division of muscle cells through mitosis to produce new cells. A decrease in size can occur in skeletal, cardiac, and smooth muscle in response to disease.

Hypertrophy and Hyperplasia

An increase in individual muscle-fiber size is referred to as **hypertrophy**. It is common in skeletal, cardiac, and smooth-muscle cells. Postnatal growth of skeletal-muscle fibers is not accomplished by an increase in the number of muscle fibers but rather by the addition of myofibrils to the periphery and of sarcomeres to the tendinous ends. An increase in the number of muscle fibers is called **hyperplasia**. Regeneration of skeletal-muscle fibers is possible from so-called **satellite cells**, but this requires an intact endomysium for successful repair. An increase in cardiac-muscle size is similar to that of skeletal muscle in that it involves hypertrophy and not hyperplasia. Regeneration of cardiac-muscle fibers does not occur because

there is no counterpart to the satellite cells of skeletal muscle. If myocardial cells die, they are replaced by fibrous, noncontractile scar tissue. Smooth-muscle organs can increase their size by hypertrophy and by hyperplasia, so smooth muscle has considerable regenerative ability.

Atrophy

A decrease in the size of a muscle is referred to as **atrophy**. When a body part has been immobilized for a period of time, the muscles become smaller (referred to as **disuse atrophy**). Loss of the nerve supply to a muscle results in **denervation atrophy**. This was formerly a common condition in harnessed draft horses. The presence of the collar presses on the suprascapular nerve that supplies the two major muscle masses of the shoulder blade (see Chapter 7). The resulting denervation causes the muscles of the shoulder to atrophy, resulting in a condition known as sweeny (also called shoulder slip).

■ SUGGESTED READING

Bailey JG. Muscle physiology. In: Reece WO, ed. Dukes' Physiology of Domestic Animals. 12th Ed. Ithaca, NY: Cornell University Press, 2004.

Cormack DC. Essential Histology. 2nd Ed. Baltimore: Lippincott Williams & Wilkins, 2001.

Frandson RD, Wilke WL, Fails AD. Anatomy and Physiology of Farm Animals. 6th Ed. Baltimore: Lippincott Williams & Wilkins, 2003.

Guyton AC, Hall JE. Textbook of Medical Physiology. 10th Ed. Philadelphia: WB Saunders, 2000.

 SELF EVALUATION—CHAPTER 8

CLASSIFICATION

1. Muscle fibers that contract more slowly and fatigue less readily are:
   a. red fibers.
   b. white fibers.

2. Cardiac-muscle cells have separations between adjacent cells known as intercalated discs. Their function is to:
   a. regenerate new cells.
   b. provide a location for neuromuscular junctions.

c. provide for low electrical resistance and thus facilitate depolarization from one cell to the next.

d. release Ca^{2+} for initiation of muscle contraction.

3. The autonomic nervous system regulates the activity of:
   a. cardiac muscle only.
   b. skeletal muscle only.
   c. smooth muscle only.
   d. both cardiac and smooth muscle.

ARRANGEMENT

4. A pelvic delivery of an unusually large calf has caused a cow to be down and unable to bring her hind legs together. Obturator nerve paralysis is suspected, and the affected muscles are classified as:
   a. abductors.
   b. adductors.
   c. extensors.
   d. flexors.

5. Muscles that pull a limb toward the median plane are:
   a. abductors.
   b. adductors.
   c. flexors.
   d. extensors.

SKELETAL-MUSCLE HARNESSING

6. The skeletal-muscle harness component most intimately associated with the sarcolemma is the:
   a. endomysium.
   b. perimysium.
   c. epimysium.

7. The part of the skeletal-muscle harness that is continuous with a tendon or an aponeurosis is the:
   a. perimysium.
   b. epimysium.
   c. endomysium.
   d. tug.

MICROSTRUCTURE OF SKELETAL MUSCLE

8. In skeletal-muscle fibers, the sarcomeres of a myofibril are in alignment with the sarcomeres of all of the other myofibrils.
   a. True
   b. False

9. Which one of the following is the smallest component of a skeletal muscle?
   a. Sarcomere
   b. Myosin
   c. Myofibril
   d. Muscle fiber

10. The sarcotubular system:
    a. is located within muscle fibers but outside of the myofibrils.
    b. is a system within each of the myofibrils.
    c. has no direct communication (openings) with extracellular fluid.
    d. consists of a nerve fiber and the muscle fibers that it innervates.

11. Conduction of depolarization from the surface of a muscle fiber to its inner aspects is accomplished by the:
    a. neuromuscular junction.
    b. actin filaments.
    c. endomysium.
    d. sarcotubular system.

12. The myofilament of skeletal muscle that is attached to the Z line is:
    a. actin.
    b. myosin.
    c. troponin.
    d. tropomyosin.

13. For skeletal muscle, the neuromuscular junction:
    a. is located on the surface at the midpoint of the muscle fiber (one for each muscle fiber).
    b. releases acetylcholine when the nerve is stimulated.
    c. release of chemical is facilitated by extracellular Ca^{2+}.
    d. all of the above.

SKELETAL-MUSCLE CONTRACTION

14. Which tubule set of the sarcotubular system releases Ca^{2+} when depolarized, for their diffusion to the myofibrils?
    a. Transverse tubules
    b. Sarcoplasmic reticulum

15. What chemical substance is released from vesicles at the neuromuscular junction on the arrival of a nerve impulse?
    a. Succinylcholine
    b. Epinephrine
    c. Acetylcholine
    d. Curare

16. Rigor mortis most probably occurs when:
    a. actin and myosin are detached.
    b. Ca^{2+} is depleted.
    c. insufficient ATP is available for relaxation.
    d. contraction frequency is rapid and sustained.

17. The function of Ca^{2+} at the level of myofilaments is to:
    a. uncover active sites on actin so that the "cocked" projections of myosin may make an attachment.
    b. depolarize the muscle-fiber membrane.
    c. initiate acetylcholine release.
    d. block pores to prevent Na^+ inrush.

18. What chemical begins the depolarization of skeletal-muscle fibers after a nerve impulse initiates its release?
    a. Ca^{2+}
    b. Acetylcholine
    c. Succinylcholine
    d. Acetylcholinesterase

19. After depolarization of the sarcoplasmic reticulum, what chemical is released that initiates the contraction process?
    a. ATP
    b. Tropomyosin
    c. Ca^{2+}
    d. ACh

20. Increased muscle strength associated with tetany is an example of:
    a. wave summation.
    b. motor-unit summation.
    c. Clostridium tetani neurotoxin activity.

21. Myosin cross-bridge heads detach from actin active sites when the cross-bridge heads bind:
    a. Ca^{2+}.
    b. ATP.
    c. creatine phosphate.
    d. ADP + Pi.

22. Rigor mortis is an example of _____, which results from a depletion of _____ and a failure of cross-bridge heads to _____ to/from actin. (Select choice below that has respective words for the blanks above.)
    a. contraction; Ca^{2+}; attach
    b. relaxation; Ca^{2+}; attach
    c. contracture; ATP; detach
    d. contraction; ATP; detach

23. The Ca^{2+} released from the sarcoplasmic reticulum begins the contraction process by:
    a. "cocking" the myosin filament cross-bridge heads.
    b. rephosphorylating ADP.
    c. exposing actin filament cross-bridge binding sites.
    d. facilitating ACH release from the neuromuscular junction.

COMPARISON OF CONTRACTION AMONG MUSCLE TYPES

24. Dense bodies (corresponding to Z lines) and intermediate filament bundles are associated with shortening of the longitudinal axis of:
    a. smooth-muscle cells.
    b. skeletal-muscle cells.
    c. cardiac-muscle cells.

25. The slower attachment-detachment of cross-bridge heads that extend from myosin to actin is advantageous for:

a. smooth muscle.
b. cardiac muscle.
c. skeletal muscle.

CHANGES IN MUSCLE SIZE

26. Muscles showing an increase in the size of their individual muscle fibers are said to have undergone:
a. atrophy.
b. treppe.

c. hypertrophy.
d. gangrene.

27. An increase in the number of muscle fibers is called:
a. atrophy.
b. hypertrophy.
c. hyperplasia.

ANSWERS TO SELF EVALUATION—CHAPTER 8

1. a	8. a	15. c	22. c
2. c	9. b	16. c	23. c
3. d	10. a	17. a	24. a
4. b	11. d	18. b	25. a
5. b	12. a	19. c	26. c
6. a	13. d	20. a	27. c
7. b	14. b	21. b	

CHAPTER 9

The Cardiovascular System

CHAPTER OUTLINE

- **HEART AND PERICARDIUM**
  Myocardium
  Heart Valves
  Blood Flow through the Heart
- **BLOOD VESSELS**
  Blood Circulatory Systems
- **LYMPHATIC SYSTEM**
- **SPLEEN**
- **CARDIAC CONTRACTILITY**
  Origin of the Heartbeat
  Conduction of the Impulse
  Cardiac Cycle
- **ELECTROCARDIOGRAM**
  Wave Forms
  Isoelectric Line
- **HEART SOUNDS**
- **HEART RATE AND ITS CONTROL**
  Metabolic Rate

  Autonomic Nervous System
  Autoregulation
  Reflexes
- **BLOOD PRESSURE**
  Pressure Generation and Flow
  Systolic and Diastolic Pressures
  Measurements
- **BLOOD FLOW**
  Autoregulation
  Cardiac Output and Blood Diversion
  Breathing and Blood Flow
  Circulation Time
- **CAPILLARY DYNAMICS**
  Diffusion and Bulk Flow
  Mechanism of Bulk Flow
  Capillary Imbalances

During early embryonic growth, dividing cells receive their nutrients and expel their wastes by diffusion from the uterine fluids that surround them. With continued development, the innermost cells become too distant from the fluids for diffusional exchange efficiency. The cardiovascular system develops to meet the needs of distant cells for nutrition and excretion. The system consists of a network of joined vessels (arteries, veins, and capillaries) for circulating the nutrient fluid (blood) and a pump (the heart) to propel the fluid through the vessels. An auxiliary system of vessels (the lymphatics) also develops to assist the return of fluids from the interstitial spaces to the blood.

■ HEART AND PERICARDIUM

1. Know the orientation of the heart within the thorax with regard to its base and apex.

2. What is the pericardial sac, and where is it attached to the heart? What is its function?

3. Know the chambers of the heart. Which chamber normally has the greatest thickness?

4. Know the location of atrioventricular and semilunar valves. What prevents eversion of atrioventricular valves when ventricles contract?

5. Follow a drop of blood from its entrance to the heart at the vena cava until its ejection from the heart into the aorta.

The heart is a cone-shaped, hollow, muscular structure located in the thorax (*Fig. 9-1*). The large arteries and veins are continuous with the heart at its base. Its **base** is directed upward (dorsal) and forward (cranial). The opposite end of the cone is known as the **apex**. During early embryonic development, the heart is pushed into a serous sac known as the **pericardium**. The part of the sac next to the heart becomes fused to the muscle of the heart and is known as the **visceral pericardium**, or **epicardium** (*Fig. 9-2*). The outer part of the sac is continuous with the epicardium and extends outward from its fusion at the base to envelop the heart completely. The apex of the heart is free (unattached) within the pericardium. This outer layer is known as the **parietal pericardium**. The **pericardial sac** is a potential space and contains a small amount of fluid to provide lubrication for the outer surface of the heart during its near-continuous motion. It is referred to as a potential space because it can increase its fluid volume during times of inflammation. A major cause of inflammation in the cow is traumatic pericarditis, such as when a foreign object (e.g., nail, wire) penetrates from the forward compartment (reticulum) of the bovine stomach (*Fig. 9-3*). A splashing sound, similar to water in a washing machine, can sometimes be heard with each beat of the heart because of the increased fluid.

Myocardium

The muscular part of the heart is known as the **myocardium**, which forms the walls for the compartments (chambers) of the heart. The muscle fibers are arranged so that, when they contract, the blood is ejected from the chambers (*Fig. 9-4*). The **heart chambers** are divided into those on the right side of the heart and

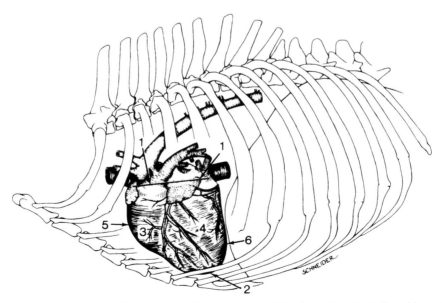

■ **FIGURE 9-1** The canine heart and its major vessels in the thorax (left lateral view). 1, Flattened base; 2, apex; 3, right ventricle; 4, left ventricle; 5, right ventricular margin; 6, left ventricular margin. (From Adams DR. Canine Anatomy: A Systemic Study. Ames, IA: Iowa State Press, 2004.)

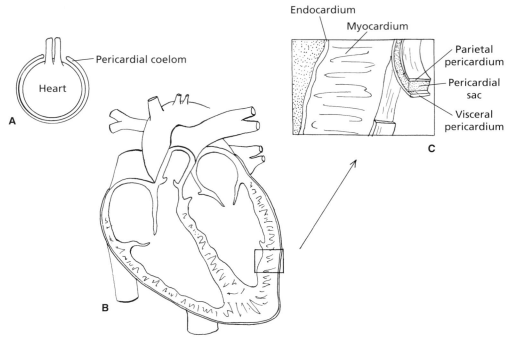

■ **FIGURE 9-2** Cross-sectional schematic representation of a mammalian heart. **A)** Embryologic invagination of heart into pericardial coelom (becomes pericardial sac). **B)** Sagittal section of heart with pericardial sac. **C)** Details of the heart wall and pericardium.

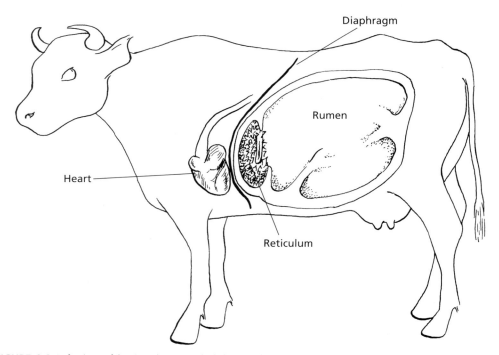

■ **FIGURE 9-3** Left view of bovine thorax and abdomen showing location of the heart relative to the reticulum. Foreign objects (nails, wire), sometimes ingested by cattle, accumulate in the reticulum (one of the bovine forestomachs). Contraction of the reticulum can force pointed objects through the reticulum wall and the diaphragm, causing final penetration of the pericardium and subsequent inflammation (pericarditis).

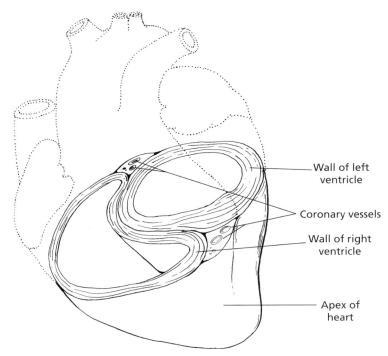

Wall of left
ventricle

Coronary vessels

Wall of right
ventricle

Apex of
heart

■ **FIGURE 9-4** Cross-sectional view of horse heart at the ventricular level showing the relative thickness of the myocardium and the orientation of the muscle fibers.

those on the left side (*Fig. 9-5*); each side has an **atrium** and a **ventricle**. To conserve space, each atrium has an extension known as an **auricle**, with a shape that conforms to that of adjacent parts. The atria receive blood from veins, and the ventricles receive blood from the atria. The right and left ventricles pump blood from the heart through the pulmonary trunk and aorta, respectively.

Heart Valves

The valves located between the atria and ventricles are known as the **atrioventricular (A-V) valves** (*Fig. 9-6A*). The valve on the right side has three cusps (flaps) and is called the **tricuspid valve**; the left A-V valve has two cusps and is called the **bicuspid**, also known as the **mitral valve**. The A-V valves prevent expulsion of ventricular blood into the atria when the ventricles contract. Because of the pressure associ-

ated with the expulsion of blood from the ventricles, the A-V valves could be everted into the atria. This is prevented by cords (**chordae tendineae**) attached to the free margin of the cusps at one end and to small muscles (**papillary muscles**) at the other end that extend from the myocardium. Papillary muscle contraction is synchronized with the myocardial contraction so that tension to the chordae tendineae is appropriately timed. Backflow of blood that has just been ejected from the ventricles is prevented by valves located at the exits of the arteries from the ventricles (*Fig. 9-6B*). The valves on both the right and left sides have three cusps and are known as the **semilunar valves**. The valve on the right side is known as the **pulmonary semilunar valve** because of its location relative to the pulmonary trunk, and the valve on the left side is known as the **aortic semilunar valve** because of its location relative to the aorta.

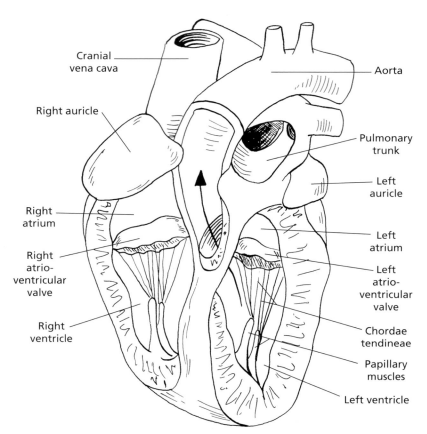

■ **FIGURE 9-5** A sagittal section of the canine heart. The right and left chambers are shown with separation of the atria and ventricles by atrioventricular valves. The auricles are extensions of the atria. The aorta is seen to be arising from the left ventricle. The pulmonary trunk arises from the right ventricle (origin not visible) and divides into right and left pulmonary arteries beyond the pulmonary semilunar valve. The cranial vena cava and caudal vena cava (not visible) deliver venous blood (unoxygenated) into the right atrium.

Blood Flow through the Heart

Blood that originally enters the heart and is finally ejected follows a specific route (*Fig. 9-7*). Blood that circulates to the tissues returns to the heart through the **cranial vena cava** (blood from forward parts of body) and the **caudal vena cava** (blood from rear parts of body). This is the venous blood. It has lost oxygen to the tissues, gained carbon dioxide, and must now be directed to the lungs, where it becomes arterial blood by gaining oxygen and losing carbon dioxide. The venous blood enters the right atrium during the atrial relax-ation phase of the cardiac cycle. At the appropriate time in the cardiac cycle, the blood is directed through the right A-V valve into the right ventricle. The ventricles contract and the blood goes through the pulmonary semilunar valves to the lungs through the pulmonary arteries. These are called arteries, even though they transport venous blood, because they transport blood away from the heart. After the blood has circulated through the lungs, it reenters the heart through the pulmonary veins (contain arterial blood). It enters the left atrium; from here the blood is directed to the left ventricle, from which it is pumped to the

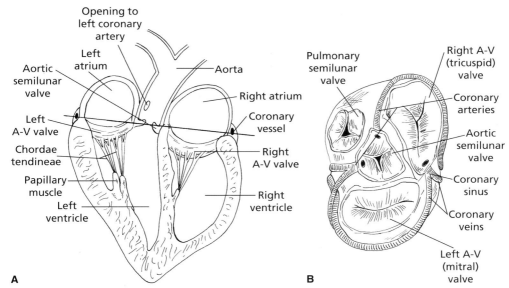

■ **FIGURE 9-6** Heart valves. **A)** Location relative to the chambers and the aorta. The pulmonary trunk and its semilunar valve are not shown. **B)** A view of the heart from above the ventricles (at the level of the straight line shown in A) to show the semilunar and atrioventricular valves. The first branches from the aorta are the coronary arteries. The coronary sinus opens into the right atrium and receives blood from the heart wall through the coronary veins.

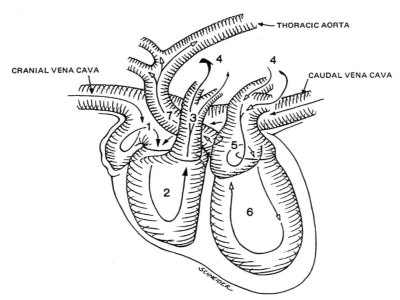

■ **FIGURE 9-7** Schematic of the blood pathway through the heart. Venous blood from the entire body (except for the lungs and some of the heart) enters the right atrium (1) and then flows sequentially through the right ventricle (2), pulmonary trunk (3), pulmonary arteries/capillary bed/pulmonary veins (4), left atrium (5), left ventricle (6), and ascending aorta (7), and into all of the body (except for the alveoli). (From Adams DR. Canine Anatomy: A Systemic Study. Ames, IA: Iowa State Press, 2004.)

systemic (whole body) circulation through the aorta. The left ventricle has the greatest muscle mass of the heart chambers because of the greater work required to pump blood throughout the entire body.

■ BLOOD VESSELS

1. What is the relationship of the blood vessel linings to the heart?
2. What is the order of blood vessels from the ventricles back to the atria? Which one of the vessel divisions permits exchange with interstitial fluid?
3. What is the function of elastic fibers in arteries?
4. What composes a capillary? Do they have muscle fibers and elastic fibers in their walls?
5. Is backflow of blood possible in veins? Do veins have muscle fibers in their walls?
6. Which blood vessels have the lowest pressure within them?
7. Differentiate between the pulmonary and systemic circulations (origin and distribution).

The inner aspect of the pericardium is described as the outer cell layer of the heart (because of fusion) and is known as the epicardium. The cardiac muscle cells of the heart occupy the middle layer of the heart, and the innermost cell layer is known as the **endocardium**. The endocardium is described here because it continues as the lining (**endothelium**) for all of the blood vessels. Endothelial cells are classified as simple (single-layered), squamous (platelike) epithelium (a primary type of tissue that also covers the body surfaces and forms active parts of glands). Simple squamous epithelium is found wherever a smooth surface is required to reduce friction. In this regard, it is ideal for lining the inner aspects of the heart, its valves, and the inner coat of the blood vessels to minimize the resistance (and hence the energy requirement) for blood flow. Inflammation of the endothelial lining in the heart is called endocarditis; if it involves the lining of valves, it is called valvular endocarditis.

The blood vessels provide a continuous route for blood leaving the heart to return to the heart. From the ventricles back to the atria they are, in order, the arteries, arterioles, capillaries, venules, and veins. An overview of the functional circulatory system is shown in *Figure 9-8*. The large arteries have a greater proportion of their mass composed of elastic tissue than do the small arteries. This elastic tissue provides for expansion as blood is pumped into them, and the expanded fibers serve as a source of energy for continuing the circulation of blood when the ventricles relax. The small arteries have some portion of their elastic fibers replaced by smooth muscle. Contraction of the smooth muscle constricts these vessels and permits reduced blood flow to a particular part and diversion of blood flow to other parts. The arterioles are muscular just before emptying into the capillaries. Changes in their muscle tone (degree of contraction) regulate blood flow to capillary beds (*Fig. 9-9*).

The volume of the capillary bed is small (4% of the total blood volume), but the vast number of capillaries provides for a large total cross-sectional area that leads to a slow rate of blood flow that favors transcapillary exchange. **Capillaries** are endothelial tubes with a diameter ranging from 5 to 10 μm. The walls are composed of endothelial cells, associated **basal lamina** (basement membrane), and pericytes. The basal lamina encloses both the endothelial cells and the **pericytes** (*Fig. 9-10*). Pericytes are undifferentiated mesenchymal cells with potential to transform into other cell types (e.g., fibroblasts, smooth-muscle cells). Also, by this means, capillaries can transform into other types of vascular tubes (i.e., arteries, veins) if the internal flow characteristics change. Capillary pericytes synthesize

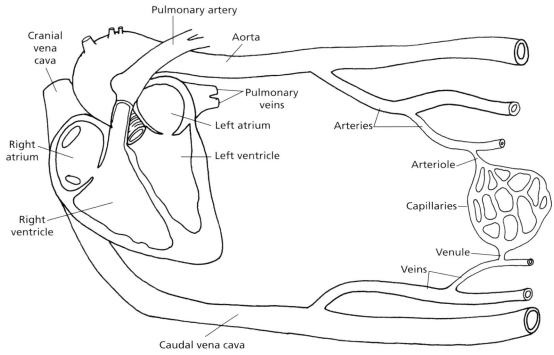

■ **FIGURE 9-8** Schematic representation of the functional circulatory system. A network of arteries, arterioles, capillaries, venules, and veins exists between the aorta and cranial and caudal venae cavae.

and release constituents of the basement membrane.

Where the endothelial cells border each other, a thin slit (slit pore) or **intercellular cleft** exists and allows for the diffusion of dissolved substances in plasma. The limited size of the slit pores inhibits the passage of large molecules (e.g., protein molecules). Pinocytotic vesicles are also present in the endothelial cells. These are formed at one surface of the cell and migrate to the opposite surface, where they discharge their contents. Many of the protein molecules are probably transported through the endothelial cells in this manner. The capillaries unite with one another to form larger vessels known as venules, and the venules unite with other venules to form the veins. The largest veins are the venae cavae, which return the blood to the right atrium of the heart.

The veins are thin-walled tubes reinforced by connective tissue, and they also contain smooth muscle fibers. Contraction of the muscle fibers increases resistance to blood flow and helps regulate the circulation. Venous constriction increases the blood pressure in all vessels that precede the veins. Valves are present in veins at irregular intervals that are directed (or opened) toward the heart (*Fig. 9-11*). External pressure on veins causes blood to advance only in a cranial direction because backflow is prevented by valve closure. Similarly, backflow does not occur when external pressure is released.

The pressures within the veins are the lowest of the vessel pressures (*Fig. 9-12*). This follows from the physical law of pressure dissipation as distance from the source (heart) increases. The pressure noted for capillaries might seem to be greater than what could be

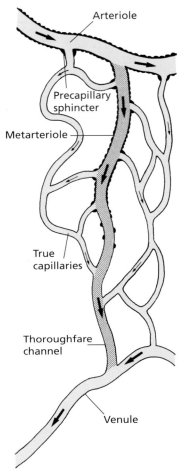

■ FIGURE 9-9 Schematic representation of a capillary bed. (From Cormack DH. Essential Histology. 2nd Ed. Baltimore: Lippincott Williams & Wilkins, 2001.)

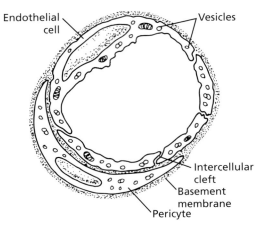

■ FIGURE 9-10 Schematic representation of a cross section through the endothelial wall of a muscle (continuous) capillary. Portions of endothelial cells are shown; these are separated from each other by intercellular clefts. Pericytes are outside of endothelial cells and are enclosed by a common basement membrane. Many pinocytotic vesicles are also shown.

Blood Circulatory Systems

The blood vessels that have been described serve two separate circulatory systems (*Fig. 9-13*). The **pulmonary system** circulates blood through the lungs (*Fig. 9-14*). The pressure providing this circulation originates from the right ventricle. The capillaries of the pulmonary system are associated intimately with the smallest terminations of the air passages, the pulmonary alveoli. Blood from this system is returned to the left atrium.

The **systemic circulation** carries blood that has returned from the lungs to all areas of the body. The pressure necessary for this circulation originates from the left ventricle. Blood that traverses this system leaves the left ventricle through the aorta and is returned to the right atrium through the venae cavae. The first branches of the aorta supply the heart muscle through the coronary arteries (*Fig. 9-15*). Within the systemic circulation are a few **portal systems**. A portal system departs from the usual pattern of circulation in that a vein returning blood to the heart branches to reform

tolerated for a single-celled tube but, because of the extremely small diameter, the tension exerted on the capillary wall is extremely low. For a given pressure within the vascular system, the wall tension increases with the radius of the vessel according to **Laplace's law**:

$$T = Pr/2$$

where T = wall tension, P = pressure in the vessel, and r = radius of the vessel.

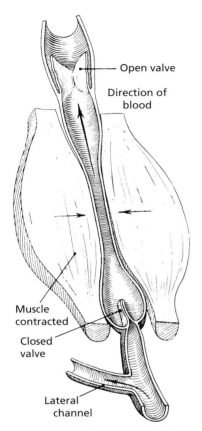

Open valve

Direction of blood

Muscle contracted

Closed valve

Lateral channel

■ FIGURE 9-11 Valves of a vein showing the pumping action of adjacent muscles. (From Grollman S. The Human Body: Its Structure and Physiology. 4th Ed. New York: Macmillan, 1978.)

capillaries, which reunite to form veins. The primary example of a portal system is the hepatic portal system in the liver (*Fig. 9-16*). The reformed capillaries are the sinusoids of the liver, which are lined by cells involved in many liver functions and by those that assist in the cleansing of blood or the removal of harmful substances by **macrophages (Küpffer cells)**.

■ LYMPHATIC SYSTEM

1. **What is meant by the lymphatic system? What is the fluid of its vessels known as?**
2. **Does protein ever leak from capillaries? What is its turnover rate?**
3. **What is the route for return of protein to the blood after it has leaked?**
4. **What is one of the most important functions of the lymphatics?**
5. **What is the location and what are the functions of lymph nodes?**

An important adjunct to the circulatory system is the lymphatic system. The lymphatic vessels have blind beginnings (lymph capillaries) in the interstitial spaces (the spaces between cells and outside of the blood vessels),

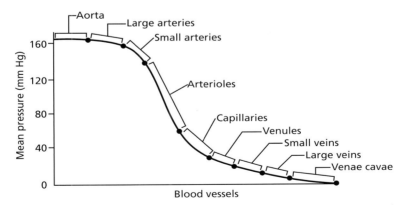

Aorta
Large arteries
Small arteries
Arterioles
Capillaries
Venules
Small veins
Large veins
Venae cavae

Blood vessels

Mean pressure (mm Hg)

■ FIGURE 9-12 Graphic illustration of decreasing pressures from major arteries to major veins. Note the sharp decrease in pressure in the arterioles, and the more gentle slope in the much wider vascular bed made up of capillaries. (Drawing made from The Dukes Physiology Film Series (DKS-15), Ames, IA: Iowa State University, 1969.)

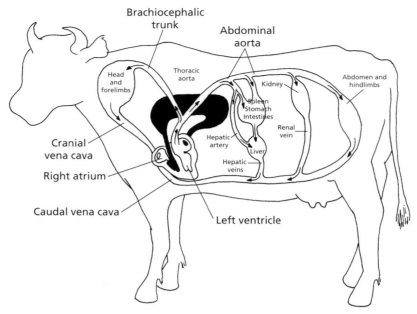

■ **FIGURE 9-13** General scheme of mammalian circulation showing the pulmonary system, which serves the lungs, and the systemic system, which serves the remainder of the body. The pulmonary circulation is shown in black.

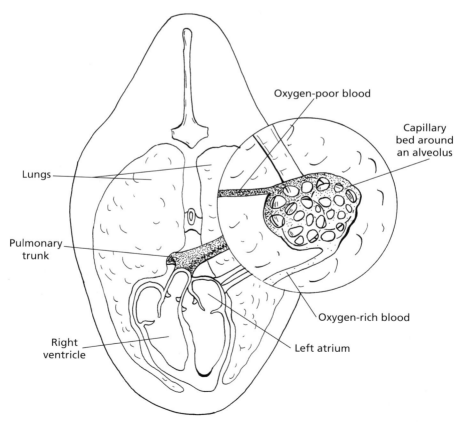

■ **FIGURE 9-14** Schematic representation of the lungs and the pulmonary circulation. The circled inset represents a functional unit of the lung, the alveolus. Mixed venous blood leaves the right ventricle through the pulmonary trunk and is oxygenated at the level of the alveoli. Oxygenated blood returns to the left atrium through the pulmonary veins.

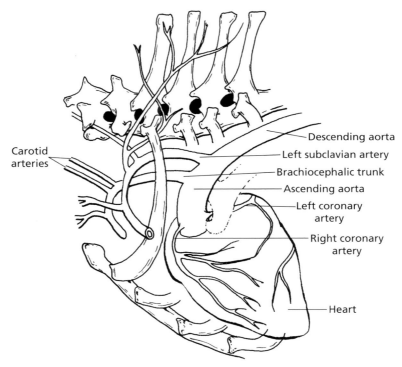

■ FIGURE 9-15 Cranial aspects of the systemic circulation. The first branches of the aorta supply the heart muscles through the coronary arteries. The descending aorta is composed of the thoracic and abdominal aorta. The main arteries to the forelimbs arise from the left subclavian artery on the left side and from the brachiocephalic trunk on the right side. The carotid arteries ascend to the head.

and the continuation vessels tend to parallel the veins (*Fig. 9-17*). Lymph vessels join with each other and eventually form a few large lymph vessels that empty directly into the large veins. The fluid of the lymph vessels is called **lymph**. There is little difference between the composition of lymph and that of interstitial fluid. Although blood capillaries permit most plasma constituents to diffuse through their endothelium, protein molecules are somewhat restrained because of their size. It is essential for proteins to enter the interstitial fluid, however, because they act as carriers for cell products or for substances needed by cells. In addition, antibodies (protein substances) are needed in the interstitial space for more intimate association with antigen. There is a complete turnover (from capillaries and return

to blood) of plasma protein once every 12 to 24 hours. Because the concentration of protein is higher in the plasma than in the interstitial space, the gradient for diffusion is to the interstitial space. Protein in the interstitial space does not diffuse back to the plasma; it can only return to the plasma through the lymphatic vessels. The blind beginnings of the lymph vessels are adapted for the intake of large molecules, and concentration and pressure gradients favor this route (*Fig. 9-18*). Anchoring filaments prevent collapse of the vessels when the tissue swells with excess fluid (**edema**). Also, the overlap of endothelial cells with each other permits easy access of interstitial fluid, but because of their valve-like arrangement, backflow is prevented. The return of protein that has leaked or that is otherwise transported

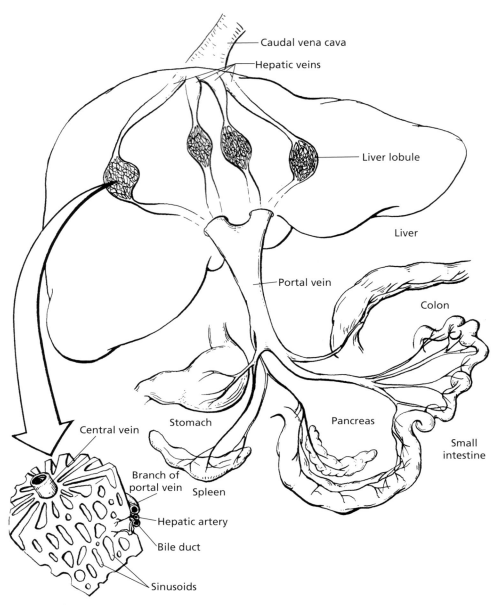

Caudal vena cava

Hepatic veins

Liver lobule

Liver

Portal vein

Colon

Central vein

Stomach

Pancreas

Branch of
portal vein

Small
intestine

Spleen

Hepatic artery

Bile duct

Sinusoids

■ **FIGURE 9-16** The mammalian hepatic portal system. Blood in the portal vein from the stomach, spleen, pancreas, and intestines goes to the liver, where it flows through the sinusoids and is reformed by the central vein of each lobule. It finally enters the caudal vena cava through the hepatic veins.

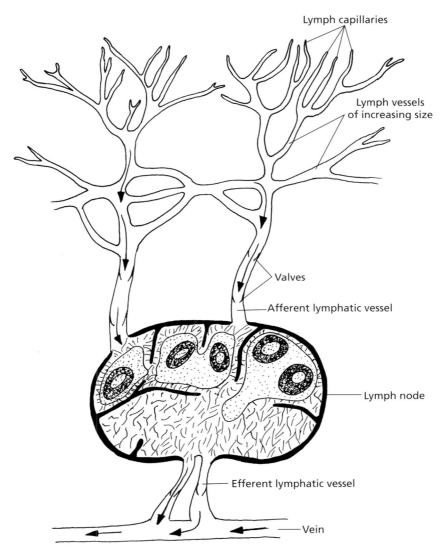

Lymph capillaries

Lymph vessels
of increasing size

Valves

Afferent lymphatic vessel

Lymph node

Efferent lymphatic vessel

Vein

■ **FIGURE 9-17** Schematic representation of lymph drainage. Interstitial fluid gains access to the blind beginnings of lymph capillaries and proceeds centrally through lymph vessels of increasing size. Lymph nodes are located along the course of lymph vessels. Lymph is returned to blood by drainage into veins.

from the blood capillaries back to the systemic circulation is one of the most important functions of the lymphatics.

Lymph nodes are nodular structures of varying sizes located along the course of lymph vessels. They contain clusters of germinal cells that reproduce to form lymphocytes (*Fig.*

9-19). The lymphocytes in turn can be of a type that produce antibodies, or they can be sensitized lymphocytes. In both cases they are highly specific against substances (antigens) that are foreign to the body. The antibodies and sensitized lymphocytes leave the lymph nodes with the lymph in the vessels and enter

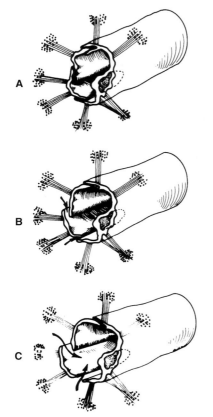

■ **FIGURE 9-18** Special structure of the lymphatic capillaries that permits passage of high–molecular-weight substances into the lymph. The structures radiating from the capillaries are anchoring filaments that give support to portions of endothelial cells where the capillaries begin. The unsupported portion of the endothelium allows fluid to flow into the capillary (arrows), as shown in B and C. Raised pressure in the capillary closes the flap against the overlapping supported endothelium, as shown in A. (From Leak LV. The fine structure and function of the lymphatic vascular system. In: Meessen H, ed. Handbüch der Allgemeinen Pathologie. New York: Springer-Verlag, 1972.)

the blood, where they can be circulated throughout the body.

Lymph nodes also contain fixed macrophages that are attached to the reticulum (inner framework) of the lymph nodes. Lymph circulating through the nodes thus is in intimate contact with the macrophages and, because the macrophages are highly phago-

cytic, foreign materials in lymph (e.g., bacteria, cellular debris) are engulfed and prevented from progressing further. Infection or inflammation of a body part often results in enlarged lymph nodes serving that part because of the entrapment and because of lymphocyte proliferation stimulated by the presence of these antigenic materials. Cancer cells might be routed from their origin and be entrapped by lymph nodes, where they can proliferate and continue into the next lymph node in the chain. Inspection of lymph nodes for enlargement is an important part of the postmortem carcass examination procedure for animals that are slaughtered for food consumption.

The lymph vessels are one-way channels that contain valves similar to those in veins, which prevent backflow of lymph once it has progressed toward the veins. Lymph progresses through the channels by contractions of the lymph vessels and by a massaging action of muscles that overlie lymph vessels. Forward movement of lymph lowers the pressure in the part of the vessel evacuated and, because there is no backflow of lymph, entry of lymph from the backward parts is favored. There is no central pump, such as the heart, to facilitate lymph circulation, and disturbances in lymph flow can cause accumulation of interstitial fluid in low-lying body parts. The return of lymph is assisted by elevation of these parts, such as the limbs, to a level higher than the centrally located veins and by muscle movement from exercise.

■ SPLEEN

1. **What are four of the functions of the spleen?**

The **spleen** is the largest lymphoid organ of the body (Fig. 9-20). It is unlike the lymph nodes in that the circulating fluid is blood instead of lymph. It is the only organ specializing in filtering blood. A section cut from the

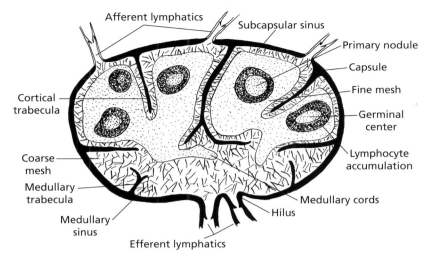

■ **FIGURE 9-19** Internal structure of a lymph node. Lymph enters through afferent lymphatics and leaves through efferent lymphatics. The lymph percolates through the coarse mesh, on which many fixed mononuclear phagocytic cells are located. Lymphocytes are produced in the primary nodules and accumulate throughout the fine mesh. A fine mesh holds small lymphocytes better than a coarse mesh.

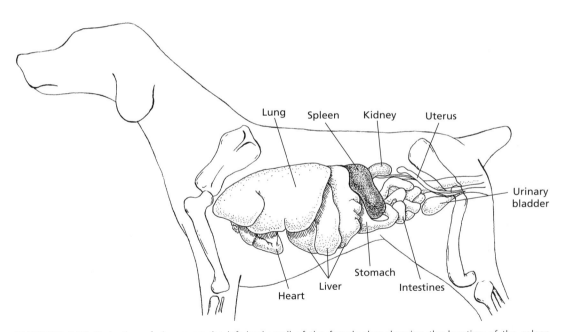

■ **FIGURE 9-20** Projection of viscera on the left body wall of the female dog showing the location of the spleen relative to other body organs. Except for the dorsal tip, the dog spleen is somewhat variable in position, and its long axis can be almost longitudinal.

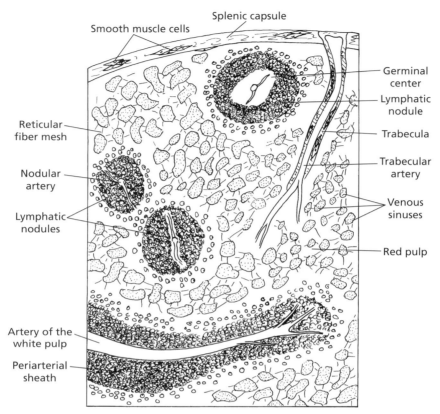

■ FIGURE 9-21 Schematic representation of the pig spleen. Multiple branches of the splenic artery enter the capsule and extend into the trabeculae. The lymphatic nodules and periarterial sheaths compose the white pulp that produces lymphocytes. The red pulp is the reticular fiber mesh that acts as a filter because of its fixed macrophages. Smooth muscle cells are present in the capsule and in the trabeculae. The venous sinuses collect filtered blood and drain into venules and finally trabecular veins (not shown).

spleen (*Fig. 9-21*) shows that it is surrounded by a capsule that has connective tissue and smooth muscle cells. The amount of smooth muscle varies with species and is quite pronounced in carnivores. **Trabeculae** extend from the capsules that are composed of elastic fibers, collagen, and smooth muscle. Arteries, veins, lymph vessels, and nerves are contained within the trabeculae. The **parenchyma** (**splenic pulp**) of the spleen is composed of **red and white pulp** and is supported by the capsule, trabeculae, and reticular fibers. Most of the splenic pulp is red because of the blood that is held within the reticular fiber mesh, which represents the part of the spleen that

acts as a filter; it has numerous fixed macrophages. The white pulp is lymphatic tissue distributed throughout the spleen as lymphatic nodules and sheaths of lymphatics around arteries and arterioles that produces lymphocytes. Blood enters the spleen via the trabeculae and is distributed either to the lymph nodules via nodular capillaries or to the red pulp or venous sinuses via terminal capillaries. Blood entering the red pulp (reticular spaces) via the terminal capillaries is then able to enter the venous sinuses through slits in the venous sinus walls. Blood entering the reticular spaces provides for greater exposure to cells of the **mononuclear phagocytic system**

(MPS). The venous sinuses collect filtered blood and drain into venules, and finally into trabecular veins.

Blood circulates through the spleen, and the spleen is active in the destruction of aged and abnormal erythrocytes by the numerous MPS cells. Also, the spleen is a storage depot of iron obtained from the destruction of erythrocytes. The spleen is an important reservoir of blood, especially of red blood cells, which accumulate within the venous sinusoids. Contraction of the spleen is possible because of the smooth muscle and occurs when more red blood cells are needed. Splenic contraction that accompanies excitement in the dog can increase the packed cell volume from 40% to more than 50%.

■ CARDIAC CONTRACTILITY

1. What is the sinoatrial node? What is its pacemaker function?
2. What are the two syncytia of the heart, and how are they separated?
3. What is the contraction sequence of the two syncytia, and what function is thereby served?
4. Describe conduction of the impulse throughout the heart. What purpose is served by fast conduction?
5. Do both atria contract at the same time? Do both ventricles contract at the same time?
6. Define diastole and systole.
7. Describe the events of the cardiac cycle.

All muscles seem to have an inherent rhythmicity of contraction. If the three muscle types (cardiac, skeletal, smooth) are removed from the nerve and blood supply and placed into physiologic fluids, contraction begins in a rhythmic manner. The frequency of contraction is greatest in cardiac muscle, followed by skeletal muscle, and finally by smooth muscle.

Origin of the Heartbeat

In cardiac muscle, the atria have a higher frequency of contraction than the ventricles. In addition, a small area of specialized cardiac muscle fibers near the junction of the cranial vena cava with the right atrium has a contraction frequency higher than that of the atria. These specialized muscle fibers constitute what is known as the **sinoatrial (S-A) node**. Impulses originating in the S-A node spread throughout the musculature of the atria, and the impulse is conducted to the ventricles by way of **internodal pathways**. Because the contraction frequency for the S-A node exceeds that of the atria and ventricles, the S-A node impulse becomes the stimulus for contraction of the atria and ventricles, whereby the contraction frequency of the S-A node becomes the contraction frequency of the atria and ventricles. The S-A node therefore serves a pacemaker function.

Conduction of the Impulse

The muscle fibers of the atria and those of the ventricles are arranged to form an atrial and a ventricular syncytium. A **syncytium** is an arrangement of muscle fibers in which the fibers form an interconnected mass of fibers. The atrial syncytium is separated from the ventricular syncytium by a fibrous ring that surrounds the A-V valves. The fibrous ring acts as an insulator between the two syncytia. An impulse that spreads throughout the atria does not spread to the ventricles, and an impulse from the ventricles does not spread to the atria. This permits independent contraction and provides an opportunity for the atria and ventricles to coordinate their function of emptying, so the ventricles are filled during their relaxation by the contraction and emptying of the atria.

It is desirable for the muscle fibers in each syncytium to contract as simultaneously as possible. All fibers contribute to the pressure increase needed for evacuation of the blood from the chambers of the syncytium. Fibers contracting at different times could not attain sufficient pressure for efficient evacuation. Because the function of the atria is to fill the ventricles before they contract, impulse conduction is completed first throughout the atria. After a slight delay, the impulse is then conducted throughout the ventricles.

To facilitate rapid conduction (and coordinated contraction), the heart has a specialized conduction system composed of specialized conduction tracts and fibers called **Purkinje fibers** (*Fig. 9-22*). The S-A node conducts the impulse throughout the atria through several small tracts of fibers called internodal pathways. Depolarization of these pathways provides the stimulus for depolarization of adjacent muscle fibers; the transmission of impulses and subsequent depolarization of other muscle fibers is facilitated by the inter-

calated disks interposed between muscle fibers. Impulse conduction by the internodal pathways is received by the A-V node, which is located at a point between the atria and ventricles. The A-V node is continued through the fibrous ring by the **A-V bundle**. A-V bundle fibers are smaller in diameter than the other Purkinje fibers, and impulse conduction is slowed to about 10% of the velocity of cardiac muscle fibers. This permits a delay of impulse to facilitate complete emptying of the atria before the ventricles contract. Conduction fibers are continued from the A-V bundle in the wall dividing the right from the left ventricles as Purkinje fibers distribute to the right ventricle (right bundle branch) and as Purkinje fibers distribute to the left ventricle (left bundle branch). These large fibers transmit impulses about two to three times faster than

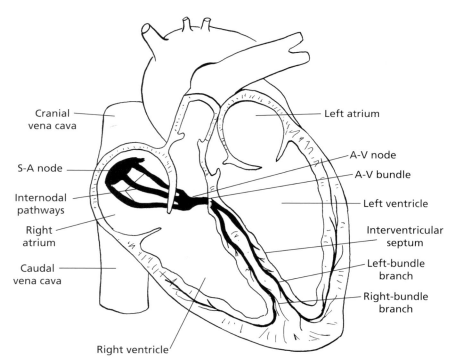

■ **FIGURE 9-22** Conduction system of the mammalian heart. Impulse originates in the S-A node located near the junction of the venae cavae with the right atrium. The internodal pathways conduct the impulse throughout the atria, and the left- and right-bundle branches of Purkinje fibers conduct the impulse throughout the ventricles. The A-V node and bundle conduct the impulse from the atria to the ventricles.

cardiac muscle fibers. The muscle in the walls of the ventricles is thicker than the muscle in the walls of the atria, and the distance of conduction is greater. Therefore, to achieve coordinated contraction of muscle fibers of the ventricles, it is essential to have a greater velocity of conduction which is provided by the Purkinje fibers.

Not only does cardiac muscle contract more slowly than skeletal muscle, but it also has a longer refractory period. A **refractory period** is the period during repolarization when a stimulus cannot evoke another depolarization. This is advantageous for the heart because, when the impulse completes its travel through each syncytium, the impulse is stopped because all the previously stimulated fibers are refractory to further stimulation. When the impulse is stopped, the muscle fibers are allowed to relax and the chambers fill with blood in preparation for the next cycle.

During this discussion about impulse conduction, it should be noted that both atria contract at the same time, which completes the filling of the ventricles, and that both ventricles contract at the same time, thus pumping blood to the pulmonary circulation and systemic circulation simultaneously. Contraction and relaxation of the muscle fibers within a syncytium are synchronized. When contraction of muscle fibers and relaxation of other muscle fibers occur at the same time in the same syncytium, the condition is referred to as fibrillation. Electrical current conducted through the heart during defibrillation causes simultaneous depolarization of all fibers, and the heart can then start a new cycle with impulses that begin in the S–A node.

Cardiac Cycle

The cardiac cycle refers to the sequence of events that occurs during one complete heartbeat. These events are continuous, and the assigned periods are arbitrary for descriptive purposes. **Diastole** refers to relaxation of a heart chamber before and during filling of the chamber. **Systole** refers to contraction of a heart chamber in the process of emptying. During atrial diastole the atria are filled with blood. After ventricular systole, and during ventricular diastole, the following sequence of events occurs (*Fig. 9-23*):

1. Volume and pressure increase in the atria as they fill by receiving blood from the venae cavae and pulmonary veins (occurs during ventricular systole); A-V valves open when atrial pressure exceeds the ventricular pressure (occurs at beginning of ventricular diastole).
2. Blood flows into relaxed ventricles (accounts for up to 70% of ventricular filling).
3. Atria contract (accomplishes complete filling or priming of ventricles).
4. Atria relax and begin refilling.
5. Ventricles begin contraction, and A-V valves are closed because ventricular pressures exceed atrial pressures.
6. Continued contraction of ventricles creates sufficient pressure to exceed arterial pressures.
7. Semilunar valves are opened.
8. Blood is ejected from ventricles.
9. Ventricles begin to relax.
10. Arterial pressures begin to exceed the ventricular pressures, and the semilunar valves close.

The cycle ends and is repeated at a frequency consistent with the heart rate for each species. The process of recording these changes is called **electrocardiography**, and the record obtained is known as the **electrocardiogram (ECG)**.

■ ELECTROCARDIOGRAM

1. What is the ECG? What are the wave forms associated with one cardiac cycle? What phase of electrical activity is associated with each wave form?
2. How are amplitudes of waves and intervals between waves measured?

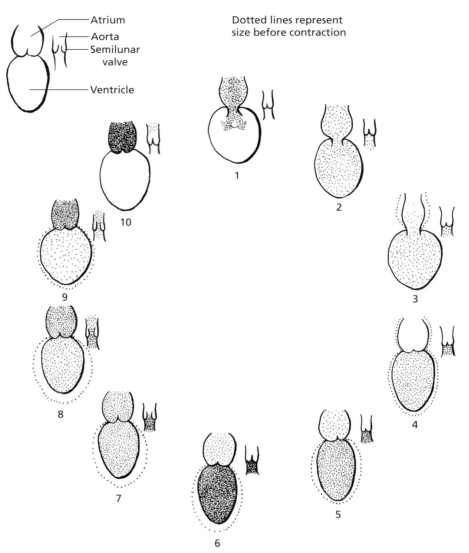

■ **FIGURE 9-23** The cardiac cycle of the mammalian heart. As shown in the key for the cycle sequence, the single chambers represent both right and left atria and ventricles. The single semilunar valve represents both the pulmonary and aortic semilunar valves that separate the ventricles from their respective pulmonary trunk and aorta. 1, A-V valves open; 2, ventricles receive blood; 3, atria contract and empty; 4, ventricles begin contraction and close A-V valves; 5, atria relax and begin to fill; 6, ventricular pressure increases; 7, semilunar valves open; 8, blood ejection begins from ventricles through semilunar valves; 9, ventricles begin relaxation; and 10, semilunar valves close, A-V valves still closed. Begin sequence 1.

When impulse conduction was explained for nerve and muscle fibers (see Chapter 4), it was noted that voltage changes occur across the nerve and muscle membranes during waves of depolarization and repolarization. The changes are relatively small and are measured in millivolts. Similar voltage changes occur when heart muscle depolarizes and repolarizes. Voltage changes that occur locally are conducted through the body fluids because body fluids are good conductors. With appropriate amplification, these voltage changes can be recorded as they occur.

Wave Forms

Connection of the amplifier with wires (known as leads) to selected body parts (usually the limbs) and to a recorder provides a characteristic wave form. The **wave form** is a recording of the electrical activity of the heart. Because the electrical activity can be changed by alterations in the heart muscle, such as thickening of the chamber walls or interruptions of current flow caused by damaged muscle, it is useful for studying heart activity in conditions of health and disease. The wave form recording is the ECG. Several leads and their characteristic wave forms are shown for the dog in *Figure 9-24*. The ECG for each cycle of the heart has characteristic deflections associated with the depolarization and repolarization of the atria and ventricles as they occur in sequence. An ECG recording, such as that which might be obtained from lead II in the dog, is shown in *Figure 9-25*. The sequence of deflections and the activity associated with them are as follows:

1. The P wave is associated with depolarization of atria; after depolarization, atrial contraction occurs.
2. The QRS wave complex represents both positive (upward) and negative (downward) deflections associated with ventricular depolarization; ventricular contraction begins after depolarization of fibers.
3. The T wave is the last wave for each heartbeat; it represents ventricular repolarization (may be positive or negative).

Because repolarization of the atria occurs during depolarization of the ventricles, a separate wave form is not observed. Instead, the voltage changes of atrial repolarization are algebraically summed into the QRS complex.

Lead	Electrode Placement		Lead Illustration	ECG Example
	Negative	Positive		
I	RA	LA		
II	RA	LL		
III	LA	LL		
aVR	LA-LL	RA		
aVL	RA-LL	LA		
aVF	RA-LA	LL		

■ **FIGURE 9-24** Examples of different electrode placements (leads) and their characteristic wave forms for the dog. (From Breazile JE. Textbook of Veterinary Physiology. Philadelphia: Lea & Febiger, 1971.)

It should now be apparent why conduction of the impulse throughout each atrial and ventricular syncytium takes place rapidly. Impulse conduction results in depolarization, which must occur before contraction proceeds. Coordinated contraction of all the muscle fibers, therefore, requires near-simultaneous depolarization.

Isoelectric Line

When viewing an ECG, it can be seen that deflections of the waves, whether positive (upward) or negative (downward), commence from a common line, known as the **isoelectric line**. Deviations from the line represent the amplitude of the wave; it is measured in millivolts and can be positive or negative. The

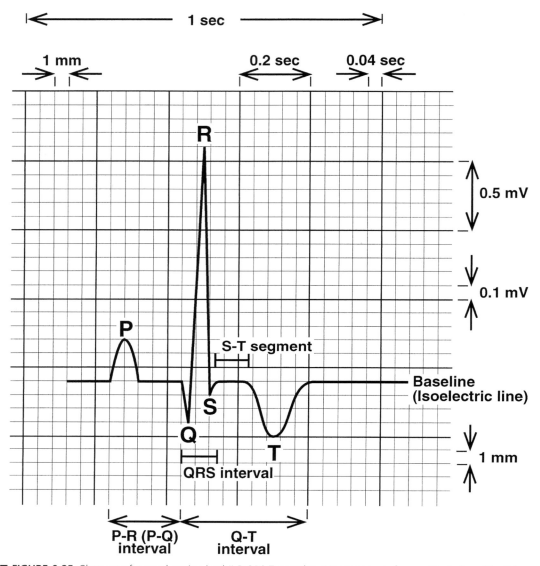

■ **FIGURE 9-25** Close-up of normal canine lead II P-QRS-T complex. Measurements for amplitude (in millivolts) are indicated by positive and negative movement; time intervals (in hundredths of a second) are indicated from left to right. There is much variation in T wave configuration, and it is shown as negative in this illustration. Paper speed, 25 mm/s; 1 cm = 1 mV. (Modified from Tilley LP. Essentials of Canine and Feline Electrocardiography. 3rd Ed. Philadelphia: Lea & Febiger, 1992.)

interval between waves is measured in hundredths of a second (see Fig. 9-25). Hypertrophy of ventricular muscle might require a greater time for depolarization, and the QRS interval (time for depolarization) would be increased. Certain heart conditions can cause the interval segment to be depressed from the isoelectric line. An S–T segment depression is observed with hypoxia (lack of oxygen) of heart muscle.

■ HEART SOUNDS

1. **What are the heart sounds, and with what are they associated?**

Listening to the heart (**cardiac auscultation**) enables the listener to hear the sounds that accompany contraction of heart muscle and the sounds associated with closure of the heart valves. These are repeated for each cardiac cycle. The more pronounced sounds are those associated with valve closings, but contracting muscle also makes a sound.

The **first heart sound** resembles the word "lub," and the **second heart sound** resembles "dub." They usually occur one after the other—lub-dub, lub-dub, lub-dub, and so on. The first sound is produced when the ventricles contract and the A-V valves close. The second sound is produced when ventricular relaxation begins and the semilunar valves close. The abrupt closing of the valves and their potential for making sounds can be visualized. A **third heart sound** can sometimes be detected on a **phonocardiogram** (recording of heart sounds); this occurs toward the end of rapid filling of the ventricles. Heart sounds are useful as diagnostic aids because the heart valves can become diseased and might not close completely. When this happens, blood leaks through the valves and the turbulence of the leakage is heard as some variation of a "shhh" sound after the lub or dub. Abnormal heart sounds are called murmurs and usually result from valve disorders. A review of the relationship of the ECG waves with ventricular systole and associated pressures and of the resulting valve closings with their associated sounds is illustrated in *Figure 9-26*.

■ HEART RATE AND ITS CONTROL

1. **What is a generalization about the relationship between heart rate and size of animal?**
2. **What are the effects of autonomic stimulation upon the heart?**
3. **What is Starling's law of the heart?**
4. **What is the response of the carotid and aortic sinus receptors to increased blood pressure?**

Heart rate refers to the frequency of cardiac cycles and is usually measured by the number of **beats per minute (bpm)**. Physiologic factors influencing the heart rate are excitement, muscular exercise, high environmental temperature, digestion, and sleep. Changes in heart rate are seen in a variety of pathologic conditions.

Metabolic Rate

In general, small animals have higher heart rates than larger animals. This is a consequence of the higher metabolic rate (and oxygen consumption) necessitated by their larger surface area per unit of body mass. The inverse relationship between heart rate and body size applies both within a species and among different species. For example, a small dog may have a resting heart rate of 120 bpm, whereas a large dog might show a resting heart rate of only 80 bpm or less. The resting heart rate of the mouse is about 600 bpm; rat, 400 bpm; guinea pig, 280 bpm; elephant, 30 bpm. Physical conditioning and the cardiac hypertrophy that occurs as a result of physical conditioning lower the resting heart rate in all animals. Young animals have a higher heart rate than mature animals, explained in part by their smaller size. Another factor is that tonic vagal inhibition is less developed in young animals. Resting heart rates for some domestic animal species and for the human are shown in *Table 9-1*.

Autonomic Nervous System

Heart rates compared among species are usually obtained with the animals being at rest. A number of factors can influence heart rate, including activity, excitement, fever,

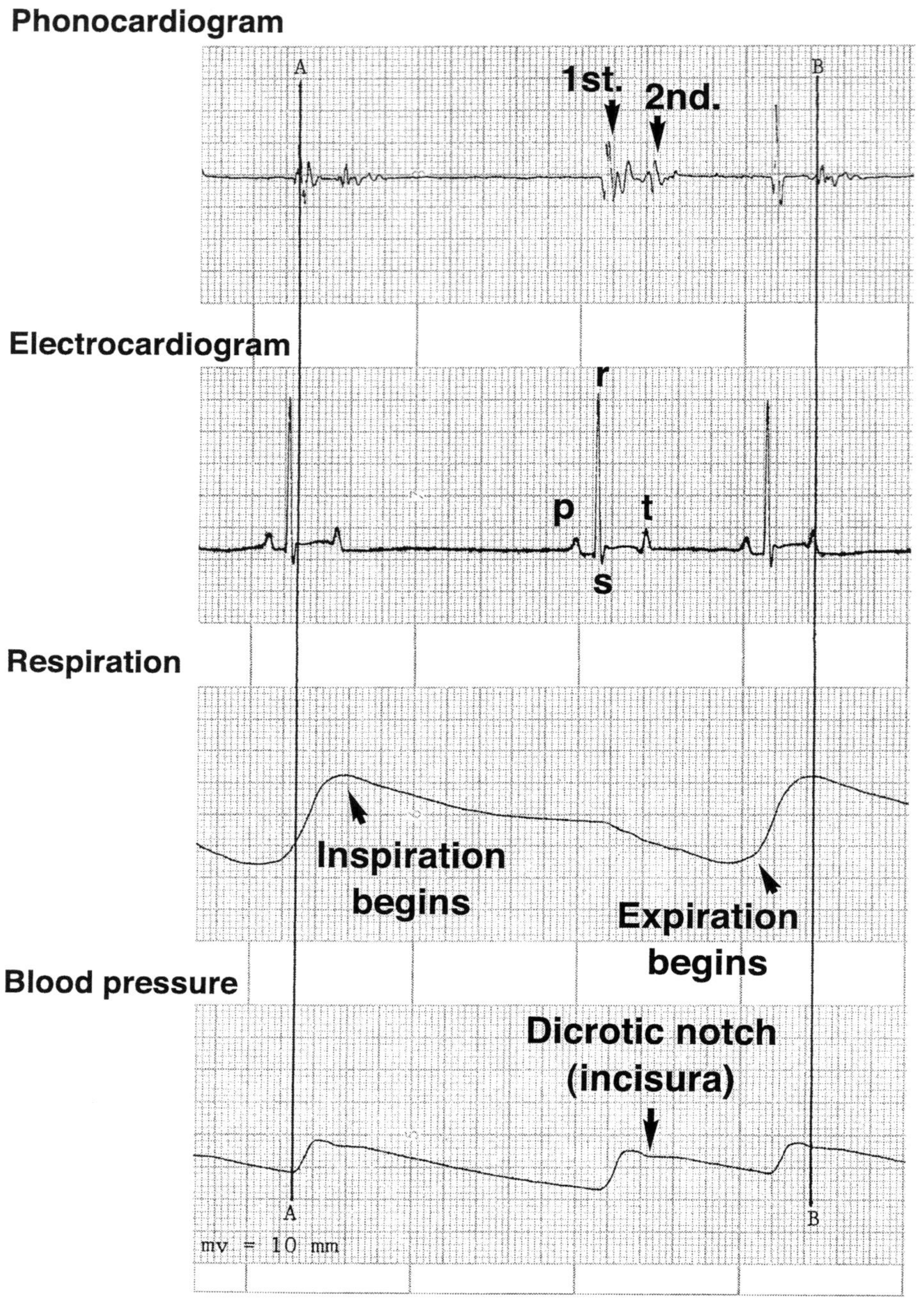

■ FIGURE 9-26 Simultaneous recording of electrocardiogram (lead II), phonocardiogram, respiration, and blood pressure of a dog. The correlation of events is represented by correlation line A (first heart sound, lub; ECG; blood pressure) and B (second heart sound, dub; blood pressure). For line A: immediately after depolarization of the ventricles, heart contraction begins, the first heart sound is perceptible, and blood pressure begins to increase. For line B: ventricular relaxation begins, blood pressure decrease begins, and semilunar valves close. Valve closure produces the second heart sound and causes a momentary blood pressure bounce upward (dicrotic notch). Respiratory sinus arrhythmia (an example of the Bainbridge reflex) is shown by correlating the inspiratory phase of the breathing cycle (blood flow to right atrium increases) with increased heart activity (R-R interval decreased). Paper speed, 25 mm/s; 1 cm = 1 mV. See Figure 9-25 for study of grid measurements.

TABLE 9-1 HEART RATES IN ADULT, RESTING ANIMALS

ANIMAL	HEART RATE (BEATS/MIN)
Horse	32–44
Horse (thoroughbred)	38–48
Dairy cow	60–70
Sheep and goat	70–80
Pig	60–80
Dog	70–120
Cat	110–130
Chicken	200–400
Human	60–90

heart disease, and altitude. The regulation of heart rate is a function of the autonomic nervous system. Sympathetic innervation to the heart occurs by way of efferent fibers from the stellate ganglia of the sympathetic trunk. Parasympathetic innervation is supplied by fibers from the vagus nerves. **Sympathetic stimulation** increases all heart activities, and **parasympathetic stimulation** decreases all heart activities (see Chapter 4). Activities of the heart that are important in this regard are: 1) rate of contraction, 2) force of contraction, 3) rate of impulse conduction, and 4) amount of coronary blood flow.

Autoregulation

In addition to the nervous regulation of heart function and output, an **autoregulation** of **cardiac output** based on the amount of blood received also exists. In other words, the more the heart is filled during diastole, the greater is the volume of blood pumped out. This is known as **Starling's law of the heart**. The heart can do this because the greater volume of incoming blood stretches the heart muscle fibers, resulting in a greater force of contraction. There are limits, however, to the amount of stretch by which the force of contraction increases. The stretch phenomenon is characteristic of all types of muscle.

Reflexes

Several important reflexes within the cardiovascular system assist in its regulation. In the arch of the aorta and where the carotid artery branches to form the internal carotid (the **aortic and carotid sinuses**, respectively), there are many receptors that respond to stretching of these vessels. Their stretch is caused by increased blood pressure from within. The receptors fire with greater frequency when stretched. The impulses from the aortic arch are transmitted to the medulla by the vagus nerves, and those from the carotids are transmitted to the medulla by the glossopharyngeal nerves. The responses of the greater number of impulses are directed toward lowering the blood pressure. This is done by greater stimulation of the **cardioinhibitory center** (which increases parasympathetic stimulation to the heart and decreases its activities) and by inhibition of the **vasomotor center** (thereby causing dilatation of the systemic blood vessels). The effects of these responses (decreased heart rate and decreased peripheral resistance) lower the blood pressure (*Fig. 9-27*). A decrease in blood pressure causes fewer impulses to be transmitted from the aortic and carotid sinuses; thus, the cardioinhibitory center receives less stimulation and the vasomotor center receives less inhibition, producing an increase in blood pressure. There are also receptors in the right atrium of the heart that are stimulated by stretch of that chamber, such as during exercise when greater amounts of blood are returned to the heart. The resulting reflex is known as the **Bainbridge reflex**. Stretch receptors transmit their impulses through the vagus nerves to the medulla of the brain. The effect of this reflex is to increase all activities of the heart to increase the circulatory effort necessary for the increased requirements.

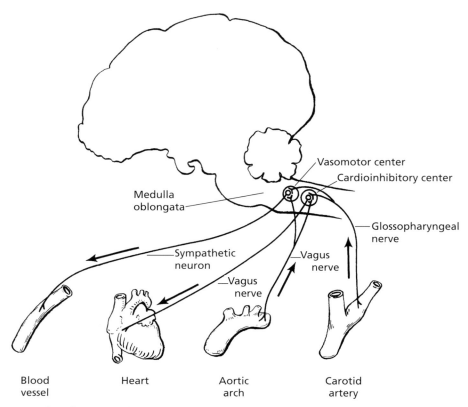

Vasomotor center
Cardioinhibitory center
Medulla oblongata
Glossopharyngeal nerve
Sympathetic neuron
Vagus nerve
Vagus nerve

Blood vessel   Heart   Aortic arch   Carotid artery

■ **FIGURE 9-27** The reflexes controlling blood pressure involve receptors in the aortic and carotid sinuses and centers in the medulla oblongata. To lower blood pressure the vasomotor center is inhibited, resulting in vasodilatation, and the cardioinhibitory center is stimulated, resulting in diminished heart activity.

■ BLOOD PRESSURE

1. Why does blood flow continuously rather than intermittently, considering that the ventricles contract intermittently?
2. Define diastolic, systolic, pulse, and mean blood pressure.

Blood is under pressure within its closed system, and the pressure varies in different parts of the circulatory system. Pressure differences can be observed when vessels are cut. Blood from the central end of a cut artery is under high pressure, and it spurts; blood from the peripheral end of a cut vein may be rapid but is under low pressure and is without pulsation. Accordingly, blood is under high pressure in arteries, moderate pressure in capillaries, and low pressure in veins. The unqualified term **blood pressure** usually refers to arterial pressure.

Pressure Generation and Flow

Blood pressure has been mentioned briefly without regard to its dynamic aspects. Because there is a pressure gradient within the circulation (highest in aorta and lowest in venae cavae), the blood flows from the left ventricle, through the vessels, and back to the right atrium. The greatest pressure develops within the aorta when the left ventricle contracts. The

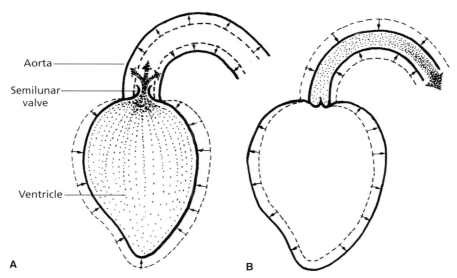

Aorta

Semilunar valve

Ventricle

A   B

■ **FIGURE 9-28** Generation of systemic blood pressure during left ventricular systole and maintenance of blood flow and pressure during diastole. A) Contraction of ventricle and stretch of elastic aorta. B) This is followed by retention of systemic blood in vessels by the closed aortic semilunar valve. Continued blood flow is provided by the elastic recoil of the aorta. Solid lines in A represent ventricular and aortic size at the end of systole. Solid lines in B represent ventricular and aortic size at the end of diastole. The stippling in the ventricle and aorta represents blood.

ventricle relaxes completely after contraction, but blood pressure in the aorta does not diminish entirely. The large arteries contain a higher number of elastic connective tissue fibers than muscle fibers. These elastic fibers permit expansion when blood advances into them from the left ventricle, and stretched elastic fibers have a rebound tendency that exerts pressure on the blood in the large vessels after the heart ceases to exert the pressure (*Fig. 9-28*). The continuous pressure in the arteries permits a continuous rather than an intermittent blood flow through the body.

Systolic and Diastolic Pressures

The high point of the arterial pressure obtained at the peak of left ventricular contraction (systole) is called the **systolic blood pressure**. The lowest pressure in the arteries occurs while the left ventricle is relaxed (diastole) and before it begins its next contraction. The low point of pressure is called the **diastolic**

pressure. Blood pressure measurements are often given as two values, one over the other (e.g., 130/70). The upper value is the systolic pressure, and the lower value is the diastolic pressure. The term **pulse pressure** refers to the difference between the systolic and the diastolic pressures; in the previous example it would be 60. The appropriate unit for expressing blood pressure values is millimeters of mercury (mm Hg) or **torr**. The **mean blood pressure** is not a value halfway between the systolic and diastolic blood pressures; it usually tends to be the diastolic pressure plus about one-third of the pulse pressure. Therefore, in the previous example, the mean blood pressure would be about 90 mm Hg. Mean blood pressure determines the average rate at which blood flows through the systemic vessels. It is closer to diastolic pressure than systolic pressure because, during each pressure cycle, the pressure usually remains at systolic levels for a shorter time than it remains at diastolic levels.

Measurements

The conformation of the body parts of animals has not been conducive to blood pressure being measured by the same noninvasive sphygmomanometric means used in humans. Instruments have been developed in recent years that now allow noninvasive means for measuring blood pressure in animals. The Doppler flow method emits an ultrasonic beam into the blood vessel; the ultrasound reflected from the moving blood changes its frequency (Doppler effect), and by proper calibration, blood pressure is being measured. Another instrument is the oscillometer, which detects oscillations of the blood flow. It can be calibrated to measure systolic, mean, and diastolic pressures. Both of these instruments require the fixation of a transducer or cuff at appropri-

ate locations on the fore- or hindlimbs or tail. The most accurate method in animals involves cannulation of arteries and measuring the pressure electronically with appropriate transducers. A blood pressure measurement taken from the carotid artery in a dog is illustrated in *Figure 9-29*. The systolic, diastolic, mean, and pulse pressures are also shown, as well as the correlation with the ECG.

Values for characteristic blood pressures in several animals are given in *Table 9-2*.

■ BLOOD FLOW

1. How is blood flow to body parts autoregulated?
2. Is blood flow to body parts constant regardless of their need?

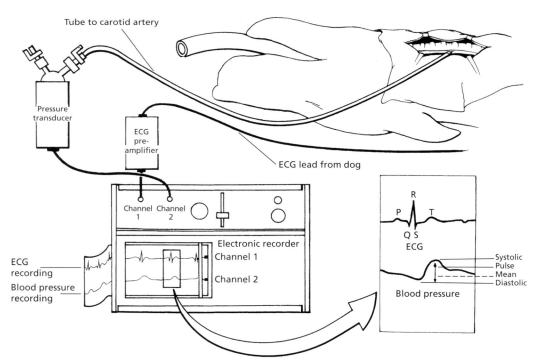

■ **FIGURE 9-29** Recording blood pressure from a surgically placed cannula and an electrocardiogram from lead II in an anesthetized dog. Note the increase in pressure that follows the QRS waves (depolarization of ventricles and subsequent contraction). Pulse pressure is represented by the double arrow between diastolic and systolic blood pressure.

TABLE 9-2 CHARACTERISTIC BLOOD PRESSURES IN ADULT, RESTING ANIMALS

SPECIES	SYSTOLIC/DIASTOLIC (MM HG)	MEAN (MM HG)
Giraffe	260/160	219
Horse	130/95	115
Cow	140/95	120
Swine	140/80	110
Sheep	140/90	114
Human	120/70	100
Dog	120/70	100
Cat	140/90	110
Rabbit	120/80	100
Guinea pig	100/60	80
Rat	110/70	90
Mouse	111/80	100
Turkey	250/170	190
Chicken	175/145	160
Canary	220/150	185

From Detweiler DK. Control mechanisms of the circulatory system. In: Swenson MJ, Reece WO, eds. Dukes' Physiology of Domestic Animals. 11th Ed. Ithaca, NY: Cornell University Press, 1993.

3. Study "Breathing and Blood Flow" very well. Visualize the expansion of the venae cavae that occurs with each inspiration. Translate expansion of the venae cavae to increased blood flow to the heart.

There must be a difference in blood pressure between intake and output for blood to flow. Blood pressure alone does not imply blood flow. The flow of blood to a body part can be changed by changing the diameter of the vessel supplying the part. Constriction of a vessel reduces the blood flow, and dilatation increases the blood flow.

Autoregulation

Generally, there is an autoregulatory mechanism affecting blood flow to a body part that is controlled by the amount of oxygen being received by the cells. When the oxygen is reduced in concentration, the blood vessels dilate and more blood is permitted to flow so that oxygen is replenished. It is also believed that more oxygen being supplied than is needed results in vasoconstriction, which would reduce blood flow and reestablish oxygen at its lower level.

Cardiac Output and Blood Diversion

Cardiac output is defined as the amount of blood pumped by the heart in a unit period of time. It is usually measured in milliliters or liters per minute. Under resting conditions, each body organ or muscle mass receives a rather constant amount. The percentage of the cardiac output that goes to the various organs or tissues changes, however, with the activity condition. At rest the muscles might receive only 20% to 25% of the cardiac output, whereas they might receive up to 75% during extreme muscular exertion. At such times there is diversion of blood flow from other organs (e.g., kidneys, intestines) so that it can be used by the muscle. This is accomplished by constriction of the arteries and arterioles supplying the kidneys and intestines and by dilatation of the vessels supplying the muscles. During muscle exertion, the cardiac output is also increased; coupled with vasodilatation, this provides adequate blood flow to the muscle to satisfy the greater oxygen needs of muscle activity (*Fig. 9-30*).

Breathing and Blood Flow

An assist to blood flow is provided during the inspiratory phase of breathing. The venae cavae course through the thorax on their way to the right atrium. More specifically, they course through the **mediastinum**, a space

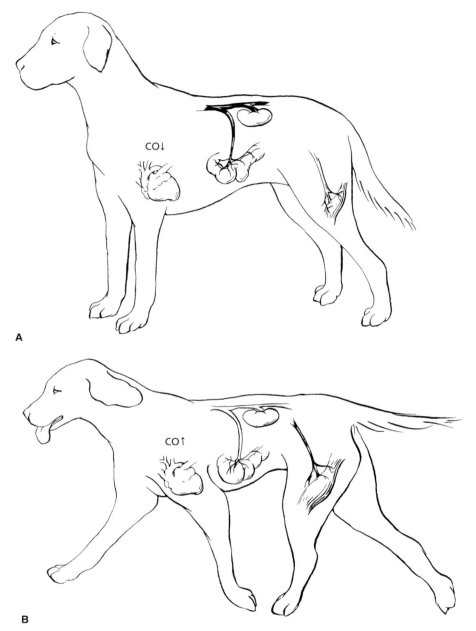

■ FIGURE 9-30 Diversion of blood flow according to need. Greater blood flow to kidneys and intestine at rest **(A)** and to muscles during exertion **(B)**. Cardiac output (CO) is greater during exertion. Blackened vessels indicate locations of greater blood flow.

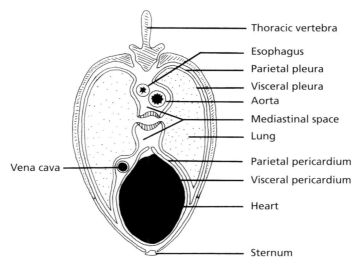

■ **FIGURE 9-31** Cross section of equine thorax at a level that shows the esophagus, caudal vena cava, aorta, and heart within the mediastinal space. Expansion of thoracic volume occurs with inspiration, which leads to lowering of pressure in the mediastinal space. This is followed by expansion of volume (and lowering of pressure) in thin-walled structures (e.g., lymphatics, venae cavae, esophagus) within the mediastinal space.

shared by the other major vessels of the heart, the large lymph vessels, the heart, and the esophagus (*Fig. 9-31*). The mediastinal space is intimately associated with the intrapleural space, a space that is in the thorax but outside the lungs. When animals inspire (inhale air), a vacuum (negative pressure) develops in the intrapleural space because of enlargement of the thorax. This vacuum provides for lung expansion. The negative pressure in the intrapleural space is also transferred to the mediastinal space because of the thin wall of separation. Any thin-walled structure within the mediastinal space responds to the developing vacuum by expansion, with the result being lowered pressure within the thin-walled structures (venae cavae, lymph vessels, and esophagus). This is helpful for the return of venous blood and lymph to the heart because it increases the pressure gradient to assist blood and lymph flow with every breath.

The above sequence of events is illustrated in *Figure 9-32*. In this laboratory model, the muscular diaphragm is represented by a rubber glove stretched over the bottom of a bell jar.

Downward traction on the glove simulates contraction of the diaphragm. The lung and caudal vena cava are represented by balloons that respond to decreasing and increasing external pressure by expansion and collapse, respectively. During inspiration the diaphragm contracts; this is followed, in order, by: 1) increased thoracic volume, 2) decreased intrapleural pressure, 3) increased volume in the lung and vena cava, 4) decreased intrapulmonic and intravenous pressures, and 5) air flow into the lung and blood flow into the thoracic part of the vena cava. During expiration the diaphragm returns to its original position, so that: 1) the volume decreases in the thorax, lung, and vena cava, and 2) the intrapleural, intrapulmonic, and intravenous pressures increase. Backflow of blood is prevented by the cranially directed valves in the vena cava, and air flows out of the lung.

Circulation Time

Circulation time refers to the time required for blood to return to the right atrium after it

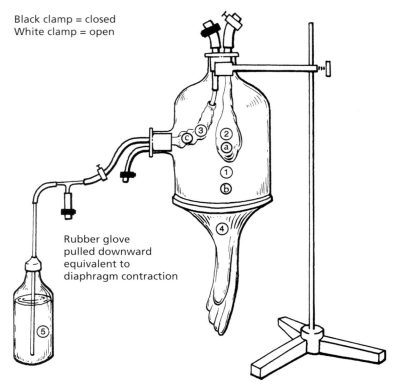

Black clamp = closed
White clamp = open

Rubber glove
pulled downward
equivalent to
diaphragm contraction

■ **FIGURE 9-32** Laboratory model of the thorax. This illustrates the mechanics of breathing and the influence of breathing on venous blood return to the heart. Structures: **1,** thorax; **2,** lung; **3,** vena cava; **4,** diaphragm; **5,** venous blood reservoir. Pressures: a, intrapulmonic; b, intrapleural; c, intravenous. During inspiration, the diaphragm (4) contracts (downward pull of glove), resulting in an increase in thoracic volume (1) and a decrease in intrapleural pressure (b). This is followed by an increase in lung volume (2) and a decrease in intrapulmonic pressure (a). Air flows into the lung. Also, there is an increase in vena cava volume (3), simultaneous with lung volume increase, and a decrease of its intravenous pressure (c). Blood flow (5) to the heart increases because of intravenous pressure decrease. During expiration the diaphragm (4) relaxes, resulting in a decrease in the volumes of the thorax (1), lung (2), and vena cava (3), and an increase in intrapleural (a), and intravenous (b), intrapulmonic (c) pressures. Air flows out of the lung. Valves in veins prevent blood from flowing backward.

has been pumped from the left ventricle. This is variable but is approximately 40 to 60 seconds. Circulation time is distinct from **mixing time**, which is the time required for a substance injected into the blood to be mixed thoroughly, with either the blood or the body fluid compartment with which it is compatible. In all cases, the mixing time exceeds the circulation time.

■ **CAPILLARY DYNAMICS**

1. Distinguish between diffusion and bulk flow.

2. What are the four pressures that are associated with bulk flow?

3. What contributes to plasma colloidal osmotic pressure?

4. Consider each of the four pressures, and determine the direction of fluid flow caused by each.

5. Study the examples given for the arterial and venous ends of a capillary that determine the extent of filtration and reabsorption.

6. Study the examples of capillary imbalance, and relate their causes to the pressure factors.

7.   Why are venous side pressure increases more conducive to imbalance caused by increased capillary pressure than arterial side pressure increases?

The topic of **capillary dynamics** refers to the physical factors associated with the exchange of fluid between the blood and interstitial fluid at the level of the capillaries. The capillaries have slit-like spaces between adjacent endothelial cells that make up the capillary wall, known as **intercellular clefts**. Although water can diffuse through all parts of the endothelium (capillary membrane), it seems to diffuse more freely through the clefts, or pores. Lipid-soluble materials (e.g., oxygen, carbon dioxide) in blood diffuse freely through the lipid portion of the capillary membrane, but lipid-insoluble substances (e.g., electrolytes, glucose, urea) must diffuse through the pores. Large lipid-insoluble molecules (e.g., protein) diffuse through the pores with difficulty.

Diffusion and Bulk Flow

The diffusion of water and its dissolved substances accounts for the greatest degree of interchange between capillaries and interstitial fluid (*Fig. 9-33*). By the time blood traverses the distance of a capillary, the water of the plasma has been exchanged with water of the interstitial fluid about 80 times. Usually the relative proportions of the extracellular water between the plasma and interstitial space are in equilibrium. In addition to **diffusional flow** of fluid, there is also a **bulk flow**; this results from osmotic and hydrostatic pressure differences between plasma and interstitial fluid. It should be noted, however, that the volume of interchange occurring by diffusion is 15,000

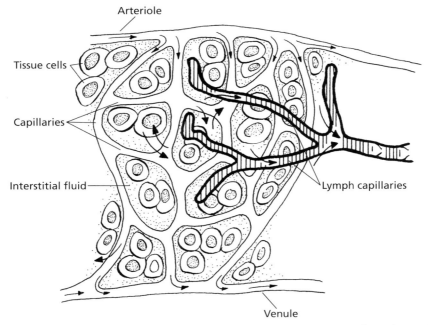

■ **FIGURE 9-33** A schematic representation of a capillary bed. Blood is supplied to capillaries by arterioles, and it leaves the capillaries through the venules. Tissue cells are surrounded by interstitial fluid (ISF). Water and dissolved substances from blood capillaries are interchanged with ISF and intracellular fluid by diffusion. ISF not returned to the blood capillaries is returned as lymph through lymphatic capillaries.

to 20,000 times greater than the volume of interchange by bulk flow. The volume of bulk flow into the interstitial space from the plasma is usually balanced by the amount returning to the capillaries from the interstitial space, coupled with that returning through the lymphatics. In certain circumstances imbalances occur and fluid can accumulate excessively in the interstitial spaces. In such cases, bulk flow into the interstitial space from the plasma exceeds the volume returned to the blood and lymph capillaries.

Mechanism of Bulk Flow

The mechanism of bulk flow is determined by a number of parameters.

Capillary Pressure

The **capillary pressure** (P_c) is the hydrostatic pressure in the capillary. It averages 17 mm Hg (25 mm Hg at the arterial end and 10 mm Hg at the venous end).

Interstitial Fluid Pressure

The **interstitial fluid pressure** (P_{if}) is the hydrostatic pressure in the interstitial fluid. It averages about −6 mm Hg. It is a negative pressure (vacuum) and is created by the return of interstitial fluids to the venous end of the capillary and to the lymphatics. This can be compared with the attachment of a device to a water faucet to create a vacuum. When water flows through its open end, a vacuum is created at its side port.

Plasma Colloidal Osmotic Pressure

The **plasma colloidal osmotic pressure** (π_c) is the effective osmotic pressure of the plasma. It occurs because of the presence of the protein molecules and cations (positive ions) retained by the net negative charge of the protein. It can also be called the oncotic pressure. It averages about 28 mm Hg.

Interstitial Fluid Colloidal Osmotic Pressure

The **interstitial fluid colloidal osmotic pressure** (π_{if}) is the effective osmotic pressure of the interstitial fluid and, like the π_c, is a result of the presence of protein molecules that have leaked from the plasma and have not yet returned to the blood through the lymphatics. The π_{if} averages about 5 mm Hg.

To understand bulk flow, it is helpful to consider these various pressures and to determine their effects, first at the arterial end of the capillary and then at the venous end. Normally, **filtration** or net outward flow occurs at the arterial end, and **reabsorption** or net inward flow occurs at the venous end of the capillary.

The arterial and venous ends of a capillary are shown in *Figure 9-34*. Each of the four pressures that influence the direction of fluid flow is shown with an arrow pointed in the direction of its influence. The effects of these four pressures are summarized in *Table 9-3*.

A filtration pressure of 8 mm Hg and reabsorption pressure of 7 mm Hg would seem to represent an imbalance (i.e., filtration exceeds reabsorption by 1 mm Hg), in which fluid would accumulate in the interstitial fluid. Accumulation does not ordinarily occur, however, because the extra filtration represented by these values is removed from the interstitial fluid by the lymphatics. In fact, some of the interstitial fluid bulk flow must be removed by the lymphatics to carry the protein that has leaked from the capillaries back to the blood. Once again, the lymphatics are the only route by which leaked protein can return.

Capillary Imbalances

An **imbalance** of bulk flow can occur; when this happens, fluid accumulates in the interstitial space. This can be seen when high capillary pressure, low blood protein concentration, lymphatic blockage, and increased porosity

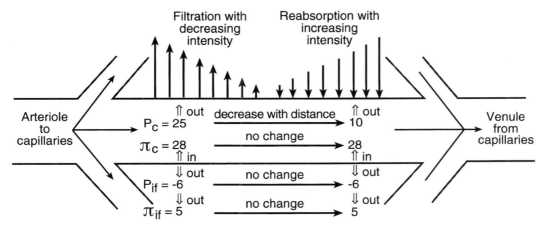

■ **FIGURE 9-34** Physical factors associated with filtration at the arterial end and reabsorption at the venous end of a capillary. Values are in millimeters of mercury (mm Hg). P_c, capillary hydrostatic pressure; Π_c, plasma colloidal osmotic pressure; P_{if}, interstitial fluid hydrostatic pressure; Π_{if}, interstitial fluid colloidal osmotic pressure. Open arrows indicate the direction of influence of P_c, Π_c, P_{if}, and Π_{if}.

TABLE 9-3 PRESSURES THAT DETERMINE FLUID FILTRATION AND REABSORPTION IN CAPILLARIES

Arterial End			
	Pressure Out (mm Hg)	Pressure in (mm Hg)	Summary
	$P_c = 25$	$\pi_c = \underline{28}$	Pressure Out = 36 mm Hg
	$P_{if}{}^a = -6$		Pressure In = <u>28</u> mm Hg
	$\pi_{if} = \underline{5}$		
Total	36	28	Filtration Pressure = 8 mm Hg
Venous End			
	Pressure Out (mm Hg)	Pressure In (mm Hg)	Summary
	$P_c = 10$	$\pi_c = \underline{28}$	Pressure Out = 28 mm Hg
	$P_{if} = -6$		Pressure In = <u>21</u> mm Hg
	$\pi_{if} = \underline{5}$		
Total	21	28	Reabsorption Pressure = 7 mm Hg

[a]A negative value of the interstitial fluid pressure favors outward flow and is the same as equivalent positive value in the capillary.

Note: P_c, capillary hydrostatic pressure; π_c, plasma colloidal osmotic pressure; P_{if}, interstitial fluid hydrostatic pressure; π_{if}, interstitial fluid colloidal osmotic pressure.

(which allows more protein to escape) are each sufficient to favor filtration over absorption and lymphatic drainage (*Fig. 9-35*). Increases in capillary hydrostatic pressure (Fig. 9-35A) can arise from either the arterial or the venous end of the capillary. High arterial blood pressure (e.g., kidney retention of salt and water) is transmitted to capillaries and

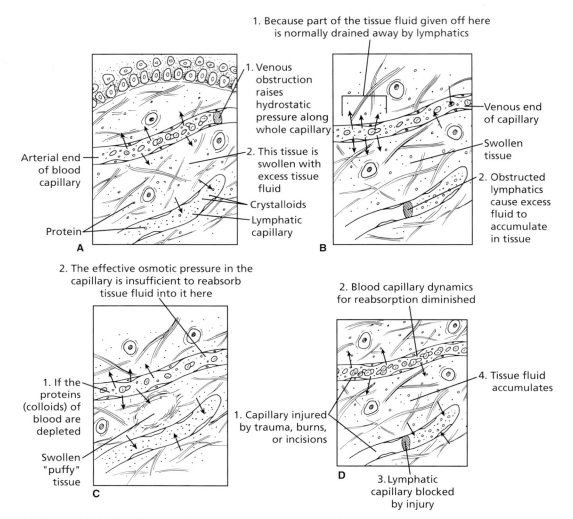

■ **FIGURE 9-35** Capillary dynamic imbalances as causes for interstitial fluid (ISF) accumulation (edema). For **A)** Venous obstruction raises hydrostatic pressure along whole blood capillary. Filtration exceeds reabsorption. For **B)** Because of lymphatic obstruction, filtration exceeds reabsorption. For **C)** Depletion of plasma proteins reduces the effective osmotic pressure in the blood capillaries. Continued filtration coupled with diminished blood capillary reabsorption exceeds lymph capillary reabsorption. For **D)** Capillary injury diminishes blood capillary dynamics for reabsorption for both blood capillary and lymph capillary dynamics. (Adapted from Ham AW. Histology. 7th Ed. Philadelphia: JB Lippincott, 1974.)

can influence capillary dynamics; however, increases of venous blood pressure are more conducive to imbalance caused by high capillary pressure than increases from the arterial side. Venous side increases transmit the increase throughout the length of the capillary, whereas the effect of an arterial side increase is minimized by its reduction in going from the arterial to the venous end. Some causes of increased venous pressures are heart failure, in which the weakened heart is unable to circulate all of the blood that is returned to it; venous blood pressure increases; venous obstruction (e.g., trauma, tight bandages); and venous pump failure (e.g., muscle paralysis, immobilized parts).

Lymphatic obstruction (Fig. 9-35B) increases Π_{if} because protein, ordinarily returned by lymphatic vessels, is retained in the interstitial fluid, thereby reducing the potential for fluid reabsorption. The failed reabsorption, in turn, causes an increase in P_{if} (from its negative value to positive) thereby contributing to increased P_c throughout the capillary and decreasing the potential for reabsorption at the venous end. Some causes of lymphatic obstruction are blockage of lymph nodes (e.g., cancer, infection), destruction of lymph vessels (e.g., surgery, trauma), and blockage of lymph vessels (e.g., obstructive devices, tumors).

A reduction of the plasma protein concentration (Fig. 9-35C) that is low enough causes an imbalance because Π_c, the reabsorption factor, is decreased to the point at which filtration exceeds reabsorption. Some causes of plasma protein depletion are renal disease (e.g., loss of protein in urine), reduced protein synthesis (e.g., liver disease, nutritional), and interstitial fluid loss (e.g., denuded skin).

Capillary injury (Fig. 9-35D) by trauma or by toxins increases the porosity of the endothelial cells, and protein is lost from the capillaries, which in turn reduces the potential for reabsorption.

In each of these examples, fluid accumulates in the interstitial space and gives it a swollen appearance, a condition known as **edema**. When it is generalized, it is referred to as **anasarca**.

■ SUGGESTED READING

Erickson HH. Heart sounds and murmurs. In: Reece WO, ed. Dukes' Physiology of Domestic Animals. 12th Ed. Ithaca, NY: Cornell University Press, 2004.

Erickson HH. Microcirculation, lymph, and edema. In: Reece WO, ed. Dukes' Physiology of Domestic Animals. 12th Ed. Ithaca, NY: Cornell University Press, 2004.

Frandson RD, Wilke WL, Fails AD. Anatomy and Physiology of Farm Animals. 6th Ed. Baltimore: Lippincott Williams & Wilkins, 2003.

Ghoshal NG. Equine heart and arteries. In: Getty R, ed. Sisson and Grossman's The Anatomy of the Domestic Animals, Vol. 1. 5th Ed. Philadelphia: WB Saunders, 1975.

Guyton AC, Hall JE. Textbook of Medical Physiology. 10th Ed. Philadelphia: WB Saunders, 2000.

 SELF EVALUATION—CHAPTER 9

HEART AND PERICARDIUM

1. An increase in the resistance to blood flow to the lungs would cause hypertrophy (because of greater work) of which one of the following chambers?
   a. Right atrium
   b. Left atrium
   c. Right ventricle
   d. Left ventricle

2. Venous blood (unoxygenated) enters the:
   a. left atrium from the vena cava.
   b. pulmonary trunk from the left ventricle.
   c. pulmonary trunk from the right ventricle.
   d. left atrium from the pulmonary veins.

3. Blood flow through the arteries is maintained during diastole because of:
   a. contraction of the ventricles.
   b. inertia.
   c. elastic fibers in large vessels.
   d. expansion of the thorax during inspiration.

4. Blood pumped from the left ventricle goes through the:
   a. aortic semilunar valve.
   b. pulmonary trunk semilunar valve.

c. right A-V valve.
d. left A-V valve.

5. Blood flow through the heart, when received from the venae cavae, proceeds in the following order:
   a. left atrium, right atrium, right ventricle, left ventricle.
   b. right atrium, left atrium, left ventricle, right ventricle.
   c. right atrium, right ventricle, left atrium, left ventricle.
   d. left atrium, left ventricle, right atrium, right ventricle.

6. Because of its greater work, the heart chamber with the greatest muscle mass is the:
   a. right ventricle.
   b. left ventricle.
   c. right atrium.
   d. left atrium.

7. During ventricular contraction (systole):
   a. the A-V valves are closed, and the semilunar valves are open.
   b. the semilunar valves are closed, and the A-V valves are open.
   c. all valves (A-V and semilunars) are open.
   d. all valves (A-V and semilunars) are closed.

BLOOD VESSELS

8. Which one of the following circulatory divisions has the lowest pressure?
   a. Capillaries
   b. Veins
   c. Arterioles
   d. Arteries

9. Smooth muscle fibers are contained within:
   a. all of the blood vessels.
   b. capillaries.
   c. capillaries and veins.
   d. veins.

LYMPHATIC SYSTEM

10. Interstitial fluid enters lymph vessels by:
    a. diffusion.
    b. inward flow through flap valves.

11. The lymphatic system:
    a. is the only route back to the blood for the return of protein that leaks from the capillaries.
    b. has a fluid in its vessels known as lymph.
    c. has a fluid in its vessels similar to interstitial fluid.
    d. has lymph nodes along the course of the lymphatic vessels that phagocytize foreign material and generate lymphocytes.
    e. all of the above.

12. Plasma proteins:
    a. never leave the blood.
    b. do leave the blood (12- to 24-hour turnover) and are returned via the lymphatics.
    c. do leave the blood, the same way as water and electrolytes, and are returned by reabsorption at the venous end of capillaries.
    d. serve no useful purpose when in the interstitial space.

SPLEEN

13. Which one of the following organs is active in the destruction of erythrocytes, stores iron, acts as a blood reservoir, phagocytizes foreign material, and produces lymphocytes?
    a. Lymph nodes
    b. Carotid body
    c. Spleen
    d. Dubissary

14. Which one of the following is NOT a true statement about the spleen?
    a. It is the largest lymphoid organ of the body.

b. It is capable of contraction, and thereby expresses RBCs into the blood vessels.

c. It is the only organ organized to filter blood.

d. Its circulating fluid is lymph.

CARDIAC CONTRACTILITY

15. A greater amount of ventricular filling results simply from blood flow into relaxed chambers than from atrial contraction.
    a. True
    b. False

16. An impulse is transmitted throughout the ventricular muscles at a rate two to three times faster than it would be transmitted through atrial muscle because of the characteristics of the:
    a. S-A node.
    b. A-V node.
    c. A-V bundle.
    d. Purkinje fibers.

17. Which of the following is the correct sequence of contraction for the heart?
    a. Simultaneous contraction of both atria followed by simultaneous contraction of both ventricles
    b. Right atrium followed by right ventricle followed by left atrium followed by left ventricle
    c. Simultaneous contraction of right atrium and right ventricle followed by simultaneous contraction of left atrium and left ventricle

18. The pacemaker of the heart is known as the:
    a. Purkinje fibers.
    b. atrioventricular node (A-V node).
    c. atrioventricular bundle (A-V bundle).
    d. sinoatrial node (S-A node).

ELECTROCARDIOGRAM

19. The QRS wave complex would immediately precede which one of the following events?

a. Atrial contraction
b. Ventricular contraction
c. The second heart sound
d. Semilunar valve closure

20. Which one of the EGG wave forms is associated with ventricular depolarization?
    a. P wave
    b. QRS complex
    c. T wave
    d. Tidal wave

21. Blood pressure begins to increase immediately and the first heart sound (lub) is produced right after the:
    a. QRS complex.
    b. P wave.
    c. T wave.

HEART SOUNDS

22. The first heart sound, lub, is caused by:
    a. closure of the semilunar valves.
    b. opening of the semilunar valves.
    c. closure of the A-V valves and contraction of the ventricles.
    d. opening of the A-V valves and contraction of the atria.

23. The second heart sound is correlated with:
    a. ventricular relaxation.
    b. closure of the semilunar valves.
    c. the incisura.
    d. all of the above.

HEART RATE AND ITS CONTROL

24. Which one of the autonomic nervous system divisions is associated with a decrease in all activities of the heart?
    a. Sympathetic
    b. Parasympathetic

25. Stimulation of the right vagus nerve (cranial nerve X; carries parasympathetic fibers) would:
    a. increase all activities of the heart.
    b. decrease all activities of the heart.
    c. have no effect on the heart because it is headed for other organs.

BLOOD PRESSURE

26. During the time between the measurements for systolic blood pressure and diastolic blood pressure, the energy for the flow of blood is derived from:
    a. the left ventricle.
    b. there is no blood flow; it is at a standstill.
    c. the right ventricle.
    d. arterial elasticity.

27. Blood pressure is being measured with an electronic recorder. The upper swing of the pen is at 130 mm Hg, and the lower swing of the pen is at 70 mm Hg. Which one of the following is the pulse pressure?
    a. 130 mm Hg
    b. 70 mm Hg
    c. 60 mm Hg
    d. 90 mm Hg

BLOOD FLOW

28. Which one of the following occurs during expansion of the thorax during inspiration?
    a. Decrease in intrapleural, mediastinal, and intravenous (venae cavae) pressure with assist to return of blood and lymph to the heart
    b. Compression of the lungs (as they fill) on the venae cavae with resistance to return of blood and lymph to the heart

CAPILLARY DYNAMICS

29. Venous obstruction of blood flow from a body part would tend to increase interstitial fluid volume of that part.
    a. True
    b. False

30. Which is favored when considering these values? (pressures in mm Hg)
    Hydrostatic pressure: $P_c = 26$; $P_{if} = -2$
    Colloidal osmotic pressure: $\pi_c = 5$; $\pi_{if} = 5$
    a. Filtration
    b. Reabsorption

31. Which one of the following would increase filtration at the capillary and tend to cause edema?
    a. Increased plasma colloidal osmotic pressure
    b. Increased venous blood pressure
    c. An increase (toward positive) of the interstitial fluid hydrostatic pressure

32. When considered as the only factor influencing bulk flow, plasma colloidal osmotic pressure (Π_c):
    a. favors filtration.
    b. favors reabsorption.

ANSWERS TO SELF EVALUATION—CHAPTER 9

1.	c	9.	d	17.	a	25.	b
2.	c	10.	b	18.	d	26.	d
3.	c	11.	e	19.	b	27.	c
4.	a	12.	b	20.	b	28.	a
5.	c	13.	c	21.	a	29.	a
6.	b	14.	d	22.	c	30.	a
7.	a	15.	a	23.	d	31.	b
8.	b	16.	d	24.	b	32.	b

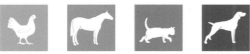
The Respiratory System

CHAPTER OUTLINE

- **RESPIRATORY APPARATUS**
  Airways to the Lungs
  Pulmonary Alveoli
  The Lungs and Pleura
- **FACTORS ASSOCIATED WITH BREATHING**
  Respiratory Cycles
  Types of Breathing
  States of Breathing
  Pulmonary Volumes and Capacities
  Respiratory Frequency
  Lung Sounds
- **RESPIRATORY PRESSURES**
  Partial Pressure
  Arterial and Venous Blood Partial
    Pressure
  Atmospheric Air versus Alveolar Air
- **PULMONARY VENTILATION**
  Dead Space ventilation
  Pressures That Accomplish Ventilation
  Pneumothorax
  Mediastinal Pressure
- **DIFFUSION OF RESPIRATORY GASES**
- **OXYGEN TRANSPORT**
  Transport Scheme
  Oxygen–Hemoglobin Dissociation Curve

- **CARBON DIOXIDE TRANSPORT**
  Hydration Reaction
  Carbamino Compounds
  Loss of Carbon Dioxide at the Alveolus
- **REGULATION OF VENTILATION**
  Neural Control
  Humoral Control
- **RESPIRATORY CLEARANCE**
  Physical Forces of Deposition
  Upper Respiratory Tract Clearance
  Alveolar Clearance
- **NONRESPIRATORY FUNCTIONS OF THE RESPIRATORY SYSTEM**
  Panting
  Purring
- **DESCRIPTIVE TERMS AND PATHOLOGIC CONDITIONS**
- **AVIAN RESPIRATION**
  General Scheme of Avian Respiratory
    Morphology
  Mechanics of Respiration and Air
    Circulation
  General Considerations

Respiration is the means by which animals obtain and use oxygen and eliminate carbon dioxide. In this chapter, the chemical factors involved in oxygen uptake and carbon dioxide production are not discussed. However, the mechanical and physical aspects of respiration that are presented are mainly concerned with the provision of oxygen to the cells, where it is taken up by the mitochondria at the end of the **electron transfer chain**. Here, the reduced cofactors of metabolism are

reoxidized and, in the process of electron transfer, hydrogen combines with oxygen to form water. This water is referred to as **metabolic water**. Generally, the mechanical and physical aspects of respiration are involved with ventilation of the lungs and with transport of gases between the lungs and blood and between the blood and tissues. The respiratory system also serves nonrespiratory functions, and some of these functions are discussed.

■ RESPIRATORY APPARATUS

1. How are the nostrils of the horse adapted to the need for greater air intake?
2. What functions are served by the conchae?
3. Where is the olfactory epithelium located?
4. List the openings to the pharynx.
5. What is the function of the pharynx and syrinx?
6. What is the function of tracheal rings? Why are they incomplete dorsally?
7. What are the subdivisions of the trachea (in order from largest to smallest)?
8. Where does most of the diffusion of gas between air and blood occur?
9. Describe the pleura and mediastinal space.
10. What structures lie within the mediastinal space?
11. What happens to mediastinal pressure when intrapleural pressure decreases?

The **respiratory apparatus** consists of the lungs and pleura and the air passages leading to the lungs, including the nostrils, nasal cavities, pharynx, larynx, trachea, bronchi, and bronchioles.

Airways to the Lungs

The **nostrils (nares)** are the paired external openings to the air passages (*Fig. 10-1*). The nostrils are the most pliable and dilatable in

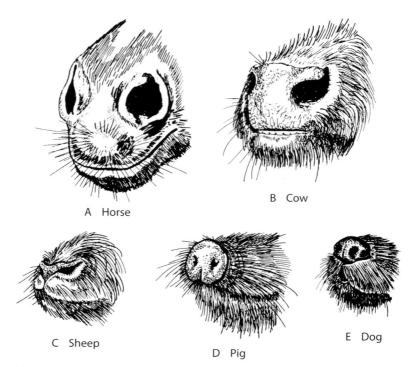

A Horse

B Cow

C Sheep

D Pig

E Dog

■ **FIGURE 10-1** The nostrils of several domestic animals. **A)** Horse. **B)** Cow. **C)** Sheep. **D)** Pig. **E)** Dog. (From Frandson RD, Wilke WL, Fails AD. Anatomy and Physiology of Farm Animals. 6th Ed. Baltimore: Lippincott Williams & Wilkins, 2003.)

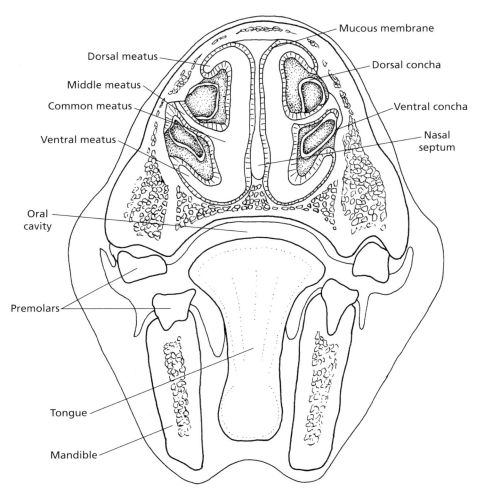

Dorsal meatus

Middle meatus

Common meatus

Ventral meatus

Oral cavity

Premolars

Tongue

Mandible

Mucous membrane

Dorsal concha

Ventral concha

Nasal septum

■ **FIGURE 10-2** Transverse section of the head of a horse showing the division of the nasal cavities. The airways are noted as the dorsal, middle, ventral, and common meatus. The conchae consist of turbinate bones covered by a highly vascularized mucous membrane. It can be seen that incoming air is exposed to a large surface area for adjustment of its temperature and humidity.

the horse and the most rigid in the pig. Nostril dilatation is advantageous when more air is required, as in running, and in situations in which breathing is not done through the mouth. The horse is a runner, and open-mouth breathing is not characteristic, therefore dilatable nostrils are advantageous.

The nostrils provide the external openings for the paired **nasal cavities**. The nasal cavities are separated from each other by the **nasal**

septum and from the mouth by the **hard** and **soft palates**. In addition, each nasal cavity contains mucosa-covered turbinate bones (**conchae**) that project to the interior from the dorsal and lateral walls, separating the cavity into passages known as the common, dorsal, middle, and ventral **meatus** (*Fig. 10-2*). The mucosa of the turbinates is well vascularized and serves to warm and humidify inhaled air. Another function, mainly for the conchae,

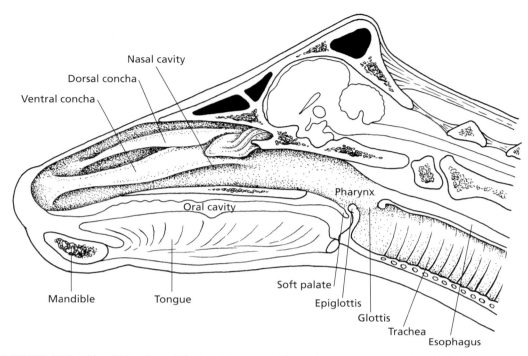

■ **FIGURE 10-3** Midsagittal section of the head of a cow with nasal septum removed. The stippled area represents the pathway for air through the nasal cavity, pharynx, larynx, and trachea. The glottis is the opening to the larynx that is continued caudally by the trachea.

that is often overlooked involves cooling the blood that supplies the brain. Arteries that supply blood to the brain divide into many smaller arteries at its base and then rejoin before entering. These smaller arteries are bathed in a pool of venous blood that comes from the walls of the nasal passages, where it has been cooled. As a result, brain temperature might be 2°C or 3°C lower than body core temperatures. The brain is the most heat-sensitive body organ, so this cooling method is particularly important during times of extreme activity. The mouth breathing that occurs when the environmental air is extremely cold seems to be reflexive, which might prevent the overcooling of the brain that could otherwise occur if all of the inhaled air traversed the meatus and had contact with the conchae. The **olfactory epithelium** is located in the caudal portion of each nasal cavity, and greater perception of odors (a non-respiratory function) is achieved by **sniffing** (i.e., fast, alternating, and shallow inspirations and expirations).

The **pharynx** is caudal to the nasal cavities and is a common passageway for air and food (*Fig. 10-3*). The openings to the pharynx include two posterior nares, two eustachian tubes, a mouth (oral cavity), a glottis, and an esophagus. The opening from the pharynx leading to the continuation of the respiratory passageway is the **larynx**, the organ of phonation (sound production) in mammals. Sound is produced by the controlled passage of air, which causes vibration of vocal cords in the larynx. The organ of phonation in birds is called the **syrinx**; this is located where the trachea divides to form the bronchi.

The **glottis** is the slit-like opening between the vocal cords and is the site for insertion of an endotracheal (within the trachea) tube when it is used for providing assisted ventilation and for administration of inhalant anesthetics. Extending craniad from the larynx is the **epiglottis**. It is a leaf-shaped plate of cartilage covered with mucous membrane. It is located at the root of the tongue, which is passively bent over the larynx during the act of swallowing, thereby preventing the entrance into the trachea of a bolus being swallowed. A cranial view of the glottis and epiglottis as they would appear with the mouth open and the tongue extended is shown in *Figure 10-4*. In this view, the soft palate (caudal extension of the hard palate) has been hyperextended with the maxilla (upper jaw). When placing an endotracheal tube, the soft palate is often seen ventral to the epiglottis with usual mouth opening and must be lifted by manipulation of the endotracheal tube to expose the glottis. *Figure 10-5* shows an endotracheal tube in place relative to the structures encountered.

The **trachea** is the primary passageway for air to the lungs. It is continued from the larynx cranially and divides caudally to form the right and left bronchi. The tracheal wall contains cartilaginous rings to prevent collapse of the tracheal airway (*Fig. 10-6*). Each **tracheal ring** is incomplete (not

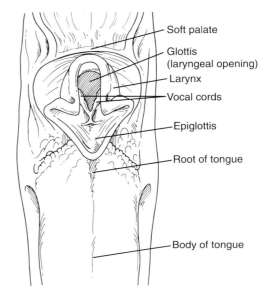

■ **FIGURE 10-4** Cranial view of canine glottis (opening to the larynx, between vocal cords) and epiglottis (cranial extension from the larynx). The soft palate is not shown in the location that would be seen with usual mouth opening techniques.

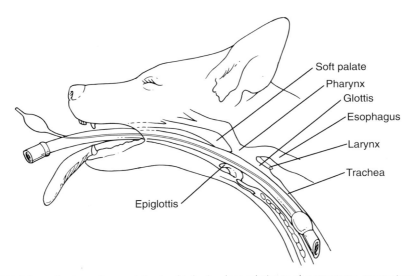

■ **FIGURE 10-5** Schematic view of an endotracheal tube in place relative to the structures encountered.

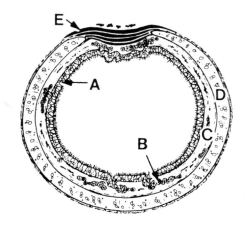

■ **FIGURE 10-6** Schematic representation of a cross section of trachea. **A)** Pseudostratified epithelium lines the lumen. **B)** Glands in the lamina propria. **C)** Glands in the submucosa. **D)** Cartilage. **E)** Band of smooth muscle. The tracheal muscle and the cartilage form most of the tracheal wall. (From Dellmann HD. Textbook of Veterinary Histology. 4th Ed. Philadelphia: Lea & Febiger, 1993.)

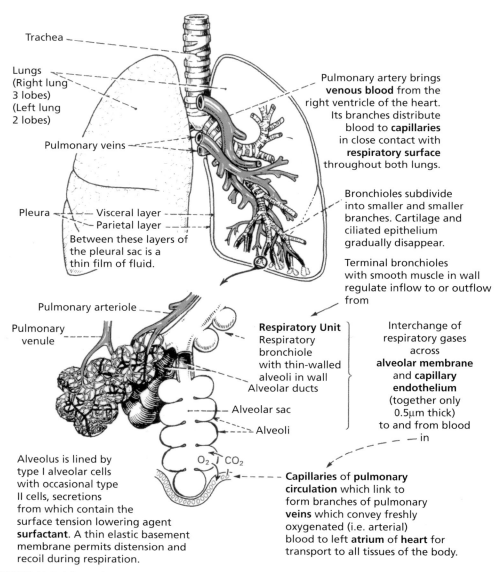

Trachea

Lungs
(Right lung
3 lobes)
(Left lung
2 lobes)

Pulmonary veins

Pleura — Visceral layer
— Parietal layer
Between these layers of
the pleural sac is a
thin film of fluid.

Pulmonary artery brings **venous blood** from the right ventricle of the heart. Its branches distribute blood to **capillaries** in close contact with **respiratory surface** throughout both lungs.

Bronchioles subdivide into smaller and smaller branches. Cartilage and ciliated epithelium gradually disappear.

Terminal bronchioles with smooth muscle in wall regulate inflow to or outflow from

Pulmonary arteriole

Pulmonary venule

Respiratory Unit
Respiratory bronchiole with thin-walled alveoli in wall
Alveolar ducts

Alveolar sac

Alveoli

Interchange of respiratory gases across **alveolar membrane** and **capillary endothelium** (together only 0.5μm thick) to and from blood — in

O_2 ↑ CO_2

Alveolus is lined by type I alveolar cells with occasional type II cells, secretions from which contain the surface tension lowering agent **surfactant**. A thin elastic basement membrane permits distension and recoil during respiration.

Capillaries of **pulmonary circulation** which link to form branches of pulmonary **veins** which convey freshly oxygenated (i.e. arterial) blood to left **atrium** of **heart** for transport to all tissues of the body.

■ **FIGURE 10-7** Schematic representation of lung subdivisions. (From Mackenna BR, Callander R. Illustrated Physiology. 6th Ed. Edinburgh: Churchill Livingstone, 1997.)

joined dorsally), which permits variations in diameter that are regulated by the tracheal smooth muscle. This diameter can increase during times of greater ventilatory requirements.

The right and left bronchi and their subdivisions continue all the way to the **alveoli**, the final and smallest subdivisions of the air passages (*Fig. 10-7*). The subdivisions of the trachea to the alveoli, from the largest to the smallest, are the: 1) bronchi, 2) bronchioles, 3) terminal bronchioles, 4) respiratory bronchioles, 5) alveolar duct, 6) alveolar sac, and 7) alveoli.

Pulmonary Alveoli

The **pulmonary alveoli** are the principal sites of gas diffusion between the air and blood. The separation of air and blood, and thus the diffusion distance, is minimal at the alveolar level. The alveolar epithelium and the capillary endothelium are intimately associated (*Fig. 10-8*). Here, venous blood from the **pulmonary arteries** becomes arterial blood and is returned to the left atrium by the **pulmonary veins**. The darker purple color of venous blood becomes bright red arterial blood during the resaturation of hemoglobin with new oxygen that has diffused from the alveoli. During the seventeenth century, Richard Lower showed that the change in blood color occurred in the lungs because of the influence of fresh air. The idea that the diffusion of oxygen and carbon dioxide between blood and air was separate from a secretion process was proven by August and Marie Krogh. (August Krogh won the Nobel prize in 1920 for his studies of the capillaries.)

The Lungs and Pleura

The lungs are the principal structures of the respiratory system. They are paired structures and occupy all space in the thorax that is not otherwise filled. When the thorax expands in volume, the lungs also expand; this provides for air flow into the lungs. Air is an excellent **radiographic contrast** media because it is radiolucent (relatively penetrable by x rays). Therefore, air-filled lungs provide good contrast for thoracic structures (normal and pathologic) that are **radiopaque** (relatively impenetrable by x rays). Dorsal-ventral and lateral view radiographs of a normal canine thorax are shown in *Figure 10-9*. The radiopaque objects (heart and blood vessels) appear superimposed on the radiolucent background of air. The heart and blood vessels are visible because the blood contained within is relatively radiopaque. The blood vessels appear as branching white tubes.

The lungs have an almost friction-free movement within the thorax because of the **pleura**, a smooth serous membrane. The pleura consists of a single layer of cells fused to the surface of a connective tissue layer. It envelops both lungs (**visceral pleura**). The pleura for the right and left lung meet near the midline, and here it reflects upward (dorsally), turns back on the inner thoracic wall, and provides for its lining (costal pleura). The space between the respective visceral pleura layers as they ascend to the dorsal wall is known as the **mediastinal space**. Within the mediastinal space are the venae cavae, thoracic lymph duct, esophagus, aorta, and trachea (*Fig. 10-10*). The mediastinal space is intimately associated with the **intrapleural space** (space between visceral and costal pleura); thus, pressure changes in the intrapleural space are accompanied by similar changes in the mediastinal space. Also, pressure changes within the mediastinal space are accompanied by changes within the mediastinal structures, provided that their walls are responsive to relatively low-pressure distensibility.

■ FACTORS ASSOCIATED WITH BREATHING

1. **What are the mechanical activities associated with inspiration? What**

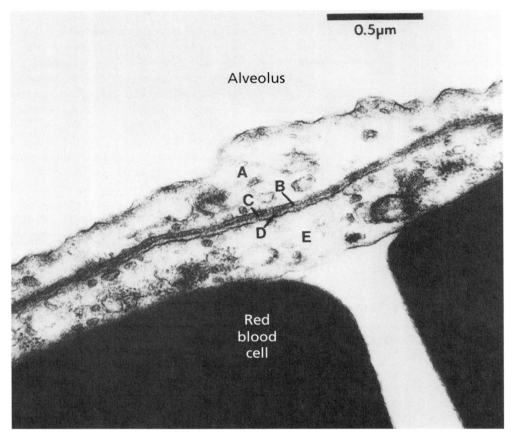

■ **FIGURE 10-8** Electron micrograph of a mouse lung showing an attenuated portion of alveolar epithelium and its proximity to capillary endothelium. The respiratory membrane (without alveolar fluid layer) is composed of the following: **A)** alveolar epithelium, **B)** alveolar epithelial basement membrane, **C)** interstitial space, **D)** capillary endothelial basement membrane, and **E)** capillary endothelium. (From Reece WO. Respiration in mammals. In: Reece WO, ed. Dukes' Physiology of Domestic Animals. 12th Ed. Ithaca, NY: Cornell University Press, 2004.)

are some conditions for active expiration?

2. Differentiate between abdominal and costal breathing. When is either accentuated?

3. What are some commonly referred to states of breathing?

4. Know the subdivisions of lung volume. What is the difference between a lung volume subdivision and a lung capacity subdivision?

5. When expansion of the lungs is restricted, how is adequate ventilation maintained?

6. What are some factors that affect respiratory frequency?

Many factors of breathing terminology must be understood for one to observe, describe, and measure individual animal behavior related to respiration.

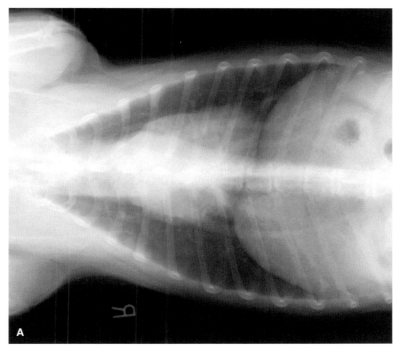

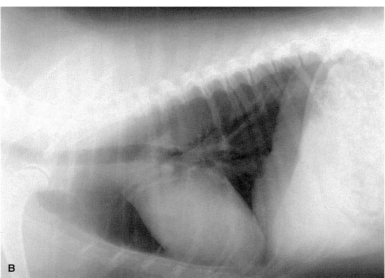

■ **FIGURE 10-9** Radiographs of healthy canine thorax. **A)** Dorsal-ventral view. Radiographs of healthy canine thorax. **B)** Lateral view. The heart and major blood vessels are visible because blood is relatively radiopaque. Blood in lesser blood vessels gives a slightly cloudy appearance to the lung field as compared with the clear appearance of air in the trachea. Radiographs courtesy of Dr. Elizabeth Riedesel, Iowa State University, College of Veterinary Medicine, Veterinary Clinical Sciences Department, Radiology Section.

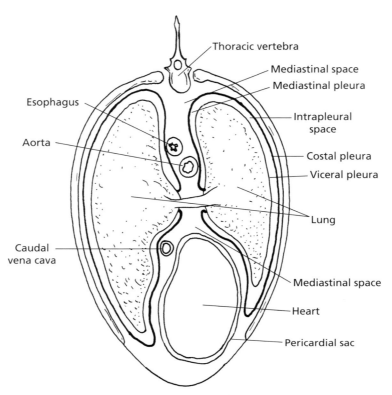

■ **FIGURE 10-10** Schematic transverse section of equine thorax showing the relationships of the visceral, costal, and mediastinal pleura. The aorta, esophagus, venae cavae, and thoracic lymph duct (not shown) are within the mediastinal space. The esophagus, venae cavae, and lymph duct (soft structures) respond by increasing and decreasing pressures within their lumens, associated with similar changes in intrapleural and mediastinal spaces.

Respiratory Cycles

A **respiratory cycle** consists of an inspiratory phase followed by an expiratory phase. **Inspiration** involves an enlargement of the thorax and lungs, with an accompanying inflow of air. The thorax enlarges by contraction of the **diaphragm** (the musculotendinous separation between the thorax and abdomen) and by contraction of appropriate **intercostal muscles** (muscles located between the ribs) (*Fig. 10-11*). Diaphragmatic contraction enlarges the thorax in a caudal direction, and intercostal muscle contraction enlarges the thorax in a craniad and outward direction. Under normal breathing conditions, inspiration requires greater effort than expiration, and sometimes expiration might seem to be passive. **Expiration** can become quite an active process, particularly during times of accelerated breathing and also when there are impediments to the outflow of air. The appropriate intercostal muscles contract to assist in expiration. Other skeletal muscles can aid in either inspiration or expiration, such as the abdominal muscles. When contracted, these muscles force the abdominal viscera forward to press on the diaphragm, which in turn decreases thoracic volume.

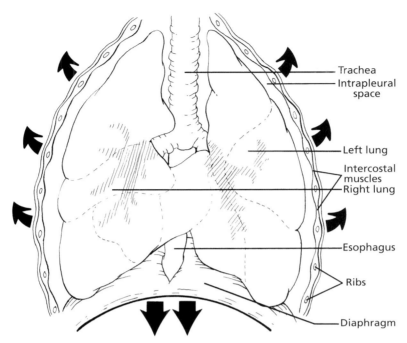

■ FIGURE 10-11 Schematic of the thorax during inspiration (ventral view). Shown are the directions of enlargement (arrows) when the diaphragm and inspiratory intercostal muscles contract during inspiration.

Types of Breathing

There are two types of breathing: abdominal and costal. **Abdominal breathing** is characterized by visible movements of the abdomen, in which the abdomen protrudes during inspiration and recoils during expiration. Normally the abdominal type of breathing predominates. The other type is called **costal breathing**; it is characterized by pronounced rib movements. During painful conditions of the abdomen, such as peritonitis, in which movement of the viscera would aggravate the pain, costal breathing can predominate. Similarly, during painful conditions of the thorax, such as pleuritis, abdominal breathing might be more apparent. Binding of the thorax to minimize the outward and craniad expansion of the thorax requires greater diaphragmatic effort, and subsequent movement of abdomi-

nal viscera accentuates the abdominal type of breathing.

States of Breathing

In addition to the different types of breathing, there are variations in breathing relating to the frequency of breathing cycles, depth of inspiration, or both. **Eupnea** is the term used to describe normal quiet breathing, with no deviation in frequency or depth. **Dyspnea** is difficult breathing, in which visible effort is required to breathe. The animal is usually aware of this breathing state. **Hyperpnea** refers to breathing characterized by increased depth, frequency, or both, and is noticeable after physical exertion. The animal is not acutely conscious of this state. **Polypnea** is rapid, shallow breathing, somewhat similar to panting. Polypnea is similar to hyperpnea in regard to frequency, but is unlike hyperpnea in regard to depth. **Apnea** refers to a cessation of breathing. However, as used clinically, it generally refers to a transient state of cessation of breathing. **Tachypnea** is excessive rapidity of breathing, and **bradypnea** is abnormal slowness of breathing.

Pulmonary Volumes and Capacities

Conventional descriptions for lung volumes are either associated with the amount of air within them at any one time or with the amount associated with a breath. **Tidal volume** is the amount of air breathed in or out during a respiratory cycle. It can increase or decrease from normal, depending on ventilation requirements. Tidal volume is probably used more frequently than other terms. **Inspiratory reserve volume** is the amount of air that can still be inspired after inhaling the tidal volume, and **expiratory reserve volume** is the amount of air that can still be expired after exhaling the tidal volume. **Residual volume** is the amount of air remaining in the lungs after the most forceful expiration. Also, some part of the residual volume remains in the lungs after they have been removed from the thorax during slaughter or for postmortem examination. Because of the remaining residual volume, excised lung sections float in water. Consolidation of lung tissue, as occurs in pneumonia, causes them to sink.

Sometimes it is useful to combine two or more of these volumes. Such combinations are called capacities. **Total lung capacity** is the sum of all volumes. **Vital capacity** is the sum of all volumes over and above the residual volume; it is the maximum amount of air that can be breathed in after the most forceful expiration. **Inspiratory capacity** is the sum of the tidal and inspiratory reserve volumes. **Functional residual capacity** is the sum of the expiratory reserve volume and the residual volume. This is the lung volume that is ventilated by the tidal volume. It serves as

the reservoir for air and helps to provide constancy to the blood concentrations of the respired gases. Relationships of pulmonary volumes and capacities are illustrated in *Figure 10-12.*

Respiratory Frequency

Respiratory frequency refers to the number of respiratory cycles each minute. It is an excellent indicator of health status, but must be interpreted properly because it is subject to numerous variations. In addition to variations observed among species, respiratory frequency can be affected by other factors, such as: 1) body size, 2) age, 3) exercise, 4) excitement, 5) environmental temperature, 6) pregnancy, 7) degree of filling of the digestive tract, and 8) state of health. Pregnancy and digestive tract filling increase frequency because they limit the excursion of the diaphragm during inspiration. When expansion of the lungs is restricted, adequate ventilation is maintained by increased frequency. For example, when cattle lie down, the large rumen pushes against the diaphragm and restricts its movement, and the respiratory frequency is seen to increase.

Respiratory frequency usually increases during disease. Thus, frequency is a useful determinant of health status, but the frequency for a species under various conditions must be known so that this parameter can be interpreted properly (*Table 10-1*). Values are meaningful only when obtained unobtrusively from animals at rest.

Lung Sounds

It is obvious from Figure 10-7 that considerable branching of the pulmonary airways occurs. Although the branches may have smaller diameters than the parent branch, the combined cross-sectional area of the branches shows an increase over that of the parent. Consequently, the velocity of air flow diminishes progressively from the trachea toward the bronchioles. Listening for lung sounds with

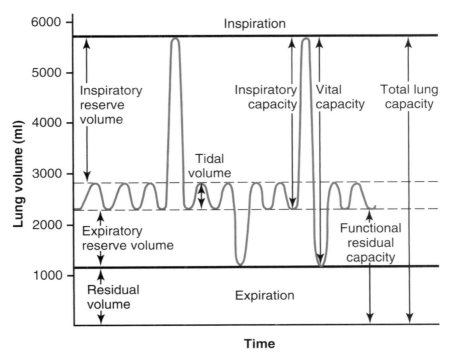

■ **FIGURE 10-12** Subdivisions of lung volume. The values shown for lung volume are those that approximate values for an average adult human male. (From Guyton AC, Hall JE. Textbook of Medical Physiology. 11th Ed. Philadelphia: Elsevier Inc. 2006.

TABLE 10-1 RESPIRATORY FREQUENCY FOR SEVERAL ANIMAL SPECIES UNDER DIFFERENT CONDITIONS

ANIMAL	NUMBER	CONDITION	CYCLES/MIN RANGE	MEAN
Horse	15	Standing (at rest)	10–14	12
Dairy cow	11	Standing (at rest)	26–35	29
	11	Sternal recumbency	24–50	35
Dairy calf	6	Standing (52 kg body weight, 3 weeks old)	18–22	20
	6	Lying down (52 kg body weight, 3 weeks old)	21–25	22
Pig	3	Lying down (23 to 27 kg body weight)	32–58	40
Dog	7	Sleeping (24°C)	18–25	21
	3	Standing (at rest)	20–34	24
Cat	5	Sleeping	16–25	22
	6	Lying down, awake	20–40	31
Sheep	5	Standing, ruminating, 1/2 inch wool 18°C	20–34	25
	5	Same sheep and conditions except 10°C	16–22	19

From Reece WO. Respiration in mammals. In: Reece WO, ed. Dukes' Physiology of Domestic Animals. 12th Ed. Ithaca, NY: Cornell University Press, 2004.

the aid of a stethoscope is termed **auscultation**. A good-quality stethoscope should be used in quiet surroundings. The high-velocity, turbulent air flow in the trachea and bronchi produces the lung sounds heard through a stethoscope in a normal animal. Laminar, low-velocity flow in the bronchioles produces no sound. To amplify the sounds, deep respiratory efforts can be produced by placing a plastic bag loosely over the muzzle of the animal.

The term **breath sound** applies to any sound that accompanies air movement through the tracheobronchial tree. Breath sounds vary randomly in intensity over a broad range depending on whether the sounds are produced over the larger airways or over the remaining lung parenchyma.

Adventitious sounds are extrinsic to the normal sound production mechanism of the respiratory tract and are abnormal sounds superimposed on the breath sounds. Adventitious sounds are further classified as crackles and wheezes. Diseases resulting in edema or exudates within the airways can result in crackles. Wheezes suggest airway narrowing (e.g., bronchoconstriction, bronchial wall thickening, external airway compression).

With the exception of laminar, low-velocity flow in the bronchioles (noted above), the absence of respiratory sounds implies that nonfunctional lung tissue is beneath the stethoscope.

■ RESPIRATORY PRESSURES

1. Define partial pressure.
2. What are the gases of the atmosphere, and what is the approximate percentage composition of each?
3. How would you determine the P_{O_2} of dry atmospheric air?
4. Why does the composition of atmospheric air differ from that of alveolar air?

Solutes and solvents diffuse from an area of their higher concentration to an area of their lower concentration, and so do gases. The concentrations of gases are usually expressed as pressures. It occasionally helps to think in terms of concentration instead of pressure when determining the diffusion of a single gas within a mixture of gases.

Partial Pressure

Usually, gas pressure is considered in terms of total pressure, regardless of whether it is a single gas or a mixture of gases. When considering the equilibrium of two gas mixtures separated by a permeable membrane, however, it is necessary to consider each gas in the mixture separately in terms of its contribution to the total pressure. The term **partial pressure** is therefore used. It is defined as the pressure exerted by a particular gas in a mixture of gases. The sum of the partial pressures of the gases within a mixture equals the **total pressure**. The physiologic notation for partial pressure is P. Specific gases are noted by their chemical symbol. Accordingly, the partial pressure of oxygen in a gas mixture is denoted by P_{O_2}. The partial pressure of oxygen in arterial blood and venous blood is given by P_aO_2 and P_vO_2, respectively, where the particularization of arterial and venous blood is noted by the subscripts a and v.

Arterial and Venous Blood Partial Pressure

Because oxygen is consumed and carbon dioxide is produced by cells, it is expected that venous blood (blood returning to the lungs after its service to the cells) will have a higher P_{CO_2} and a lower P_{O_2} than arterial blood (blood that has been replenished by the lungs and is on its way to the cells). Arterial blood taken from one part of the body will have approximately the same gas content as arterial blood from another part of the body because none of it has reached capillary systems where the exchange (loss of O_2 and gain of CO_2) takes place. Venous blood from different parts of the body may vary, however, because of different metabolism associated with the function of the body part. A more active location would consume more O_2 and produce more CO_2 than less active locations. Because of these differences, the jugular vein blood may not be representative of whole body venous blood (i.e., blood from the right atrium).

Atmospheric Air versus Alveolar Air

The total pressure of **one atmosphere (1 atm)** of air under conditions of standard temperature and pressure is **760 mm Hg**. The appropriate composition of dry atmospheric air (and corresponding partial pressures) is as follows: 21.0% O_2 (PO_2; about 159 mm Hg); 0.03% CO_2 (PCO_2; about 0.23 mm Hg); 79.0% N_2 (PN_2; about 600 mm Hg). The total pressure is approximately 760 mm Hg. CO_2 is almost absent in the atmospheric air. This explains the effective diffusion gradient for CO_2 from the body (where it is produced) to the air around us. Note that this is the composition of dry air. Any amount of humidification is represented by a **water vapor** partial pressure value (PH_2O). Its presence would cause a dilution of the other gases, and thus their partial pressures would be lowered to maintain the total pressure at 760 mm Hg.

It might be supposed that the composition of alveolar air is the same as atmospheric air because it represents the transfer of air from one place to another. However, the ventilation process does not evacuate the alveoli completely with each breath, but rather it is a gradual replenishment and evacuation. The approximate composition of alveolar air, measured in partial pressure, is as follows (dry atmospheric air partial pressures are in parentheses): PO_2 = 104 mm Hg (159); PCO_2 = 40 mm Hg (0.23); PN_2 = 569 mm Hg (600); PH_2O = 47 mm Hg (0.00). The differences from

atmospheric air are apparent. The total pressure of alveolar air is equal to 760 mm Hg, and all of its components are diluted by water vapor, which is equal to 47 mm Hg. A PH_2O of 47 mm Hg represents 100% humidification of alveolar air at body temperature (37°C for humans). In addition, the PO_2 is lower and the PCO_2 is higher than their respective atmospheric pressures because oxygen is continually diffusing from alveolar air to the tissues (where it is used) and CO_2 is continually diffusing from the tissues (where it is produced) to the alveolar air (where it is expelled). The PN_2 of alveolar air is lower than its value in atmospheric air primarily because of its dilution by water vapor.

■ PULMONARY VENTILATION

1. What makes up dead space ventilation?
2. Is physiologic dead space volume less than anatomic dead space volume?
3. What are the components of tidal volume?
4. What functions are served by dead space ventilation?
5. How do intrapulmonic and intrapleural pressures change during a respiratory cycle? Study Figure 9-32 (Laboratory model of the thorax).
6. How could a condition of pneumothorax be corrected?
7. How does a decrease in mediastinal pressure (as occurs during inspiration) assist in the return of blood and lymph to the heart?

Ventilation is generally regarded as the process by which gas in closed places is renewed or exchanged. As it applies to the lungs, it is a process of exchanging the gas in the airways and alveoli with gas from the environment. The main function of breathing is to provide for ventilation. When cattle are stunned at the time of slaughter, it has been observed that breathing often stops. The heart continues to beat for 4 to 10 minutes longer, but it also stops when the oxygen available from the functional residual capacity has been depleted. Therefore, a non-breathing animal still has resuscitation potential if the heart continues to beat.

Dead Space Ventilation

The tidal volume is used to ventilate not only the alveoli, but also the airways leading to the alveoli. Because there is little or no diffusion of oxygen and carbon dioxide through the membranes of most of the airways, they compose part of what is called **dead space ventilation**. The other part of dead space ventilation is made up of alveoli with diminished capillary perfusion. Ventilating these alveoli is ineffective in producing changes in the blood gases. Ventilation of nonperfused alveoli and the airways, because neither accomplishes exchange of the respiratory gases, is referred to as physiologic dead space. **Physiologic dead space** is defined as the volume of gas that is inspired but takes no part in gas exchange in the airways and alveoli. Therefore, the tidal volume (V_T) has a dead space component (V_D) and an alveolar component (V_A), or $V_T = V_D + V_A$.

Dead space ventilation is a necessary part of the process of ventilating the alveoli and is not totally wasted. It assists in tempering and humidifying inhaled air and in cooling the body under certain conditions, such as when panting is necessary. During panting, the respiratory frequency increases and the tidal volume decreases so that alveolar ventilation remains approximately constant.

Pressures That Accomplish Ventilation

The pressure within the lungs is referred to as **intrapulmonic pressure**, and the pressure outside the lungs but within the thoracic cavity (between the visceral and parietal pleura) is referred to as **intrapleural pressure**. Air flows into the lungs during inspiration because the pressure within the lung, the intrapulmonic pressure, becomes lower than the atmospheric pressure. Similarly, air flows out of the lungs during expiration because the intrapulmonic pressure exceeds atmospheric pressure at that time. The intrapleural and intrapulmonic pressures associated with inspiration and expiration are shown in *Figure 10-13*.

The intrapulmonic pressure decreases during inspiration because the volume of the lungs increases. The lungs can increase in volume because they are elastic structures that can stretch. Also, the pressure around them, the intrapleural pressure, is being reduced because the volume of the intrapleural space increases in response to contraction of the diaphragm and intercostal muscles (see *Fig. 10-11*). When contraction of the inspiratory muscles ceases, expiration begins.

To permit air to flow out of the lungs during expiration, the intrapulmonic pressure must become positive. Positive pressure is primarily generated by the recoil tendency of the lungs, which were previously stretched during inspiration. The **recoil tendency** is produced not only by the **elastic fibers** within the lung, but also by the **surface tension** of the fluid that lines the alveoli. Retraction of the lungs can also be assisted by expiratory muscles. The diaphragm is an inspiratory muscle, and its contraction assists only inspiration; conversely, its relaxation permits expiration. During eupnea the intrapulmonic pressure can be about −1 mm Hg (below atmospheric) during inspiration, and it can be +1 mm Hg during expiration. During this time, the intrapleural pressure changes from −2 mm Hg at the end of expiration to about −6 mm Hg at the end of inspiration. Thus, the intrapleural pressure changes slightly more than the intrapulmonic pressure changes.

Intrapleural pressure (pressure in a closed space) is normally lower than atmospheric pressure, even at the end of expiration and

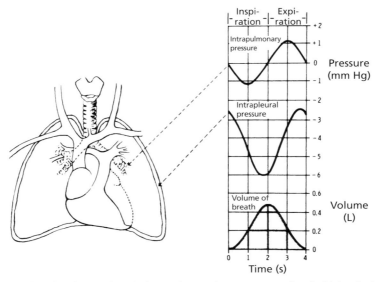

■ **FIGURE 10-13** Intrapleural and intrapulmonic (intrapulmonary) pressures associated with inspiration and expiration. (Reproduced with permission from Ganong WF. Review of Medical Physiology. 20th Ed. New York: McGraw-Hill, 2001.)

before inspiration. This is a result of the constant recoil tendency of the lungs and of the absorption of gases from closed spaces caused by the existence of a diffusion gradient between the closed space and venous blood. The total pressure in the intrapleural space is in equilibrium with venous blood. It is lower than atmospheric pressure because the reduction of PO_2 caused by oxygen absorption is greater than the increase in PCO_2. The reduced total pressure of the intrapleural space is comparable with that of a slight vacuum.

Pneumothorax

If the intrapleural space is opened to the atmosphere (e.g., during certain surgical procedures), it would not be possible for diaphragmatic contraction to generate a greater vacuum in the intrapleural space, and the lungs would not inflate (*Fig. 10-14*). This condition is known as pneumothorax. A respirator would be necessary to ventilate the lungs, or the animal would die. Correction of pneumothorax involves effecting final closure

of the unnatural opening simultaneously with full inflation of the lungs. Normal lung retraction could then reestablish the normal negative intrapleural pressure. The next inspiration would generate negative pressure in the intrapleural space, and the lungs would expand because the trachea would be the only passageway available for air intake.

Mediastinal Pressure

During inspiration, when the intrapleural pressure is reduced, the mediastinal space pressure is also reduced. Reduction of the mediastinal space pressure is followed by the expansion of volume and reduction of pressure within the distensible structures of the mediastinal space (venae cavae, thoracic lymph duct, esophagus). This reduction in pressure assists in the return of blood and lymph to the heart. During regurgitation in ruminants (see Chapter 12), reduced pressure in the esophagus, associated with an exaggerated inspiration with a closed glottis, also assists in this process.

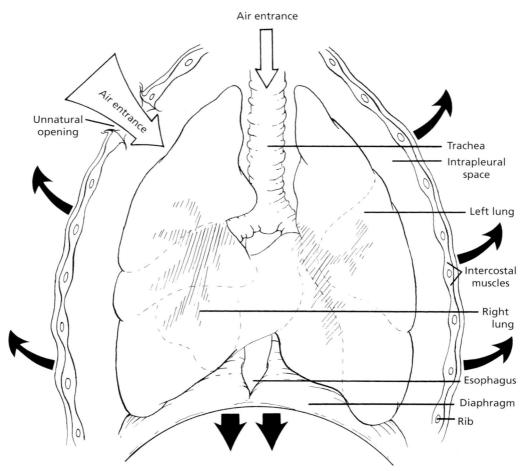

■ **FIGURE 10-14** Pneumothorax (ventral view). The volume of air that enters at the unnatural opening exceeds that which enters the trachea when the intrapleural volume is increased during inspiration. The intrapleural pressure reduction is then not sufficient to permit lung inflation. The dark arrows show the directions of thoracic enlargement when the diaphragm and inspiratory intercostal muscles contract during inspiration.

■ DIFFUSION OF RESPIRATORY GASES

1. Which one of the respiratory gases, O_2 or CO_2, diffuses more readily through cell membranes?
2. Read the text to understand Table 10-2 and Figure 10-15.

The respiratory gases diffuse readily throughout the body tissues. Because of its greater lipid solubility, carbon dioxide diffuses about 20 times more readily than oxygen through membranes. Also, as the distance of diffusion increases, as in **pulmonary interstitial edema**, the diffusion rate decreases. Under this condition, one may notice greater ventilation efforts in an attempt to compensate for the **hypoxemia** (decreased O_2 concentration in arterial blood) that has developed because of the reduced rate of diffusion. Blood-gas analysis shows reduced partial

TABLE 10-2 TOTAL AND PARTIAL PRESSURES (IN MM HG) OF RESPIRATORY GASES IN HUMANS AT REST (SEA LEVEL)

GASES	VENOUS BLOOD	ALVELOR AIR	ARTERIAL BLOOD	TISSUES
Oxygen	40	109	100	30 or less
Carbon dioxide	45	40	40	50 or more
Nitrogen	569	564	569	569
Water vapor	47	47	47	47
Total	701	760	756	696

From Reece WO. Respiration in mammals. In: Reece WO, ed. Dukes' Physiology of Domestic Animals. 12th Ed. Ithaca, NY: Cornell University Press, 2004.

pressures for both O_2 and CO_2. Because of the decrease in diffusion rate caused by distance, one might have expected an increase in P_{CO_2} in view of its reduced elimination. Its diffusion coefficient is much greater than that for O_2, however, so that the increased ventilation overcompensates for diffusion decrease caused by distance. The thicker membrane (and thus greater diffusion distance) does impair O_2 diffusion, however, resulting in reduced arterial P_{O_2} and hypoxemia.

Table 10-2 presents information to help explain the movement of gases from alveoli to blood to tissues and from tissues to blood to alveoli. Ventilation brings O_2 to the alveoli and removes CO_2. Because O_2 is being consumed in the tissues, a pressure difference exists for its diffusion from alveoli to venous blood (which then becomes arterial) and from arterial blood to the tissues. Because CO_2 is being produced in the tissues, a pressure difference exists for its diffusion from tissue to arterial blood (which then becomes venous) and from venous blood to the alveoli. Table 10-2 indicates that little change occurs in P_{H_2O} and P_{N_2}. The aqueous environment of the body ensures a constant P_{H_2O} and, because N_2 is neither produced nor consumed, its pressure also remains constant. Nitrogen acts only as a filler. The total pressure in venous blood is somewhat less than atmospheric pressure (760 mm Hg) because the volume of CO_2 produced is lower than the volume of O_2 consumed; in other words, the added P_{CO_2} is less than the subtracted P_{O_2}. This is also true for O_2 and CO_2 in the tissues but is only true to a slight degree in arterial blood because not all of the blood going to the lungs is arterialized (**nonperfused alveoli**). The **intraperitoneal pressure** (pressure in the abdomen, a closed space) is similarly affected. The inrush of air into the abdomen can be heard faintly when an incision is first made.

The direction of diffusion in response to differences in partial pressures is shown for oxygen and carbon dioxide in *Figure 10-15*.

■ OXYGEN TRANSPORT

1. What volume of oxygen is normally transported in 100 mL of arterial blood?

2. Why does O_2 diffuse from alveoli to hemoglobin? Why does O_2 diffuse from hemoglobin to tissue cells (see *Fig. 10-16*)?

3. When the P_aO_2 is 100 mm Hg, what is the saturation of Hb?

4. When P_vO_2 is 40 mm Hg, what is the saturation of Hb?

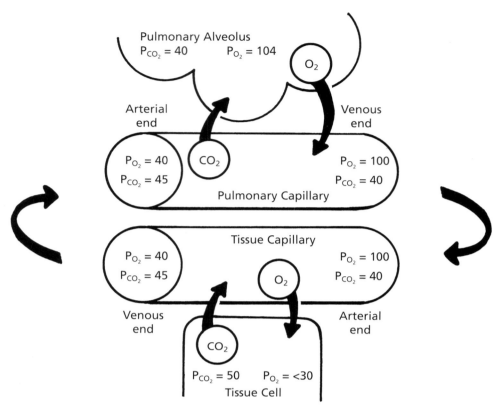

■ **FIGURE 10-15** Direction of diffusion for oxygen (O_2), and carbon dioxide (CO_2), as shown by arrows. In the pulmonary alveolus the P_{CO_2} is 40 mm Hg and the P_{O_2} is 104 mm Hg; at the arterial end of the pulmonary capillary the P_{O_2} is 40 mm Hg and the P_{CO_2} is 45 mm Hg, whereas at the venous end the P_{O_2} is 100 mm Hg and the P_{CO_2} is 40 mm Hg; at the venous end of the tissue capillary the P_{O_2} is 40 mm Hg and the P_{CO_2} is 45 mm Hg, whereas at the arterial end the P_{O_2} is 100 mm Hg and the P_{CO_2} is 40 mm Hg; and in the tissue cell the P_{CO_2} is 50 mm Hg and the P_{O_2} is <30 mm Hg.

5. **Regardless of the amount of Hb in blood, would its saturation be dependent only on P_{O_2} exposure?**

Under normal circumstances there are about 20 mL of molecular oxygen in each deciliter of arterial blood (20 mL/dL, or 20 volumes %). With normal activity, mitochondria consume about 25% of that amount (see Chapter 1) as the blood is circulated to the tissues. The remainder is available as reserve for times of greater activity. The 25% value is referred to as the utilization coefficient; with

strenuous activity, the utilization coefficient is increased.

Transport Scheme

The **transport of oxygen** is illustrated in *Figure 10-16*. The procession of oxygen during its uptake by hemoglobin is from air in the alveolus to successive solution in interstitial fluid (1), in plasma (2), and in erythrocyte fluid (3), and finally to combination with hemoglobin (4). For oxygen yield to the cells, the procession of oxygen is from interstitial fluid (1), followed by that which is from plasma (2), and

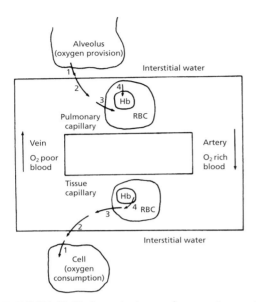

■ FIGURE 10-16 General scheme of oxygen transport showing oxygen procession. Procession occurs because of the presence of pressure gradients. In this diagram, blood is oxygenated at the top and deoxygenated at the bottom; blood flow is clockwise. See text for further explanation. (From Reece WO. Respiration in mammals. In: Reece WO, ed. Dukes' Physiology of Domestic Animals. 12th Ed. Ithaca, NY: Cornell University Press, 2004.)

from erythrocyte fluid (3), which in turn is replenished by the oxygen that is combined with hemoglobin (4). Diffusion of oxygen away from interstitial fluid lowers the PO_2 of the erythrocyte fluid and, just as an increased PO_2 increases the saturation of hemoglobin with oxygen, decreased PO_2 causes desaturation of hemoglobin.

Oxygen–Hemoglobin Dissociation Curve

Oxygen dissolves in blood only slightly. If blood contained O_2 only in solution, there would need to be about 60 times more blood to transport the 20 volumes % present. Transport is accomplished with the available volume of blood because of the O_2 transport potential

of the hemoglobin contained in erythrocytes. Oxygen in solution only needs to diffuse into and out of the erythrocytes to be associated with or dissociated from hemoglobin, respectively.

The relationship between the PO_2 of blood and the percentage saturation of hemoglobin with oxygen is shown by the **oxygen–hemoglobin dissociation curve** (*Figure 10-17*). Note that hemoglobin is nearly 100% saturated when the PO_2 of the blood is 100 mm Hg. This is the normal PO_2 of arterial blood. Also, at the PO_2 of mixed venous blood (about 40 mm Hg), hemoglobin is still about 75% saturated with oxygen. The 25% that has been lost (dissociated from hemoglobin) corresponds to the utilization coefficient. Regardless of the hemoglobin concentration (15 g/dL or 7.5 g/dL, as shown in Figure 10-17), the percentage saturation of hemoglobin is identical for the same PO_2 exposure, i.e., the uptake of O_2 by hemoglobin (regardless of its concentration) is in equilibrium with the partial pressure of O_2. Figure 10-17 illustrates the effect of a lowered hemoglobin concentration (15 g/dL, normal; 7.5 g/dL, 50% normal) on the volume of O_2 transported and illustrates that PO_2 analysis does not reveal the amount of oxygen present in blood. There would be twice the amount of oxygen in blood having 15 g/dL hemoglobin than there would be for blood having 7.5 g/dL at any particular PO_2. Anemic animals, with low hemoglobin concentration, may have normal P_aO_2, but the amount of oxygen in each increment of blood is reduced. To compensate, the heart beats faster to increase blood flow (i.e., more blood [with its reduced oxygen] presented per time period). Figure 10-17 also shows that the rate of oxygen dissociation from hemoglobin increases sharply as the PO_2 decrease approaches the middle and lower ends of the PO_2 scale. This characteristic of hemoglobin facilitates the provision of oxygen at the capillary level by supplying greater amounts with less lowering of PO_2, thus maintaining an adequate pressure difference for diffusion to the cells.

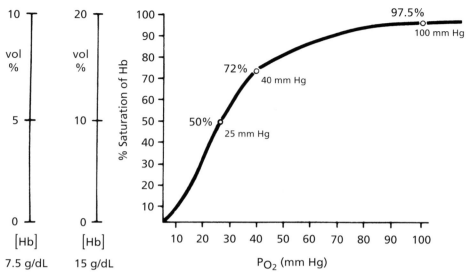

■ **FIGURE 10-17** The oxygen–hemoglobin dissociation curve. See text for explanation. (From Reece WO. Respiration in mammals. In: Reece WO, ed. Dukes' Physiology of Domestic Animals. 12th Ed. Ithaca, NY: Cornell University Press, 2004.)

■ CARBON DIOXIDE TRANSPORT

1. What is the relationship of CO_2 transport to the hydration reaction?
2. Why is venous blood more acidic than arterial blood?
3. What is the most plentiful compound available for buffering H^+ formed during the hydration reaction?
4. What is a carbamino compound?

The **transport of carbon dioxide** is facilitated by several reactions that effectively provide other CO_2 forms in addition to that which is in solution. Even though CO_2 is more soluble in water than O_2, the amount produced exceeds the amount that can be carried in solution. The general scheme for CO_2 transport is shown in *Figure 10-18*.

Hydration Reaction

About 80% of carbon dioxide transport occurs in the form of bicarbonate (HCO_3^-). Its formation results from the hydration reaction (*Equation 10-1*):

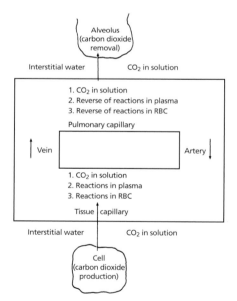

■ **FIGURE 10-18** General scheme of carbon dioxide transport showing carbon dioxide procession. Procession occurs because of the presence of pressure gradients. In this diagram, flow is clockwise; carbon dioxide is taken up from cells at the bottom and removed from blood at the top. Items are numbered in the order of their occurrence. (From Reece WO. Respiration in mammals. In: Reece WO, ed. Dukes' Physiology of Domestic Animals. 12th Ed. Ithaca, NY: Cornell University Press, 2004.)

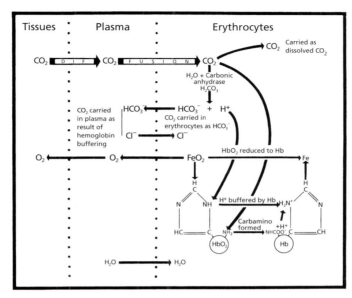

■ **FIGURE 10-19** Schematic representation of the processes that occur when carbon dioxide diffuses from tissues into erythrocytes. (From Davenport HW. The ABC of Acid-Base Chemistry. 6th Ed. Chicago: University of Chicago Press, 1974.)

$$CO_2 + H_2O \rightleftarrows H_2CO_3 \rightleftarrows H^+ + HCO_3^-$$
Eq. 10-1

The equilibrium of the hydration reaction is far to the left in plasma, and the plasma reaction accounts for little transport of CO_2. The reaction is favored within the erythrocytes because of the presence of the enzyme carbonic anhydrase and it proceeds with ease, forming H^+ and HCO_3^-. It would be a rate-limited reaction, however, if the reaction products were not removed. Removal is accomplished by chemical buffering of the H^+ and by diffusion of HCO_3^- out of the erythrocytes into the plasma. Not all of the hydrogen ions are buffered, so venous blood has a lower pH than arterial blood. Also, because of the diffusion of HCO_3^- from erythrocytes to plasma, venous blood has a higher HCO_3^- concentration than arterial blood.

The most plentiful compound available for buffering H^+ formed during the hydration reaction is hemoglobin. When hemoglobin is deficient, as in **anemia**, buffering of H^+ from all sources is jeopardized and acidemia (increased H^+ concentration in blood) results during periods of increased H^+ production, such as exertion.

The erythrocyte processes involved in carbon dioxide transport are shown in *Figure 10-19*.

Carbamino Compounds

Another reaction accounting for CO_2 transport involves the combination of CO_2 with terminal amino groups on the proteins of plasma and hemoglobin to form **carbamino compounds** (*Equation 10-2*).

$$\underset{\underset{COOH}{|}}{R-NH_2} + CO_2 \longleftrightarrow \underset{\underset{COO^- + H^+}{|}}{R-N} \longleftrightarrow R$$
Eq. 10-2

The amount produced with hemoglobin exceeds that produced with plasma proteins because there are fewer terminal amino groups on plasma proteins.

Loss of Carbon Dioxide at the Alveolus

When the venous blood reaches the alveoli and the CO_2 pressure difference favors diffusion of CO_2 in solution from the plasma to the alveoli, there is a prompt reversal of the hydration reaction (see *Fig. 10-18*) and of the reaction that forms carbamino compounds (return of CO_2 to solution). The effect is loss of the CO_2 that was transported from the tissues.

■ REGULATION OF VENTILATION

1. Where is the respiratory center for the regulation of ventilation located?
2. What are the Hering-Breuer reflexes? Give three additional examples of neural mechanisms that modify the basic rhythm of respiration.
3. What are the three humoral factors that influence ventilation?
4. Where are the receptors located for the detection of O_2 lack?
5. Why is there no increase in ventilation when there is O_2 lack caused by carbon monoxide poisoning?

Pulmonary ventilation is regulated closely to maintain the concentrations of H^+, CO_2, and O_2 at relatively constant levels while meeting the needs of the body under varying conditions. If either the H^+ or the CO_2 concentration increases or if the O_2 concentration decreases, their levels will be returned to normal by increasing ventilation. Conversely, if either the H^+ or CO_2 concentration decreases or if the O_2 concentration increases, pulmonary ventilation will be decreased. This regulatory mechanism is controlled by changes in tidal volume, frequency of respiratory cycles, or both. The central mediator of these changes is the respi-

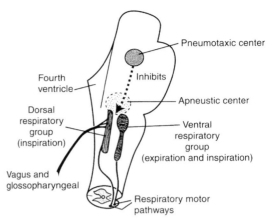

■ **FIGURE 10-20** Components of the respiratory center. The pneumotaxic and apneustic centers are located in the pons, and the dorsal and ventral respiratory groups are located in the medulla. (From Guyton AC, Hall JE. Textbook of Medical Physiology. 10th Ed. Philadelphia: WB Saunders, 2000.)

ratory center in the brain stem, which has four specific regions (*Fig. 10-20*):

1. Pneumotaxic center: believed to modulate respiratory center sensitivity to inputs that activate termination of inspiration and facilitate expiration
2. Apneustic center: believed to be associated with deep inspirations, such as the sigh
3. Dorsal respiratory group: group of neurons predominately associated with inspiratory activity (particularly involved in lung inflation-induced termination of inspiration)
4. Ventral respiratory group: group of neurons containing inspiratory and expiratory neurons (assist in inspiration begun by those in the dorsal respiratory group and also provide for assisted expiration)

A **central pattern generator** has been hypothesized; it is believed to be the neural network that provides for rhythmicity. This central pattern generator is also thought to be in the brain stem. It is influenced by inputs from the vagus and glossopharyngeal nerves and by chemoreceptors.

Neural Control

Impulses going to the respiratory center (afferent impulses) from several receptor sources have been identified. The **Hering-Breuer reflexes** are probably the most noteworthy. The receptors for these reflexes are located in the lungs, particularly in the bronchi and bronchioles. The nerve impulses generated by the receptors of the Hering-Breuer reflexes are transmitted by fibers in the vagus nerves to the respiratory center. The effect of inflation-receptor stimulation is to inhibit further inspiration (stimulation of neurons in the dorsal respiratory group) and to stimulate expiratory neurons in the ventral respiratory group. Tidal volume can be increased, however, by pneumotaxic center modulation. Another component of the Hering-Breuer reflexes is activated at some particular point of deflation. The deflation receptors might not be activated to bring about the next inspiration during eupnea, but they might be active when deflation is more complete.

In addition to lung receptors, there are other peripherally located receptors that modify the basic rhythm. Stimulation of **receptors** in the skin are excitatory to the respiratory center, and deeper than usual inspiration can be noted. Their excitation to the inspiratory area might be through the apneustic area because inspiratory gasps are occasionally noted. Advantage is taken of these receptors when breathing stimulation is desired in newborn animals. Rubbing the skin with a rough cloth often initiates the breathing cycles. It is also believed that, when impulses descend from the **cerebral cortex** to the skeletal muscles, a branch might also go to the respiratory center to increase ventilation. This mechanism could explain changes that occur during exercise, in which increases in ventilation occur that are not explainable merely by observing changes in the CO_2, O_2, and H^+ concentrations in the blood.

Several respiratory reflexes originate from receptors in the **upper air passages**. Stimulation of the mucous membranes in these regions causes reflex inhibition of breathing. A striking example of this reflex is the inhibition of breathing that occurs during swallowing; also, in diving birds and mammals, there is a reflex inhibition of breathing when they submerge. Stimulation of the laryngeal mucous membrane in the unanesthetized animal causes not only inhibition of breathing, but also usually powerful expiratory efforts (coughing). Similarly, sneezing can be observed after stimulation of the nasal mucous membrane by various mechanisms. The function of all of these latter reflexes is protection of the delicate respiratory passages and the alveoli of the lungs from harmful substances (e.g., irritating gases, dust, smoke, food particles) that might otherwise be inspired. To ensure protection, the glottis is closed and the bronchi can be constricted.

Ordinary respirations proceed involuntarily. It is generally true, however, that they can be altered voluntarily within wide limits—they can be hastened, slowed, or stopped altogether, for a while. Phonation and use of the abdominal press in the expulsive acts of defecation, urination, and parturition are all examples of (more or less) complete **voluntary control** of the respiratory movements. These acts, however, are not concerned with gas exchange between the organism and its environment, but represent secondary functions of the respiratory apparatus.

Afferent impulses from pressure receptors in the **carotid and aortic sinuses** have as their principal function a role in the regulation of circulation, but impulses from these receptors also go to the respiratory center. The impulses are inhibitory in nature—the higher the blood pressure, the greater the inhibition to respiration. Because of the influence of inspiration on return of blood to the heart, it can be seen that the reduction in inspirations would slow down the return flow of blood to the heart and thus help to lower blood pressure.

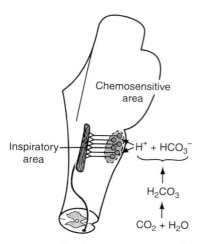

■ **FIGURE 10-21** The chemosensitive area of the brain stem respiratory center. The chemosensitive area is stimulated by hydrogen ions, which are formed by the conversion of carbon dioxide through the hydration reaction. (From Guyton AC, Hall JE. Textbook of Medical Physiology. 10th Ed. Philadelphia: WB Saunders, 2000.)

Humoral Control

Humoral control refers to those factors in the body fluids that influence ventilation: carbon dioxide, hydrogen ions, and oxygen. Because these are constituents of the body fluids, it seems natural that they should exert the greatest influence on ventilation in maintaining constancy. Their concentrations in the blood affect alveolar ventilation in several ways:

1. Carbon dioxide increase causes alveolar ventilation to increase; its decrease causes alveolar ventilation to decrease.
2. Hydrogen ion increase causes alveolar ventilation to increase; its decrease causes alveolar ventilation to decrease.
3. Oxygen decrease causes alveolar ventilation to increase; its increase causes alveolar ventilation to decrease.

Influences of Carbon Dioxide and Hydrogen Ions

The effects of carbon dioxide and hydrogen ions are mediated through bilateral chemosen-

sitive areas beneath the ventral surface of the medulla (*Fig. 10-21*). Because of the much greater diffusibility of carbon dioxide, as compared with H^+, it is distributed more quickly from the blood to the interstitial fluid of the medulla and to the cerebrospinal fluid than hydrogen ions. It is believed, however, that the H^+ concentration of the interstitial fluid of the brain stem is the deciding stimulus for respiratory drive. The influence of CO_2 is exerted by its conversion to H^+ through the hydration reaction (Equation 10-1; see previous section).

Influences of Oxygen

The influence of oxygen is transmitted from the carotid and aortic bodies to the respiratory center. The carotid and aortic body receptors also respond to carbon dioxide and hydrogen ion concentration, but the effectiveness of the carotid and aortic body response to carbon dioxide and hydrogen ions is far less than the response from the brain stem. Thus, the carotid and aortic bodies are considered to be the most influential for the regulation of oxygen. These bodies are distinct structures with an abundant blood supply located just outside the aortic arch, at the division of the carotid arteries. They respond to changes **in the P_aO_2 of blood.** Blood with **reduced amounts** of hemoglobin, and consequently less oxygen, has the same P_aO_2 as blood with normal hemoglobin and oxygen (see Fig. 10-17), and thus no ventilation response would be elicited because there is no change in P_aO_2. Also, blood in which oxygen has been displaced from hemoglobin by carbon monoxide has the same P_aO_2 as normal blood, and there would be no increase in ventilation. The P_aO_2 would remain the same because it is an expression of alveolar PO_2 (which has not changed) and represents the PO_2 of oxygen in solution. In the case of decreased hemoglobin (e.g., as in anemia) ventilation might be increased, not because of less oxygen, but because of greater hydrogen ion concentra-

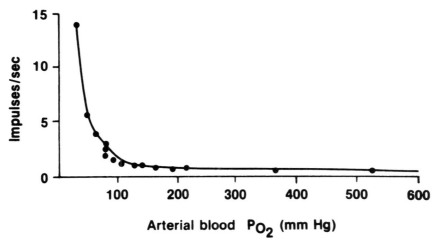

■ **FIGURE 10-22** Effect of arterial oxygen partial pressure on the number of impulses per second from the carotid body to the respiratory center. The impulses are excitatory. (From Reece WO. Respiration in mammals. In: Reece WO, ed. Dukes' Physiology of Domestic Animals. 12th Ed. Ithaca, NY: Cornell University Press, 2004.)

tion caused by reduced buffering associated with the hemoglobin decrease. In the case of carbon monoxide poisoning and lack of oxygen carried by hemoglobin, ventilation is not increased, not only because the P_aO_2 is normal, but also because there is adequate hemoglobin present for buffering hydrogen ions.

Arterial blood PO_2 must be in the range of 30 to 60 mm Hg for the respiratory center to receive stimulation to ventilation from the carotid and aortic bodies (*Fig. 10-22*). This seems to be an appropriate range, because hemoglobin is still about 90% saturated with oxygen at a PO_2 of 60 mm Hg. Also, the slowing effect of an increased arterial PO_2 is subtle and would not normally be observed in animals breathing atmospheric air because the arterial PO_2 seldom increases above 100 mm Hg. The slowing effect is noted, however, in anesthetized animals breathing an oxygen-enriched atmosphere, in which the arterial PO_2 could increase to 350 to 400 mm Hg (*Fig. 10-23*).

Importance of Oxygen Regulation

The regulation of ventilation by oxygen is not ordinarily thought to be important. There is usually no problem in maintaining arterial blood PO_2 in the range of 80 to 100 mm Hg, and it is not advantageous to have it higher than 100 mm Hg because hemoglobin is almost saturated at that partial pressure. Ventilation could even be reduced to about 50% of normal and hemoglobin still would be considerably saturated. Accordingly, the most important chemical factor in the regulation of ventilation is the concentration of carbon dioxide; relatively small changes can have an effect. The regulation of ventilation by oxygen becomes more important in such conditions as pneumonia and pulmonary edema, in which gases are not diffused as readily through the respiratory membrane. Decreased diffusion is more noticeable for oxygen than for carbon dioxide (see previous section) because of the smaller diffusion coefficient for oxygen. Hyperventilation

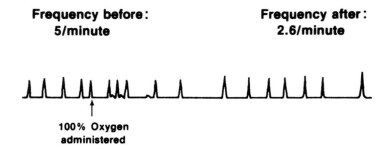

Frequency before:
5/minute

Frequency after:
2.6/minute

↑
100% Oxygen
administered

■ **FIGURE 10-23** Pneumogram showing the effect of oxygen enrichment on respiratory frequency. An oxygen atmosphere was provided to a pentobarbital-anesthetized dog. Note the decreased respiratory frequency after administration of oxygen (drawn from actual recording). (From Reece WO. Respiration in mammals. In: Reece WO, ed. Dukes' Physiology of Domestic Animals. 12th Ed. Ithaca, NY: Cornell University Press, 2004.)

caused by oxygen lack can therefore reduce the carbon dioxide concentration (because CO_2 readily diffuses) and thus the consequent reduced formation of hydrogen ions (see Equation 10-1) so that they become ineffective in stimulating increased ventilation. The **oxygen deficiency mechanism** (originating from the carotid and aortic bodies) continues to function and provides the drive to increase ventilation.

Braking Effect

The effect of decreased concentrations of H^+ and CO_2 and increased concentration of O_2 to slow down ventilation is referred to as a **braking effect**. The braking effect of O_2 was shown to be unimportant, but it is important for CO_2 and H^+ to decrease ventilation because they are both involved in maintaining the acid-base equilibrium of the body fluids. The uncontrolled lowering of either CO_2 or H^+ would result in some degree of **alkalemia** (decreased H^+ concentration in blood). A braking effect can be observed when anesthetized animals being hyperventilated with a respirator are removed suddenly from the respirator. A minute or more might be required for CO_2 and H^+ to accumulate to a level at which they no longer exert their braking effect and breathing finally resumes. In this example, oxygen lack

is apparent, and it could also be a contributory factor in the resumption of breathing.

The factors that influence ventilation are summarized in *Figure 10-24.*

■ RESPIRATORY CLEARANCE

1. Define respiratory clearance.
2. What are the physical factors that affect particle deposition?
3. What is the moving mucous blanket, and what is its rate of moving mucus and contained particles?
4. What is the size of particles that reach the alveoli?
5. What are the mechanisms of alveolar clearance?

The surface area of the inner aspects of the lungs is about 125 times larger than the surface area of the body, and therefore the lungs represent an important route of exposure for many environmental substances. The inhalation of certain agricultural chemicals is a significant health hazard for which precautionary measures to prevent inhalation have been developed. The removal of particles that have been inhaled into the lungs is called **respiratory clearance**. There are two types, **upper respiratory clearance** and **alveolar clearance**,

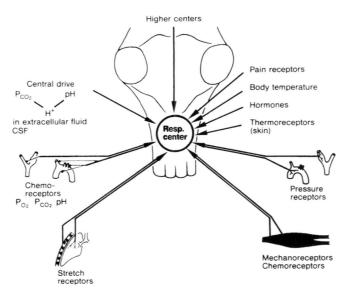

■ **FIGURE 10-24** Summary of factors that influence pulmonary ventilation. (From Schmidt PS, Thews G, eds. Human Physiology. Berlin: Springer-Verlag, 1989.)

and each depends on the depth to which particles have been inhaled. Inhaled particles that settle out onto a membrane of the respiratory tract are said to have been **deposited**.

Physical Forces of Deposition

The physical forces that affect deposition are gravity, inertia, and brownian movement. **Gravitational settling** (sedimentation) causes deposition of particles simply because of the force of gravity and the mass of the particle. Particles of greater mass settle out more rapidly than those with lesser mass. **Inertia** accounts for the deposition of particles when, because of their mass, they continue forward as the air in which they are suspended makes a turn. Considering the branching of the bronchioles, there is considerable opportunity for inertial deposition. **Brownian motion** accounts for the deposition of submicronic particles (less than 0.3 μm), which show a random motion that is imparted by air molecule bombardment. Deposition by brownian motion is most significant

in extremely small airways where the surface area is large relative to the airway diameter. The percentage of particles deposited according to their size is shown in *Figure 10-25*.

Upper Respiratory Tract Clearance

Removal of particles deposited cranial to the alveolar ducts is accomplished by the **moving mucous blanket**. This blanket of mucinous fluid is located on the surface of the epithelial cells lining the airways and is derived from alveolar fluid and mucus-secreting cells along the airways (*Fig. 10-26*). The mucous blanket contains the deposited particles and is moved toward the pharynx at a rate of about 15 mm/min by cilia of the epithelial cells. Mammals swallow the mucinous fluid and particles after they reach the pharynx.

Alveolar Clearance

Particles can escape gravitational and inertial forces and be deposited in the alveoli. These

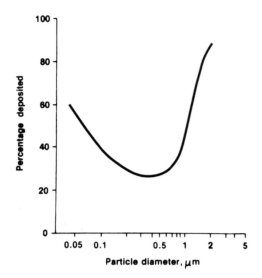

■ **FIGURE 10-25** Percentage of inhaled particles of unit density deposited in the lung according to their size. Particles in the range of 0.1 to 1.0 μm are those least affected by combined brownian motion, sedimentation, and inertial impaction. (Redrawn with permission from Morrow PE. Some physical and physiological factors controlling the fate of inhaled substances—I. Health Physics 1960;2:372.)

particles are usually smaller than 1 μm in diameter. The mechanisms of alveolar clearance of these particles can be summarized as follows:

1. After their deposition in the alveoli, they can be **phagocytized** by a macrophage or can continue as free particles. The "dust"-laden macrophage or free particles might be directed to the moving mucous blanket along with the alveolar fluid film.
2. Particles might enter the interstitial space of the alveoli and be **transported** to lymph nodes in series with the lungs.
3. Particles might be dissolved and transferred in **solution**, either into the lymph or into the blood.
4. Some particles might not be phagocytized or might be insoluble. Instead, they could stimulate a local connective tissue reaction and be **sequestered** (isolated) within the

lung. Examples of this include the conditions known as **asbestosis** and **silicosis**. Dogs and cats living in highly industrialized areas can show signs of **anthracosis** caused by inhalation of coal dust.

The importance of respiratory clearance is apparent when considering the exposure of livestock to the aerosols emanating from feedlot dust or other confinement sources. The aerosols can be combined with bacteria and viruses, so their prompt removal can help to prevent diseases caused by them. Similarly, the removal of irritant substances prevents lung disease and protects lung efficiency.

■ NONRESPIRATORY FUNCTIONS OF THE RESPIRATORY SYSTEM

1. What function is served by panting?
2. Is alveolar ventilation increased by panting?
3. Visualize the three patterns of panting in the dog.
4. How do cats purr?
5. What possible function might be served by purring?
6. Does purring signify wellness?

The respiratory system has functions other than providing for alveolar ventilation, and this was noted for respiratory clearance, in which the function was to remove inhaled particles. Also of particular interest among animals are panting and purring. Panting provides for body cooling, and the reason for purring is not known.

Panting

Panting is prevalent among many animal species and has been best described in the dog. It is probably similar for the other animals in which it is observed.

The respiratory center of the dog responds not only to the usual stimuli, but also to body

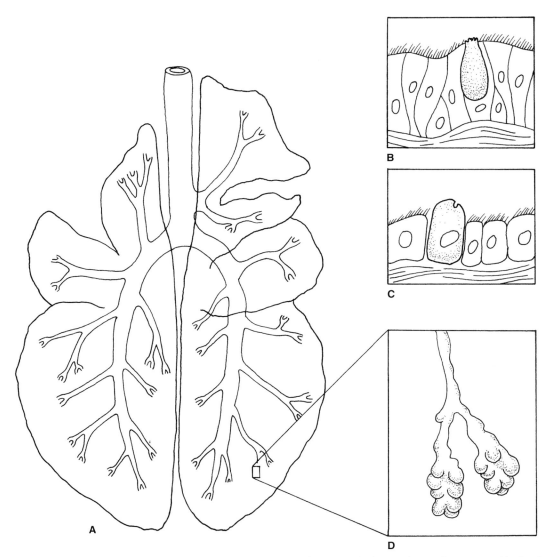

■ **FIGURE 10-26** Contributors to the moving mucous blanket of the bronchial tree. The moving mucous blanket is directed toward the pharynx by the action of the ciliated cells, and the secretion is provided by the goblet cells of the bronchi, the Clara cells of the bronchioles, and alveolar fluid. **A)** Outline of the bovine lung superimposed over the bronchial tree. **B)** Pseudostratified epithelium of the bronchi, composed of secretory (goblet) cells, ciliated cells, and basal cells. **C)** Cuboidal epithelium of the terminal bronchioles, composed of ciliated cells and secretory (Clara) cells. **D)** The terminal bronchiole is the most distal air passage free of alveoli.

core temperature. When these inputs are integrated, the dog's body responds to metabolic needs by regulating alveolar ventilation and to dissipation of heat by regulating dead space ventilation. Dead space ventilation is increased by panting, which provides for body cooling by evaporation of water from the mucous membranes of the tissues involved.

Studies have shown that the three **patterns of panting** are: 1) inhalation and exhalation through the nose, 2) inhalation through the nose and exhalation through the nose and mouth, and 3) inhalation through the nose and mouth and exhalation through the nose and mouth. The least amount of cooling is accomplished by inhaling and exhaling through the nose (pattern 1) because the heat and water added to the air during inhalation are partially regained during exhalation. Pattern 2 is more effective because air entering the nose is exposed to a large surface area (nasal conchae) as compared with the mouth, and water is added by the nasal mucosa and nasal glands. This combination picks up a considerable amount of heat, which is then dissipated mainly by exhalation through the mouth. Pattern 3 is somewhat similar to pattern 2, except that inhalation through the mouth and the nose permits a greater tidal volume, which might be required during times of exertion. The advantage of changing the relative amount of air exhaled through either the nose or the mouth is that the dog can modulate the amount of heat dissipated without changing the frequency or tidal volume associated with panting. Energy is conserved by not changing the frequency (300 pants/min), and hyperventilation (and thus alkalemia) is prevented by keeping the tidal volume constant.

Purring

Purring is noted in some members of the feline family and is both audible and palpable in most domestic cats. Studies in the domestic cat have shown that the purr results from a highly regular, alternating activation of the diaphragm and of the intrinsic laryngeal muscles (those within the larynx) at a frequency of 25 times/sec during both inspiration and expiration. Contraction of the laryngeal muscles closes the vocal cords. The laryngeal muscles then relax while the diaphragm contracts. Contraction of the diaphragm accomplishes air inflow, which vibrates the vocal cords and results in the purring sound while they are opening (no longer closed by laryngeal contraction), and also contributes to a fraction of the inspiratory phase of the respiratory cycle. The diaphragm then relaxes and the laryngeal muscles contract; this is again followed by their relaxation and diaphragm contraction. The entire process is repeated 25 times/sec until inspiration is completed. The accumulation of small sounds produced with each opening of the vocal cords makes the **purring sound**. The same sequence occurs during expiration, except that the diaphragm does not contract, and air outflow and hence vibration of the vocal cords is accomplished by recoil of the lungs.

The reason for purring in cats is not known. Cats purr when they are contented, sick, and asleep. Purring might provide for more effective ventilation during periods of shallow breathing because of the intermittent inspiration and expiration that is provided.

■ DESCRIPTIVE TERMS AND PATHOLOGIC CONDITIONS

1. Define hypoxia, hypercapnia, cyanosis, and asphyxia.
2. What is pulmonary surfactant?
3. What characterizes pneumonia, emphysema, and atelectasis?

Many terms associated with respiration have been defined in this chapter. The following terms are also commonly used.

Anoxia literally means without oxygen, and it should not be used when the condition is one of decreased oxygen. In such a case, **hypoxia** is more appropriate.

Hypercapnia and **hypocapnia** refer to excess and reduced amounts of carbon dioxide, respectively, in the blood.

Cyanosis refers to a bluish or purplish coloration of the skin and mucous membranes. The intensity of the color is a result of the degree of deoxygenation of hemoglobin. As observed systemically, it relates to inadequate oxygenation of blood. When seen locally, it is probably caused by blood flow obstruction.

Asphyxia is a condition of hypoxia combined with hypercapnia. Hypoxia and hypercapnia can occur as separate entities, but only their combination results in asphyxia. Breathing into a closed space is an example, resulting in what is commonly called **suffocation**.

Three pathologic conditions often referred to when discussing respiratory physiology are emphysema, pneumonia, and atelectasis. **Emphysema** is a condition in which destruction of alveolar membranes has occurred, resulting in a smaller area available for gas diffusion. It is often coupled with other conditions, such as **chronic bronchitis**, that increase the positive pressure within alveoli that is needed for the expiratory phase of the respiratory cycle. **Pneumonia** is an inflammatory condition of the lungs in which the alveoli fill with fluid and cell debris. Atelectasis is a collapse of alveoli. This can result from airway obstruction and from lack of surfactant. **Pulmonary surfactant** is a surface tension–reducing substance produced by the alveolar epithelial cells. The alveolar surface is compressed during expiration, which concentrates surfactant at the surface. The concentration of surfactant reduces the surface tension and makes beginning inspiration easier. At the end of inspiration the **surfactant** is spread out because of enlargement of the alveoli and surface tension increases, which assists expiration.

■ AVIAN RESPIRATION

1. What respiratory structures account for ventilation of the avian lungs, which are fixed in position?
2. Describe the relationship of the bronchi to the lungs and air sacs.
3. Where are the air sacs located? What are the two major groups?
4. Could smoke enter a broken wing bone (humerus) and exit the trachea?
5. What are the parabronchi? Name their extensions, which compose the parabronchial mantle.
6. Where does gas exchange occur in the avian lung?
7. Is there significant gas exchange in air sacs?
8. Where would blood perfusion be more abundant, in the air sacs or the air capillaries?
9. Is diaphragm contraction a factor in avian inspiration?
10. Describe how body volume changes influence inspiration and expiration.
11. Has air that enters the caudal and cranial air sacs been through a parabronchial mantle?
12. Does air that leaves the caudal air sacs go through parabronchial mantles?
13. Does air that leaves the cranial air sacs go through parabronchial mantles?
14. Study Figure 10-30, and understand how blood leaving the lung can have a lower Pco_2 and a higher O_2 than gas that leaves the parabronchi. Can blood leaving the mammalian lung (arterial blood) have a lower Pco_2 and a higher Po_2 than alveolar gas?
15. Compare the hemoglobin saturation of arterial and venous blood between birds and mammals.

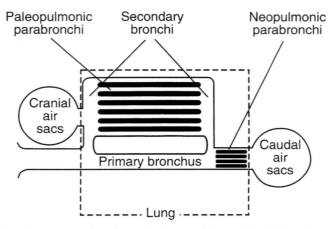

■ **FIGURE 10-27** A schematic representation of the avian lung and air sacs. The blackened areas correspond to blood capillaries, and the white areas adjacent to the blood capillaries correspond to tertiary bronchi (parabronchi). The air sacs are extensions from the lungs, acting as bellows to create air flow. (Modified from Fedde MR. Respiration in birds. In: Swenson MJ, Reece WO, eds. Dukes' Physiology of Domestic Animals. 11th Ed. Ithaca, NY: Cornell University Press, 1993.)

16. How can blowing off excess CO_2 during heat stress lower bicarbonate concentration (think hydration reaction)?

17. What is meant by a statement that notes that the utilization coefficient for most birds is about one-half, versus one-fourth for mammals?

Aside from subtle differences, many basic features of respiration in mammals apply to birds (e.g., respiratory pressures, oxygen t transport, carbon dioxide transport, regulation of respiration). The description of avian respiration that follows assumes familiarity with basic features and addresses major differences.

General Scheme of Avian Respiratory Morphology

The respiratory apparatus of birds is decidedly different than that of mammals. It was mentioned (see previous section) that the organ of phonation, the **syrinx**, is located at the bifur-

cation of the trachea, near the lungs, rather than near the pharynx. Also, the **tracheal rings** are complete, rather than incomplete as in mammals. Beyond the trachea, more striking differences are apparent. The **lungs** continue to be the gas exchange structures, but they do not expand and contract during respiratory cycles. They are relatively small and are fixed in position by their attachment to the ribs. Their ventilation depends on bellows-like extensions from the lungs known as **air sacs**, which do expand and contract during respiratory cycles, as will be described later. The lungs and air sacs are served by airway divisions from the trachea known as primary, secondary, and tertiary **bronchi**. The tertiary bronchi are also known as **parabronchi**. The relationship of the bronchi to each other and to the air sacs is shown in *Figure 10-27*. There are nine air sacs that are divided into a cranial group (two cervical, two cranial thoracic, and one clavicular) and a caudal group (two caudal thoracic and two abdominal). The air sacs occupy space in the thoracic and abdominal cavities, and many have diverticula (extensions) into many of the bones, causing them

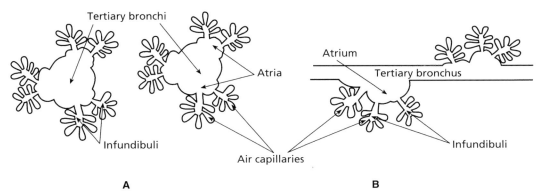

■ **FIGURE 10-28** Schematic representation of tertiary bronchi and their extensions. **A)** Transverse section. **B)** Sagittal section. The atria are outpocketings from the tertiary bronchi. The infundibuli extend from the atria, and they have a number of extensions known as air capillaries. The air capillaries are in intimate contact with the blood capillaries. The association of air capillaries with blood capillaries is known as the parabronchial mantle.

to be pneumatic. In the domestic species, the most prominent **pneumatic bone** is the humerus. It is not known what function is served by pneumatic bones.

The parabronchi give rise to outpocketings (**atria**), to extensions from the atria (**infundibuli**), and finally to extensions from the infundibuli known as **air capillaries** (*Fig. 10-28*). The structures arising from the parabronchi are known as its **mantle**. The blood capillaries make intimate contact with the air capillaries and provide for the gas exchange that occurs in the mantle of the lung. In most avian species, there are two sets of parabronchi and they are known as the **paleopulmonic parabronchi** and the **neopulmonic parabronchi**. The latter set is caudal to the former and exists just cranial to the caudal air sacs (see Fig. 10-27).

The air sacs are mucoserous sacs regarded as continuations of secondary bronchi beyond the lungs. Their walls are thin and have a poor blood supply. Because of their poor blood supply, air sacs are vulnerable to infection and to a condition known as air sacculitis. There is no significant gas exchange taking place in the air sacs. They do change volume during respiratory cycles and thereby function to increase pulmonary ventilation.

Mechanics of Respiration and Air Circulation

Birds have no diaphragm, therefore, there is no separation between the abdominal and thoracic cavities. Accordingly, the entire body volume is changed during each respiratory cycle. The energy for the body volume change is derived from skeletal muscles in the body wall. During expiration the body wall muscles contract, causing the body volume to decrease. The decrease in body volume increases air sac pressure, forcing the air within to flow back through the lungs and into the environment. Inspiration follows when the body wall muscles relax and body volume increases. Body volume increase is followed by a decrease in its pressure that is followed by expansion of the air sacs and a decrease in their pressure. The decreased pressure allows air to flow through the lungs and into the air sacs. Air flows through avian lungs during both phases of the respiratory cycle. During inspiration, air moving to cranial air sacs goes through a large set of parabronchi (paleopulmonic) before getting to the sacs. Air moving to the caudal air sacs goes through a smaller set of parabronchi (neopulmonic) before getting to the sacs. During expiration, gas from the caudal air sacs passes again through the neopulmonic para-bronchi and then through paleopulmonic parabronchi (directed to cranial air sacs). Gas from the cranial air sacs moves into secondary bronchi and out of the lungs through primary bronchi and the trachea without passing through gas exchange surfaces (parabronchial mantles). Air flow as described previously is illustrated in *Figure 10-29*. One bolus of air is followed through two respiratory cycles, from its entrance during inspiration of the first cycle to its exit during expiration of the second cycle. Notice that air entering the caudal air sacs during inspiration has already been sub-jected to gas exchange and it is again aerating the lungs during expiration. The cranial air sacs receive gas that has passed through the parabronchial mantles during inspiration and expel the gas into the environment during expiration without sending it through the parabronchial mantles.

Gas exchange between blood capillaries and air capillaries is illustrated in *Figure 10-30*. Air moves through the parabronchi by con-vection and into the air capillaries by diffu-sion. Blood perfusing a parabronchial mantle is partitioned so that each increment perfuses separate air capillaries throughout the length of the parabronchus. This arrangement, whereby the gas flows through a parabronchus at right angles to the flow of blood, is known as **cross-current flow**. As gas flows through the parabronchus, CO_2 is continuously diffusing from the blood and O_2 is continuously diffus-ing to the blood. Although the air capillaries that progress to the parabronchial outflow have an increasing P_{CO_2} and a decreasing P_{O_2}, the potential for gas diffusion is maintained because each increment of blood perfusing the air capillaries has the same high P_{CO_2} and low P_{O_2}. Because of this arrangement, the continu-ous loss of CO_2 and gain of O_2 causes the P_aCO_2 leaving the lung to be lower and the P_aO_2 to be higher than the gas leaving the parabronchus. This cannot be the case for venous blood exposed to alveolar gas in mammals, in which blood leaving alveolar exposure (arterial blood) has either equal or higher P_aCO_2 and equal or lower P_aO_2 than alveolar gas. The cross-current arrangement is more efficient than gas exchanges in the mammalian lung and is most apparent when ventilation is increased in response to low oxygen (i.e., high altitude). Under these conditions arterial P_{O_2} may be only a few millimeters of mercury less than air entering the parabronchi.

General Considerations

1. Valves to direct air flow have not been found in birds, and it is believed that air flow dynamics are in response to smooth muscle contraction that constricts bronchi.
2. Birds have a respiratory center and, similar to mammals, have chemoreceptors for CO_2 and O_2 that influence the response of the respiratory center.
3. Unlike mammals, birds have CO_2 recep-tors in their lungs that detect the CO_2 levels in lung air. There is maximum receptor activity when CO_2 is low, and this causes inhibition to respiration.
4. Oxygen saturation of hemoglobin of arte-rial blood (approximately 90%) and of venous blood (approximately 40%) in the chicken is lower than in mammalian blood (arterial blood approximately 97.5% and venous blood approximately 72%).
5. The P_{CO_2} of avian blood is lower than for mammals (28 to 34 mm Hg versus 40 to 45 mm Hg, respectively).
6. The utilization coefficient for most birds is about one-half, versus about one-fourth for mammals.
7. Diving ducks (not dabbling) have respira-tory center sensitivity to postural changes (stretching of the neck, experimentally or naturally, as in diving, produces apnea).
8. Ventilation of the lungs can be impaired by restricting movement of the sternum

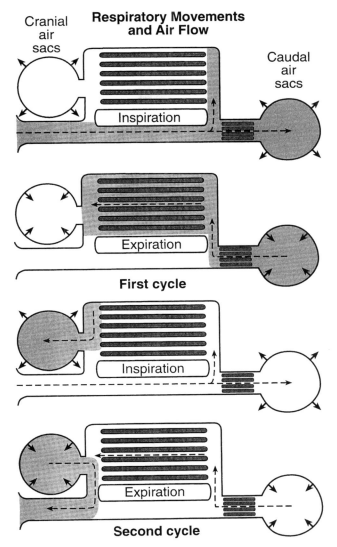

FIGURE 10-29 Pathway of air flow associated with inspiration and expiration in birds. The same bolus of air (darkened area) is followed through two respiratory cycles. It can be seen that ventilation of the parabronchial mantle is accomplished during inspiration and during expiration. Air going to the caudal air sacs ventilates the neopulmonic mantle, and as it leaves it ventilates both neopulmonic and paleopulmonic mantles. When the cranial air sacs expand during inspiration, they are filled by air that has passed through the parabronchial mantles. Cranial air sac air is then directed to the exterior during expiration without ventilating parabronchial mantles. (Modified from Scheid P, Slama H, Piiper J. Mechanisms of unidirectional flow in parabronchi of avian lungs: measurements in duck lung preparations. Respir Physiol 1972;14:83–95.)

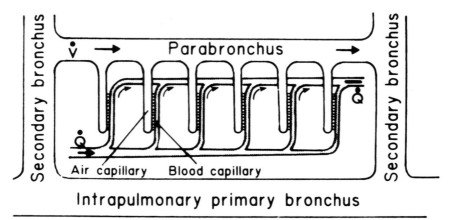

■ **FIGURE 10-30** Schematic model of the cross-current gas exchange system in the avian lung. Q̇ is the blood perfusion of the parabronchial mantle, and V̇ represents the convective flow of gas through the parabronchus. Because of this arrangement, blood leaving the parabronchial mantle has a higher P_{O_2} and a lower P_{CO_2} than air leaving the parabronchus. (From Fedde MR. Respiration in birds. In: Swenson MJ, Reece WO, eds. Dukes' Physiology of Domestic Animals. 11th Ed. Ithaca, NY: Cornell University Press, 1993.)

because the sternum must have downward and forward movement to assist body volume increase. This is an important consideration during bird restraint.

9. Air sac infections can seriously impair ventilation, particularly if exudate plugs the entry from air sacs to lungs (common in aspergillosis, a fungus infection).

10. Hyperventilation caused by heat stress reduces the P_{CO_2} and bicarbonate concentration. The loss of bicarbonate causes egg shells to be thinner, and greater breakage occurs.

■ SUGGESTED READING

Ganong WF. Review of Medical Physiology. 20th Ed. New York: McGraw-Hill, 2001.

Guyton AC, Hall JF. Textbook of Medical Physiology. 10th Ed. Philadelphia: WB Saunders, 2000.

Ludders JW. Respiration in birds. In: Reece WO, ed. Dukes' Physiology of Domestic Animals. 12th Ed. Ithaca, NY: Cornell University Press, 2004.

Powell FL. Respiration. In: Whittow GC, ed. Sturkie's Avian Physiology. 5th Ed. New York: Academic Press, 2000.

Reece WO. Respiration in Mammals. In: Reece WO, ed. Dukes' Physiology of Domestic Animals. 12th Ed. Ithaca, NY: Cornell University Press, 2004.

 SELF EVALUATION—CHAPTER 10

RESPIRATORY APPARATUS

1. Which respiratory structures serve to warm and humidify inhaled air and also to cool blood going to the brain?
   a. Larynx
   b. Nares
   c. Conchae
   d. Syrinx

2. Diffusion of gases between air and blood occurs mostly in the:
   a. respiratory bronchioles.
   b. alveoli.

c. conchae.

d. heart.

3. The aorta, venae cavae, esophagus, and large lymph vessels occupy a space within the thorax known as the:
   a. intrapleural space.
   b. mediastinal space.
   c. intrapulmonic space.
   d. outer space.

FACTORS ASSOCIATED WITH BREATHING

4. A condition of pleuritis would accentuate:
   a. abdominal breathing.
   b. costal breathing.

5. A difficult, labored state of breathing is termed:
   a. eupnea.
   b. dyspnea.
   c. hyperpnea.
   d. polypnea.

6. The amount of air breathed in or out during a respiratory cycle is known as the:
   a. vital capacity.
   b. residual volume.
   c. tidal volume.
   d. functional residual capacity.

7. The functional residual capacity in an animal is composed of the:
   a. inspiratory reserve volume and the tidal volume.
   b. expiratory reserve volume and the tidal volume.
   c. residual volume and the expiratory reserve volume.
   d. residual volume only.

8. Generally speaking, which one of the domestic animals has a resting respiratory frequency of 10 to 16 cycles/min?
   a. Cow
   b. Pig
   c. Dog

d. Horse

e. Cat

RESPIRATORY PRESSURES

9. The P_{O_2} of dry atmospheric air approximates:
   a. 40 mm Hg.
   b. 100 mm Hg.
   c. 160 mm Hg.
   d. 760 mm Hg.

10. The P_{CO_2} of dry atmospheric air approximates:
    a. 0.23 mm Hg.
    b. 23 mm Hg.
    c. 40 mm Hg.
    d. 45 mm Hg.

11. The total pressure of a gas mixture is 400 mm Hg. Twenty-five percent of the mixture is oxygen. What is the P_{O_2} of oxygen?
    a. 25 mm Hg
    b. 400 mm Hg
    c. 100 mm Hg
    d. 250 mm Hg

12. As compared with atmospheric air, alveolar air has:
    a. higher P_{O_2}, lower P_{CO_2}, higher P_{N_2}.
    b. lower P_{O_2}, higher P_{CO_2}, lower P_{N_2}.

PULMONARY VENTILATION

13. During inspiration:
    a. intrapleural and intrapulmonic pressures are decreased.
    b. intrapleural and intrapulmonic pressures are increased.
    c. intrapleural pressure is decreased and intrapulmonic pressure is increased.
    d. intrapleural pressure is increased and intrapulmonic pressure is decreased.

14. During inspiration the pressure within the mediastinal space:
    a. increases.
    b. decreases.
    c. remains the same.

15. During expiration the intrapulmonic pressure:
    a. increases.
    b. decreases.
    c. goes bonkers.

16. Return of blood to the right atrium is assisted when:
    a. the thorax is expanded (intrapleural pressure decreased from normal) during inspiration.
    b. the thorax is contracted (intrapleural pressure returned to normal) during expiration.

17. A pulmonary physiologic dead space is:
    a. the total volume of airways (anatomic volume).
    b. the total volume of airways and alveoli.
    c. one composed only of nonperfused alveoli.
    d. that part of the tidal volume that is inspired but takes no part in gas exchange.

18. When the lungs are expanded during inspiration:
    a. the pressure inside the venae cavae is increased.
    b. the pressure inside the venae cavae is decreased.
    c. there is no change in the pressure inside the venae cavae.

19. Which one of the ventilation subdivisions is normally increased during panting?
    a. Alveolar ventilation
    b. Dead-space ventilation

DIFFUSION OF RESPIRATORY GASES

20. Alveolar P_{CO_2} is measured to be 45 mm Hg. Considering this value, one would expect atmospheric P_{CO_2} to be _____ than 45 mm Hg and venous blood P_{CO_2} to be _____ than 45 mm Hg. (Select the respective words from the sets below that complete the above blanks.)
    a. greater, less
    b. less, less

    c. less, greater
    d. greater, greater

21. The P_{O_2} of blood in the pulmonary arteries is higher than the P_{O_2} of blood in the pulmonary veins.
    a. True
    b. False

22. The P_{CO_2} in the interstitial fluid compartment is higher than the P_{CO_2} of blood in the capillaries.
    a. True
    b. False

OXYGEN TRANSPORT

23. How does an animal with a P_aO_2 of 400 mm Hg compare with that animal when it had a P_aO_2 of 100 mm Hg, with respect to amount of oxygen being transported (assume equal concentration of Hb for both situations)?
    a. Four times more
    b. Two times more
    c. Slightly more because of the additional amount in solution and complete saturation of hemoglobin (100% versus 97.5%)

24. Most of the oxygen transported in the blood is that which is:
    a. in solution.
    b. associated with plasma proteins.
    c. associated with carbon dioxide.
    d. associated with hemoglobin.

25. A decrease of P_{O_2} from 100 mm Hg to 40 mm Hg for blood leaving the left ventricle and returning to the right atrium represents an approximate desaturation of hemoglobin of:
    a. 60%.
    b. 25%.
    c. 40%.
    d. 50%.

CARBON DIOXIDE TRANSPORT

26. The chemical form that accounts for the greatest amount of carbon dioxide transport is:
    a. CO_2 associated with amino groups of hemoglobin.
    b. CO_2 in solution (dissolved).
    c. HCO_3^- (bicarbonate).

27. The most plentiful compound available for buffering hydrogen ions formed during the hydration reaction (carbon dioxide transport) is:
    a. bicarbonate.
    b. plasma proteins.
    c. hemoglobin.

28. As a result of carbon dioxide transport, venous blood has a lower pH than arterial blood.
    a. True
    b. False

REGULATION OF VENTILATION

29. The PO_2 of arterial blood during the development of carbon monoxide poisoning is:
    a. normal.
    b. greater than normal.
    c. less than normal

30. Which one of the following causes increased ventilation of the lungs?
    a. Decreased CO_2 concentration in the blood
    b. Increased CO_2 concentration in the blood
    c. Increased PO_2 of arterial blood
    d. Increased pH of the blood (decreased H^+ concentration)

31. Where is the respiratory center for the regulation of ventilation located?
    a. Brain stem
    b. Lungs
    c. Cerebral cortex
    d. Hypothalamus

32. Receptors for the detection of changes in arterial blood PO_2 are located in the:
    a. lungs.
    b. brain stem respiratory center.
    c. carotid and aortic bodies.
    d. heart.

33. During the development of carbon monoxide poisoning or as observed in anemic (nonexerted) animals:
    a. ventilation of the lungs is not increased because the PO_2 of arterial blood remains normal.
    b. ventilation of the lungs is increased because of hypoxemia.
    c. carbon monoxide does not interfere with oxygen transport and there is no deficiency of hemoglobin, respectively.

34. A calf breathing room air has a pulmonary ventilation rate of 26 L/min. It is placed on a gas mixture, and the rate becomes 22 L/min. The gas mixture most likely is:
    a. oxygen enriched.
    b. carbon dioxide enriched.

RESPIRATORY CLEARANCE

35. Deposition of inhaled particles by brownian movement is most likely to occur in the:
    a. trachea.
    b. bronchi.
    c. terminal bronchioles.
    d. alveolar ducts.

36. Inhaled particles that are deposited and not cleared, but rather stimulate a local connective tissue reaction, are those that become:
    a. dissolved.
    b. sequestered.
    c. phagocytized.

NONRESPIRATORY FUNCTIONS OF THE RESPIRATORY SYSTEM

37. When cats purr, which one of the following is false?

a. The muscles of the larynx that close the vocal cords and the diaphragm contract simultaneously during inspiration.
b. Sound is produced by the vocal cords while they are opening.
c. The vocal cords open and close 25 times each second to produce the purring sound.

38. Which component of ventilation is significantly increased when animals pant?
a. Alveolar ventilation
b. Dead-space ventilation

DESCRIPTIVE TERMS AND PATHOLOGIC CONDITIONS

39. Hypercapnia refers to:
a. an excess of carbon dioxide in the blood.
b. an excess of carbon monoxide in the blood.
c. increased frequency and depth of breathing.

40. Atelectasis refers to:
a. a condition in which destruction of alveolar membranes has occurred.
b. an inflammatory condition of the lungs in which the alveoli fill with fluid and cell debris.
c. a collapse of alveoli.

AVIAN RESPIRATION

41. The bronchi that correspond to parabronchi are the:

a. primary.
b. secondary.
c. tertiary.

42. The air capillaries are immediate extensions of:
a. parabronchi.
b. air sacs.
c. infundibuli.
d. atria.

43. Compression of air sacs is associated with:
a. inspiration.
b. expiration.

44. Ventilation of the lungs occurs during:
a. inspiration.
b. expiration.
c. both inspiration and expiration.

45. Gas exchange occurs between the interface of:
a. air capillaries and blood capillaries.
b. air sacs and blood capillaries.
c. both a and b.

46. Both cranial and caudal air sacs ventilate the parabronchial mantles during expiration.
a. True
b. False

47. Because of cross-current ventilation, it is possible to have a lower P_{CO_2} and a higher P_{O_2} in arterial blood than in gas leaving the parabronchial mantles.
a. True
b. False

ANSWERS TO SELF EVALUATION—CHAPTER 10

1. c	7. c	13. a	19. b
2. b	8. d	14. b	20. c
3. b	9. c	15. a	21. b
4. a	10. a	16. a	22. a
5. b	11. c	17. d	23. c
6. c	12. b	18. b	24. d

25.	b	31.	a	37.	a	43.	b
26.	c	32.	c	38.	b	44.	c
27.	c	33.	a	39.	a	45.	a
28.	a	34.	a	40.	c	46.	b
29.	a	35.	d	41.	c	47.	a
30.	b	36.	b	42.	c		

CHAPTER 11

The Urinary System

CHAPTER OUTLINE

- **GROSS ANATOMY OF THE KIDNEYS AND URINARY BLADDER**
- **THE NEPHRON**
  Nephron Components
- **FORMATION OF URINE**
  Distribution of Blood at the Glomerulus
- **GLOMERULAR FILTRATION**
  Dynamics of Filtration
  Filtration Factors
  Autoregulation
- **TUBULAR REABSORPTION AND SECRETION**
  Reabsorption of Na$^+$, Cl$^-$, Glucose, and
    Amino Acids
  Reabsorption of Water and Urea
  Secretion of H$^+$, K$^+$, NH$_3$, and Organic
    Molecules
  Transport Maximum
- **COUNTERCURRENT MECHANISM**
  Countercurrent Multiplier System
  Countercurrent Exchanger System
  Role of Urea
- **CONCENTRATION OF URINE**
  Antidiuretic Hormone and
    Osmoregulation
  Concentration Failure
- **EXTRACELLULAR FLUID VOLUME REGULATION**
- **ALDOSTERONE**
- **OTHER HORMONES WITH KIDNEY ASSOCIATION**
  Parathyroid Hormone
  Erythropoietin
  Prostaglandins
- **MICTURITION**
  Transfer of Urine to the Urinary Bladder
  Micturition Reflexes
  Descriptive Terms
- **CHARACTERISTICS OF MAMMALIAN URINE**
- **RENAL CLEARANCE**
  Creatinine Clearance
- **MAINTENANCE OF ACID-BASE BALANCE**
  Relationship of pH to H$^+$ Concentration
  Mechanism of H$^+$ Secretion by the
    Kidneys
  Role of Respiratory System
  Chemical Buffer Systems
- **AVIAN URINARY SYSTEM**
  Anatomic Features
  Renal Portal System
  Uric Acid Formation and Excretion
  Concentration of Avian Urine
  Modification of Ureteral Urine
  Urine Characteristics and Flow

The kidneys are usually thought to have the excretion of metabolic waste products as their only function. Another function, which is at least equally important, is the regulation of the volume and composition of the body's internal environment, the extracellular fluid (ECF). It has been said that the composition of the body fluids is determined not by what the mouth takes in, but by what the kidneys keep. Both functions—excretion of metabolic waste products and regulation of volume and composi-

tion of ECF—are performed by the kidneys because of their perfusion with blood, resulting in the formation of urine, a fluid of varying composition.

■ GROSS ANATOMY OF THE KIDNEYS AND URINARY BLADDER

1. Study the shape of kidneys of different species.

2.   What is the location of the kidney cortex and medulla? What is the renal hilus and renal pelvis?

3.   What is the difference between the ureter and the urethra?

4.   What is the relationship between the ureterovesicular junction and prevention of backflow of urine from the bladder to the kidney?

5.   Describe the innervation to the kidneys.

The kidneys are paired organs suspended from the dorsal abdominal wall by a peritoneal fold and the blood vessels that serve them.

They are located slightly cranial to the mid-lumbar region (*Fig. 11-1*). Because they are separated from the abdominal cavity by their envelopment of peritoneum, they are called **retroperitoneal** structures. Blood is carried to each kidney by a renal artery, and venous blood is conveyed away from each kidney by a renal vein. The renal artery arises directly from the aorta, and the renal vein empties directly into the caudal vena cava (*Fig. 11-2*).

The kidney is described as a bean-shaped structure for most domestic animals. In the horse, however, it is described as heart-shaped, and in cattle it is lobulated (*Fig. 11-3*). If a midsagittal cut is made through the kidney (*Fig. 11-4*), an outer cortex and an inner

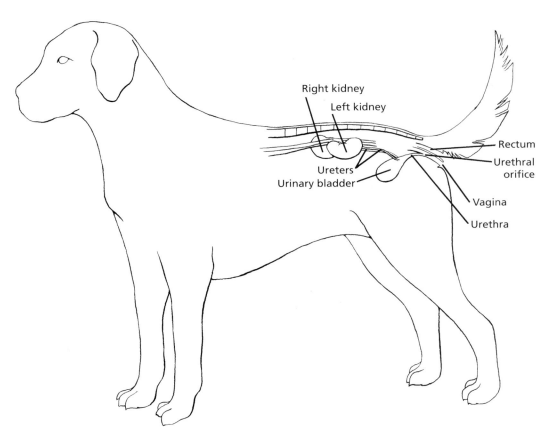

■ **FIGURE 11-1** Side view of female dog showing general location of kidneys, ureters, urinary bladder, urethra, urethral orifice, and vagina.

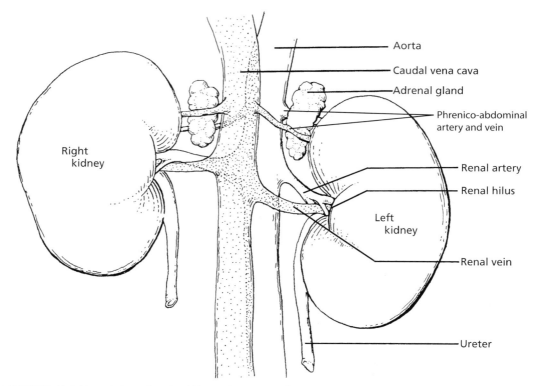

■ **FIGURE 11-2** Ventral view of canine kidneys showing renal arteries, veins, and ureters and their positions relative to the aorta, vena cava, and adrenal glands.

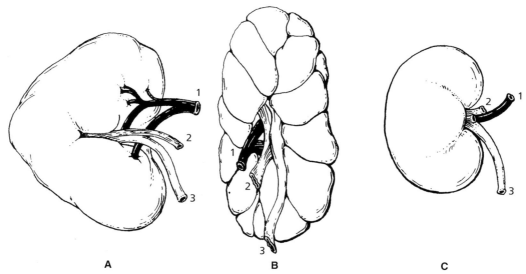

A   **B**   **C**

■ **FIGURE 11-3** Right kidney, ventral view. **A)** Horse. **B)** Cow. **C)** Sheep. These represent heart-shaped, lobulated, and bean-shaped kidneys, respectively. 1) Renal artery; 2) renal vein; 3) ureter.

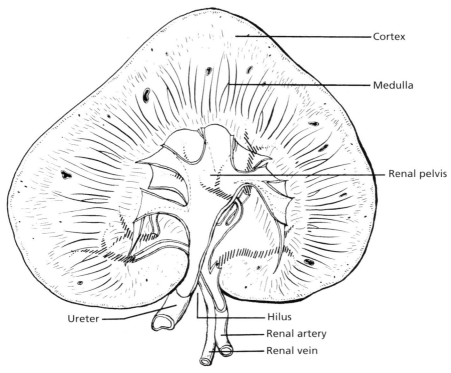

Cortex

Medulla

Renal pelvis

Hilus

Ureter

Renal artery

Renal vein

■ **FIGURE 11-4** Midsagittal plane of horse kidney showing cortex, medulla, renal pelvis, hilus, ureter, renal artery, and renal vein.

medulla are visible. The striations of the medulla are formed by the anatomic arrangement of the major parts that occupy the medulla, the **loop of Henle** of long-looped nephrons and the medullary portion of the **collecting tubules** (see later section on the nephron). The medullary portions of the collecting tubules are known as **collecting ducts**. The **renal hilus** is the indented area on the concave edge of the kidney through which the ureter, blood vessels, nerves, and lymphatics enter or leave. The **renal pelvis** (see Fig. 11-4) is the expanded origin of the ureter within the kidney. The final discharge of urine from the many collecting ducts is received by the renal pelvis. Innervation to the kidney is provided by the sympathetic (adrenergic) division of the autonomic nervous system. The postganglionic renal nerves enter the hilus of the kidney

in association with the renal artery and vein and provide adrenergic innervation to the renal vasculature, all segments of the nephron, and the juxtaglomerular (JG) granular cells. The **ureter** is a muscular (smooth muscle) tube that conveys urine from the renal pelvis to the urinary bladder. The ureter enters the bladder at an oblique angle (**ureterovesicular junction**), thus forming a functional valve to prevent backflow when the bladder is filling (*Fig. 11-5*). The urinary bladder is a hollow, muscular (smooth muscle) organ that varies in size depending on the amount of urine it contains at any one time. The smooth muscle of the urinary bladder is known as the **detrusor muscle**. The epithelial cell lining of the bladder accommodates for the change in size and is known as **transitional epithelium** (see Chapter 1). When the bladder is empty, the

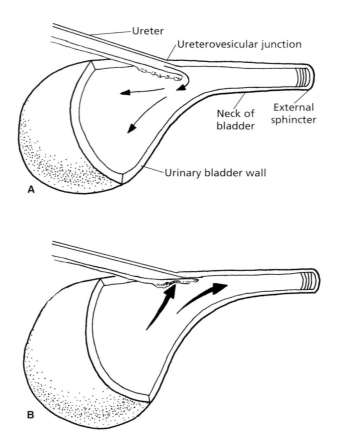

■ **FIGURE 11-5** Ureterovesicular junction (oblique entrance of ureter into the urinary bladder). **A)** Urine is conveyed to the urinary bladder from the renal pelvis by peristalsis and enters at the ureterovesicular junction. **B)** During micturition (emptying of the urinary bladder), urine is directed through the neck of the bladder to the urethra. Urine does not reenter the ureter because the ureterovesicular junction is closed by the hydrostatic pressure of urine associated with contraction of the detrusor muscle of the bladder wall.

cells appear to be piled on one another, giving it a stratified (layered) appearance. A transition occurs on filling so that the piled-up appearance gives way to a thinner epithelial stratification.

The **neck of the bladder** is the caudal continuation of the bladder leading to the urethra. The smooth muscle in the neck is mixed with a considerable amount of elastic tissue and functions as an **internal sphincter**.

The **urethra** is the caudal continuation of the neck of the bladder. It conveys the urine from the bladder to the exterior (*Fig. 11-6*). The **external sphincter** lies beyond the neck;

it is composed of skeletal muscle that encircles the urethra at this point. The functional boundary between the bladder and the urethra is represented by this sphincter.

Prevention of urine escape while the bladder is filling is provided for by contraction of the external sphincter and by tension passively exerted by the elastic elements in the neck of the bladder. When urine is expelled from the bladder, the external sphincter relaxes and the bladder muscles contract. The bladder muscle contraction opens its neck into a funnel shape. The contraction not only forces urine into the urethra but, because of the muscle fiber

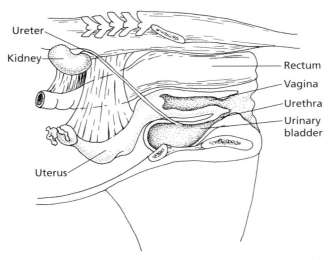

■ FIGURE 11-6 Midsagittal plane of the cow pelvis showing positions of the urinary bladder and urethra relative to other organs.

arrangement, widens the beginning of the urethra.

■ THE NEPHRON

1. Do large-breed dogs have significantly greater numbers of nephrons in their kidneys than small-breed dogs?
2. What is the difference between a cortical nephron and a juxtamedullary nephron?
3. What are the components of the nephron (in order) from the glomerulus to the inner medullary-collecting duct?
4. What are the components of the JG apparatus?

TABLE 11-1 APPROXIMATE NUMBER OF NEPHRONS IN EACH KIDNEY FOR SEVERAL DOMESTIC ANIMALS AND HUMANS

SPECIES	NEPHRONS/KIDNEY
Cattle	4,000,000
Pig	1,250,000
Dog	415,000
Cat	190,000
Human	1,000,000

The functional unit of the kidney is the **nephron**. An understanding of nephron function is essential for understanding kidney function. Nephron numbers vary considerably among species, and approximate numbers for several species are given in *Table 11-1*. Within a species the nephron numbers are relatively constant. Considering the differences in size among various breeds of dogs, it might be thought that the kidneys of large-breed dogs would contain more nephrons than the kidneys of small-breed dogs. This is not the case, however, and the larger kidney size in large dogs is compensated for by their having larger nephrons rather than more nephrons.

The mammalian kidney has two principal types of nephrons, identified by: 1) the location of their glomeruli and 2) the depth of penetration of the loops of Henle into the medulla. Those nephrons with glomeruli in the outer and middle cortices are called cortical or **corticomedullary nephrons**. They are associated with a loop of Henle that extends to the junction of the cortex and medulla or into the outer zone of the medulla. Those nephrons with glomeruli in the cortex close to the medulla are known as **juxtamedullary nephrons**. Juxtamedullary nephrons are associated with loops of Henle that extend more deeply into the medulla; some extend as deep as the renal pelvis. The relationship of each nephron type to the cortex and medulla is shown in *Figures 11-7* and *11-8*. The juxtamedullary nephrons are those that develop and maintain the osmotic gradient from low to high in the outer medulla to the inner medulla, respectively. The percentage of nephrons having long loops of Henle (juxtamedullary nephrons) varies among animal species and ranges from 3% in the pig to 100% in the cat. In humans the percentage of long-looped nephrons is about 14%. The tubular

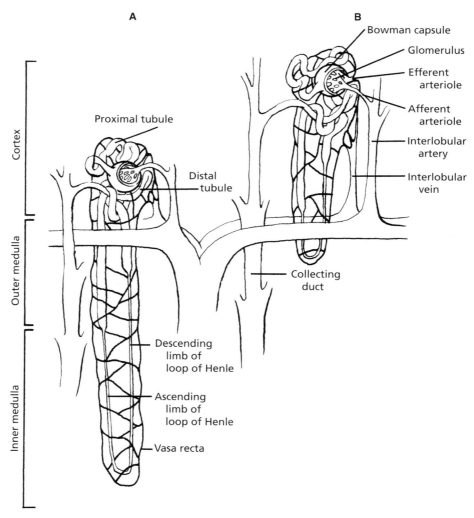

■ **FIGURE 11-7** Types of mammalian nephrons. **A)** Juxtamedullary (long-looped) nephron. **B)** Cortical nephron.

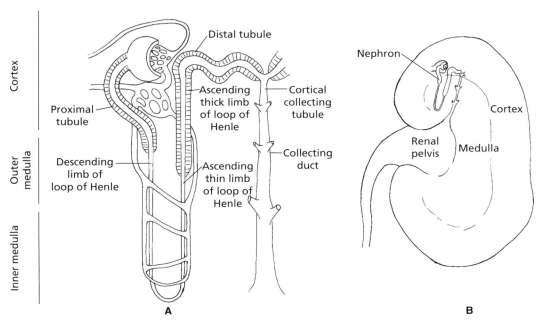

■ **FIGURE 11-8 A)** Component parts of a juxtamedullary nephron (mammalian) relative to their locations in the cortex and medulla. **B)** Midsagittal section of the kidney showing the location of a juxtamedullary nephron (exaggerated size) relative to the cortex, medulla, and renal pelvis.

fluid from both nephron types enters the collecting tubules and collecting ducts, where it is exposed to the effects of medullary osmotic gradients as it proceeds to the renal pelvis.

Nephron Components

A typical nephron and its component parts are shown in *Fig. 11-9*. The **glomerulus** is the tuft of capillaries through which filtration is accomplished. The **afferent arteriole** conducts blood to the glomerulus, and the **efferent arteriole** conducts blood away from the glomerulus. Blood leaving through the efferent arterioles is redistributed into another bed of capillaries known as the **peritubular capillaries**; these perfuse the nephron tubules. The **vasa recta** are capillary branches from the peritubular capillaries associated with the long-looped nephrons. After perfusion of the kidneys, blood is returned to the caudal vena cava by the renal veins.

Nephron Tubules and Ducts

Filtrate from the glomerulus is collected by the **Bowman capsule** and is subsequently directed through the **proximal tubule**, **loop of Henle**, and **distal tubule**. The distal tubule empties into a cortical collecting tubule. A **cortical collecting tubule** is not unique to a single nephron because it receives tubular fluid from the convoluted portion of several distal tubules. When the collecting tubule turns away from the cortex and passes down into the medulla, it is known as a **collecting duct**. Successive generations of collecting ducts coalesce to form progressively larger collecting ducts. The tubular fluid is finally discharged from the larger collecting ducts into the pelvis of the kidney, and is conveyed from there by the ureters to the urinary bladder for storage until discharge through the urethra. A summary of nephron component parts encountered by glomerular filtrate as it becomes tubular fluid and

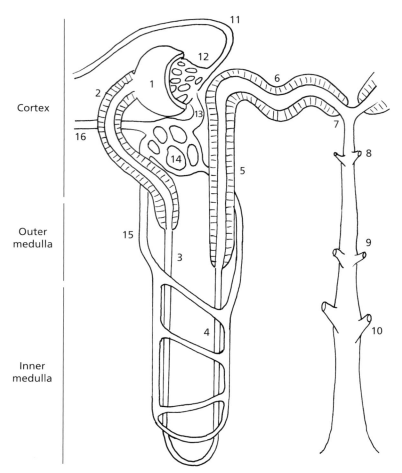

■ **FIGURE 11-9** The functional nephron with blood supply. **1)** The Bowman capsule; **2)** proximal tubule; **3)** descending limb of loop of Henle; **4)** thin ascending limb of loop of Henle; **5)** thick ascending limb of loop of Henle; **6)** distal tubule; **7)** connecting tubule; **8)** cortical collecting tubule; **9)** outer medullary collecting duct; **10)** inner medullary collecting duct; **11)** afferent arteriole; **12)** glomerulus; **13)** efferent arteriole; **14)** peritubular capillaries; **15)** vasa recta; **16)** to renal vein. Thick ascending limb of loop of Henle becomes distal tubule when it passes between the afferent and efferent arteriols at the glomerulus (location of macula densa).

finally urine with final discharge through the urethra is shown in *Figure 11-10*.

Loop of Henle

The loop of Henle is composed of three segments: the **thin descending limb**, the **thin ascending limb**, and the **thick ascending limb**. Their relative thicknesses are a result of differences in the epithelial cells and do not refer to

changes in lumen diameter. The thin segment for each loop is continuous with the thin segment of the other at the hairpin curve. The descending limbs of cortical nephrons only go as deep as the outer aspect of the outer medulla. The juxtamedullary nephrons have descending limbs of loops of Henle that can extend to the renal pelvis. The thin segment of the descending limb is a straight tubule continuous from the proximal tubule and is followed after its hairpin

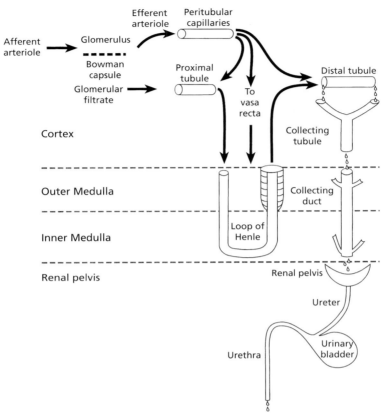

■ FIGURE 11-10 Summary of kidney blood flow and tubular fluid flow as it applies to the nephron. After removal of the filtration fraction of plasma at the glomerulus, the remaining blood that enters the efferent arteriole is distributed via peritubular capillaries to the nephron as shown. The fraction of plasma filtered at the glomerulus enters Bowman's capsule as glomerular filtrate. It continues through the nephron tubules and ducts as tubular fluid. The tubular fluid is subjected to reabsorption and secretion and enters the renal pelvis as urine. Urine is finally evacuated from the urinary bladder by micturition.

turn by the thin ascending limb. The thick segment of the ascending limb is a straight tubule continuous from the thin ascending limb. The thick segment of the ascending limb of the loop of Henle returns in its ascent to its glomerulus of origin, passes between the afferent and efferent arteriole, and proceeds from there as the distal tubule to its cortical collecting tubule.

Juxtaglomerular Apparatus

The junction of the distal tubule and glomerulus is known as the juxtaglomerular (JG) appa-

ratus (*Fig. 11-11*). There are characteristic cell types at this location. In the tubule, the cells are collectively known as the **macula densa**; in the afferent and efferent arterioles, they are called the JG cells; and the cells located between the macula densa and the arterioles are known as extraglomerular mesangial (lacis) cells. The JG apparatus is associated with regulating the amount of blood flowing to the kidney, the amount of filtration, and the secretion of **renin**, an enzyme involved in the formation of the hormone **angiotensin II** (a vasoconstrictor).

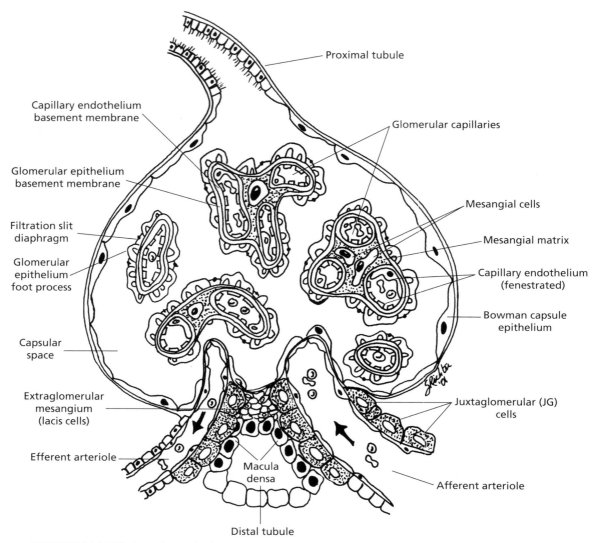

Proximal tubule

Capillary endothelium
basement membrane

Glomerular capillaries

Glomerular epithelium
basement membrane

Mesangial cells

Mesangial matrix

Filtration slit
diaphragm

Glomerular
epithelium
foot process

Capillary endothelium
(fenestrated)

Bowman capsule
epithelium

Capsular
space

Extraglomerular
mesangium
(lacis cells)

Juxtaglomerular (JG)
cells

Efferent arteriole

Macula
densa

Afferent arteriole

Distal tubule

■ **FIGURE 11-11** The juxtaglomerular (JG) apparatus. The JG apparatus is located at the junction of the distal tubule and its glomerulus of origin. It is associated with regulation of blood flow and filtration fraction for the nephron and with the secretion of renin, an enzyme involved in the formation of angiotensin II. Structures within capsular space (the Bowman capsule) appear as independent structures because of the transverse section view. Structurally, they are continuous with each other and with the afferent and efferent arterioles. (From Reece WO. Kidney function in mammals. In: Reece WO, ed. Dukes' Physiology of Domestic Animals. 12th Ed. Ithaca, NY: Cornell University Press, 2004.)

■ FORMATION OF URINE

1. What is the difference between plasma, glomerular filtrate, tubular fluid, and urine?
2. Be able to follow fluid from plasma in the afferent arteriole through the several components of the nephron to its final discharge from the urethra.
3. Define RBF, RPF, GFR, and FF. Which variable (RBF, RPF, or GFR) represents the largest volume? What is an approximate value for the percentage of glomerular filtrate that is excreted as urine?
4. What are the three processes associated with urine formation?

The three processes involving the nephrons and their blood supply in urine formation are: 1) glomerular filtration, 2) tubular reabsorp- tion, and 3) tubular secretion. As a result of glomerular filtration, an ultrafiltrate of plasma known as **glomerular filtrate** appears in the Bowman capsule. Glomerular filtrate becomes **tubular fluid** when it enters the nephron tubules because of the compositional changes that begin to occur immediately as a result of reabsorption from the tubular lumen and secre- tion into the tubular lumen (*Fig. 11-12*). Tubular reabsorption and tubular secretion continue throughout the length of the nephron and collecting duct so that tubular fluid does not become urine until it enters the renal pelvis. With the possible exception of mucus addition in the horse, there are no compositional changes in urine beyond the collecting ducts.

Distribution of Blood at the Glomerulus

Renal blood flow (RBF) refers to the rate at which blood flows to the kidneys (in milliliters

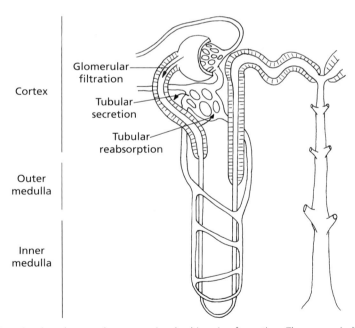

■ **FIGURE 11-12** Functional nephron and processes involved in urine formation. The arrows indicate the origins and destinations of the three processes associated with the formation of urine. After glomerular filtration, glomerular filtrate enters the proximal tubule and becomes tubular fluid. Tubular secretion is directed from the peritubular capil- laries into the tubules, and tubular reabsorption is directed from the tubules into the peritubular capillaries. Tubular reabsorption and tubular secretion occur throughout the length of the nephron.

per minute). Inasmuch as plasma is the fluid part of the blood, from which the glomerular filtrate is formed, **renal plasma flow (RPF)** refers to that part of the RBF that is plasma. As long as there continues to be an RBF, a glomerular filtrate will be formed from the plasma at the glomerulus. The rate at which it is formed is known as the **glomerular filtration rate (GFR)** and is measured in milliliters per minute. RBF and RPF are also measured in milliliters per minute, and the ratio of GFR to RPF (GFR:RPF) is referred to as the **filtration fraction (FF)**. The FF is the fraction (or percentage) of plasma flowing through the glomerulus that becomes glomerular filtrate. The blood that continues into the efferent arterioles has an increased value for packed cell volume and protein concentration because a fraction of the plasma has been filtered and has entered the tubules. The protein concentration is higher because it is virtually prevented from being filtered with the other plasma components (see upcoming section).

An example for the relationships of RBF, RPF, GFR, FF, and the percentage of urine formed relative to the amount of filtrate formed in 24 hours is shown in *Table 11-2*.

■ GLOMERULAR FILTRATION

1. What are the two capillary beds that perfuse the nephrons? Which one resembles the arterial end of a muscle capillary, and which one resembles the venous end?
2. Study the capillary dynamics associated with filtration at the glomerulus.
3. How does efferent arteriolar constriction increase the FF?
4. What are the factors associated with autoregulation of RBF and GFR?

The kidneys have the functional counterpart of two capillary beds, represented by the glomeruli and the peritubular capillaries. The

TABLE 11-2 APPROXIMATE VALUES FOR SEVERAL KIDNEY FUNCTION VARIABLES IN AN 11.35-kg (25-lb) DOG IN A NORMAL STATE OF HYDRATION

VARIABLE	VALUE
Cardiac output (mL/min)	1,500
Blood flow to kidneys (% of cardiac output)	20
Renal blood flow (mL/min)	300
Renal plasma flow[a] (mL/min)	180
Glomerular filtration rate (mL/min)	45
Filtration fraction (decimal equivalent)	0.25
Urine volume in 24 hr[b] (mL)	681
Glomerular filtrate volume in 24 hr (mL)	64,800
Volume of urine as percent of filtrate	1.05
Filtrate reabsorbed (%)	98.95

[a]Based on plasma portion of hematocrit being approximately 60%.
[b]Calculated from average rate for dogs being 60 mL/kg/24 hr.

glomeruli are considered to be a high-pressure system (high hydrostatic pressure [HP], favoring filtration), and the peritubular capillaries, which are perfused with blood coming from the glomerular capillary bed, are considered to be a low-pressure system (low HP, favoring reabsorption). As such, the glomeruli are similar to the arterial end of a typical muscle capillary and the peritubular capillaries are similar to the venous end (see Chapter 9). It seems that the capillary endothelium of the glomerulus is slightly more porous than muscle capillary endothelium and larger molecules are filtered more readily.

Dynamics of Filtration

The barriers to filtration from glomerular capillaries to the capsular space (the **glomerular membrane**) are the fenestrated capillary endothelium basement membrane and the filtration slit diaphragm, shown in Figure 11-11. The dynamics of filtration through the glomerular membrane are illustrated in *Figure 11-13*. No

colloidal osmotic pressure is shown on the Bowman capsule side. Although some filtration of protein (a potential source of colloidal osmotic pressure) occurs (as in muscle capillaries), the filtrate does not accumulate as it does in muscle because the HP in the Bowman capsule causes the filtrate to flow away from the capsule and through the nephron tubules. Therefore, the colloidal osmotic pressure in

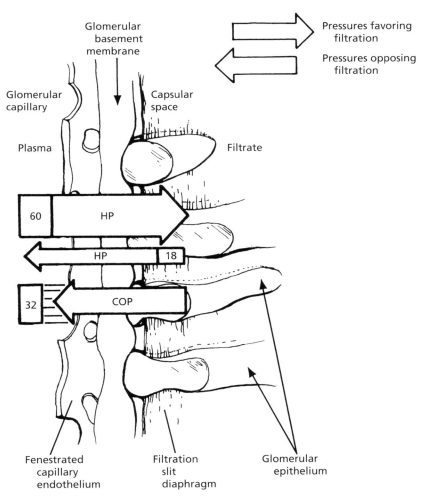

■ **FIGURE 11-13** Dynamics of glomerular filtration in mammals. The Bowman capsule is separated from the glomerulus by a glomerular membrane, through which filtration occurs. The extent of filtration is determined by the difference between the pressures favoring filtration and those opposing filtration. In this illustration, filtration occurs because 60 − (32 + 18) = 10 mm Hg. Values greater than or less than 10 mm Hg would correlate with more or less filtration, respectively. Pressure values (60, 32, 18) are in mm Hg. HP, hydrostatic pressure; COP, colloidal osmotic pressure.

the Bowman capsule urinary space is negligible.

Filtration Factors

The GFR can be varied by changing the diameter of the afferent or efferent arterioles. Dilatation of the afferent arteriole increases the blood flow to the glomerulus, which in turn increases the HP and potential for filtration. Constriction of the efferent arteriole increases the glomerular HP, just as blockage of a vein increases the HP in capillaries behind it. Even though RBF to the glomerulus is reduced because of the decreased outflow caused by efferent arteriole constriction, the GFR is maintained (because of the greater HP) and this allows for a continued FF.

For any given molecular size, positively charged molecules are more readily filtered than negatively charged molecules. This happens because there are negatively charged (anionic) sites (mostly proteoglycans) in the glomerular basement membrane that repel similarly charged molecules. Accordingly, plasma albumin molecules are relatively restricted from filtration (might not be excluded altogether) because, coupled with their large molecular size, they are polyanionic in the physiologic pH range. In kidney disease, in which poor perfusion may become a factor, the electrostatic charge of the glomerular membrane can change, and molecules previously restricted from filtration can be filtered and gain entrance to the capsular space.

Autoregulation

A feedback mechanism, known as the tubuloglomerular feedback mechanism, performs the function of autoregulation. It has two components that act together to control GFR: 1) an afferent arteriolar feedback mechanism and 2) an efferent arteriolar feedback mechanism. Macula densa cells sense changes in volume delivery to the distal tubules. Decreased GFR slows the flow rate in the loop of Henle that allows for increased reabsorption of sodium and chloride ions in the ascending limb of the loop of Henle, thereby decreasing the concentration of sodium chloride at the macula densa cells. This results in a signal from the macula densa decreasing resistance to blood flow in the afferent arterioles which raises glomerular HP, helping to return GFR to normal. The signal from the macula densa also increases release of renin from the JG cells of the afferent and efferent arterioles (major storage sites for renin). Renin, an enzyme, increases the formation of angiotensin I, which is converted to angiotensin II by angiotensin converting enzyme (ACE).

Angiotensin II constricts the efferent arterioles, thereby increasing glomerular HP and assisting the return of GFR toward normal. The production of angiotensin II continues because of the conversion of plasma angiotensinogen (produced in the liver) to angiotensin I by renin and its subsequent conversion to angiotensin II by ACE (*Fig. 11-14*). Although ACE is derived mainly in the capillary endo-

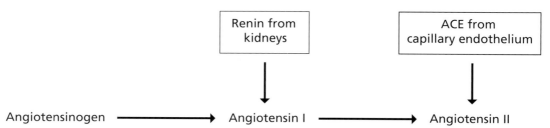

■ **FIGURE 11-14** The conversion of angiotensinogen to angiotensin II. Plasma angiotensinogen is produced in the liver. Its conversion to angiotensin II begins in the kidney by renin release from juxtagtomerular cells of the afferent and efferent arterioles of the glomerulus.

thelium of the lung, because of its vascularity, it is also derived in the kidney endothelium and other organ beds.

Next to vasopressin, angiotensin II is the second most potent vasoconstrictor produced in the body. It is rapidly destroyed in the peripheral capillary beds by a number of enzymes called angiotensinases. Although not related to autoregulation, angiotensin II stimulates the secretion of aldosterone, which causes reabsorption of [Na^+]. This becomes a factor in (ECF) volume regulation.

■ TUBULAR REABSORPTION AND SECRETION

1. What nephron part accounts for the greatest amount of reabsorption?
2. What is meant by transport maximum, and how does it differ from renal threshold?

For reabsorption to occur, a substance must pass from the tubular lumen through the tubular epithelial cells, diffuse through the interstitial fluid (ISF), and enter the capillary. A substance to be secreted must leave the capillary, diffuse through the ISF, and pass through the tubular epithelial cell into the tubular lumen. A sagittal section of tubular epithelium and its relationship to the tubular lumen and peritubular capillary are shown in *Figure 11-15*.

Reabsorption of Na^+, Cl^-, Glucose, and Amino Acids

Substances important to body function, such as glucose and amino acids, enter tubular fluid by filtration at the glomerulus. Because of their relatively small molecular size, they pass easily through the glomerular membrane, and their concentration in the glomerular filtrate is equal to their concentration in plasma. Unless

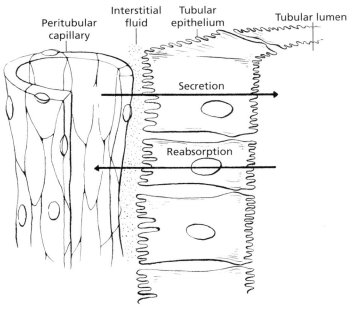

■ **FIGURE 11-15** Structures that separate tubular fluid in the tubular lumen from plasma in peritubular capillaries. The energy requirement for reabsorption and secretion processes is provided by the Na^+-K^+-ATPase ("sodium pump") located in the basolateral membrane of proximal tubule epithelial cells.

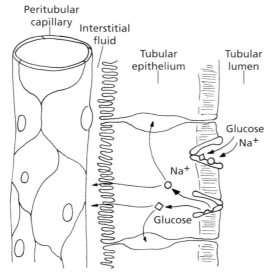

■ **FIGURE 11-16** Transport of Na⁺ from tubular lumen into the tubular epithelial cell and its cotransport with glucose. The protein carrier conformation permits reception of Na⁺ and glucose from the lumen. Carrier conformational change permits Na⁺ and glucose release into the epithelial cytoplasm. Once released, the carrier returns to its original conformation for the reception of more Na⁺ and glucose. The Na⁺ released into the tubular epithelial cytoplasm is actively transported through the basal and lateral borders of the cells into the ISF and diffuses from there into the capillaries. Glucose follows the same pathways except that it is not actively transported. Amino acids are also cotransported with Na⁺ similar to that of glucose.

these substances are returned to the blood, they are excreted in the urine and lost from the body. In the epithelial cells of the proximal convoluted tubules, glucose and amino acids are transferred from the tubular lumen to the ISF, from which they diffuse into the peritubular capillaries. Their transport from the tubular lumen into the tubular epithelial cell is coupled with the transport of Na⁺. For example, Na⁺ and glucose (or an amino acid) are coupled to the same carrier when moving through the brush border of the epithelial cell from the lumen to the cytoplasm of the cell (*Fig. 11-16*). The energy for transport is associated with the active transport of Na⁺ through the basal and lateral membranes of the tubular

epithelial cells. The active transport of Na⁺ out of the cell at the basal and lateral borders creates a chemical gradient for diffusion of Na⁺ from the tubular lumen, where its concentration is higher, into the cell cytoplasm. The transport of glucose and amino acids does not require additional energy because of their transport with Na⁺. Once glucose and amino acids are inside the cell, and are uncoupled from their carrier, they diffuse through the basal and lateral borders into the ISF and from there into the capillaries. The protein carrier on which they were transported from the lumen into the cell with Na⁺ returns to its previous conformation to transport more glucose, amino acids, and Na⁺.

Because Na⁺ is transported from the tubular epithelial cells to the ISF, an electrical gradient is established between the ISF and the tubular lumen (lumen negative). The Cl⁻ diffuses through membranes easily and its diffusion from the lumen follows the transport of Na⁺ into the tubular epithelium to maintain electrical neutrality. Consequently the lumen has a low negativity in the proximal tubule, where much of the Na⁺ is reabsorbed.

Reabsorption of Water and Urea

The removal of Na⁺, glucose, amino acids, and other substances from the lumen into the ISF and capillaries increases the concentration of water within the lumen, and water is reabsorbed by osmosis into the ISF and capillaries. Reabsorption of water into the peritubular capillaries from the ISF is favored because of the relatively low HP and because of the increased colloidal osmotic pressure (loss of water, but not protein, at the glomerulus) in the peritubular capillaries. This situation is similar to that at the venous end of a muscle capillary (see Chapter 9).

The removal of water from the tubular lumen increases the concentration of diffusible substances (particularly urea), and they move from the lumen to the ISF and capillaries by simple diffusion. The proximal tubules reabsorb about 65% of H_2O, Na^+, Cl^-, and HCO_3^- and 100% of the glucose and amino acids that were previously filtered at the glomerulus.

Secretion of H^+, K^+, NH_3, and Organic Molecules

The transfer of substances from the capillaries into the ISF and hence to the tubular lumen—tubular secretion—occurs for several substances. The secretion of H^+ occurs throughout the length of the nephron tubules (except in the thin limb of loops of Henle) and is coupled with the reabsorption of HCO^-. The secretion of K^+ occurs in the distal convoluted tubule and collecting tubules and ducts and is coupled with the reabsorption of Na^+. Ammonia is secreted by the nephron tubules. Its rate of secretion varies, depending on the acid-base equilibrium of the body fluids (see later text). Several organic molecules are also secreted by the tubular epithelial cells into the tubular lumen. A substance similar to penicillin is lost from the body fluids because of tubular secretion. Penicillin-like substances have been developed that persist in the body fluids for longer periods of time because their rate of secretion has been slowed.

Transport Maximum

Substances such as glucose that are associated with a carrier or that have active transport mechanisms for their reabsorption have a maximum rate at which they can be reabsorbed, known as the **tubular transport maximum** (T_M). When the T_M for the substance is exceeded, the substance will appear in the urine. In the disease known as **diabetes mellitus**, insulin is either deficient or lacking, and the movement of glucose from the plasma into body cells is impaired. Glucose concentration in the plasma therefore increases, causing the plasma and tubular loads of glucose to increase. The increased tubular load exceeds the availability of carrier

molecules for its transport and reabsorption, and excess glucose continues its flow through the tubules into the urine. Because it is retained within the tubules, it contributes to the effective osmotic pressure of the tubular fluid, and water is also retained. In diabetes mellitus, glucose is detected in the urine and a greater volume of urine is formed. Greater amounts of water are lost from the body in the urine, so the afflicted animal drinks more water to compensate for the urine loss. Increased urine formation is known as **diuresis**. When it is caused by retention of water because of greater effective osmotic pressure in the tubular lumen, it is known as **osmotic diuresis**.

Not all of the hundreds of thousands of nephrons have the same T_M. The first appearance of glucose in the urine does not represent the T_M for the kidney, it represents the **renal threshold** (the plasma concentration of a substance when it first appears in the urine). The T_M for the kidney is reached when all nephrons are reabsorbing to their maximum ability. For glucose, the renal threshold (its plasma concentration when glucose first appears in urine) is about 180 mg/dL and the T_M (its plasma concentration when further increments of glucose increase in the plasma result in similar increments of glucose increase in the urine) is about 260 mg/dL.

■ COUNTERCURRENT MECHANISM

1. What is the function of the countercurrent mechanism?
2. Differentiate between the countercurrent multiplier and countercurrent exchange systems.
3. What is the tone of tubular fluid as it enters the distal tubule?
4. What functions are served by the recirculation of urea?

Preparation of the tubular fluid (after it leaves the proximal tubule) for the conservation or elimination of water depends on the existence of a very high osmolality in the ISF of the renal medulla. The osmolality increases with distance from the cortex, reaching a maximum in the innermost aspects of the medulla. The maximum value varies by species. In the dog, it is about 2,400 mOsm/kg H_2O, compared with plasma osmolality of about 300 mOsm/kg H_2O. The high osmolality exists because of the **countercurrent mechanism**. It is established by the activities of the loops of Henle and is maintained by the special characteristics of the blood supply to the medulla (**the vasa recta**).

A countercurrent system of tubules or vessels exists where the inflow of fluid runs parallel to, counter (opposite) to, and close to the outflow for some distance. These characteristics are common to the anatomic arrangements of the loops of Henle and the vasa recta. Accordingly, the countercurrent mechanism in the kidney comprises two countercurrent systems: the **countercurrent multiplier (loops of Henle)** and the **countercurrent exchanger (vasa recta)**.

Countercurrent Multiplier System

The countercurrent multiplier is represented in *Figure 11-17* by the: 1) descending limb, 2) thin segment of the ascending limb, and 3) thick segment of the ascending limb of the loop of Henle. Osmolality changes of the tubular fluid occur as it progresses through the loop of Henle because of the permeability characteristics of the loop of Henle limbs and segments coupled with an active cotransport of NaCl in the thick segment of the ascending limb. In the descending limb (impermeable to solutes, permeable to water), water diffuses by osmosis to the higher osmotic pressure of the ISF, and solute concentration (mostly NaCl) increases while approaching the hairpin turn of the loop of Henle. The thin segment of the ascending limb is permeable for NaCl and impermeable for H_2O. Therefore, water remains in the tubule and NaCl diffuses (because of

concentration gradient) to the ISF. In the thick segment of the ascending limb, NaCl is actively transported (cotransport) to the ISF, and water continues to be retained. Whereas the osmolality of the tubular fluid entering the descending limb was 300 mOsm/kg H_2O, the tubular fluid leaving the ascending limb and entering the distal tubule has been diluted (osmolality 185 mOsm/kg H_2O). Tubular fluid osmolality changes (described in upcoming sections) that determine whether the urine is dilute or concentrated occur in the distal tubule and collecting ducts.

The vertical osmotic gradient in the ISF (lower in outer medulla, higher in inner medulla and at hairpin turn) is established and maintained by: 1) continued active transport of NaCl by the thick segment of the ascending limb, 2) concentration of tubular fluid in the descending limb, and 3) passive diffusion of NaCl from the lumen of the thin segment of the ascending limb into the inner medullary ISF.

Countercurrent Exchanger System

A countercurrent exchanger is a countercurrent system in which transport between outflow and inflow is entirely passive. The vasa recta act as countercurrent exchangers (*Fig. 11-18*). They are permeable to water and solutes throughout their length. In the descending limbs, water is drawn by osmosis from the plasma of the vasa recta to the hyperosmotic ISF (created by countercurrent multiplier), and the solutes diffuse from the ISF into the vasa recta. In the ascending limbs, solutes diffuse back into the ISF, and water is drawn by osmosis back into the vasa recta. The net result is that the solutes responsible for the vertical medullary gradient are mostly retained in the ISF of the medulla. The vasa recta carry away slightly more solutes than are brought into them.

An increased rate of medullary blood flow would reduce the time for diffusion of solute from the ascending limb back to the ISF, and

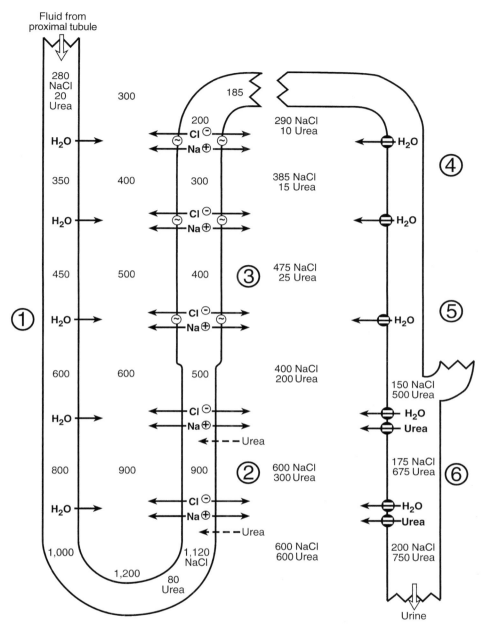

FIGURE 11-17 Countercurrent multiplication in the loop of Henle and recirculation of urea. Values shown (in milliosmoles per kilogram H_2O) are hypothetical but approximate those of humans under conditions of low water intake. Single numbers represent total osmolality. Identified numbers (NaCl, urea) represent specific contribution to total osmolality. Transport of NaCl and urea at the level of the thin segment of the ascending limb of the loop of Henle is by simple diffusion. Active transport of Na^+ in the ascending thick limb is coupled with the transport of Cl^- (cotransport). Water channels (also urea) on the right are open (influence of antidiuretic hormone). In this example, urine is being concentrated. Circled numbers identify locations as follows: 1) descending limb of the loop of Henle; 2) thin segment of ascending limb of loop of Henle; 3) thick segment of ascending limb of loop of Henle; 4) cortical collecting duct; 5) outer medullary collecting duct; 6) inner medullary collecting duct. See text for details. (From Reece WO. Kidney function in mammals. In: Reece WO, ed. Dukes' Physiology of Domestic Animals. 12th Ed. Ithaca, NY: Cornell University Press, 2004.)

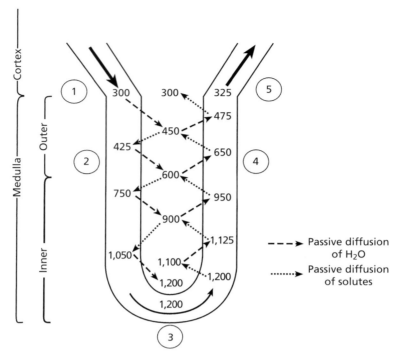

■ **FIGURE 11-18** Countercurrent exchange in vasa recta. Values shown (milliosmoles per kilogram H_2O) approximate those of humans. Blood enters from the cortex near circled number 1 with a milliosmolality of about 300 and descends through an increasingly hypertonic peritubular fluid in the medulla (circled number 2). Water diffuses out and solute diffuses in until the hairpin turn is reached (circled number 3). The blood then ascends through decreasing hypertonicity, and water diffuses in and solute diffuses out (circled number 4). When blood returns to the cortex (circled number 5), the milliosmolality is only slightly higher than when it entered the vasa recta. (From Reece WO. Kidney function in mammals. In: Reece WO, ed. Dukes' Physiology of Domestic Animals. 12th Ed. Ithaca, NY: Cornell University Press, 2004.)

the blood leaving the ascending limb would have higher concentration of solute. The result would be a gradual loss or washout of the medullary gradient, referred to as **medullary washout**. Medullary loss of solute is normally prevented because the blood flow to the vasa recta is reduced (vasa recta compose 10% to 20% of kidney blood flow) and it is often characterized as sluggish. All of the excess salt removed from the medullary ISF by the vasa recta must be replaced by the loops of Henle for the osmotic gradient to be maintained. If countercurrent blood flow in the vasa recta did not exist, and blood from the descending limbs of the vasa recta returned directly to the renal

vein instead of counterflowing into the ascending limb, the solute of the renal medulla would be quickly removed instead of being retained.

Role of Urea

In addition to NaCl, urea also contributes to the high solute concentration in the ISF of the kidney medulla. Urea presence is accomplished by a recirculation mechanism for urea between the collecting ducts and the loop of Henle (see Fig. 11-17). **Recirculation** means that urea diffuses from the inner medullary collecting ducts into the ISF, and from there diffuses into the lumen of the thin segment of the ascending limbs of the loops of Henle. Diffusion occurs because of the permeability of these nephron parts for urea and because of concentration differences (high to low concentration). After the entrance of urea into the loops of Henle, it is retained there because of membrane impermeability until it again arrives at the inner medullary collecting ducts, which have a variable permeability depending on the amount of **antidiuretic hormone** (**ADH**). See following section. The recirculation mechanism and high concentration of urea in the medulla not only assist the countercurrent multiplier system and osmotic gradient, but also ensure excretion of urea when urine output is low. For example, if urine is formed at the rate of 2 mL/min and it has a urea concentration of 2 mg/mL, then 4 mg of urea would be excreted each minute. If, however, urine formation is reduced to 1 mL/min (greater reabsorption of water), the concentration of urea is increased to 4 mg/mL and excretion is maintained at 4 mg/min. The concentration of urea remains high in the collecting ducts because the concentration is also high in the ISF (diffusion from the collecting duct limited by concentration difference).

■ CONCENTRATION OF URINE

1. Where is the degree of dehydration of the ECF detected?
2. Where does ADH exert its influence?
3. What is the direction of water diffusion (i.e., collecting duct to medullary ISF or vice versa) when ADH secretion is increased?
4. What blood vessels collect water reabsorbed into the interstitial space of the medulla?
5. What is the approximate urine-to-plasma osmolal ratio in the dog? How does this compare to that of humans? Would greater urine concentration be possible where the ratio is increased?
6. How do diabetes insipidus and diabetes mellitus differ regarding cause of observed polydipsia and polyuria?
7. What are reasons for concentration failure in chronic renal failure disease?

There is continued active transport of NaCl and low permeability for water and urea in the distal tubule. At the end of the distal tubule, and before the fluid enters the cortical collecting tubules and ducts, the osmolality is about 150 mOsm. Tubular fluid entering the distal tubules has an osmolality lower than that of plasma because of the removal of Na^+ and Cl that occurred in the ascending limb of the loops of Henle along with the simultaneous retention of water.

Antidiuretic Hormone and Osmoregulation

The epithelial cells of the collecting tubules and collecting ducts have a variable permeability for water, depending on the amount of ADH that has been secreted from the posterior pituitary gland. ADH increases the permeability of these cells for water. Significant changes occur in the rate of ADH secretion when there are deviations in the plasma osmolality of as little as 2% in either direction.

The degree of hydration of the ECF is detected by **osmoreceptor cells** in the hypothalamus. The osmoreceptors of the hypothalamus respond to effective osmotic pressure; hence, osmolality increase must be caused by substances restricted from diffusion into the osmoreceptor cells. For this reason, the osmoreceptor cells are often considered to be Na^+ receptors because Na^+ is the nondiffusible cation with the greatest concentration in the ECF. Osmolality increase as a result of urea (freely diffusible) does not stimulate the receptors. When the cells detect increased plasma osmolality (hyperosmolality), they stimulate the posterior pituitary to secrete more ADH and, when decreased plasma osmolality (hypoosmolality) is detected, the rate of ADH

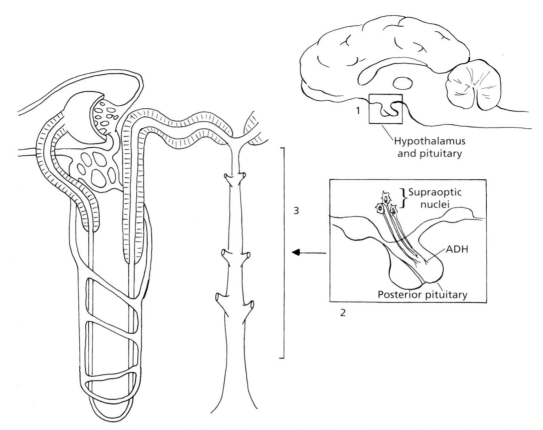

■ **FIGURE 11-19** Relationships among the hypothalamus, posterior pituitary, and kidneys in the regulation of extra cellular hydration. 1) Extracellular dehydration detected by osmoreceptors in the hypothalamus. Boxed area in 1 shows location in the brain of the boxed area in 2. 2) ADH (neurosecretion of supraoptic nuclei in hypothalamus) secreted into blood in response to dehydration. 3) Cortical collecting tubules and medullary collecting ducts are targets of ADH, causing increased reabsorption of H_2O.

release is decreased. The secreted ADH is circulated by the blood to the kidney tubules, where the water permeability changes take place (*Fig. 11-19*). The thirst center, also located in the hypothalamus, is stimulated by hyperosmolality. A water deficit requires water intake for correction, and animals seek water. The responses to increased plasma osmolality are summarized in *Figure 11-20*.

Hypotonic tubular fluid entering the collecting tubules and ducts could be excreted as urine if water was not reabsorbed. This happens in **diabetes insipidus**, in which there

is either an absence of ADH or severely decreased amounts of ADH. Animals with this condition have clinical signs of **polyuria** (formation and excretion of a large volume of urine) and **polydipsia** (excessive thirst manifested by excessive water intake). The urine formed is dilute and has a lower-than-normal specific gravity. Animals with diabetes mellitus may also show polyuria and polydipsia. Polyuria in this disease is caused by an osmotic diuresis because of the presence of glucose in the urine (failed to be reabsorbed) and is not caused by a lack of ADH. The urine

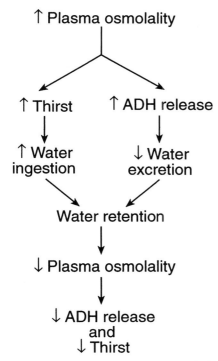

↑ Plasma osmolality

↑ Thirst   ↑ ADH release

↑ Water   ↓ Water
ingestion   excretion

Water retention

↓ Plasma osmolality

↓ ADH release
and
↓ Thirst

■ **FIGURE 11-20** Cycle of events for the relief of hyper-osmolality. Increased thirst is the predominant factor for the correction of hyperosmolality. ADH, antidiuretic hormone. (From Reece WO. Kidney function in mammals. In: Reece WO, ed. Dukes' Physiology of Domestic Animals. 12th Ed. Ithaca, NY: Cornell University Press, 2004.)

region of the medulla. In the dog, this would approach 2,400 mOsm and the urine-to-plasma osmolal ratio (2,400 : 300) would be approximately 8 : 1. The urine would have a concentration eight times that of plasma. Some desert rodents attain a urine-to-plasma osmolal ratio of about 16 : 1. This ratio represents an extreme adaptation for body water conservation. Environmental water is not available for desert animals (water gain mostly metabolic water), and water losses are minimized for survival. *Table 11-3* compares the percentage of long-looped nephrons (loops of Henle extending deeply into the medulla) and **relative medullary thickness** of different animals. The relative medullary thickness is derived from measurements of the depth of the medulla from the corticomedullary junction to its innermost depth, which protrudes into the renal pelvis. Relative medullary thickness is believed to be a better predictor of urine concentrating ability than percentage of long-looped nephrons. As judged by freezing point depression (solute particles lower the freezing point of solutions), the kangaroo rat has the greatest concentrating capacity for urine. As compared with humans, it seems that its innermost medullary osmolality would be about four times that of humans, or about 4,800 mOsm.

Other Factors Affecting ADH Release

ADH release from the posterior pituitary is influenced by other factors in addition to hydration of the ECF. Cold environments inhibit ADH release, so urine production and water intake increase. The need for water intake results from thirst induced by water loss from diuresis. The need for water availability in cold weather is apparent.

Ethyl alcohol inhibits ADH secretion, and dehydration is a consequence of alcohol consumption (not a factor for domestic animals).

Concentration Failure

In addition to diabetes insipidus, other kidney disease processes are characterized

specific gravity would likely be higher than normal and would test positive for glucose. As in diabetes insipidus, polydipsia is a compensation for the polyuria to overcome the water deficit.

In healthy animals, when tubular fluid enters the collecting tubules and ducts, water is reabsorbed as it proceeds to the renal pelvis because it is exposed to effective osmotic pressures of increasing magnitudes in the ISF of the kidney medulla, as established by the counter-current mechanism. ADH secretion is consistent with the need for water conservation. In extreme cases of water conservation, it would be possible for the osmolality of the tubular fluid, and hence that of the urine, to approach the osmolality of the ISF in the innermost

TABLE 11-3 RELATIONSHIP OF STRUCTURE TO CONCENTRATING CAPACITY IN MAMMALIAN KIDNEYS

ANIMAL	KIDNEY SIZE[a] (MM)	LONG-LOOPED NEPHRONS (%)	RELATIVE MEDULLARY THICKNESS[B]	MAXIMUM FREEZING POINT DEPRESSION IN URINE (°C)
Beaver	36	0	1.3	0.96
Pig	66	3	1.6	2
Human	64	14	3	2.6
Dog[c]	40	100	4.3	4.85
Cat	24	100	4.8	5.8
Rat	14	28	5.8	4.85
Kangaroo rat	5.9	27	8.5	10.4
Jerboa	4.5	33	9.3	12
Psammomys	13	100	10.7	9.2

[a]Kidney size = cube root of the product of the dimensions of the kidney.
[b]Relative medullary thickness = medullary thickness in millimeters = 10 ÷ kidney size.
[c]Beeuwkes and Bonventre have shown (1975) that the dog kidney does contain short-looped or corticomedullary nephrons; therefore, long-looped nephrons compose fewer than 100% of the nephrons.
From Schmidt-Nielsen B, O'Dell R. Am J Physiol 1961;200:1119–1124.

by decreased concentrating ability. Impaired concentrating ability is notable in **chronic renal** failure. Reasons cited are as follows:

1. More solute than usual is presented to the remaining functional nephrons, whereby the high solute content in the tubules contributes to osmotic diuresis.
2. Hypertonicity in the medullary ISF is not maintained because of: a) loss of medullary tissues or decreased blood flow in the vasa recta, and b) decreased Na^+ and Cl^- transport from the thick segment of the ascending limb of the loop of Henle.
3. Damage to cells in the collecting tubules and collecting ducts makes them less responsive to ADH.

■ **EXTRACELLULAR FLUID VOLUME REGULATION**

1. How do osmoregulation and volume regulation differ?
2. Where are the receptors located that respond to blood volume changes?
3. What are the graded responses to efferent renal sympathetic nerve activity?

In **osmoregulation** (regulation of ECF osmolality), the ratio of Na^+ to water (osmoconcentration) is being regulated, and in **volume regulation** (regulation of ECF volume and hence blood volume), the absolute amounts of Na^+ and water that are present are being regulated. The principal receptors responding to acute changes in blood volume are those in the left atrium of the heart. Vagal nerve afferents from these receptors provide a neural link between the heart as a sensor of blood volume and the kidneys as effector organs. In hypovolemia (abnormally decreased volume of circulating fluid in the body), there is decreased left atrial filling that is followed by decreased vagal afferent stimulation and responses that are summarized in *Figure 11-21*.

Stimulation to the kidneys is provided by **efferent renal sympathetic nerve activity**

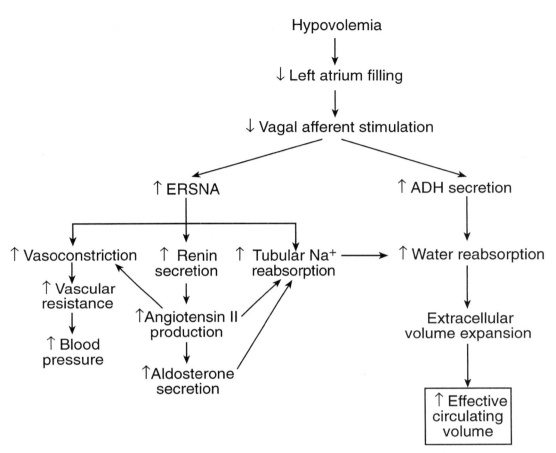

■ **FIGURE 11-21** Renal and cardiovascular responses induced by the sympathetic division of the autonomic nervous system in response to reduced circulating volume (hypovolemia). Efferent renal sympathetic nerve activity (ERSNA) responses are graded depending on the severity of hypovolemia. Accordingly, renin secretion is the first response, followed by tubular Na^+ reabsorption, and finally vasoconstriction to alleviate declining blood pressure associated with hypovolemia. ADH, antidiuretic hormone. (From Reece WO. Kidney function in mammals. In: Reece WO, ed. Dukes' Physiology of Domestic Animals. 12th Ed. Ithaca, NY: Cornell University Press, 2004.)

with innervation to the JG granular cells, the nephron tubules, and the renal vasculature. Each of these groups is innervated by functionally specific groups of the sympathetic nerves. Accordingly, the responses to the groups are graded and with increasing intensity, renin secretion from the JG granular cells increases first, followed by increased renal tubular reabsorption of sodium, and lastly by renal vasoconstriction with decreases in RBF and increased vascular resistance.

These effects can override autoregulatory responses.

■ ALDOSTERONE

1. **What is the function of aldosterone? How does aldosterone secretion assist in restoring blood volume?**

2. **Does aldosterone regulate ECF Na^+ concentration?**

It is noted in Figure 11-21 that angiotensin II production not only increases tubular Na^+ reabsorption, but also increases aldosterone secretion, which in turn also increases tubular Na^+ reabsorption. **Aldosterone** is a hormone of the adrenal cortex (see Chapter 6) and is more particularly involved with the regulation of K^+ concentration in the ECF and promotes the secretion of K^+. The mechanism of K^+ secretion, however, involves the reabsorption of Na^+. Therefore, the secretion of aldosterone in response to angiotensin II has as its function the reabsorption of Na^+.

Aldosterone regulates the K^+ concentration of the ECF by its activity in the cortical collecting tubules and in medullary collecting ducts. In this regard, aldosterone is secreted in response to elevated K^+ concentrations in the ECF. Although Na^+ reabsorption is coupled with K^+ secretion (not a 1:1 exchange), aldosterone is not involved with the regulation of Na^+ concentration. The ADH thirst mechanism (osmoregulation) regulates the concentration of Na^+ concentration in the ECF.

■ OTHER HORMONES WITH KIDNEY ASSOCIATION

1. What is the relationship of parathyroid hormone, the kidneys, and calcium ion homeostasis?
2. What is the function of erythropoietin? Where is it produced?

Angiotensin II, ADH, and aldosterone have been mentioned because of their direct association with the functions of the kidney. There are others that have an intermediate association with the kidney as a part of their overall function or that are produced in the kidney with functions elsewhere. Parathyroid hormone exemplifies the former and erythropoietin (EPO) the latter.

Parathyroid Hormone

Parathyroid hormone, secreted by the parathyroid glands (see Chapter 6), acts on the kidney tubules to increase reabsorption of Ca^{2+}, while at the same time promoting the excretion of phosphorus. Parathyroid hormone is secreted in response to low concentrations of Ca^{2+} in the ECF. Another role of the kidney in response to a decreasing Ca^{2+} concentration in the ECF involves the formation of the **active form of vitamin D** (1,25-dehydroxycholecalciferol), also known as **calcitriol** (*Fig. 11-22*). Active vitamin D promotes Ca^{2+} absorption from the intestine. Parathyroid hormone controls the formation of active vitamin D by the kidney.

Erythropoietin

Erythropoietin (EPO) is a hormone produced in response to the tissue need for oxygen and stimulates the production of new erythrocytes by its activity in the bone marrow (see Chapter 3). The kidney is the major site (the only site in dogs) of EPO production in adult mammals. EPO is produced by peritubular interstitial cells located within the inner cortex and outer medulla of the kidney. The liver is an extrarenal source of EPO in adults (the major site in the mammalian fetus). Extrarenal EPO production in certain animals and humans helps to maintain erythropoiesis during anemia caused by severe kidney diseases. Anemia is a common sequelae of chronic interstitial nephritis in dogs because of the lack of an extrarenal source of EPO.

Prostaglandins

The space between the macula densa and the afferent and efferent arterioles, as well as the space between the glomerular capillaries, is known as the mesangial region, and it consists of mesangial cells and mesangial matrix (see Fig. 11-11). **Mesangial cells** secrete the matrix, secrete the glomerular basement membrane, provide structural support, have phagocytic activity, and secrete prostaglandins. **Prostaglandins** are secreted by almost all body tissues and have diverse functions. More detail is provided in Chapter 6. The function of the

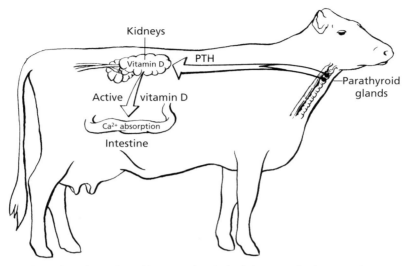

■ **FIGURE 11-22** Relationship of parathyroid hormone (PTH), the kidneys, and calcium ion homeostasis in the cow. PTH from the parathyroid gland activates vitamin D in the kidney; activated vitamin D promotes absorption of Ca^{2+} from the intestine.

prostaglandins at this location has not been described but may be related to the contractile activity of the mesangial cells, and also to their influence on blood flow through glomerular capillaries.

■ MICTURITION

1. **What is meant by micturition?**
2. **Where are the reflex control centers located for micturition?**
3. **Talk through the events involved in filling of the urinary bladder and micturition.**
4. **Which division of the autonomics is involved in micturition?**
5. **Be familiar with the descriptive terms associated with micturition.**

During the formation of urine, the tubular fluid flows through the tubules because of a HP difference that exists between the Bowman capsule and the renal pelvis. The HP in the Bowman capsule is about 15 to 20 mm Hg, and there is almost no HP in the renal pelvis.

Transfer of Urine to the Urinary Bladder

Urine is transported from the renal pelvis to the urinary bladder by peristalsis in the ureters. The ureters enter the urinary bladder at an oblique angle to form a functional valve, the **ureterovesicular valve** (see Fig. 11-5). Once urine has entered the bladder, its backflow into the ureters is prevented as the bladder fills.

Micturition Reflexes

Micturition is the physiologic term for empty-ing of the bladder. The bladder is allowed to fill before emptying because of reflexes having control centers in the sacral spinal cord and brain stem. Receptors in the bladder wall are stretched during filling and have the reflex ability (activation of sacral spinal cord reflex center) of allowing urine to be evacuated through the neck of the bladder and external sphincter. The brain stem reflex center, however, prevents the contraction of the bladder and relaxation of the external sphincter that would otherwise occur. Normal filling occurs, and the cerebral cortex is aroused when the bladder is sufficiently full. Voluntary control intervenes, and micturition is permitted when appropriate. Once micturition proceeds, complete emptying is ensured because of another reflex (brain stem) activated by flow receptors in the urethra. As long as urine is flowing, bladder contraction continues until there is no further flow (the bladder is empty).

The parasympathetics are the sole motor nerve supply to the detrusor muscle of the bladder. The sympathetics have no effect on micturition, but seem to constrict the neck of the bladder during ejaculation, thus directing the ejaculate through the penile urethra rather than having backflow into the bladder.

Descriptive Terms

Urinary continence is the normal condition of storing urine in the bladder while it fills. Continence is maintained by continuous tone of the external sphincter muscle and by closure of the neck of the bladder, which is augmented by elastic tissue. An incontinent animal dribbles urine at frequent intervals instead of permitting the bladder to fill. Spinal injuries cranial to the sacrum are frequently the cause; in such injuries, the brain stem reflexes do not effectively prevent emptying, and thus emptying is initiated by the sacral reflexes as the bladder fills. **Polyuria** refers to increased urine output, **oliguria** means decreased output, and **anuria** describes the condition of no output. **Dysuria** is a term used to describe difficult or painful micturition. **Stranguria** is slow, dropwise, painful discharge of the urine caused by spasm of the urethra and bladder. Stranguria is a clinical sign of **feline urologic syndrome**, caused by obstruction of the urethra by a plug consisting of struvite (magnesium ammonium phosphate) crystals and mucoid material.

■ CHARACTERISTICS OF MAMMALIAN URINE

1. **Make a statement about the composition, color, odor, consistency, nitrogenous component, and amount and specific gravity of mammalian urine. How would you respond if asked about any one of these variables?**

Urinalysis is a very important diagnostic procedure consisting of an evaluation of several physical and chemical properties of urine, estimation of its solute concentration, and microscopic examination of urine sediment. It requires a mastery of laboratory techniques and thoughtful interpretation. It is beyond the scope of this book to provide detailed information for urinalysis, and only some general characteristics of urine are considered.

Composition. Urine is formed to keep the composition of the ECF constant, and, generally, most substances that are present in ECF are also present in urine. Also, the composition of urine varies depending on whether substances are being conserved or excreted.

Color. Urine is usually yellow in color. The yellow color is derived from bilirubin that was excreted into the intestine and reabsorbed into the portal circulation as urobilinogen. Much of the urobilinogen is reexcreted by the liver into the intestine, but urobilinogen that bypasses the liver can be excreted by the kidneys into the urine. The various bilinogens are colorless but are spontaneously oxidized on exposure to oxygen. Thus urobilinogen, when partially oxidized, is known as **urobilin**, and it is largely responsible for the yellow color of urine.

Odor. The odor of urine is characteristic for a species and is probably influenced by diet. For example, the characteristic odor imparted to human urine after the ingestion of asparagus is caused by the formation of asparagine (the amide form of the amino acid, aspartic acid).

Consistency. Urine has a watery consistency in most species. Horse urine is somewhat thick and syrupy, however, because of the secretion of mucus from glands in the pelvis of the kidneys and the upper part of the ureters. The urine of the horse has high concentrations of carbonates and phosphates, which seem to precipitate on standing. The secretion of mucus provides a carrier for the precipitated carbonates and phosphates and prevents their collection in the renal pelvis.

Nitrogenous component. The principal nitrogenous constituent of mammalian urine is urea. Urea is formed by the liver from ammonia, which is produced during amino acid metabolism. The body expends considerable energy in producing urea so that the toxicity of ammonia can be avoided. As compared with ammonia, urea is relatively nontoxic at normal concentrations.

Amount and specific gravity. The amount of urine excreted daily varies with diet, work, external temperature, water consumption, season, and other factors. Marked pathologic variations may occur. The specific gravity of urine varies with the relative proportion of dissolved matter and water. In general, the greater the volume, the lower the specific gravity. Volume and specific gravities for several domestic animals and humans are shown in *Table 11-4*.

■ RENAL CLEARANCE

1. What is meant by renal clearance?
2. Can renal clearance be an index for kidney function?
3. How can renal clearance be used to establish values for GFR, RPF, FF, and RBF?
4. With normal kidney function there is total reabsorption of glucose. What would the renal clearance be for glucose with normal kidney function?

TABLE 11-4 VOLUMES AND SPECIFIC GRAVITIES OF URINE

ANIMAL	VOLUME (mL/ KG BODY WEIGHT/DAY)	SPECIFIC GRAVITY MEAN AND RANGE
Cat	10–20	1.030 (1.02–1.040)
Cattle	17–45	1.032 (1.030–1.045)
Dog	20–100	1.025 (1.016–1.060)
Goat	10–40	1.030 (1.015–1.045)
Horse	3–18	1.040 (1.025–1.060)
Sheep	10–40	1.030 (1.015–1.045)
Swine	5–30	1.012 (1.010–1.050)
Human	8.6–28.6	1.020 (1.002–1.040)

From Reece WO. Kidney function in mammals. In: Reece WO, ed. Dukes' Physiology of Domestic Animals. 12th Ed. Ithaca, NY: Cornell University Press, 2004.

5. Be familiar with the determination of GFR by creatinine clearance.

Study of the renal clearance concept is useful for understanding basic elements of kidney function. Renal clearance measurements are made for determining RPF and GFR. Values for GFR and RPF are used to determine FF, and the value determined for RPF, when coupled with the packed cell volume, can be used to calculate the RBF.

Renal clearance is a measurement of the kidney's ability to remove substances from the plasma. It can be determined by the formula:

$$C_x = (U_x \dot{V})/P_x \qquad Eq.\ 11\text{-}1$$

where C_x = clearance of substance x (mL/min), U_x = concentration of x in urine (mg/mL), $\dot{V}$ = rate of urine formation (mL/min), and P_x = concentration of x in plasma (mg/mL). Thus, if U_x = 130 mg/mL, $\dot{V}$ = 1 mL/min, and P_x = 2 mg/mL, then C_x = (130 × 1) ÷ 2 = 65 mL/min.

$U_x \dot{V}$ (130 mg/mL × 1 mL/min = 130 mg/min) is the rate at which substance x is excreted. Accordingly, dividing the excretion rate by the concentration of the substance in plasma (130 mg/min ÷ 2 mg/mL = 65 mL/min) gives the amount of plasma that would be needed each minute to provide the quantity that is excreted. Only a few substances are removed completely from the blood as it circulates through the kidney, so the renal clearance measurement does not actually describe an event, but only provides values for comparison. For example, a renal clearance value for urea of 50 mL/min does not mean that 50 mL of the RPF is completely cleared of urea and that the remainder continues through the kidney, with none extracted. Rather, it means that each milliliter of the RPF contributes urea to that which is excreted, but the amount

excreted in the urine each minute would require all of the urea in 50 mL of the RPF.

A substance such as inulin in the plasma is filtered freely at the glomerulus. It is not reabsorbed from the tubular fluid, nor is it secreted into the tubular fluid from the peritubular capillaries. All that is filtered is excreted. Because it is filtered freely, any increase in plasma concentration results in a similar excretion rate. Plasma clearance does not change (*Fig. 11-23*). A substance such as glucose is filtered freely at the glomerulus and, as long as the renal threshold is not reached, all that is filtered is reabsorbed and the renal clearance is zero. If the plasma concentration is increased to the point at which the renal threshold is surpassed, however, part of the filtered glucose is excreted and renal clearance values begin to increase. These values can never equal the renal clearance

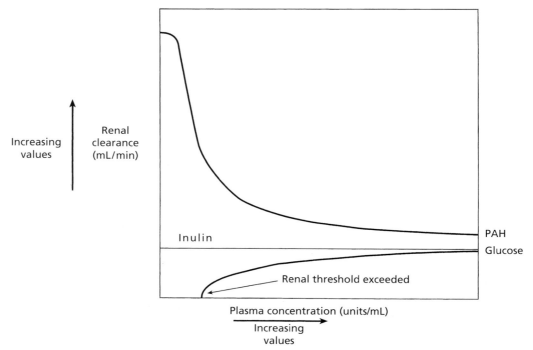

■ **FIGURE 11-23** Effect of tubular reabsorption and tubular secretion on renal clearance. Glucose represents a substance that is reabsorbed from the tubules, p-aminohippuric acid (PAH) represents a substance that is secreted into the tubule but not reabsorbed, and inulin represents a substance that is neither reabsorbed nor secreted by the renal tubules. All of these substances are freely filtered at the glomerulus and enter the tubules. The decrease for renal clearance of PAH and the increase of renal clearance for glucose indicates a point at which their renal clearance is changed as their plasma concentration increases. See text for details.

values for inulin because some of the glucose filtered will always be reabsorbed (see Fig. 11-23). A plasma substance such as p-aminohippuric acid, which is filtered freely and is not reabsorbed from the tubules, but is secreted into the tubules (increases the tubular load), will always have a renal clearance value greater than that of inulin because a greater proportion of the plasma load is excreted (filtration plus secretion versus filtration only; see Fig. 11-23).

Thus, by comparison with inulin, information can be obtained about how different substances are handled by the kidney. Also, the health status of the kidneys can be assessed by these measurements. For example, diseased kidney has a lower renal clearance value for inulin than a normal kidney because the excretion rate is diminished, as a result of reduced filtration (fewer functional nephrons) and because it is not cleared, the plasma concentration would be correspondingly higher. Renal clearance measurements are also used pharmacologically to determine how certain drugs alter kidney function and how they are handled by the kidney. A drug with a renal clearance value higher than inulin would indicate that it is secreted into the tubules at a rate greater than it is reabsorbed or excreted, and one with a value lower than inulin would indicate that it is reabsorbed at a rate greater than it is secreted or excreted.

Creatinine Clearance

Creatinine clearance is a useful clinical assessment for the evaluation of kidney disease. In many animals (e.g., the dog) creatinine is cleared in a manner similar to inulin (i.e., filtered freely, not reabsorbed, not secreted). Its measurement provides an estimate of GFR. The **endogenous creatinine clearance method** is most often used for this purpose. It is endogenous in that it uses the amount that is normally present in blood and does not require the infusion of creatinine to complement the amount normally present. When creatinine is infused for the purpose of determining the GFR, it is termed the **exogenous creatinine clearance method**.

Creatinine is a nitrogenous byproduct of muscle metabolism. The major reaction that produces creatinine is the spontaneous loss of phosphoric acid from creatine phosphate in muscle. Creatinine production is independent of protein metabolism. The amount produced depends on the mass of muscle in the body and is very constant from day to day. Because it is constantly produced, it is constantly excreted, and normal plasma creatinine concentrations are 0.5 to 2.0 mg/dL.

Creatinine clearance as a measurement of GFR can be used clinically for the assessment of kidney function because creatinine clearance is directly related to the functional renal mass. Accordingly, a loss of nephron numbers by kidney disease can be confirmed by a corresponding decrease in GFR. Normal values for endogenous creatinine clearance in the dog are between 2 and 4 mL/min/kg body weight.

To understand creatinine clearance as a measure of GFR, consider the following:

1. The concentration of creatinine in the glomerular filtrate is the same as the concentration of creatinine in the plasma (because it is filtered freely).
2. Water is reabsorbed from the tubules but creatinine stays (also, no creatinine is added by tubular secretion) and becomes more concentrated.
3. The excreted creatinine represents all that was present when filtered.
4. The plasma concentration of creatinine represents its concentration in the filtrate as the filtrate was formed.
5. The filtrate volume can be determined by dividing the urine concentration of creatinine by its plasma concentration.
6. The volume per unit of time (mL/min) is obtained by appropriate application of the urine flow rate.

Creatinine clearance (C_{cr}) as determined by the endogenous method would consider the following:

1. Collection of urine for a 24-hour period
2. Volume collected divided by 1,440 (number of minutes in 24 hours) to determine urine flow rate ($\dot{V}$) in milliliters per minute
3. Determination of creatinine concentration for urine [U_{cr}] and for plasma [P_{cr}]
4. The product of the urine concentration [U_{cr}] and the $\dot{V}$ provides the excretion rate ([U_{cr}] $\dot{V}$)
5. The quotient obtained from [U_{cr}] $\dot{V} \div$ [P_{cr}] is further divided by the animal's weight in kilograms to provide an estimation of GFR in milligrams per minute per kilogram
6. Increasing values for [P_{cr}] result in decreasing values for C_{cr}

An example for the determination of GFR by the endogenous creatinine clearance method is provided in *Table 11-5*.

■ MAINTENANCE OF ACID-BASE BALANCE

1. **Study the secretion of H⁺ by the kidney.**
2. **Does the secretion of H⁺ result in reclaiming bicarbonate for the ECF?**
3. **Would greater H⁺ production and secretion involve greater reabsorption of HCO₃⁻?**
4. **Is pulmonary ventilation increased when the Pco₂ of ECF increases? Does this result in the greater elimination of H⁺?**
5. **Is hemoglobin a chemical buffer of the body?**

The relatively constant [H⁺] in ECF is the result of a balance between acids and bases. **Acids** are substances that donate hydrogen ions to a solution; **bases** are substances that accept and bind hydrogen ions from a solution. A disturbance to this balance occurs when acids or bases are added to or removed from the body fluids. A depression of blood pH to below the normal range is known as

TABLE 11-5 DETERMINATION OF GFR BY THE ENDOGENOUS CREATININE CLEARANCE METHOD IN A HEALTHY 14-kg DOG[a]
Collected data:
$\dot{V}$ = urine flow rate = 280 mL ÷ 1,440 minutes = 0.194 mL/min
[U_{cr}] = urine creatinine concentration = 150 mg/dL = 1.5 mg/mL
[P_{cr}] = plasma creatinine concentration = 0.6 mg/dL = 0.006 mg/mL
Calculations:
[U_{cr}] $\dot{V}$ = creatinine excretion rate = 1.5 mg/mL × 0.194 mL/min = 0.291 mg/min
C_{cr} = [U_{cr}] $\dot{V}$/[P_{cr}] = 0.291 mg/min ÷ 0.006 mg/mL = 48.5 mL/min
GFR = C_{cr}/kg body weight = 48.5 mL/min ÷ 14 kg = 3.46 mL/min/kg

[a]Normal values for endogenous creatinine clearance in dogs: 2.98 ± 0.96 mL/min/kg body weight.

acidemia; a value above the normal pH is called **alkalemia**. The disturbance caused by the addition of excess acid or the removal of base from ECF is known as **acidosis**. If it is caused by the addition of excess base or the loss of acid, the disturbance is called **alkalosis**.

Under normal conditions, acids or bases are added continuously to the body fluids, either because of their ingestion or as the result of their production in cellular metabolism. In disease, an unusual loss or gain of acid or base may occur as a result of insufficient respiratory ventilation, vomiting, diarrhea, or renal insufficiency. Three basic mechanisms are involved in the correction of these disturbances: 1) chemical buffering, 2) respiratory adjustment of blood carbon dioxide concentration, and 3) excretion of hydrogen ions or bicarbonate ions by the kidney.

Relationship of pH to H⁺ Concentration

In their role of regulating the composition of the ECF, the kidneys are important in maintaining a constant hydrogen ion concentration. The pH (negative log of H^+ concentration) of the ECF seldom varies from the normal value of about 7.4. A pH change of 0.3 units doubles or halves the H^+ concentration. For example, a pH of 7.4 represents a H^+ concentration of 40 nEq/L. A pH of 7.1 and 7.7 represents H^+ concentrations of 80 and 20 nEq/L, respectively. In these examples the H^+ has doubled or halved from the normal pH of 7.4. A pH of 7.1 represents severe acidemia, and a pH of 7.7 represents severe alkalemia.

Mechanism of H⁺ Secretion by the Kidneys

The epithelial cells throughout the length of the nephron (except the thin segment of the loop of Henle) secrete H^+, but about 85% is secreted by the proximal tubule. The mechanism associated with H^+ secretion is shown in *Figure 11-24*. The hydration reaction, $CO_2 + H_2O \div H_2CO_3 \div H^+ + HCO_3^-$ (see Chapter 10), occurs in the cytoplasm of the tubular epithelial cell and is accelerated by the presence of carbonic anhydrase (an enzyme) within the cytoplasm. CO_2 in the ECF diffuses freely into the cells. Increased amounts of CO_2 promote more hydration, and decreased amounts reduce hydration. After hydration, the H^+ formed is secreted into the tubular lumen in exchange for a Na^+ (countertransport). The H^+ that is secreted combines with the bicarbonate tubular buffer to form H_2CO_3, which is further dehydrated to the CO_2 and H_2O that become a part of urine. Dehydration at this location is facilitated by **carbonic anhydrase** located on the brush border. The HCO_3^- formed from hydration within the cell diffuses into the ECF, accompanied by the Na^+ exchanged for the H^+. The ECF loses a H^+ and gains a HCO_3^-. The gain of HCO_3^- (into the ECF) and the loss of HCO_3^- (from the tubular fluid) just about balance each other so that pH equilibrium is maintained. When excess hydrogen ions are produced, the phosphates, another tubular buffer, are used for the exchange with H^+ (*Fig. 11-25*). If acidosis persists, the formation and secretion of ammonia by the tubular epithelial cells (*Fig. 11-26*) increases so that the H^+ can continue to be secreted without lowering the pH of the tubular fluids.

An increase in intracellular pH of the tubular epithelial cells, as might be caused by acidosis not related to increased CO_2, is also a stimulus for increased secretion of H^+ by the tubular epithelial cells.

Role of Respiratory System

Equally important in maintaining acid-base equilibrium in the ECF is the respiratory system. During transport from the body cells to the lungs, CO_2 diffuses into the erythrocytes and is hydrated under the influence of carbonic anhydrase. The H^+ that is formed is buffered, and HCO_3^- diffuses into the plasma. When blood passes through the pulmonary capillaries, the diffusion of CO_2 to the alveoli is favored and the hydration reaction (see previous text and Eq. 10-1) is reversed quickly so that H^+ is lost from the ECF. Increases in unbuffered H^+ cause ventilation of the lungs to increase. Accordingly, the gradient for loss of CO_2 into the pulmonary alveoli increases and hydrogen ions are lost at an increased rate. Furthermore, increases in CO_2 also increase ventilation so that extra hydrogen ions from increased hydration are lost at the lungs. The role of pulmonary ventilation in regulating H^+ concentration can thus clearly be seen.

Chemical Buffer Systems

Chemical buffer systems constitute the first line of defense in maintaining constant pH of the ECF. The principal chemical buffer systems are the bicarbonate, phosphate, and protein systems.

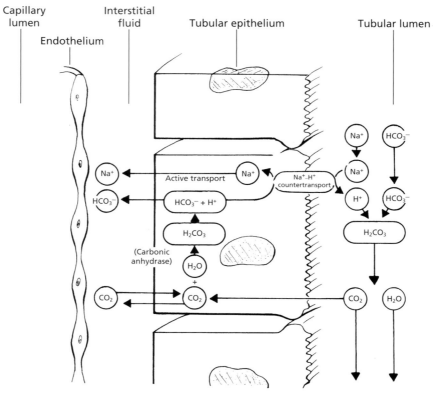

■ **FIGURE 11-24** Mechanism for the renal secretion of H⁺ associated with the bicarbonate buffer system in the tubular fluid.

Mechanisms of Action

The **bicarbonate system** is represented by $NaHCO_3$ and H_2CO_3; they react with acid and base as follows:

$$HCl + NaHCO_3 \rightarrow H_2CO_3 + NaCl$$

Eq. 11-2

$$NaOH + H_2CO_3 \rightarrow NaHCO_3 + H_2O$$

Eq. 11-3

In Equation 11-2, the basic component of the system reacts with an acid to form a weaker acid and a salt. In Equation 11-3, the weak acid component reacts with a base to form a weaker base and H_2O.

The **phosphate buffer system** is represented by NaH_2PO_4 and Na_2HPO_4. They react similarly to acid and base, respectively:

$$HCl + Na_2HPO_4 \rightarrow NaH_2PO_4 + NaCl$$

Eq. 11-4

$$NaOH + NaH_2PO_4 \rightarrow Na_2HPO_4 + H_2O$$

Eq. 11-5

Proteins act as buffers because their molecules contain a large number of acidic and basic groups. The basic groups (R-NH₂) act as buffers by taking up H⁺ and forming cations (R-NH₃⁺). The acidic groups (R-COOH) act as buffers by losing H⁺ and forming anions (R-COO⁻).

Relative Merits of Buffer Systems

The bicarbonate buffer system is rather weak because: 1) the pH of the body fluids is about 7.4 and the pK (negative logarithm of the dissociation constant) of the system is 6.1 (buff-

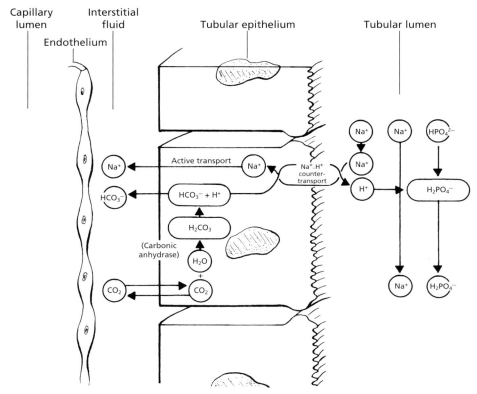

■ **FIGURE 11-25** Mechanism for the renal secretion of H$^+$ associated with the phosphate buffer system in the tubular fluid.

ering power greatest when pH = pK), and 2) the concentration of the buffering elements is not high. The bicarbonate system is unique, however, because it can be adjusted by the respiratory system and the kidneys (i.e., the components are elements of the hydration reaction).

The concentrations of the phosphate buffer components are relatively low in the ECF, but are higher in the intracellular fluids. Accordingly, the phosphate buffer system is more important as an intracellular buffer, not only because of concentration, but also because its pK (6.8) is closer to intracellular pH. Phosphate buffer is also important as a buffer in the kidney tubular fluids when H$^+$ is secreted.

Because of their abundance, the proteins of the body cells, plasma, and hemoglobin (protein of red blood cells) are important

chemical buffers. Anemic animals (low hemoglobin concentration) quickly become acidic when they are exerted. Hemoglobin is normally the most plentiful chemical buffer in the body.

The various buffer systems are not isolated from each other in the body. According to the isohydric principal, any condition causing H$^+$ change results in a balance of all the buffer systems, so they change at the same time (the buffers buffer the buffers).

■ **AVIAN URINARY SYSTEM**

1. Understand the division of the kidneys of birds into lobes and lobules and the structural detail of a lobule.

2. What are the two nephron types associated with avian kidneys?

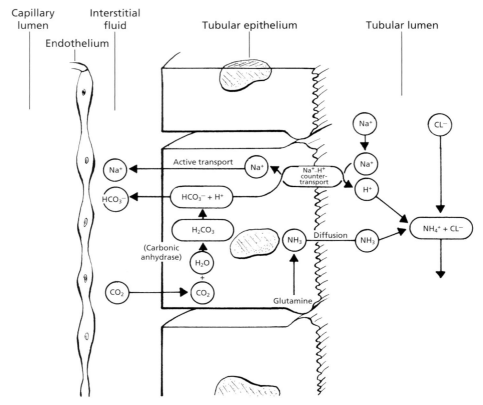

■ **FIGURE 11-26** Mechanism for the secretion of H⁺ associated with the secretion of ammonia by the tubular epithelial cells.

3. What is the location of each nephron type within a lobule?

4. What is lacking in the reptilian nephron that makes it incapable of concentrating urine?

5. Where are the loops of Henle of the mammalian nephrons located within a lobule?

6. What structures are located in the medullary cone?

7. Would the tubular fluid from reptilian nephrons be exposed to the osmotic gradient in the medullary cone on its exit from the kidney?

8. What is the exit route for ureteral urine?

9. What is the cloaca?

10. Avian kidneys can alternate between reptilian and mammalian nephron types. Which nephron type would promote greater water conservation?

11. Describe the renal portal system.

12. Where does renal portal blood enter the vascular supply that perfuses the renal tubules?

13. What is the value of two sources of blood perfusing the tubules?

14. What is the value of having uric acid precipitated in the tubules?

15. What is the principal nitrogenous component of avian urine?

16. What organs in birds are sites for the conversion of ammonia to uric acid?

17. What is the principal site for the post renal modification of ureteral urine?

18. What is the extent of urine concentration in birds (osmolality maximum)?

19. What color is bird urine, and what is the function of its being mixed with mucus?

20. How much urine could be produced by a 3-kg hen in a 24-hour period?

There are many similarities between birds and mammals in urine formation and elimination. Also, there are many differences. Similarities include the three phenomena of urine formation, glomerular filtration, tubular reabsorption, and tubular secretion. Also, birds are able to modify the concentration of ureteral urine so that it may have an osmolality that is above or below that of plasma. Differences between mammals and birds include: in birds, the presence of two major nephron types, the presence of a renal portal system, formation of uric acid instead of urea as the major end product of nitrogen metabolism, and postrenal modification of ureteral urine.

Anatomic Features

Avian kidneys are paired retroperitoneal structures that are fitted closely to the bony depressions on the dorsal wall of the fused pelvis. Each kidney has **cranial**, **middle**, and **caudal lobes**. Ureters transport urine from the kidneys to the cloaca (mammalian urinary bladder not present). The **cloaca** is a common collection site, not only for the urinary organs, but also for the digestive and reproductive organs (*Fig. 11-27*). Each lobe has lobules (*Fig. 11-28*), and a lobule gives the appearance of a *mushroom*, with its *cortex* corresponding to the cap of the mushroom and the *medulla* corresponding to the stem.

Avian kidneys are characterized by having two nephron types, **reptilian** and **mammalian** (*Fig. 11-29*). The reptilian types lack loops of Henle and are located in the cortex. They are not capable of concentrating urine. Mammalian-type nephrons have well-defined loops of Henle that are grouped into a **medullary cone** (see Fig. 11-27), the part of the lobule that

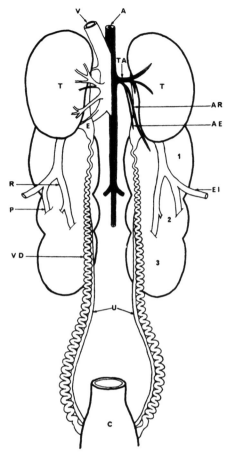

■ **FIGURE 11-27** Ventral view of organs and associated structures of the dorsal abdominal cavity of a rooster (male chicken). A, abdominal aorta; AE, epididymal artery; AR, cranial renal artery; C, cloaca; E, epididymis; EI, external iliac vein; P, caudal renal portal vein; R, renal vein; T, testis; TA, testicular artery; U, ureters; V, caudal vena cava; VD, ductus deferens; 1, 2, and 3, cranial, middle, and caudal lobes of the left kidney, respectively. (From Hodges R. The Histology of the Fowl. New York: Academic Press, 1974.)

corresponds to the stem of a mushroom. Other structures in the medullary cone are those that would be found in the medulla of a mammalian kidney, the collecting ducts, and vasa recta. The medullary structures enter at the wider cortical end of the cone. The extent of the vasa recta is shown in *Figure 11-30*. Osmolality of the medullary ISF increases from its

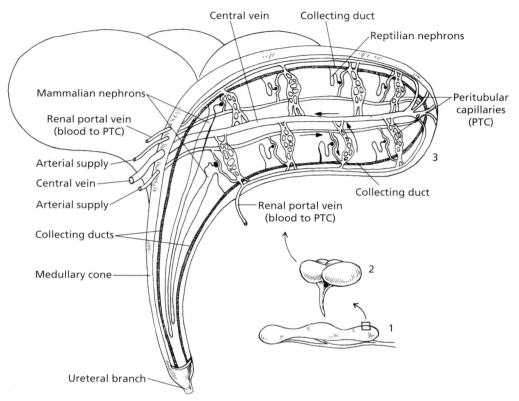

■ **FIGURE 11-28** Arrangement of reptilian and mammalian nephrons within a lobule. 1) An avian kidney with its three lobes. 2) A number of lobules from a lobe. 3) The inner structure of a lobule. Reptilian nephrons do not have loops of Henle. Mammalian nephrons are located near the medullary cone and extend their loops of Henle into the cone. The tubular fluid from both nephron types is received by common collecting ducts that also extend into the medullary cone, where it is exposed to ISF concentration gradients similar to mammalian kidneys. All urine from a lobule leaves by a common ureteral branch.

beginning near the cortex to the tip of the cone. The osmotic gradient is established by the loops of Henle and is maintained by the vasa recta as in mammalian kidneys, and permits the excretion of urine that has an osmolality greater than that of plasma. All tubular fluid, whether from nephrons of the reptilian or the mammalian type, is exposed to the osmotic gradient because of the exit of the collecting tubules and ducts through the cone to join the common ureteral branch (see Fig. 11-27).

Avian kidneys can alternate between the use of reptilian-type and mammalian-type nephrons, depending on the need for water conservation. Greater use of mammalian-type nephrons would promote greater water conservation. When both nephron types are functional, 25% of the filtrate comes from mammalian-type nephrons and 75% from reptilian-type nephrons.

Renal Portal System

A unique feature of the avian kidney is its **renal portal system** for part of the blood supply that perfuses the tubules. The renal portal blood is venous blood that comes to the kidney from the hindlimbs via the external iliac and sciatic veins (*Fig. 11-31*). This venous

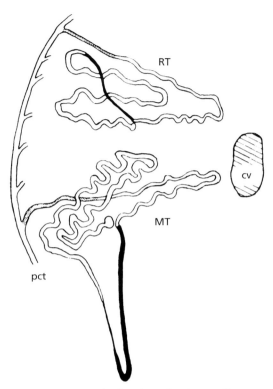

■ **FIGURE 11-29** The location of avian reptilian-type (RT) and mammalian-type (MT) nephrons relative to an intralobular central vein (cv) and a perilobular collecting tubule (pct). The intermediate segment of the RT nephron and the nephron loop of the MT nephron are shown in black. The finely stippled areas are beginning collecting tubules. (From Johnson O. Urinary organs. In: King A, McClelland J, eds. Form and Function in Birds. San Diego: Academic Press, 1979.)

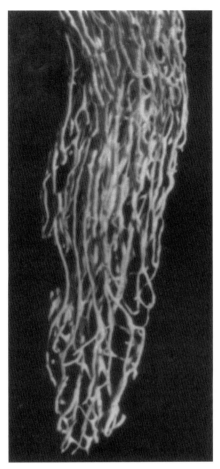

■ **FIGURE 11-30** The vasa recta and associated capillary plexus from an avian kidney medullary cone. Microfill injection via ischiadic artery. (From Johnson O. Urinary organs. In: King A, McClelland J, eds. Form and Function in Birds. San Diego: Academic Press, 1979.)

blood enters the kidney from its periphery, supplying afferent blood to the peritubular capillaries. Within the peritubular capillaries, it is mixed with efferent arteriolar blood coming from the glomeruli (*Fig. 11-32*). The mixture perfuses the tubules and proceeds to the central vein of the lobule. The renal portal system supplies one-half to two-thirds of the blood to the kidneys. There is a valve, known as a **renal portal valve**, located at the juncture of the right and left renal veins and their associated iliac veins (see Fig. 11-30). Closure of the valve would have the potential of diverting more blood to the renal portal system. Respective adrenergic and cholinergic innervation affect valve closure and opening.

Uric Acid Formation and Excretion

The metabolism of proteins and amino acids results in the production of nitrogenous end products. Among each of the many different kinds of animals, either ammonia, urea, or uric acid accounts for two-thirds or more of the

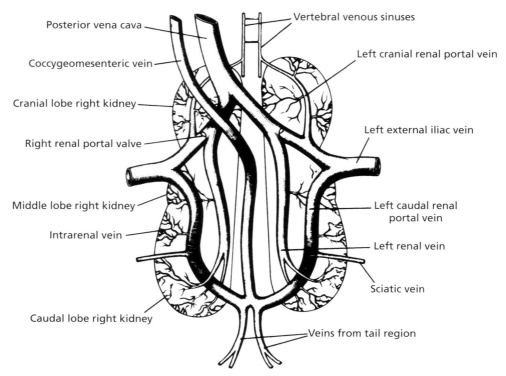

■ **FIGURE 11-31** The veins associated with the renal portal system of birds. Blood arrives from the hindlimbs via the external iliac and sciatic veins. Also shown is a renal portal valve. Its closure has potential for diverting more blood to the renal portal system. (From Sturkie PD. Kidneys, extrarenal salt excretion, and urine. In: Sturkie PD, ed. Avian Physiology. 4th Ed. New York: Springer-Verlag, 1986.)

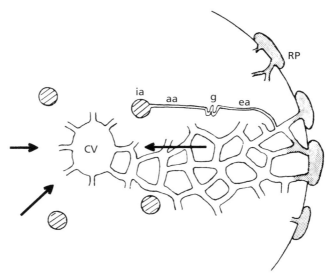

■ **FIGURE 11-32** Intralobular blood flow. Intralobular artery (ia) blood supplies afferent arterioles (aa) going to glomeruli (g). Blood leaving the glomeruli via efferent arterioles (ea) enters the peritubular capillaries and mixes with blood from branches of the renal portal (RP) veins. Peritubular blood enters the central vein (CV) of each lobule. Arrows indicate direction of blood flow. (From Johnson O. Urinary organs. In: King A, McClelland J, eds. Form and Function in Birds. Academic Press: San Diego, 1979.)

total nitrogen excreted. Accordingly, animals are divided into three groups depending on whether their main nitrogenous excretory product is ammonia, urea, or uric acid. Because ammonia is a very toxic substance, it must be either excreted rapidly or converted to a substance that is less toxic, such as urea or uric acid. **Ammonia excretion** is encountered only in animals that are entirely aquatic, in which the ammonia can be quickly discharged into their aquatic environment. The **urea excreting group** is found among mammals and among amphibians.

In reptiles and birds, **uric acid** is formed instead of urea because these animals develop in eggshells that are impervious to water. The excretion of urea obligates water excretion (because of its effective osmotic pressure) and, because there is only limited water in eggs, it must be conserved. Uric acid reaches a certain concentration, and it precipitates. As a precipitate (no effective osmotic pressure), there is no water obligated in its excretion. If urea were excreted it would be necessary to eliminate the liquid urine formed, and this is not possible within eggs.

Just as urea is formed in the liver of mammals from ammonia, so is uric acid formed in the liver of birds from ammonia. The kidneys of birds are also a site for the formation of uric acid. Uric acid precipitates in the tubules because the extra blood from the renal portal system that perfuses the tubules leads to greater tubular secretion and consequently greater tubular concentration. The greater amounts in the tubules exceed uric acid solubility, and it precipitates. Uric acid continues in the tubules in its precipitated form and appears in the urine as a white coagulum. Because uric acid is no longer in solution, it does not contribute to the effective osmotic pressure of the tubular fluid, and obligatory water loss is avoided.

Concentration of Avian Urine

The permeability of the collecting tubules and collecting ducts responds to ADH as in mammals. Accordingly, with a need for water conservation, the tubular fluid reaches osmotic equilibrium with the ISF surrounding the tubules, and it becomes hyperosmotic to plasma as collecting tubules and ducts pass through the medullary cone. The hypertonicity of the ISF of the medullary cone is created by NaCl transport from the ascending limbs of the loops of Henle. The maximum concentration of urine that is attainable in birds is much less than for mammals and is about 540 mOsm/kg H_2O, which is the concentration of the ISF at the tips of the medullary cones. A maximum urine-to-plasma osmolal ratio would be about 1.58:1.

Modification of Ureteral Urine

After presentation of ureteral urine to the cloaca, there may be retrograde flow into the colon. In the colon, Na^+ is reabsorbed and water is reabsorbed by osmosis. The same phenomenon could occur in the ceca if retrograde flow occurred to that level. There is no water reabsorbed from the cloaca even though there may be some Na^+ reabsorption.

Urine Characteristics and Flow

Bird urine is cream-colored and contains thick mucus. The precipitated uric acid is mixed with the mucus, whereby the mucus secretion facilitates transport of the precipitate, similar to the mucus in equine urine that facilitates the transport of the carbonates and phosphates that precipitate. Urine flow for hydrated chickens is reported to be about 18 mL/kg/hr, and for hydrated turkeys it is about 30 mL/kg/hr.

■SUGGESTED READING

Cormack DH. Essential Histology. 2nd Ed. Baltimore: Lippincott Williams & Wilkins, 2001.

Frandson RD, Wilke WL, Fails AD. Anatomy and Physiology of Farm Animals. 6th Ed. Baltimore: Lippincott Williams & Wilkins, 2003.

Goldstein DL, Skadhauge E. Renal and extrarenal regulation of body fluid composition. In: Whittow GC, ed. Sturkie's Avian Physiology. 5th Ed. San Diego: Academic Press, 2000.

Guyton AC, Hall JE. Textbook of Medical Physiology. 10th Ed. Philadelphia: WB Saunders, 2000.

Henrickson C. Urinary system. In: Dellmann HD, Eurell JA, eds. Textbook of Veterinary Histology. 5th Ed. Baltimore: Lippincott Williams & Wilkins, 1998.

Reece WO. Kidney function in mammals. In: Reece WO, ed. Dukes' Physiology of Domestic Animals. 12th Ed. Ithaca, NY: Cornell University Press, 2004.

 SELF EVALUATION—CHAPTER 11

GROSS ANATOMY OF THE KIDNEYS AND URINARY BLADDER

1. What prevents the backflow of urine from the bladder into the ureters?
   a. Angle of ureter entrance at the ureterovesicular junction
   b. A discrete muscular sphincter
   c. Constant peristaltic waves toward the bladder
   d. There is nothing to prevent it.

2. Which one of the following structures conveys urine from the renal pelvis to the urinary bladder?
   a. Urethra
   b. Distal tubule
   c. Ureter
   d. Loop of Henle

3. A heart-shaped kidney is characteristic of:
   a. dogs.
   b. horses.
   c. pigs.
   d. cattle.

4. Innervation to the kidneys is provided by:
   a. sympathetic division of autonomics.
   b. parasympathetic division of autonomics.
   c. cranial nerves.
   d. spinal nerves.

THE NEPHRON

5. Which one of the following nephron parts is first encountered by blood entering from the afferent arteriole?
   a. Bowman capsule
   b. Glomerulus
   c. Proximal convoluted tubule
   d. Loop of Henle

6. Where would one expect to find the lowest hydrostatic pressure?
   a. Glomerulus
   b. Peritubular capillaries
   c. Renal vein
   d. Renal artery

FORMATION OF URINE

7. The composition of glomerular filtrate is the same as tubular fluid.
   a. True
   b. False

8. Which one of the following measurements would be the least at any one time?
   a. Renal plasma flow
   b. Renal blood flow
   c. Glomerular filtration rate

GLOMERULAR FILTRATION

9. The counterpart to the venous end of a muscle capillary (favors reabsorption) would be the:
   a. glomerulus.
   b. peritubular capillaries.
   c. vasa recta.
   d. renal vein.

10. Renin secretion in response to detection by macula densa cells of reduced [Na^+] leads to:
    a. the formation of angiotensin II.
    b. glomerular efferent arteriolar constriction.

c. an increased filtration fraction.

d. all of the above.

TUBULAR REABSORPTION AND SECRETION

11. Which one of the following nephron parts accounts for the largest amount of water, glucose, amino acid, and vitamin reabsorption?
    a. Glomerulus
    b. Distal tubule
    c. Proximal tubule
    d. Collecting tubule

12. The plasma concentration at which glucose first appears in the urine would be defined as its:
    a. downfall.
    b. transport maximum.
    c. renal threshold.

13. The greatest part of Na^+ reabsorption occurs in the:
    a. proximal tubule.
    b. loop of Henle.
    c. cortical collecting tubules and medullary collecting ducts.

COUNTERCURRENT MECHANISM

14. Which one of the following nephron parts is associated with the establishment of a high salt concentration in the medulla of the kidney?
    a. Bowman capsule
    b. Proximal tubule
    c. Loop of Henle
    d. Distal tubule

15. Loss of solute (Na^+, Cl^-) and retention of H_2O that occurs in the ascending limb of the loop of Henle causes the tubular fluid to be _____ as compared with plasma.
    a. hypotonic
    b. hypertonic
    c. isotonic

16. With regard to the tubular transport of urea:
    a. it is actively transported from the proximal tubule so that about one-third to one-half of its presence continues to the loop of Henle.
    b. it is essentially trapped within the nephron tubules throughout their length so that it can be excreted.
    c. it plays no part in the osmoconcentration of the ISF of the renal medulla.
    d. during the process of its being excreted, there is a recirculation of some urea from the inner medullary collecting ducts to the ascending thin limb of the loop of Henle.

CONCENTRATION OF URINE

17. Which one of the following is not associated with diabetes mellitus?
    a. Increased urine formation
    b. Renal threshold for glucose is exceeded.
    c. Increased thirst
    d. Lack of antidiuretic hormone (ADH)

18. When antidiuretic hormone from the posterior pituitary is released in greater amounts, what will happen to the fluid in the collecting ducts of the kidney?
    a. It will become more dilute.
    b. It will remain the same.
    c. It will become more concentrated.

19. If excess glucose fails to be reabsorbed (renal threshold exceeded), the effective osmotic pressure in the tubular lumen:
    a. increases.
    b. decreases.
    c. becomes ineffective.

20. Detection of increased osmoconcentration of the ECF by osmoreceptors in the hypothalamus would result in:
    a. more concentrated urine.
    b. more dilute urine.
    c. no change in urine concentration.

EXTRACELLULAR FLUID VOLUME REGULATION

21. Receptors responding to acute changes in blood volume are:
    a. macula densa cells.
    b. in the left atrium of the heart.
    c. in the hypothalamus.
    d. in the renal pelvis.

22. The first of the graded responses to decreased left atrial filling (hypovolemia) is:
    a. renin secretion from JG granular cells.
    b. increased renal tubular reabsorption of Na^+.
    c. renal vasoconstriction.

ALDOSTERONE

23. Which one of the following hormones promotes the tubular reabsorption of Na^+ and the tubular secretion of K^+?
    a. Antidiuretic hormone
    b. Secretin
    c. Aldosterone
    d. Oxytocin

24. Aldosterone, secreted by the adrenal cortex, regulates:
    a. plasma $[K^+]$.
    b. plasma $[Na^+]$.
    c. both $[Na^+]$ and $[K^+]$ of plasma.

OTHER HORMONES WITH KIDNEY ASSOCIATION

25. What hormone acts on the kidney to activate vitamin D, which in turn increases Ca^{2+} absorption from the intestine?
    a. Calcitonin
    b. Thyroxine
    c. Aldosterone
    d. Parathyroid hormone

MICTURITION

26. The physiologic term for emptying the bladder is:

a. parturition.
b. micturition.
c. defecation.
d. ammunition.

27. Tubular fluid is transported from the Bowman capsule to the renal pelvis by:
    a. action of cilia.
    b. peristalsis.
    c. hydrostatic pressure gradient.
    d. bucket brigade.

CHARACTERISTICS OF MAMMALIAN URINE

28. The principal nitrogenous constituent of mammalian urine is:
    a. amino acids.
    b. uric acid.
    c. urea.
    d. ammonia.

29. Mucus in the urine of horses:
    a. prevents infection.
    b. slows micturition.
    c. provides a carrier for precipitated carbonates and phosphates and prevents their collection in the renal pelvis.
    d. prevents splashing.

RENAL CLEARANCE

30. A renal clearance value for urea of 50 mL/min means that:
    a. 50 mL of the RPF are completely cleared of their urea, and the remainder continues through the kidney with none extracted.
    b. 50 mL of filtrate are formed each minute, and all of the urea is excreted.
    c. each mL of the RPF contributes urea to that which is excreted, but the amount excreted in the urine each minute would require all of the urea in 50 mL of the RPF.

31. Creatinine clearance provides information about:

a. renal plasma flow.
b. glomerular filtration rate (and hence functional renal mass).
c. renal blood flow.
d. all of the above.

MAINTENANCE OF ACID-BASE BALANCE

32. The kidneys and lungs have no role in the maintenance of body acid-base balance.
    a. True
    b. False

33. Increases in P_{CO_2} from poor ventilation would increase the secretion of H^+s by the kidney.
    a. True
    b. False

34. Increased $[H^+]$ because of poor kidney function and consequent reduced H^+ secretion would stimulate ventilation and increase CO_2 loss, which would assist in lowering $[H^+]$.
    a. True
    b. False

AVIAN URINARY SYSTEM

35. Which one of the following nephron components is lacking in reptilian nephrons?
    a. Proximal tubule
    b. Loop of Henle
    c. Distal tubule
    d. Collecting tubule

36. Renal portal system blood is:
    a. venous blood.
    b. arterial blood.

37. Reptilian nephron tubular fluid goes directly to the ureters and escapes the medullary cones, where it could become concentrated.

a. True
b. False

38. The avian nephron type that provides for water conservation is the:
    a. reptilian nephron.
    b. mammalian nephron.

39. Renal portal blood enters the vascular supply perfusing the renal tubules at the level of the:
    a. glomerulus.
    b. peritubular capillaries.
    c. vasa recta.
    d. vena cava.

40. The principal nitrogenous component of avian urine is:
    a. ammonia.
    b. urea.
    c. uric acid.

41. Uric acid precipitates in the renal tubules to:
    a. avoid ammonia toxicity.
    b. avoid obligation of water excretion.
    c. make it more slippery.
    d. have a better mix with feces.

42. Ammonia is converted to uric acid in birds:
    a. in the liver.
    b. in the kidneys.
    c. in the liver and kidneys.

43. Water reabsorption from urine deposited in the cloaca may occur in the:
    a. cloaca.
    b. colon.
    c. colon and cecum.

44. A urine-to-plasma osmolal ratio of $3:1$ is not uncommon in birds.
    a. True
    b. False

ANSWERS TO SELF EVALUATION—CHAPTER 11

1.	a	12.	c	23.	c	34.	a
2.	c	13.	a	24.	a	35.	b
3.	b	14.	c	25.	d	36.	a
4.	a	15.	a	26.	b	37.	b
5.	b	16.	d	27.	c	38.	b
6.	c	17.	d	28.	c	39.	b
7.	b	18.	c	29.	c	40.	c
8.	c	19.	a	30.	c	41.	b
9.	b	20.	a	31.	b	42.	c
10.	d	21.	b	32.	b	43.	c
11.	c	22.	a	33.	a	44.	b

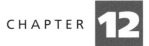

Digestion and Absorption

- **INTRODUCTORY CONSIDERATIONS**
- **THE ORAL CAVITY AND PHARYNX**
  Teeth
  Tongue
  Pharynx
- **THE SIMPLE STOMACH**
  Esophagus
  Stomach
- **INTESTINES**
  Small Intestine
  Large Intestine
- **ACCESSORY ORGANS**
- **COMPOSITION OF FOODSTUFFS**
  Carbohydrates
  Proteins
  Lipids
  Accessory Foods
- **PREGASTRIC MECHANICAL FUNCTIONS**
  Prehension
  Mastication
  Deglutition
- **GASTROINTESTINAL MOTILITY**
  Segmentation and Peristalsis
- **MECHANICAL FUNCTIONS OF THE STOMACH AND SMALL INTESTINE**
  Delay of Gastric Emptying
  Emesis
  Mechanical Functions of the Small Intestine

- **MECHANICAL FUNCTIONS OF THE LARGE INTESTINE**
  Defecation
  Intestinal Transport of Electrolytes and Water
- **DIGESTIVE SECRETIONS**
  Saliva
  Gastric Secretions
  Pancreatic Secretions
  Biliary Secretions
- **DIGESTION AND ABSORPTION**
  Carbohydrates
  Proteins
  Fats
  Microbial Digestion in the Large Intestine
- **THE RUMINANT STOMACH**
  Structure and Function
- **CHARACTERISTICS OF RUMINANT DIGESTION**
  Rumination
  Gas Production and Eructation
- **CHEMISTRY AND MICROBIOLOGY OF THE RUMEN**
- **RUMINANT METABOLISM**
  Gluconeogenesis
  Energy Production
  Ruminant Ketosis and Bloat
- **AVIAN DIGESTION**

The maintenance of life requires that animals obtain nutrients essential for the body processes from food. Animals can live for a period of time without food; in such a situation, the body stores of energy and finally the tissues themselves are broken down and metabolized through biochemical conversion. During prolonged and continued deprivation of food, however, death finally ensues as a result of starvation.

It is generally believed that food is in the body after its acquisition and ingestion, but the digestive tract is a hollow, tubelike structure that extends from the mouth to the anus, so materials within its lumen are still, strictly speaking, outside the body. Therefore, the acquisition of food must be followed by processes that divide food into smaller parts through both physical and chemical means, so that the structural units or other simple chemical compounds can finally enter the body by crossing the intestinal barrier. The process associated with this division (or, as often stated, degradation of food to more basic units) is called digestion, and the process of crossing the intestinal epithelium and entering the blood is called absorption. The reactions and conversions necessary to provide energy, build tissues, and synthesize secretions constitute intermediary metabolism. The continuance of intermediary metabolism in the body depends on digestion and absorption.

■ INTRODUCTORY CONSIDERATIONS

1. **Know the order of the principal parts of the digestive tract. What are the accessory organs of the digestive tract?**

Animals are classified, according to the diet in their natural state, as carnivorous, omnivorous, or herbivorous. The extremes are represented by the **carnivorous**, or **flesh-eating**, animals and by the **herbivorous**, or **plant-eating** animals. Those subsisting on both flesh and plants are **omnivorous** animals. Because of the diversity of diet, various parts of the digestive system developed in different ways. Whereas the dog, a carnivorous animal, has an inconspicuous cecum, the horse, a herbivorous animal, has a voluminous cecum. The cecum of the horse facilitates the digestion of coarse plant materials by microbial fermentation. Only minimal fermentation is necessary in the dog, so its cecum is minimally developed. Whatever fermentation is required in the dog occurs mainly in the colon. The pig is an omnivorous animal. It not only has a relatively long small intestine for digesting and absorbing foodstuffs not requiring fermentation, but it also has an expanded part of its colon in which fermentation of the fibrous parts of its diet takes place. A comparison of the gastrointestinal tracts of the dog, horse, and cattle (a ruminant) is shown in *Figure 12-1*.

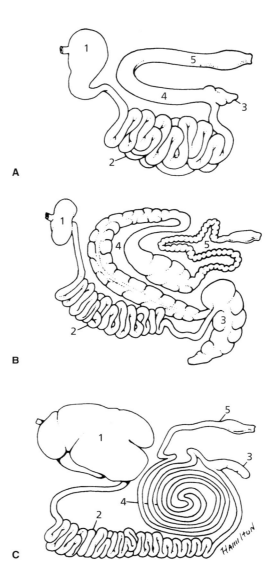

■ **FIGURE 12-1** Comparisons of gastrointestinal tracts of the dog (**A**), of the horse (**B**), and of cattle (**C**). **1)** Stomach; **2)** small intestine; **3)** cecum; **4)** ascending colon in dog, large colon in horse, coiled colon (ansa spiralis) in cattle; **5)** descending colon. (From Dyce KM, Sack WO, Wensing CJG. Textbook of Veterinary Anatomy. 2nd Ed. Philadelphia: WB Saunders, 1996.)

The principal parts of the digestive tract as it courses through the body are the mouth, teeth, tongue, pharynx, esophagus, stomach, small intestine, and large intestine. The salivary glands, liver, and pancreas serve as accessory organs of the digestive tract. Generally, the digestive tract among the various animal species has the same parts, but the size and function of the parts for any one species differ according to the characteristics of the natural diet.

■ THE ORAL CAVITY AND PHARYNX

1. **What are the components of a dental formula? How does one read a dental formula?**
2. **Define the various exposed surfaces of a tooth.**
3. **How do points develop on the upper and lower arcades of cheek teeth in the horse (see Fig. 12-2)?**
4. **What is meant by the terms "full mouth," "in wear," and "smooth mouth" when determining the age of a horse by examination of its teeth?**
5. **What is the unique characteristic of muscle fiber direction in the tongue? What purpose is served?**
6. **What function is served by the papillae of the tongue? What sensory organs are located in the vicinity of certain papillae?**

The oral cavity is the most cranial part of the digestive tract and is often referred to as the mouth. It is where food is first received and where reduction in the size of food particles begins. Associated with reduction in size, the food particles are mixed with saliva so that subsequent swallowing of the food mass (**bolus**) is facilitated. The teeth and tongue are structures within the oral cavity that assist digestion.

Teeth

The teeth mechanically reduce the size of ingested food particles by grinding, and at the same time increase the surface area of the food for chemical and microbiologic degradation. Teeth are also used for cutting; in this way food can be first presented to the mouth. In some species, the teeth serve a protective function when used to inflict wounds and a food gathering function when used to capture and kill other animals.

The four types of teeth are described according to their location and function. The **incisors** are the most forward teeth in the mouth and are used principally for cutting; they are sometimes called nippers. Next to the incisors are the **canine teeth**, also known as fangs, eye teeth, and tusks. The shape of the canines permits their use for tearing and separation of a food mass. The **premolars** are located caudal to the canines, and their shape and size are more suitable for grinding. This function is also carried out by larger teeth located caudal to them, the **molars**. The molars and premolars are collectively called **cheek teeth**.

A **dental formula** indicates the numbers of incisors (I), canines (C), premolars (P), and molars (M) on one side of the mouth. For the permanent teeth of the cow, the dental formula is I 0/4 C 0/0 P 3/3 M 3/3. The numerator of the fraction represents the teeth in the upper jaw, and the denominator represents the teeth in the lower jaw. The formula represents the number of teeth on one side of the mouth, so the total number is twice that shown. For the cow the total number of teeth is 32. The cow has a firm **dental pad** in place of the upper incisors, which provides for the compression necessary to shear forage against the lower incisors. The first appearance of a tooth is referred to as **eruption**. Dental formulas and eruption times for **permanent teeth** of various species are listed in *Table 12-1*.

Several terms are used to describe the exposed surfaces of a tooth. The **grinding (table) surface** makes contact with a tooth

TABLE 12-1 DENTAL FORMULAS AND ERUPTION TIMES FOR PERMANENT TEETH

TEETH	HORSE	COW	SHEEP	PIG	DOG
		PERMANENT FORMULA			
UJ (Number)	3 1 3 or 4 3	0 0 3 3	0033	3 1 4 3	3 1 3 2
	2 (I-C-P-M)	2 (I-C-P-M)	2 (I-C-P-M)	2 (I-C-P-M)	2 (I-C-P-M)
LJ (Number)	3 1 3 3	4 0 3 3	4 0 3 3	3 1 4 3	3 1 4 3
		PERMANENT ERUPTION			
Incisors					
I1	2-1/2 yr	1-1/2–2 yr	1–1-1/2 yr	1 yr	3–5 mo
I2	3-1/2 yr	2–2-1/2 yr	1-1/2–2 yr	16–20 mo	3–5 mo
I3	4-1/2 yr	3 yr	2-1/2–3 yr	8–10 mo	4–5 mo
I4		3-1/2–4 yr	3-1/2–4 yr		
Canines					
C	4–5 yr			9–10 mo	4–6 mo
Premolars					
P1	5–6 mo	2–2-1/2 yr	1-1/2–2 yr	12–15 mo	4–5 mo
P2	2-1/2 yr	1-1/2–2-1/2 yr	1-1/2–2 yr	12–15 mo	5–6 mo
P3	3 yr	2-1/2–3 yr	1-1/2–2 yr	12–15 mo	5–6 mo
P4	4 yr			12–15 mo	5–6 mo
Molars					
M1	9–12 mo	5–6 mo	3–5 mo	4–6 mo	5–6 mo
M2	2 yr	1-1/2 yr	9–12 mo	8–12 mo	6–7 mo
M3	3-1/2–4 yr	2–2-1/2 yr	1-1/2–2 yr	18–20 mo	6–7 mo

Note: I, incisors; C, canines; P, premolars; M, molars; UJ, upper jaw; LJ, lower jaw.
From Frandson RD, Spurgeon TL. Anatomy and Physiology of Farm Animals. 5th Ed. Philadelphia: Lea and Febiger, 1992.

from the opposite jaw and is the principal wearing surface. The side of the tooth next to the tongue is called the **lingual surface**. The outer surface is **labial** if next to the lips and **buccal** if next to the cheek. The **contact surface** is next to a neighboring tooth of the same **arcade (row)**. The upper arcades of cheek teeth (molars and premolars) are slightly wider apart than the lower arcades of cheek teeth. Also, the upper cheek teeth have a wider table surface than the lower cheek teeth. The rota-

tion of the jaw associated with chewing usually provides for even wear of the table surfaces, but uneven wear can develop, particularly in horses, in which points are formed that inflict injury to the buccal or lingual membranes (*Fig. 12-2*). Eating becomes painful, and the points must be filed off with a dental rasp. The procedure of removing the points is referred to as floating the teeth.

The **age of horses** can be approximated by examining the lower incisors, determining

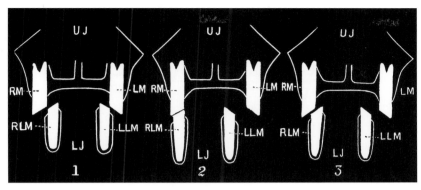

■ **FIGURE 12-2** Schematic transverse section of the upper and lower jaws of the horse between the third and fourth molars showing the position of the tables of the teeth during rest and mastication. **1)** Position of the teeth during rest. The outside edge of the lower row is in apposition with the inside edge of the upper. **2)** Jaws fully crossed, masticating from left to right (lower jaw movement). The tables of both right upper and lower molars now rest on each other. **3)** Position halfway through mastication. The outer half of the right lower tooth wears against the inner half of the right upper. Note the potential for developing "points" on the cheek side of the uppers and on the tongue side of the lowers. Right lower jaw movement followed by left lower jaw movement. UJ, upper jaw; LJ, lower jaw; RM, right molar; LM, left molar; RLM, right lower molar; LLM, left lower molar. (From Smith F. Manual of Veterinary Physiology. 5th Ed. Chicago: Alexander Eger, 1921.)

whether the permanent incisors have erupted, and examining for characteristics associated with wear. The three pairs are the **central** (I1), **intermediate** (I2), and **corner** (I3) **incisors**, respectively, according to their location from the midline to the outside. A rule of thumb for their eruption is 2-1/2, 3-1/2, and 4-1/2 years for I1, I2, and I3, respectively. A horse is said to have a **full mouth** when all three pairs of permanent incisors have erupted.

Wear characteristics are related to tooth structure (*Fig. 12-3*). The progression of wear is shown in Figure 12-3C. A mouth is said to be **in wear** when two complete enamel rings are present on the table surface of each incisor. Approximate ages for each pair to be in wear are 6, 7, and 8 years for I1, I2, and I3, respectively. Finally, a judgment is made about disappearance of the **infundibulum** (which eliminates the inner enamel ring) and appearance of the **pulp cavity (dental star)**. The loss of the inner enamel ring and appearance of the dental star occur at about 11, 12, and 13 years of age for each pair of I1, I2, and I3, respectively; a horse has a **smooth mouth** when these occur in all three pairs of incisors. A rough

approximation of age in a horse as determined by the incisors is 5, 10, and 15 years for full mouth, in wear, and smooth mouth, respectively. Much variation occurs naturally, depending on diet and associated wear. The practice of aging horses by "mouthing" was more common when dealers abounded in the draft horse market. Similar practices occur in cattle and sheep husbandry and are related more to eruption than to wear characteristics.

Tongue

The **tongue** is a muscular organ used to maneuver the food mass within the mouth. The tongue can be differentiated microscopically from other muscle tissues because it has fibers oriented in three directions. The multidirectional orientation attests to its extreme mobility. The tongue not only moves food to the table surfaces of the cheek teeth, but also serves as a plunger to move food into the esophagus. It assists some animals in seizing food and bringing it to the mouth.

The rough surface of the tongue is provided for by numerous projections, known as

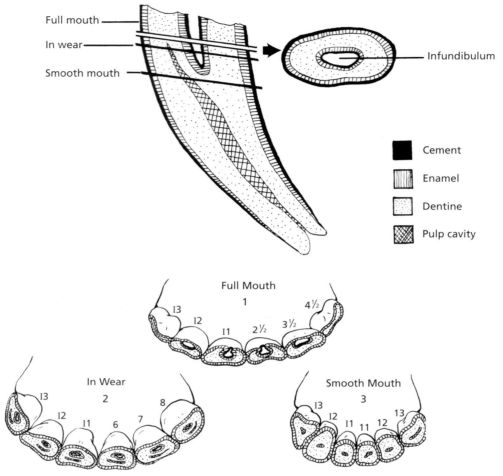

■ **FIGURE 12-3** Incisors of the horse showing wear characteristics. **A)** Longitudinal section. **B)** Transverse section. **C)** Table surfaces. **1** = Full mouth; **2** = In wear; **3** = Smooth mouth. I1 = Central incisors, I2 = Intermediate incisors, I3 = Corner incisors. Approximate age of appearance shown in years by corresponding numbers on right.

papillae. These provide traction for moving the food within the mouth of the animal and help in grooming their own or their offspring's hair surface (*Fig. 12-4*).

The digestive process is assisted by the discriminatory taste buds located on the tongue surface within the **vallate** and **fungiform papillae** (see Chapter 5). Discrimination is a more significant factor when food is obtained in its native (unprocessed) state. Distinction can then be made between harmful and proper foods.

Pharynx

The **pharynx** is the common passageway for food and air and is located caudal to the oral and nasal cavities (*Fig. 12-5*) (see Chapter 10). The pharynx opens into the oral and nasal cavities, eustachian tubes, larynx, and esophagus. During its passage through the pharynx, food is prevented from entering the glottis and nasal cavities because of reflex and mechanical factors associated with deglutition (swallowing) (see Deglutition, this chapter). The eusta-

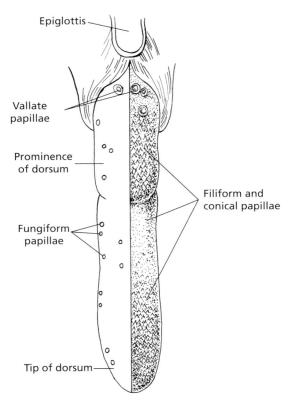

Epiglottis

Vallate
papillae

Prominence
of dorsum

Filiform and
conical papillae

Fungiform
papillae

Tip of dorsum

■ **FIGURE 12-4** A view of the dorsal surface (dorsum linguae) of a bovine tongue with special emphasis on its roughness provided by the papillae. Conical papillae are dominant on the prominence. Rostral to the prominence are large and horny filiform and conical papillae with sharp points directed caudally. These papillae impart to the tip its rasp-like roughness and make it very efficient in the prehension of food. One-half of tongue shown without filiform and conical papillae for contrast.

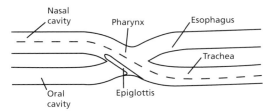

A. Normal Respiration

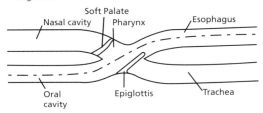

B. Deglutition

■ **FIGURE 12-5** The respective relationship of the nasal and oral cavities to the pharynx during respiration and deglutition. Reflexes associated with deglutition facilitate the safe passage of food from the oral cavity pharynx into the esophagus. Modified from Frandson RD, Spurgeon TL. Anatomy and Physiology of Farm Animals. Malvern, PA: Lea & Febiger, 1992.

chian tubes are air passages leading from the pharynx to the middle ear that provide for air pressure within the middle ear to be equalized to atmospheric pressure. Distortions of the tympanic membrane (eardrum) that might otherwise occur are thereby prevented.

■ THE SIMPLE STOMACH

1. What is the principal tissue of the esophagus? Describe its principal features (consider accommodation of a large bolus or other object). On which side of the neck could a bolus in the esophagus be observed?
2. What are the glandular regions of the stomach, and what are their secretions?
3. Note the extent of the esophageal region (see Fig. 12-7). Is it glandular?
4. What are the forestomachs of the ruminant? What is their function?

Regarding stomach structure and function, domestic animals are represented by two general classes, **ruminants** and **nonruminants**. Cattle, sheep, and goats belong to the former class; the other domestic animals belong to the latter. The stomach of nonruminants is relatively simple, consisting of only one compartment. For this reason it is frequently referred to as the simple stomach. The stomach of birds is unique and will be described separately. That of ruminants is more complex, consisting typically of four compartments, only one of which secretes gastric juice. Digestion in the simple stomach will be described first, with some references to ruminants, but the major aspects of ruminant digestion are described separately.

Esophagus

The **esophagus** is a muscular tube extending from the pharynx to the stomach. During its course to the stomach, the esophagus enters the thorax at the thoracic inlet and travels within the mediastinal space, in which it is subjected to pressure changes associated with that space. The esophagus finally passes through its opening in the diaphragm and enters the stomach within the abdominal cavity. Food and water are moved from the pharynx to the stomach by contraction waves in the muscular wall. Esophageal sphincters have not been morphologically shown, but have been suggested by functional studies (points at which flow is impeded). Muscle activity can constrict the lumen of the esophagus at certain locations. Accordingly, the esophagus is normally closed at the pharyngeal end by tonic muscle activity providing for a **cranioesophageal sphincter**. Although a thickening, suggestive of a sphincter, occurs at the junction of the esophagus with the stomach (**the cardia**), the opening remains closed, not because of an anatomic sphincter, but because of a closure that is functional in nature. The lumen of the esophagus is normally closed, which produces folds in its inner surface. During passage of a bolus the folds are extended so that a minimum of stretch is necessary. Unusually large objects extend the folds and stretch the mucosal and submucosal layers, and they can become lodged at points of narrowing (e.g., the thoracic inlet).

The pharyngeal opening to the esophagus lies just above the **glottis**, which is the opening to the trachea. On its way to the stomach the esophagus courses along the left side of the trachea. Bolus transport can be observed by watching the left side of the neck (this is particularly apparent in cattle).

The muscle fibers of the esophagus are arranged circularly and longitudinally. In most animals they are striated, but a part of the caudal portion is smooth muscle in some. Because of the muscular nature of the esophagus, it is recovered at slaughter as an edible source for certain meat products.

Stomach

Food is received by the stomach for storage (pending further digestion) and for the beginning of digestion. Because the stomach serves a storage function, it is a dilated portion of the digestive tube. As viewed from the outside (*Fig. 12-6*), it is seen to be subdivided into parts, which are continuous with one another. The **cardia** (entrance area) is located nearest the esophagus and is continued by the **fundus**, which is the dome-shaped part of the stomach. The fundus is adjacent to the **body**, which is the large middle portion. It extends from the fundus to the pyloric antrum. The **pyloric antrum** is the constricted part of the stomach that joins with the duodenum via the **pylorus** (a sphincter muscle that controls stomach emptying). The **lesser curvature** is the very short side of the stomach between the cardia

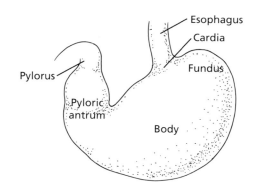

■ **FIGURE 12-6** Parts of the canine stomach.

and pylorus. The greater curvature defines the much longer convex opposite side.

The inner aspect of the stomach has specific regions according to cell type: the esophageal, cardiac gland, fundic gland, and pyloric gland regions. The several regions of the stomach lining for the horse, pig, and ruminant are shown in *Figure 12-7*. The **fundic gland region** includes the entire space between the **cardiac gland** (nearest the cardia) and **pyloric gland regions** (near the pylorus); these glands are sometimes called the **gastric glands**. The cardiac, gastric, and pyloric glands all secrete mucus. In addition, the gastric glands secrete hydrochloric acid (HCl) and pepsinogen by their parietal and neck chief cells, respectively. The pyloric glands also secrete the hormone **gastrin**.

The **esophageal region** is the area immediately around the cardia. The epithelium of the esophageal region is continuous with the lining of the esophagus. It varies in size, depending on the species, and is nonglandular. Notice the differences for the ruminant. The **ruminant forestomachs** (the rumen, reticulum, and omasum) are followed by the true stomach, or **abomasum**. The forestomachs comprise the entire esophageal region, and the epithelium of the abomasum consists mostly of the fundic gland region and pyloric gland region. The cardiac gland region occupies a very small area adjacent to the opening into the abomasum from the omasum.

■ INTESTINES

1. What part of the small intestine receives the pancreatic and bile duct?
2. For those animals not requiring extensive fermentation of their food, where does most of the digestion and absorption take place?
3. Study Figures 12-9, 12-10, 12-11, 12-12, and 12-13. These explain and illustrate the functional aspects of small intestine morphology. Read the text that accompanies the above figures.

4. How is the surface of the small intestine amplified?
5. How are epithelial cells for the villi renewed? What is their replacement time?
6. How does blood and lymph return from the intestines differ?
7. Is fermentation common to the large intestine of all animals? What is the location difference for fermentation between ruminant and nonruminant herbivores?
8. Are the microbes of fermentation available for their own digestion in both ruminant and nonruminant herbivores?
9. Note the differences of the digestive tract between the cecum and transverse colon among the domestic animals. Which animals have an ansa spiralis? Which animal has the double horseshoe (ventral and dorsal large colon)?
10. What is the function of the sacculations (haustra) in the cecum and colon of the pig and horse?
11. What is the rectum?

Stomach content leaving the stomach and entering the intestine is known as **chyme**. Its consistency is fluid or semifluid, and its reaction is acid. The composition of chyme depends on the diet and feeding habits of the animal. In the intestine, chyme undergoes important changes, which constitute intestinal digestion.

Small Intestine

The small intestine is composed of three sections as it proceeds caudally from the pylorus: the **duodenum**, **jejunum**, and **ileum**. The duodenum makes a loop as it turns to cross from the right to the left side. Closely related to the duodenum is the pancreas. The duodenum receives pancreatic secretions involved in

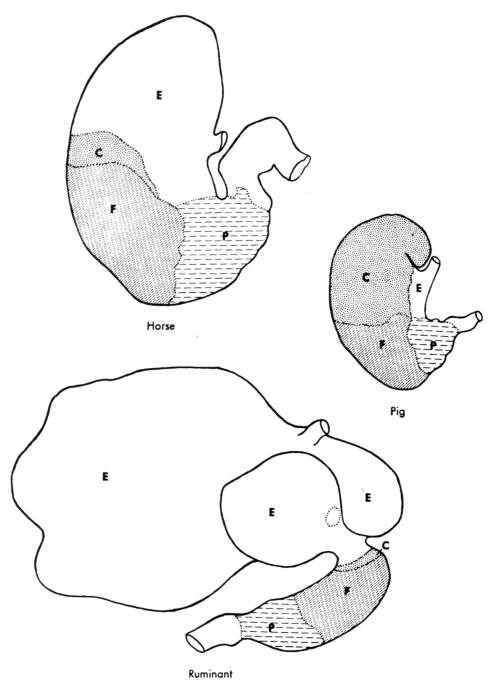

■ **FIGURE 12-7** Inner regions of the stomach in the horse, pig, and ruminant. E, Esophageal region; C, cardiac gland region; F, fundic gland region; P, pyloric gland region. (From Frandson RD, Wilke WL, Fails AD. Anatomy and Physiology of Farm Animals. 6th Ed. Baltimore: Lippincott Williams & Wilkins, 2003.)

digestion through two pancreatic ducts for most species and one for others (*Fig. 12-8*). The duodenum also receives bile formed in the liver through the common bile duct, which transports bile from the liver or gallbladder to the intestine. Most digestion and absorption takes place in the small intestine for those animals not requiring extensive fermentation of their ingested food. A cross section of the small intestine is shown in *Figure 12-9*.

The inner layer of the small intestine, having intimate contact with the contents of the lumen, is composed of an epithelial cell layer known as the **mucosa**. The **submucosa** is a connective tissue layer that provides space for blood vessels, lymph vessels, and nerve fibers. In addition, a sparse layer of smooth muscle fibers is in the submucosa, known as the **muscularis mucosae**. The muscularis mucosae produce folds in the mucosa, thereby increasing surface area. These folds change location to bring different parts of the intestine into more intimate contact with the luminal contents. Individual fibers from the muscularis mucosae attach to villi and cause villus movement when contracting. This facilitates lymph movement and placement of the villus into new areas of luminal fluid. Beneath the submucosa are circular and longitudinal muscle layers composed of smooth muscle fibers. Contraction of these muscles is associated with mixing and propulsive movements of intestinal content.

A nerve network (**Meissner plexus**) in the submucosa is important in controlling secretions of the epithelial cells and blood flow. This network (plexus) also serves a sensory function—it receives signals from stretch receptors (pain perception) and from the gut epithelium. Another nerve plexus (**Auerbach plexus**), between the inner circular and outer longitudinal muscle layers, is important in controlling gastrointestinal movements. These two nerve plexuses are referred to as the enteric nervous system, and extend from the esophagus to the anus. Although the enteric nervous system has its own "pacemakers" and conduction fibers similar to those of the heart, it also has connections with the autonomic nervous system (sympathetic and parasympathetic fibers) that can alter the degree of activity of the enteric nervous system.

The outer layer of the intestine is the **serosa**. It covers the intestine and is continuous with the **mesentery**, which is the suspension for the intestine within the abdominal cavity. The mesentery in turn is continuous with the lining of the abdominal cavity, the peritoneum (see Chapter 1).

A large surface area is presented to the lumen of the small intestine (*Fig. 12-10*). The small intestine has considerable length; average

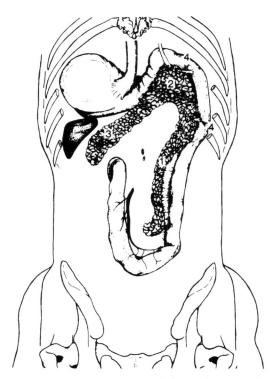

■ **FIGURE 12-8** Dorsal view of the canine stomach, duodenum, and pancreas. **1)** Right lobe of pancreas; **2)** body of the pancreas; **3)** left lobe of pancreas; **4)** pancreatic ducts. The common bile duct is received into the duodenum in close association with the anterior pancreatic duct. (From Adams DR. Canine Anatomy: A Systemic Approach. Ames, IA: Iowa State University Press, 1986.)

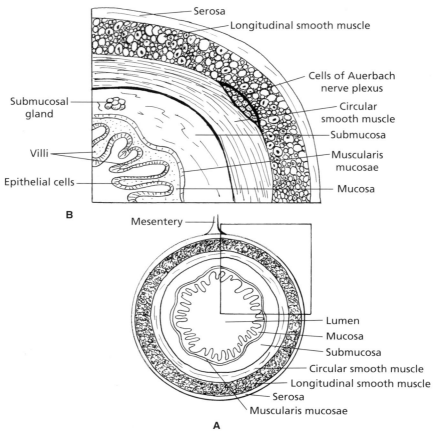

■ **FIGURE 12-9** Schematic representation of the general organizational features of the mammalian gastrointestinal tract. **A)** Cross section of small intestine with its mesenteric suspension that envelops the intestine as its serosa. **B)** Boxed section from A to show greater detail. The Auerbach nerve plexus controls gastrointestinal movements. The Meissner plexus (not shown) is in the submucosa, and it controls secretions and blood flow. The muscularis mucosae produces folds in the mucosa for amplification of surface area.

lengths for several species are given in *Table 12-2.* Its length is accommodated within the abdomen by looping and coiling. Another feature is the unfolding of the intestinal surface, which can be observed when the intestine is opened for inspection. The folds, or plications, are covered with **villi**, and the individual epithelial cells that cover the villi have their own **microvilli** on the luminal surface. The microvilli provide for the greatest amplification of surface area and constitute the brush border (*Fig. 12-11*). The amplification just described provides the small intestine with about 600

times more surface area than that of a smooth cylinder (of comparable volume).

Figure 12-12 illustrates the epithelial surface of the small intestine in more detail. The **crypts of Lieberkühn** are cloistered groups of undifferentiated cells between adjacent villi. These are the only cells of the villi that undergo cell division. Renewal of cells for the villi is provided by the migration of new cells from the crypts toward the tips of the villi. The migration of new cells occurs simultaneously with the continued loss or extrusion of older cells from the villi tips. Moderate physical or

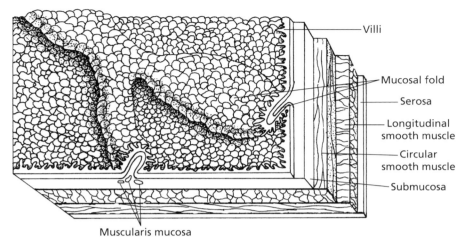

Villi

Mucosal fold

Serosa

Longitudinal smooth muscle

Circular smooth muscle

Submucosa

Muscularis mucosa

■ **FIGURE 12-10** A layered section of intestine as viewed from its inner surface. The folds are produced by strategic contraction of the muscularis mucosae. The projections from the surface represent the villi, another means of surface amplification.

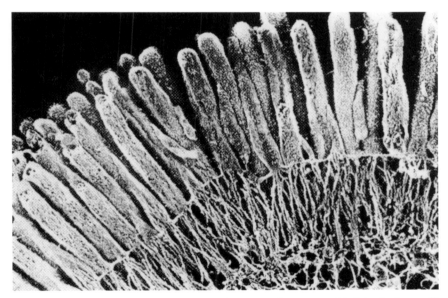

■ **FIGURE 12-11** Photomicrograph of microvilli extending from a small intestine epithelial cell. The cordlike structures extending downward from the microvilli are contractile actin filaments. (From Fawcett DW. Bloom & Fawcett: A Textbook of Histology. 11th Ed. Philadelphia: WB Saunders, 1986. Courtesy of N. Hirokawa and J. Heuser.)

functional loss of villus cells, either through attrition or disease, can be replaced by the dividing cells at the crypt. The normal villous epithelial cell replacement time (migration from crypt to tip) is faster in younger than in older animals (about 2 to 4 versus 7 to 10 days). The undifferentiated cells can become absorptive, mucus-producing, or endocrine cells, which then perform the necessary functions of the small intestine.

TABLE 12-2 LENGTHS OF INTESTINAL PARTS FOR SEVERAL SPECIES

ANIMAL	PART OF INTESTINE	RELATIVE LENGTH (%)	AVERAGE ABSOLUTE LENGTH (M)	RATIO OF BODY LENGTH TO INTESTINE LENGTH
Horse	Small intestine	75	22.4	1:12
	Cecum	4	1.00	
	Large colon	11	3.39	
	Small colon	10	3.08	
	Total	100	29.91	
Ox	Small intestine	81	46.00	1:20
	Cecum	2	0.88	
	Colon	17	10.18	
	Total	100	57.06	
Sheep and goat	Small intestine	80	26.20	1:27
	Cecum	1	0.36	
	Colon	19	6.17	
	Total	100	32.73	
Pig	Small intestine	78	18.29	1:14
	Cecum	1	0.23	
	Colon	21	4.99	
	Total	100	23.51	
Dog	Small intestine	85	4.14	1:6
	Cecum	2	0.08	
	Colon	13	0.60	
	Total	100	4.82	
Cat	Small intestine	83	1.72	1:4
	Large intestine	17	0.35	
	Total	100	2.07	
Rabbit	Small intestine	61	3.56	1:10
	Cecum	11	0.61	
	Colon	28	1.65	
	Total	100	5.82	

From Argenzio RA. General functions of the gastrointestinal tract and their control and integration. In: Swenson MJ, Reece WO, eds. Dukes' Physiology of Domestic Animals. 11th Ed. Ithaca, NY: Cornell University Press, 1993.

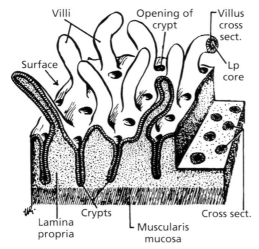

■ **FIGURE 12-12** Three-dimensional representation of the small intestine lining. The villi are fingerlike processes with cores of lamina propria that extend into the lumen. The crypts of Lieberkühn are depressions into the lamina propria (Lp). (From Ham AW. Histology. 7th Ed. Philadelphia: JB Lippincott, 1974.)

The blood supply and lymphatic vessels for a villus are shown in *Figure 12-13*. The arrangement of capillaries and lymph vessels provides for capillary exchange of nutrients and fluids and for lymphatic removal of large molecules not accommodated by return to the capillaries. For substances to be absorbed into the blood from the epithelial cells, they must traverse the epithelial cell membrane, basement membrane, interstitial fluid, and capillary membrane. Large molecules not entering the capillaries enter the **central lacteals**. Blood from the veins of the intestine enters the liver through the portal vein before it returns to the right ventricle of the heart. Lymph from the central lacteals bypasses the liver and reenters the blood through the thoracic duct.

Large Intestine

Contents from the terminal part of the ileum enter the large intestine at the cecum (ileocecal junction), as in the horse; at the colon

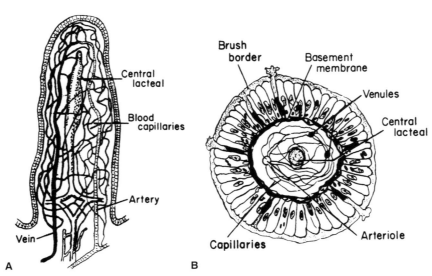

■ **FIGURE 12-13** Functional organization of the villus: **A)** Longitudinal section. **B)** Cross section showing the epithelial cells and basement membrane. (From Guyton AC. Textbook of Medical Physiology. 8th Ed. Philadelphia: WB Saunders, 1991.)

(ileocolic junction), as in the dog and cat; or at the cecum and colon (ileocecocolic junction), as in the ruminant and pig.

The large intestine consists of the **cecum** and **colon**. Development of the large intestine varies among animals according to diet. Fermentation occurs to some extent in the large intestine of all animals but is a more widespread process in the cecum and colon of herbivorous animals. In ruminants, the forestomachs constitute the principal location for fermentation; in nonruminant herbivores (simple herbivores), the cecum and colon provide fermentation. Enzymatic digestion occurs after fermentation in ruminants, and the bacterial and protozoan cells are themselves digested. In simple herbivores enzymatic digestion precedes fermentation, so only

fermentation products and not microbes are available for digestion and absorption.

Food requiring further digestion by fermentation usually enters or is diverted into the cecum unless it is developed poorly, as in the dog. The colon continues from the cecum to its termination at the anus; it consists of **ascending**, **transverse**, and **descending** parts. All animals have a transverse and descending colon, but the arrangement between the cecum and transverse colon differs among species. The dog and cat have an ascending colon between the cecum and transverse colon (*Fig. 12-14*), but the horse, pig, and ruminant have a counterpart to the ascending colon. In the pig and ruminant this is known as the **ansa spiralis (coiled colon)**, and in the horse the ascending colon is replaced

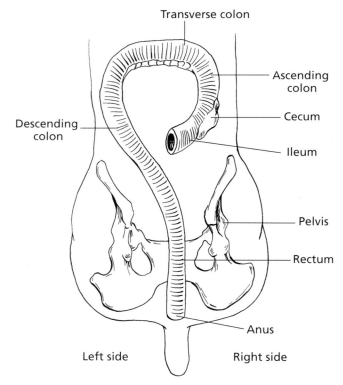

■ **FIGURE 12-14** Dorsal view of the dog cecum and colon (large intestine). The dog, a carnivore, has no special arrangement for its ascending colon. The rectum is the pelvic portion of the descending colon that terminates at the anus.

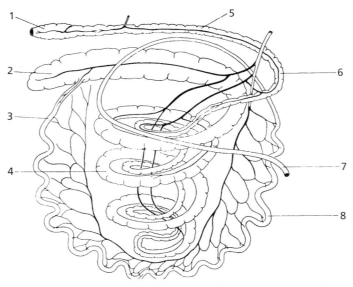

■ FIGURE 12-15 Schematic representation of the intestinal tract of the pig. **1)** Rectum; **2)** cecum; **3)** ileum; **4)** ansa spiralis (coiled colon); **5)** descending colon; **6)** transverse colon; **7)** second curve of duodenum; **8)** jejunum. (From Engel HH, St. Clair LE. Anatomy. In: Leman AD, et al, eds. Diseases of Swine. 6th Ed. Ames, IA: Iowa State University Press, 1986.)

by the **large colon**, which consists of a **ventral colon** and a **dorsal colon**. The ansa spiralis of the pig, which resembles a coiled bedspring, is shown in *Figure 12-15*. The coil is directed downward as it leaves the cecum and returns upward, coiled inside the downward coil. The coiled colon for ruminants (*Fig. 12-16*) resembles a cartwheel. When the colon leaves the cecum it is coiled to the hub; it then reverses at the hub to be recoiled to the rim, and from there proceeds to the transverse colon.

In the horse the cecum is a large, comma-shaped structure that extends from the pelvic inlet to the abdominal floor, with its tip just behind the diaphragm (*Fig. 12-17*). It is mainly located on the right side of the horse. The ventral colon continues craniad from the base of the cecum, which is near the pelvic inlet, to the diaphragm, where it turns caudad and returns to the pelvic inlet. Another turn is made cranially, and it continues as the dorsal colon, located above the ventral colon. The ventral and dorsal colons can be described as

double horseshoes because one seems to be on top of the other. A turn is made at the diaphragm, and the dorsal colon continues for a short distance and joins the transverse colon, which is directed toward the left side of the horse. The descending colon in the horse is called the **small colon**.

The cecum and colon of the pig and horse are sacculated as a result of the presence of longitudinal bands of muscle. The sacculations, called **haustra**, seem to act as buckets. By accommodating extra volume, they can help to prolong the retention of contents, thus allowing more time for microbial digestion (see Figs. 12-15 and 12-17).

The descending colon terminates at the **anus**. The part of the descending colon located within the pelvis is known as the **rectum**. It is relatively dilatable, and serves to store feces prior to its expulsion.

The anus is the junction of the terminal part of the digestive tract with the skin. It closes by means of a muscular sphincter composed of smooth and striated muscle fibers.

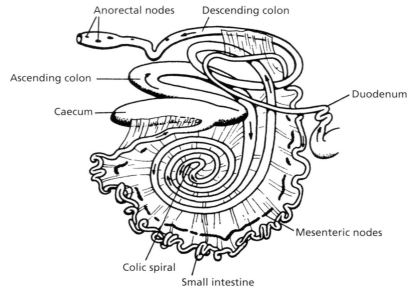

■ **FIGURE 12-16** Gastrointestinal tract of the cow showing the colic spiral (ansa spiralis). (From Dyce KM, Wensing CJG. Essentials of Bovine Anatomy. Philadelphia: Lea & Febiger, 1971.)

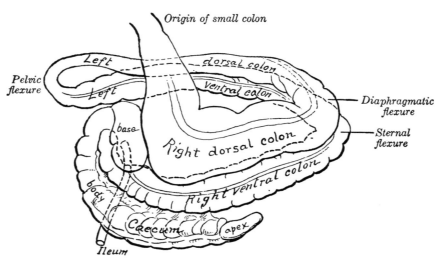

■ **FIGURE 12-17** Schematic representation of the cecum and colon of the horse. (From Getty R. Sisson & Grossman's Anatomy of the Domestic Animals. 5th Ed. Philadelphia: WB Saunders, 1975.)

■ ACCESSORY ORGANS

1. What are the names of the three pairs of salivary glands? Where are their openings? How are their secretions described?

2. Describe the location of the pancreas. What are its secretions?

3. Which animal has clearly visible connective tissue septa surrounding each lobule of the liver?

4. Study the triad of vessels and ducts present in a liver lobule (Fig. 12-21). What is the name of the large phagocytic cells that line the sinusoids of the liver lobules?

The **salivary glands**, pancreas, and liver supply secretions to the digestive tract and provide for digestion within the lumen. These secretions are in addition to those supplied by the many glands of the stomach and intestine and include electrolytes, water, digestive enzymes, and bile salts. This combination of secretions causes dietary substances to be degraded within the lumen so that the new substances can interact with the epithelial enzymes.

The salivary glands consist of three pairs of well-defined glands and some lesser-defined scattered salivary tissue. The larger glands are known as the **parotid**, **mandibular**, and **sublingual** salivary glands. These are connected to the oral cavity by one or more excretory ducts that have openings through the cheeks or tongue. The general location of the salivary glands is shown in *Figure 12-18* for the dog.

Salivary glands are serous, mucous, or mixed, depending on their secretion. A **serous secretion** is a watery, clear fluid as compared with **mucus**, which is a viscid, tenacious material that acts as a protective covering throughout the digestive tract. A mixed gland secretes both serous and mucous fluids. Blood vessels and nerves enter each gland where the ducts exit. Innervation is provided by the sympathetic and parasympathetic divisions of the autonomic nervous system.

The **pancreatic gland** has both **endocrine** and **exocrine** functions: it produces hormones (endocrine) and digestive secretions (exocrine). The pancreas is always located near the first part of the duodenum and appears as an elongated gland of loosely connected aggregated nodules. The main pancreatic duct enters the first part of the duodenum close to the common bile duct, which comes from the liver (see Fig. 12-8). In sheep and goats, a single

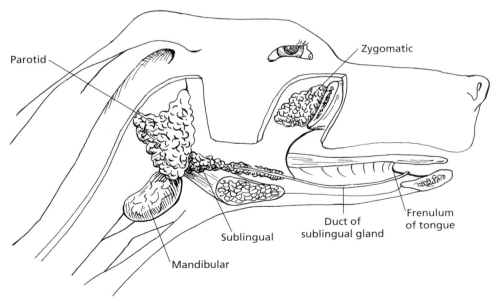

Parotid

Zygomatic

Sublingual

Duct of sublingual gland

Frenulum of tongue

Mandibular

■ **FIGURE 12-18** Location of salivary glands in the dog. They are paired glands, and only those on the right side are shown. The right mandible has been removed to show the sublingual salivary gland and its duct. The duct empties on a small papilla located near the anterior end of the frenulum (midventral fold of the tongue).

pancreatic duct empties directly into the common bile duct so that a mixture of bile and pancreatic juice enters the duodenum. The accessory duct, if present, opens a short distance from the main duct. The endocrine portions of the pancreas, the **pancreatic islets** (formerly called islets of Langerhans), are isolated groups of cells scattered throughout the gland. The **beta cells** produce **insulin**, and the **alpha cells** produce **glucagon**. Secretions from the alpha and beta cells are made directly into the blood (ductless secretions). Islet cells are clearly visible with a microscope (*Fig. 12-19*).

The **liver** is a multipurpose organ; its production of **bile** and **bile salts** is only one of its many important functions. The epithelial cells of liver lobules are metabolically active in synthesis, storage, and metabolic conversions. The location of the liver varies among species, but it is always located immediately behind the diaphragm. In ruminants it tends to be on the right side. The lobules of the liver are clearly demarcated; in the pig they are surrounded by visible connective tissue septa. Other animals have fewer connective tissue divisions and accordingly cannot be seen. The liver and its location in a pig are shown in *Figure 12-20*.

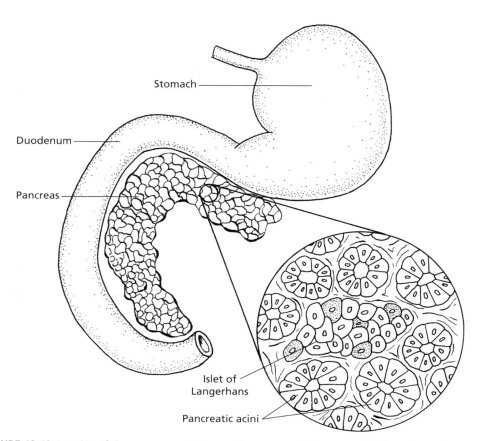

Stomach

Duodenum

Pancreas

Islet of Langerhans

Pancreatic acini

■ **FIGURE 12-19** Location of the pancreas and its general appearance. The pancreas is always located near the first part of the duodenum and appears as an elongated gland of loosely connected aggregated nodules. The inset from the pancreas shows an islet of Langerhans (endocrine) situated among a number of pancreatic acini, the exocrine (digestive secretions) portion.

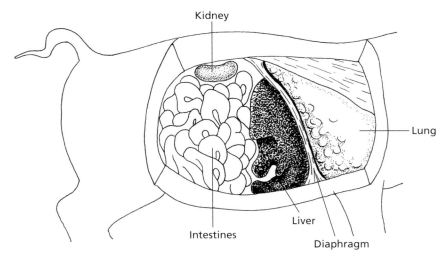

■ **FIGURE 12-20** The pig liver and its location relative to other organs. Because of the large amount of interlobular connective tissue, the lobules are mapped out sharply. For this reason, the liver is much less friable (easily broken) than that of other animals.

The liver receives arterial blood for its many cells from the hepatic artery and venous blood through the portal vein from the stomach, spleen, pancreas, and intestines. Blood from both sources is circulated through the **sinusoids** (second capillary bed of the hepatic portal system). Here it is detoxified and modified before reentering the central vein (second venous drainage of hepatic portal system) for return to the hepatic veins; and from there it proceeds to the heart through the caudal vena cava. The arrangement of a liver lobule with its triad of vessels and ducts (branches of portal vein, hepatic artery, and bile duct) is shown in *Figure 12-21*. Bile flows opposite to the direction of blood flow in the hepatic artery and portal vein branch.

The largest part of the macrophage system is present in the liver and is represented by the fixed macrophages, the **Küpffer cells**. Küpffer cells are highly phagocytic and remove foreign materials entering the blood from the stomach and intestines. They also remove tissue debris, such as old and fragile erythrocytes.

■ COMPOSITION OF FOODSTUFFS

1. From a diet standpoint, what is the difference between roughages and concentrates?
2. How are carbohydrates classified?
3. What are the principal monosaccharides and disaccharides?
4. What are the polysaccharides that are important to animals? How do they differ?
5. What are the products of complete protein hydrolysis?
6. How are amino acids linked to form a protein? Differentiate among dipeptides, oligopeptides, polypeptides, and proteins.
7. Differentiate among neutral fats, phospholipids, and cholesterol. What happens to most of the cholesterol formed in the body?
8. Are water, minerals, and vitamins proper foods or accessory foods? What distinguishes proper foods from accessory foods?

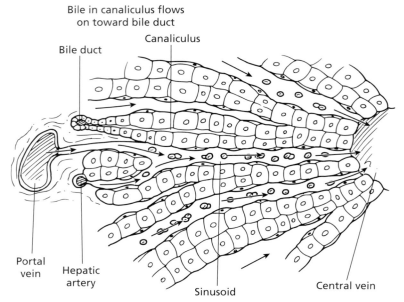

■ FIGURE 12-21 Portion of a liver lobule (highly magnified). Blood from the portal vein and hepatic artery flows into sinusoids (lined with Kupffer cells) and empties into the central vein. Bile travels in the opposite direction in canaliculi to empty into bile ducts in the triad areas. (From Ham AW. Histology. 7th Ed. Philadelphia: JB Lippincott, 1974.)

The six basic foodstuffs are classified chemically as carbohydrates, proteins, lipids, water, inorganic salts, and vitamins. These are found in varying amounts in the foods that are ingested; a balanced diet must contain some proportion of each. Herbivorous animals can have a diet consisting of roughages and concentrates. **Roughages** are foods that contain a high percentage of cellulose; they generally have a low digestibility. **Concentrates** are composed of seeds from plants and most of their by-products, and are more digestible than roughages. Feeding practices help dictate whether animals receive a high-roughage or a high-concentrate diet.

Carbohydrates

Carbohydrates are classified as monosaccharides, disaccharides, or polysaccharides, depending on the number of five-carbon (pentose) or six-carbon (hexose) units they

contain. The **monosaccharides** include ribose (a five-carbon sugar), glucose, fructose, and galactose (*Fig. 12-22*). The **disaccharides** are chemical combinations of two molecules of monosaccharides and include sucrose, maltose, and lactose (*Fig. 12-23*). Disaccharides are degraded (broken down) to monosaccharides through the process of **hydrolysis**. Hydrolysis involves the cleavage of a compound by the addition of water, the hydroxyl group being incorporated in one fragment and the hydrogen atom in the other. The hydrolysis of sucrose yields one molecule each of glucose and fructose; the hydrolysis of maltose yields two molecules of glucose; and the hydrolysis of lactose yields one molecule each of glucose and galactose. The **polysaccharides** are molecules that contain multiple (more than two) numbers of simple sugars, most of which are hexoses. Polysaccharides important to animals are starch, glycogen, and cellulose. **Starch** is a food reserve of most plants; when eaten it serves as

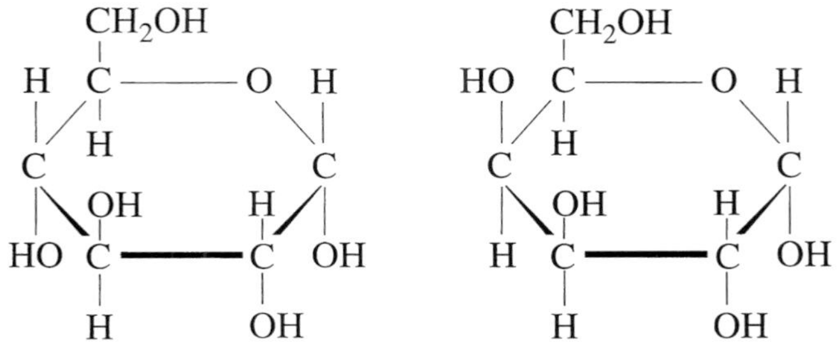

CH₂OH

α–D–glucose α–D–galactose

■ **FIGURE 12-22** Chemical structure of monosaccharides are represented by glucose and galactose.

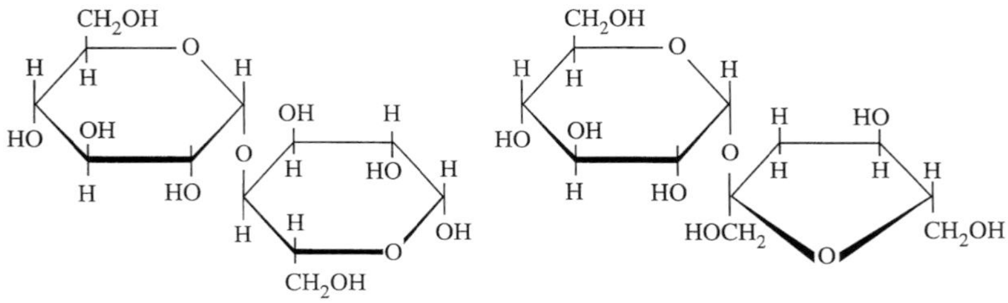

Maltose   Sucrose

■ **FIGURE 12-23** Chemical structure of disaccharides as represented by maltose and sucrose.

an excellent source of energy. Starch is degraded through hydrolysis to maltose, a disaccharide, and finally to glucose, a monosaccharide, so it can be absorbed. **Glycogen** represents the principal carbohydrate reserve in animals; it is stored in the liver and in muscles. It is a highly branched molecule of glucose units (*Fig. 12-24*) and can be degraded as needed to glucose, and thereby used for energy. **Cellulose** is the structural component of plants. It can be digested only by enzymes of cellulose-splitting microorganisms that function mainly in herbivorous animals (forestomachs of ruminants, cecum and colon of simple herbivores). Cellulose is similarly hydrolyzed to glucose.

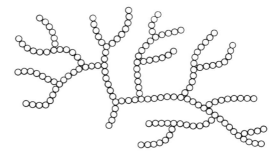

■ **FIGURE 12-24** Schematic representation of the highly branched glycogen molecule. Each bead of the chain represents a glucose molecule. (From Conn EE, Stumpf PK. Outlines of Biochemistry. New York: John Wiley & Sons, 1963.)

Proteins

Proteins are complex, high–molecular-weight, large, colloidal molecules that contain a high percentage of amino acids. In addition to

carbon, hydrogen, and oxygen, proteins also contain nitrogen. Hydrolysis of proteins yields **amino acids**, the building blocks of protein. The coupling of amino acids to form proteins occurs at the carboxyl group of one amino acid with the amino group of another, accompanied by the loss of a water molecule. The degradation of proteins involves the addition of water and the reforming of the amino acids (hydrolysis).

The linkage of amino acids (called the **peptide bond**) to form a protein is shown in *Figure 12-25*. **Dipeptides** consist of two amino acids. **Oligopeptides** consist of more than two, but not more than 10, amino acids. **Polypeptides** consist of more than 10, but not more than 100, amino acids. Polypeptides are classified as proteins when they contain more than 100 amino acids. The **essential amino acids** are those that cannot be synthesized either at all or rapidly enough to permit normal growth; they must therefore be provided for in the diet. The nonessential amino acids are those that can be synthesized by the animal in sufficient quantities to ensure normal growth. **Protein quality** is important; the highest-quality protein is one that provides all of the essential amino acids in the exact proportions required. A lower-quality protein either lacks essential amino acids or does not supply them in proper proportions. Manufacturing processes can change a high-quality protein to one of lower quality.

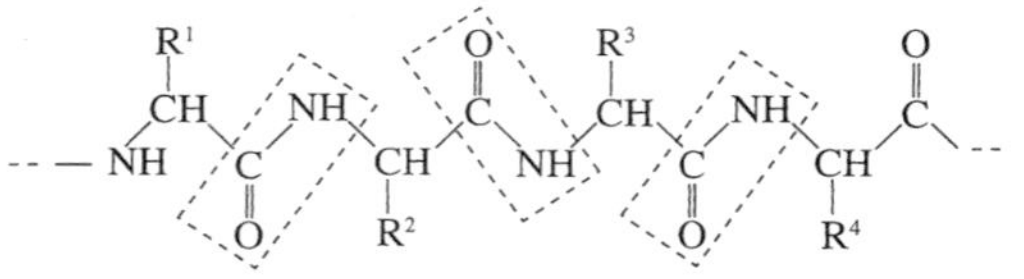

Lipids

The lipids include fats and related substances. **Neutral fats** (triglycerides) are esters (formed by the reaction between an acid and an alcohol) produced by three molecules of fatty acids combining with one molecule of glycerol (*Fig. 12-26*). **Phospholipids** are complex lipids that contain phosphate (*Fig. 12-27*); in addition, they usually contain glycerol, fatty acids, and a nitrogenous base. Phospholipids are important structural elements of cell membranes and of sphingomyelin (a phospholipid), which occurs in myelin sheaths of nerves. Thrombo-

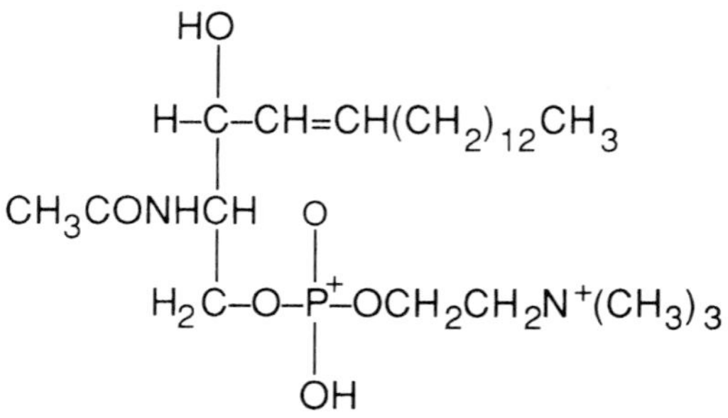

■ FIGURE 12-25 A polypeptide chain, the basic primary structure of a protein. The peptide bonds are shown by the areas boxed by dashed lines.

■ FIGURE 12-27 Sphingomyelin. This phospholipid is common to myelin sheaths of nerve fibers.

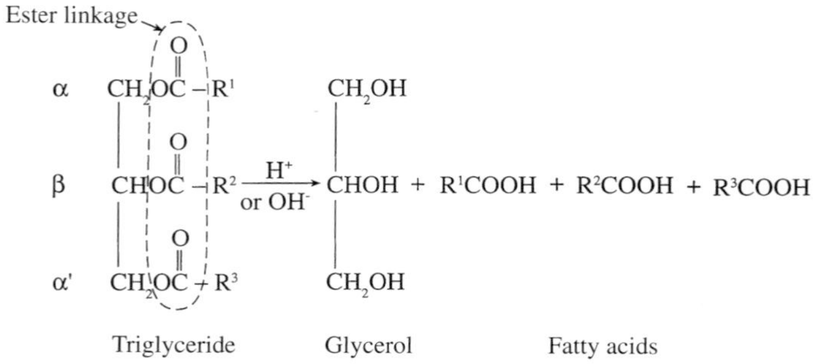

■ FIGURE 12-26 Hydrolysis of a simple lipid. Three molecules of long-chain fatty acids and one molecule of glycerol are released when a triglyceride molecule is hydrolyzed. The great majority of lipids are triglycerides. Lipids are esters of glycerol and fatty acids. The ester linkages are shown within the area circumscribed by the dashed lines.

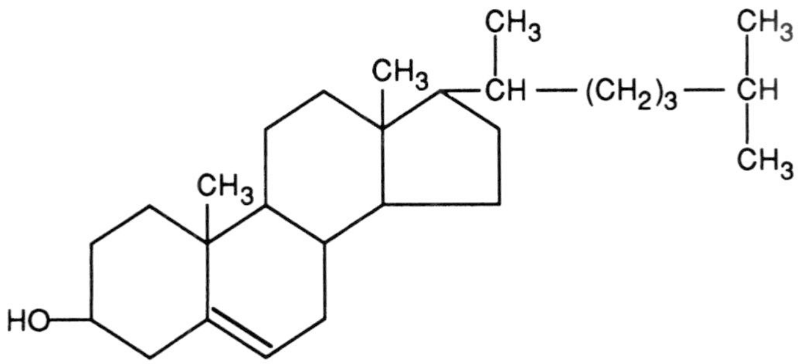

■ **FIGURE 12-28** Chemical structure of cholesterol.

plastin, another phospholipid, is involved in blood coagulation.

Cholesterol (*Fig. 12-28*) is a fatty substance derived from triglycerides. It is a high–molecular-weight alcohol; its sterol nucleus is synthesized from degradation products of fatty acid molecules. Approximately 80% of all cholesterol formed in the body is conjugated in the liver to form bile salts, which are then transported to the intestine for use in digestion. Cholesterol is also an important structural component of cell membranes.

Accessory Foods

Minerals, vitamins, and water are considered to be **accessory foods**; and carbohydrates, fats, and proteins are called **proper foods**. The principal distinction is that proper foods supply energy, whereas accessory foods are essential for life but do not supply energy. The role of water as an accessory food has been described (Chapter 2).

Minerals

Minerals are inorganic foodstuffs. The combined amount in a diet can be determined by burning; when this is done, the mineral is referred to as ash. Minerals are essential for normal growth and reproduction of animals. Those required in greater quantities are referred to as **macrominerals**, and this group includes calcium, phosphorus, sodium, chlorine, potassium, magnesium, and sulfur. These elements are important structural components of bone and other tissues and serve as important constituents of body fluids. As noted in earlier chapters, they play vital roles in the maintenance of acid-base balance, osmotic pressure, membrane electrical potential, and nerve transmission. The elements required in much smaller amounts are referred to as **trace minerals**. This group includes cobalt, copper, iodine, iron, manganese, molybdenum, selenium, zinc, chromium, and fluorine. Macro minerals (e.g., calcium and phosphorus) might be required for diets in substantial amounts, but trace minerals (e.g., cobalt and manganese) might be required only in minute amounts. Minerals can be actual components of body chemicals or act as catalysts for chemical reactions. Their presence in plasma is only a reflection of their presence in cells and other body fluids. It is beyond the scope of this book to discuss mineral functions, deficiencies, toxicities, and interrelationships. An excellent reference for this purpose (Goff JP. Minerals.) is listed under Suggested Reading at the end of this chapter.

Vitamins

The **vitamins** are a group of chemically unrelated organic compounds essential for life. They function as metabolic catalysts or regulators, and can be classified on the basis of their solubility as **fat-soluble vitamins** (A, D, E, and K) or **water-soluble vitamins** (B vitamins and C). All of the vitamins are required for normal function in all animals, and for most, the diet must supply them if the animal is to function normally. In some animals, there is no dietary requirement for some because they are synthesized within that animal's body, e.g., in ruminants, microbes are capable of producing many of the water-soluble B vitamins needed to support their needs.

As was also noted for minerals, an excellent reference relating to vitamin functions, deficiencies, toxicities, and syndromes of concern (Goff JP. Vitamins.) is listed under Suggested Reading at the end of this chapter.

■ PREGASTRIC MECHANICAL FUNCTIONS

1. What is meant by prehension? What are the principal prehensile structures?
2. Why are cattle prone to tongue injuries? What assists sheep in their ability to graze close to the ground?
3. Observe how different animals drink water. What is an important prehensile organ in the horse?
4. What is accomplished by mastication?
5. Is there a voluntary phase to deglutition? Can an anesthetized or sleeping animal swallow?
6. Study Fig. 12-29 to better visualize the swallowing reflexes. Talk through the events of swallowing.

The stomach is the first major organ associated with digestion. Before food can be received by the stomach, important pregastric functions are performed to receive, prepare, and deliver a bolus to the stomach. Performance of these functions varies among the animals and depends mostly on adaptations associated with their diet.

Prehension

The first mechanical function necessary for the digestive process is **prehension**, the seizing and conveying of food into the mouth. The lips, teeth, and tongue are the principal prehensile structures in domestic animals. The highly mobile upper lip is a useful prehensile organ in the horse, especially when eating from a feedbox containing grain. When pasturing, the horse draws the lips back and uses the incisor teeth to sever grass.

The upper lip of cattle is rather immobile, and the tongue is used as a prehensile organ. The tongue is highly mobile and can grasp grass (aided by the papillae), bringing it to the mouth between the lower incisors and upper dental pad. An upward movement of the head accomplishes shearing of the grass. Because of its use as a prehensile organ, the tongue is vulnerable to injury by sharp or pointed objects that might be in the way of the grasping movement. "Wooden tongue" in cattle is a chronic inflammation caused by an organism introduced through an eating-associated injury.

The tongue is also an active prehensile organ in sheep. The cleft upper lip of sheep facilitates grazing close to the ground. Close shearing is particularly useful when grass is in short supply.

The heavy snout and pointed lower jaw of pigs are adaptations for rooting. Characteristic head movements of rooting are retained by pigs when grain is eaten from a feeder.

Dogs and cats convey liquids to the mouth with the tongue, whereby the free end is contracted to form a ladle. Other domestic animals drink water by suction. Most birds fill the beak with water by dipping and then lifting the head to allow the water to enter the esophagus by gravity. The pigeon, however, drinks by suction.

Mastication

Mastication refers to the mechanical breakdown of food in the mouth. It is commonly called chewing and is carried out to varying degrees by different animals. The fibrous nature of the diet of herbivores requires more chewing than the meat diet of carnivores. In the latter, chewing is of short duration; the teeth are used mostly for tearing and for gnawing on bones in a more leisurely fashion. The table surfaces of the cheek teeth of herbivores wear unevenly, which facilitates more efficient mastication of their diet.

A bolus of food (rounded or oblong) is formed by the mastication process. The bolus might be imperfectly formed by animals that gulp their food. The food material of the bolus is mixed with saliva. The mucous secretion of saliva provides a certain adhesiveness and, coupled with its serous secretion, lubricates the food mass for easier transport through the esophagus.

Deglutition

Deglutition is the act of swallowing or conveying the food mass from the mouth to the stomach. This complex process involves a number of reflexes that are coordinated by a swallowing center in the brain. There are three stages of swallowing: 1) through the mouth (voluntary), 2) through the pharynx (reflex), and 3) through the esophagus (reflex). Swallowing begins as a voluntary activity and is followed by reflex activity. Some degree of consciousness is required for swallowing because of the voluntary stage. Unconscious animals can inhale vomitus because of lack of the voluntary state and because the reflex centers are depressed and do not respond to receptor stimulation in the mouth and pharynx. The reflexes move the food and close the glottis and nasal cavity, thereby preventing food from entering these parts. The sequence of reflexes is as follows:

1. Respiration is inhibited, and the danger of inhaling food is minimized.
2. The glottis (opening to the larynx) is closed.
3. The larynx is pulled upward and forward.
4. The root of the tongue can now fold the epiglottis (forward projection from the glottis) over the glottis as the tongue

plunges the bolus from the mouth into the pharynx.
5. The soft palate is elevated, which closes the nasal cavity from the pharynx.
6. A peristaltic contraction of the pharynx directs food into the esophagus.
7. A reflex peristaltic wave in the esophagus is initiated, which transports the bolus into the stomach.

A representation of food about to be forced into the esophagus and the associated displacement of the soft palate, epiglottis, pharynx, and tongue is shown in *Figure 12-29*.

■ GASTROINTESTINAL MOTILITY

1. **Study Fig. 12-30 and review nerve impulse transmission to understand changes in intestinal motility.**
2. **What is the basic difference between segmentation and peristalsis? How would you define peristalsis?**
3. **Would peritonitis (e.g., from hardware disease in cattle) inhibit intestinal activity?**
4. **How do gastrin, cholecystokinin, and secretin affect gastrointestinal motility?**

Once food reaches the stomach, its movement is controlled by the activity of the smooth muscle in the wall of the stomach and intestine. Muscle activity is spontaneous (myogenic) and is modulated by the autonomic nervous system. Smooth muscle is an excitable tissue, and the resting membrane potential of about 50 mV is subject to fluctuation (*Fig. 12-30*). The fluctuations are represented by slow waves characterized by slow, transient, undulating changes of the resting membrane potential that are propagated for varying distances. When the peak (toward positive) of a slow wave reaches **threshold** (membrane potential at which an action potential is produced), a **spike potential** (true action potential) is

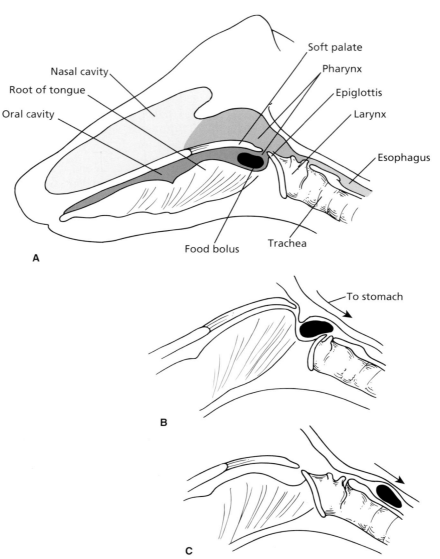

■ **FIGURE 12-29** Displacement of structures associated with swallowing a food bolus. **A)** A food bolus is moved through the oral cavity and plunged into the pharynx near the root of the tongue during the voluntary stage of swallowing. This begins the reflex stages. **B)** Pharyngeal stimulation leads to inhibition of respiration and closing of the glottis (opening to the larynx and trachea). The caudal direction of the root of the tongue elevates the soft palate, closing off the nasal cavity, and the epiglottis, closing off the glottis. Pharyngeal contraction forces the food bolus into the esophagus. **C)** A peristaltic reflex is initiated by presence of the food bolus in the esophagus; the bolus is transported to the stomach by peristalsis; pharyngeal structures return to the normal position.

observed, and muscle contraction follows. The greater the encroachment of the peaks of slow wave potentials on the threshold potentials, the greater the frequency of the spike poten-

tials, and gastrointestinal muscle contraction is sustained for a longer period.

The duration of spike potentials is longer in gastrointestinal smooth muscle than in

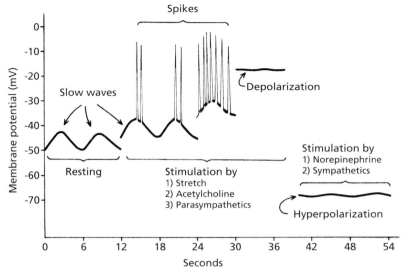

■ **FIGURE 12-30** Membrane potentials in mammalian intestinal smooth muscle. Note the slow waves, spike potentials, and directions of depolarization and hyperpolarization. (From Guyton AC, Hall JE. Textbook of Medical Physiology. 10th Ed. Philadelphia: WB Saunders, 2000.)

nerve fibers because, in addition to the inflow of Na^+ associated with depolarization, there is also an inflow of Ca^{2+}; the "channels" that permit Ca^{2+} to enter are slower to open and close than the Na^+-only channels of nerve fibers. In addition, the calcium ions that enter are associated with the actin and myosin interaction of contraction. A representation of spikes superimposed on slow waves is shown in Figure 12-30. Less-negative values (toward positive) are associated with depolarization, and more-negative values (further from threshold) are associated with hyperpolarization. The rhythmical frequencies of the slow waves represent the maximum frequency for contraction and act as pacemakers. Parasympathetic stimulation causes the resting membrane potential to approach threshold, resulting in depolarization, and increases spiking that results in more vigorous gastrointestinal activity, whereas sympathetic stimulation hyperpolarizes and reduces spiking that results in decreased gastrointestinal activity.

Segmentation and Peristalsis

Two important intestinal reflexes are segmentation and peristalsis. Segmentation movements are myogenic (i.e., property of smooth muscle cells) and do not depend on a nervous mechanism. **Segmentation** causes back-and-forth mixing as a result of intermittent circular muscle contractions occurring at different sites on an intestinal segment (*Fig. 12-31*). Contraction is initiated by distention and chyme is moved in both directions, creating new distentions that are followed by contractions. Segmentation movements promote digestion and absorption by mixing chyme and bringing it into contact with the epithelial cells lining the intestinal lumen.

Peristalsis is characterized by unidirectional, usually aboral (toward the anus) waves of contraction that are propulsive in nature. These movements are neurogenic and are carried out through local reflexes mediated through intrinsic nerve plexuses within the

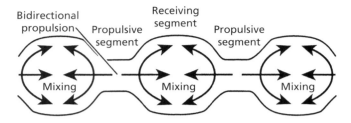

Same length of intestine later in time

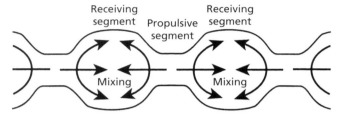

■ **FIGURE 12-31** Segmentation contractions of the small intestine. Movement of chyme into the receiving (relaxed) segment by the propulsive (contracting) segment results in mixing. The receiving segment then becomes the propulsive segment, and mixing continues. (From Rhoades RA, Tanner GA. Medical Physiology. 2nd Ed. Baltimore: Lippincott Williams & Wilkins, 2003.)

wall of the structure where they occur. The peristaltic reflex is initiated by distention of the bowel, which activates local reflexes and causes stimulation of activity cranial to and inhibition of activity caudal to the distention. The cranial activity creates a zone of higher pressure that drives contents into the relaxed area caudal to the distention. The moving contents propagate the reflex and provide for movement of the contents aborally (*Fig. 12-32*). There is also an extrinsic reflex for the small intestine that responds to gas distention, pain, and peritonitis, which can inhibit gastrointestinal motility.

■ **MECHANICAL FUNCTIONS OF THE STOMACH AND SMALL INTESTINE**

1. **How do the stomach parts serve their mechanical functions?**
2. **How do the parasympathetics increase the number of contractions?**
3. **Does a hyperosmotic solution in the stomach become isotonic by withdrawal of water from the blood?**
4. **What factors delay gastric emptying?**
5. **What animals vomit easily? Is there a vomiting center? What interferes with vomiting in the horse? Why is vomiting not observed in cattle?**
6. **Why must the flow of contents in the small intestine be controlled? Where does the greatest delay occur?**

The most important functions of the stomach are storage of ingested food, mixing of the food with secretions, and control of the emptying of its contents. The parts of the stomach mentioned above (fundus, corpus, and antrum) are suited to these functions. The fundus receives and stores contents by adapting its volume so that excessive pressure does not develop. The corpus serves as the mixing vat for saliva, food, and gastric secretions. The antrum serves as the pump by regulating the propulsion of food past the pyloric sphincter into the duodenum. The antrum contractions, together with a contracted pyloric sphincter, cause the contents to return to the corpus for

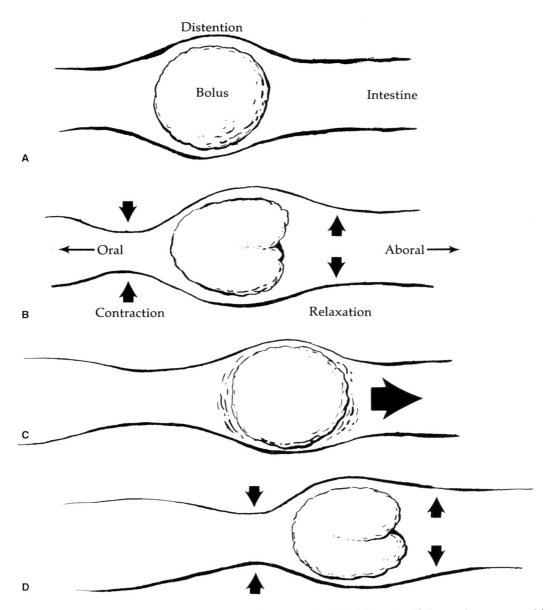

■ **FIGURE 12-32** Intestinal peristalsis and movement of contents. **A)** Original distention. **B)** Contraction occurs cranial to the distention and relaxation caudal to the distention. **C)** Contraction and relaxation followed by movement of contents in an aboral direction. **D)** A new distention point initiates a new locus of contraction and relaxation, which continues aborally as a wave.

additional mixing. Liquid leaves the stomach at a faster rate than solid materials, so adequate time is given for required solubilization and beginning digestion of solid materials.

The maximum number of contractions of the antrum is controlled by the slow waves. For the stomach, these occur at the rate of four or five each minute. The slow waves do not, however, necessarily result in contraction. Contraction depends on the superimposition of spikes that are created when the stomach is distended with food. Stomach distention causes receptors in the stomach wall to be activated; this in turn increases vagal tone (parasympathetic tone) so that the slow waves are closer to threshold and spike more readily. The spikes (action potentials) are followed by contraction waves.

Delay of Gastric Emptying

Inhibition to emptying is produced through a neural mechanism (**enterogastric reflex**) and an endocrine mechanism (**enterogastrone reflex**). The receptors for these mechanisms are present in the duodenum. The **osmoreceptor**, an important receptor in this regard, monitors the osmotic pressure of the material entering the duodenum. The gastric contents could be hyperosmotic and, if emptied into the duodenum, would result in fluid being withdrawn from the blood to achieve osmotic equilibrium of the contents. This does not occur in the stomach because of its lower permeability to water. The osmoreceptors detect the hypertonicity and inhibit gastric emptying via a neural mechanism so that slow emptying occurs and rapid loss of water from the blood is prevented.

Excess protein or carbohydrate is also effective in inhibiting gastric emptying. It is believed that their influence is mediated through the osmoreceptor neural mechanism. Other receptors respond to high hydrogen ion concentrations and cause delays in gastric emptying until the gastric content previously emptied into the duodenum has been neutralized by secretions from the pancreas and liver. These two reflexes are mediated by a neural mechanism. A hormonally mediated delay to gastric emptying occurs in response to lipids entering the duodenum. **Cholecystokinin** is released in response to the presence of lipids, and delayed emptying provides sufficient time for fat digestion. Another hormone, **gastric inhibitory polypeptide (GIP)**, is secreted by the jejunal mucosa in response to the presence of lipids and carbohydrate, and it also delays gastric emptying.

The following list summarizes the factors that delay gastric emptying and thus permit time for adequate digestion:

1. Enterogastric reflexes (neural mechanisms)
   a. Osmoreceptors in the duodenum respond to hypertonic content (hypertonicity can be caused by the presence of products of protein and carbohydrate digestion as well as electrolytes).
   b. Hydrogen ion receptors in duodenum respond to high hydrogen ion concentration.
2. Enterogastrone reflexes (endocrine mechanisms)
   a. Cholecystokinin released from duodenal mucosa in response to lipids
   b. GIP released from jejunal mucosa in response to lipids and carbohydrate

Emesis

Emesis (vomiting) is an emptying of the cranial part of the duodenum and stomach in an orad (toward the mouth) direction. A series of reflexes is involved to initiate antiperistalsis and closure of the glottis and nasal cavity. Swine, dogs, and cats vomit easily. Vomiting is a protective mechanism that helps prevent absorption of noxious substances. Vomiting in ruminants occurs as an ejection of abomasal content into the forestomachs; thus, ejection from the mouth does not occur. Vomiting in the horse is rare because of the difficulty in opening the cardia from a reverse direction.

Dilatation of the horse's stomach because of pressure from attempted vomiting can occur to the point of rupture. The reflexes of vomiting are controlled by a vomiting center in the brain.

Mechanical Functions of the Small Intestine

The small intestine provides movements that both mix the contents and propel the contents aborally as digestion proceeds. The flow of contents must be controlled for two major reasons: 1) to provide proper mixing of luminal contents with pancreatic enzymes and bile; and 2) to provide time for luminal digestion of carbohydrates, fat, and proteins and for maximum exposure of digested nutrients to the mucosa of the small intestine. One means of delaying transport is to delay transit time in the ileum. This can occur because of the greater number of segmental contractions and fewer peristaltic contractions at that location.

Small intestine activity can be increased or decreased by parasympathetic and sympathetic stimulation, respectively. Also, the hormone secretin inhibits and cholecystokinin and gastrin stimulate small intestine motility. These hormones control the rate of passage of intestinal content.

■ MECHANICAL FUNCTIONS OF THE LARGE INTESTINE

1. What are the functions of the large intestine? Is greater time required for these functions?
2. Why is increased colonic activity associated with constipation and decreased activity associated with diarrhea?
3. Why is the reabsorption of water from the intestine an important function? Where are the major sites that this occurs?
4. Note the frequency of defecation in cattle, horses, and carnivores. Note the transit times of food in pigs, horses, and cattle.

The large intestine provides for microbial digestion and for reabsorption of electrolytes and water. Both of these functions take longer than the digestion and absorption that occurs in the small intestine. Fermentation of the magnitude that occurs in the large intestine of the horse requires a large volume of buffered fluid to neutralize the acidic end-products of microbial digestion. The motor activity of the large intestine provides for the delay time. Cecal contractions help to mix the contents and remove gas, with controlled emptying into the colon. Haustral contractions are isolated events in the colon and help to mix the contents. The stationary haustral contractions increase resistance to flow in either direction.

Peristaltic movements in the colon occur in either an oral or an aboral direction. In an oral direction they produce retrograde flow, which delays movement of ingesta. Retrograde flow coupled with anatomic narrowing delays filling of various parts of the colon. Anatomic narrowing occurs at the pelvic flexure in the horse, where the ventral colon turns to become the dorsal colon. Accordingly, filling of the dorsal colon is delayed. The frequency of slow wave activity in the small intestine decreases in the aboral direction, but the frequency of slow waves in the colon decreases in the oral direction for the first half of the colon and accounts for the retrograde movement of contents (see previous text). Mass movement of ingesta in the aboral direction is accomplished by prolonged bursts of spikes migrating in the aboral direction that are independent of slow wave activity. The bursts of spikes are followed by prolonged and powerful contractions of the circular smooth muscle, which results in mass movement of the ingesta.

Much of the activity of the colon is thus directed toward the delay of transit and filling of its parts (reservoir function). Increased colonic activity is therefore associated with constipation, and decreased activity is associated with diarrhea.

Defecation

Defecation is a complex reflex act in which feces are evacuated from the terminal colon and rectum. The frequency of defecation varies among animals but can occur 5 to 10 times daily in vigorous horses, 10 to 20 times daily in cattle, and 2 to 3 times daily in carnivores. The reflex can be assisted or inhibited by certain voluntary muscles.

The time required for food to pass through the digestive tract varies among species. Studies were carried out in various species using dye-stained (marked) food. The average time for food passage was determined because ingested food that is marked is mixed with food ingested at other times. The average time for pigs was found to be 48 hours, and for horses it was 24 to 48 hours. Because of the voluminous forestomach in cattle, the dilution of marked food with other food is increased and makes its initial appearance in feces in 12 to 24 hours. About 80% of the initial amount is passed by 3 to 4 days, and final evacuation is complete by 7 to 10 days.

Intestinal Transport of Electrolytes and Water

The secretion of water and electrolytes into the digestive tract has many purposes. These secretions are derived from the extracellular fluids. They are particularly voluminous in herbivorous and omnivorous animals. An important function of the intestine is the return of water and electrolytes to the extracellular fluid before they are lost in the feces. The major reabsorption sites for these substances are the distal small intestine and the large intestine. Reabsorption of secretions is compromised in diarrhea and other conditions and, if the problem is not corrected or the secretions are not replenished, an animal can soon die because of blood volume loss and circulatory collapse.

■ DIGESTIVE SECRETIONS

1. What is an approximate volume for salivary secretion in a cow?
2. What function of saliva is served in ruminants?
3. Is salivary amylase an important component of domestic animal saliva?
4. In addition to mucus, what are the gastric secretions?
5. What is the function of pepsin?
6. Why would the pH of blood increase (become more alkaline) after ingestion of food? Where is the situation reversed?
7. What factors regulate gastric secretions?
8. Contrast the pancreatic flow rates between the horse and the dog. Why is there a difference?
9. How is trypsinogen activated? Where does this occur? What activates the other proenzymes?
10. What stimulates the secretion of secretin and cholecystokinin? What is the effect of their secretion?
11. What is bile? Are bile salts a component of bile? What is meant by recirculation of bile salts? What is the relationship of bile salts to cholesterol? What are gallbladder stones (gallstones)?
12. What controls the contraction of the gallbladder and relaxation of the sphincter of Oddi?
13. Is bicarbonate from the liver (biliary bicarbonate) an important source of bicarbonate for the intestines of some species?
14. What substances from bile emulsify fats?
15. Study Figure 12-35 for summary of gastrointestinal hormones and association with gastric, pancreatic, and biliary secretions.

In addition to the secretions of the salivary glands, pancreas, and liver, there are those supplied by the many glands of the stomach and intestines that include mucus, hormones, and digestive enzymes. All of these secretions assist the degradation of dietary substances to forms that can be absorbed.

Saliva

In all animal species, salivary secretions facilitate mastication and deglutition because of their watery nature and the lubrication that is provided. The volume of the salivary secretion varies, but is greatest in herbivorous animals. In addition to its lubrication function, saliva increases the potential for evaporation and cooling for panting animals. Saliva has an additional important function in ruminants, in which large volumes of buffered fluid are needed to support microbial fermentation in the rumen and to neutralize the large amounts of acids that are produced as a result of fermentation. To meet the buffering demand, ruminant saliva contains bicarbonate and phosphate buffers. Phosphates are particularly supportive of bacterial growth. In ruminants, salivary secretion is continuous, but the flow of saliva varies with activity and increases with feeding and rumination. Saliva has important antifoaming characteristics and might play a role in reducing the foaming tendency of certain diets. Consequently, increased salivary flow during eating might help to prevent dietary bloat. In cattle, about 80% of the water entering the stomach is provided by salivary flow derived from extracellular fluid. The need for reabsorption of the water from the large intestine is obvious (see previous section, Intestinal Transport of Electrolytes and Water).

The major digestive enzyme produced by the salivary glands is **amylase**. Among the domestic animals, amylase is most abundant in the saliva of pigs. In contrast, the amount of amylase in human saliva is 100 times that present in pigs.

In addition to the spontaneous secretion of saliva from certain glands in some species (parotid glands in ruminants), secretion is controlled by the autonomic nervous system. Parasympathetic stimulation increases salivary flow that is low in protein (more watery). Sympathetic stimulation, however, has less effect on flow rate, but increases the amount of protein and mucin and renders saliva more tenacious. The increase in flow rate is brought about by central stimulation from the salivary center and by the mechanical stimulation of receptors in the mouth and stomach. The central component is sometimes referred to as the psychic component (e.g., when an animal salivates in anticipation of food).

Gastric Secretions

In addition to mucus, which is usually secreted throughout the length of the digestive tract, the stomach secretes **pepsinogen**, **HCl**, and **gastrin**. Pepsinogen and HCl are secreted into the lumen of the stomach, and gastrin (a hormone) is secreted into the blood. Specific glandular regions are identified within the stomach; their extent varies among species (see Fig. 12-7). Generally, the cardiac region secretes only mucus. The fundic gland region secretes HCl and pepsinogen (HCl by parietal cells and pepsinogen by neck chief cells), and the pyloric gland region secretes mucus and gastrin. A variable amount of surface (depending on species) around the cardia has epithelium similar to that of the skin (stratified squamous). This area serves a protective function in the same sense that mucus protects other parts of the digestive tract.

HCl and pepsinogen initiate the digestion of protein. **Pepsinogen** is a precursor of pepsin, a proteolytic enzyme. Conversion of the precursor to its active form in the lumen prevents proteolytic digestion of the producing cell. The conversion of pepsinogen to pepsin occurs in the lumen under the influence of HCl and begins at about pH 5. Optimal activity of pepsin occurs at pH 1.8 to 3.5 and initiates gastric protein digestion.

When H^+ is secreted into the lumen by the gastric cell, HCO_3^- is simultaneously secreted into the blood. H^+ is formed in the cell from CO_2 according to the hydration reaction:

$$CO_2 + H_2O \leftrightarrow H_2CO_3 \leftrightarrow H^+ + HCO_3^-$$

H^+ is secreted into the stomach lumen, and HCO_3^- is secreted into the blood in exchange for Cl^-. The chloride ion is subsequently secreted into the stomach lumen with H^+ (*Fig. 12-33*). The increase in plasma bicarbonate concentration that occurs after a meal is known as the **alkaline tide**, in which the blood pH increases. It is a transient situation that lasts until the pancreas becomes active in secreting HCO_3^-. An amount equivalent to the amount of HCO_3^- that entered the blood from the gastric parietal cells is returned to the duodenum by the pancreatic cells.

Because of the high H^+ concentration in the stomach, a barrier exists to prevent diffusion of H^+ back to the blood. The tight junction between cells is extremely effective and even prevents diffusion of H_2O through the epithelium. This is why highly hypertonic solutions can enter the duodenum—they are not diluted by the diffusion of water into the stomach.

Gastric acid secretion is stimulated by acetylcholine, gastrin, and histamine. **Acetylcholine** is the parasympathetic secretion; it acts directly on the parietal cells to secrete HCl and on the gastrin cells to secrete gastrin. **Gastrin** in turn stimulates HCl and pepsinogen secretion. Chemical releasers of gastrin are digested proteins and amino acids in the stomach. **Histamine** is an amino acid derivative present in most body tissues. It is believed that the local gastric mucosal histamine stimulates HCl secretion by potentiating the action of gastrin or by direct stimulation.

Inhibition of gastric acid secretion occurs when the pH of the gastric contents decreases to pH 2 or lower. The acid acts directly on the gastrin cells. Inhibition to gastric acid secretion also originates from the intestine in response to acidic, fatty, and hypertonic solutions entering the duodenum from the stomach. These same substances are also effective in

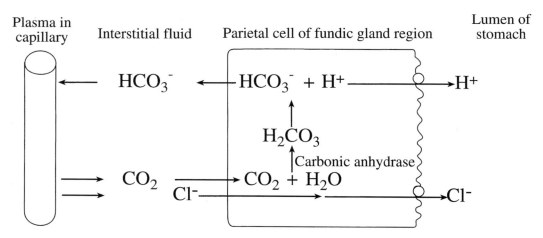

■ **FIGURE 12-33** Mechanism of hydrochloric acid secretion by parietal cells of the gastric mucosa. Carbonic anhydrase facilitates the formation of H_2CO_3 from CO_2 that diffuses into the cells from the interstitial fluid. H_2CO_3 dissociates into H^+ and HCO_3^-. H^+ and Cl^- are actively secreted by the parietal cells into the lumen of the stomach, and this causes a gradient for diffusion of Cl^- from the plasma. The loss of Cl^- from plasma is followed by diffusion of HCO_3^- into plasma so that electrical neutrality is maintained. Accordingly, plasma bicarbonate concentration increases after ingestion of food, associated with the secretion of HCl into the lumen of the stomach.

inhibiting gastric emptying. The inhibition is mediated by neural or hormonal mechanisms. The neural mechanism provides inhibitory neurons that synapse with the parasympathetic fibers going to the gastrin cells. The hormones released into the blood from intestinal cells in response to acidic, fatty, and hypertonic solutions are secretin and cholecystokinin (CCK). When secreted, these circulate to the stomach and occupy the site on the parietal cells that gastrin would have occupied, thus preventing gastrin stimulation of HCl secretion.

The secretion of pepsinogen is stimulated by the same stimuli as those for HCl, except that secretin enhances pepsinogen secretion (but inhibits HCl secretion). It would seem that there is less need for inhibiting pepsinogen secretion inasmuch as protein digestion is to be favored.

Intrinsic factor is a mucoprotein secreted by the gastric mucosa. It interacts with vitamin B_{12} to form a complex that binds to receptors in the ileum to facilitate vitamin B_{12} absorption. The secretion of intrinsic factor is correlated closely with H^+ secretion, and it is also secreted by the parietal cells.

In addition to the gastric secretions mentioned above, the young ruminant secretes an enzyme called rennin. This enzyme is a milk-coagulating enzyme; in the presence of Ca^{2+} it forms a coagulum from milk. This coagulum delays the passage of milk so that more protein digestion occurs in the stomach. The offspring of other animals do not secrete rennin; it is thought that HCl accomplishes the needed coagulation. The need for rennin in ruminants might relate to their proportionately larger intake of milk at a single nursing than is observed for other animals.

The factors that regulate gastric secretions can be summarized as follows:

1. Stimulation
   a. Acetylcholine
   b. Gastrin
   c. Histamine
   d. Secretin (pepsinogen only)

2. Inhibition
   a. Within stomach: decrease of pH to 2
   b. From duodenum: presence of acidic, fatty, and hypertonic solutions
      (1) Neural mechanism—inhibitory neurons to parasympathetic fibers that stimulate gastrin cells
      (2) Hormonal mechanism—secretion of secretin and cholecystokinin, which then occupy gastrin sites on parietal cells (HCl secretors); gastric inhibitory polypeptide (GIP) is released in response to fat or glucose and inhibits all gastric secretions

Pancreatic Secretions

Only the exocrine secretions (HCO_3^- and digestive enzymes or precursors) of the pancreas are involved in the digestive process. The secretion of HCO_3^- is needed to neutralize the HCl concentration of the stomach contents that enter the duodenum and also for neutralization of acids produced from fermentation in the large intestine. Enzymes and enzyme precursors are needed for digestion in the intestinal lumen so that the products of degradation can be absorbed. These secretions are somewhat more unique in omnivores and nonruminant herbivores. In these animals, a large volume of buffered fluid is needed for the microbial digestion that occurs in the cecum and colon. The digestive enzymes provide for small intestine digestion, and the larger volume of fluid and HCO_3^- serves a function similar to that of saliva in the ruminant. In the horse, the rate of enzyme secretion is low in comparison with that of other species. This might occur because a greater proportion of the horse's ingested food is of a type that requires microbial digestion beyond the small intestine.

There is a continuous flow of pancreatic fluid in the horse, even under basal (nonfeeding) conditions. This ensures that an adequate volume of buffered fluid (containing HCO_3^-) is present for the continuous fermentation in the cecum and colon. The rate can be increased under stimulation. In contrast, the dog might have almost no fluid flow from the pancreas under basal conditions, but high rates of flow are produced under stimulation. This pattern is appropriate because the dog eats less frequently, and because little fermentation occurs in the large intestine and a large volume of buffered fluid is not needed.

The pancreas secretes all of the enzymes and enzyme precursors (proenzymes) necessary for the digestion of proteins, fats, and carbohydrates. The proteases are secreted in proenzyme form and include trypsinogen, chymotrypsinogen, elastase, and carboxypeptidases A and B. **Trypsinogen** is activated by **enterokinase** (present in the intestinal epithelium) to form **trypsin** only after it reaches the intestinal lumen, and the reaction occurs at the brush border. Trypsin then becomes the activator for the other proenzymes. Digestion of the pancreas is prevented because the proteolytic enzymes are secreted as proenzymes. Spontaneous conversion of trypsinogen to trypsin is prevented in the pancreas by the presence of trypsin inhibitor.

Pancreatic lipase hydrolyzes dietary triglycerides into substances that can then be absorbed. Bile salts are needed to activate pancreatic lipase.

Pancreatic amylase is secreted in its active form. This carbohydrate enzyme hydrolyzes starch to maltose, a disaccharide. No free glucose is formed by pancreatic amylase hydrolysis.

The exocrine secretions of the pancreas are controlled by autonomic nerves as well as by the gastrointestinal hormones gastrin, CCK, and secretin. Parasympathetic stimulation increases the secretion of enzymes and proenzymes, with little secretion of electrolytes and water in most species. Increased water and electrolyte secretion, however, does accompany parasympathetic stimulation in the pig and horse (these animals need large volumes of water and HCO_3^- for large intestine fermentation). Gastrin that is secreted when the parasympathetics are stimulated can also stimulate the pancreas to release enzymes and proenzymes, so the parasympathetic effect on the pancreas is potentiated. Two hormones secreted when the stomach contents enter the intestine are secretin and CCK. Secretin release is stimulated by acid perfusion of the duodenum and causes the pancreas to secrete HCO_3^-. Secretin was the first hormone discovered (in 1902, as the result of work by Bayliss and Starling). The hormone CCK is secreted in response to the presence of protein and fat in the duodenum and causes the pancreas to secrete enzymes and proenzymes. Secretin and CCK are synergistic to each other—that is, the presence of one enhances the effect of the other.

Biliary Secretions

Bile is a greenish-yellow solution of bile salts, bilirubin, cholesterol, lecithin, and electrolytes (Na^+, K^+, Cl^-, and HCO_3^-). Bile salts are synthesized continuously by hepatic cells, but the quantity needed for digestion far exceeds the rate of production by the liver. Therefore, bile salts are recirculated from the intestine (after being used in the intestine) to the hepatic cells, where they are resecreted (enterohepatic circulation). Because of this reuse of bile salts, an adequate amount is available for efficient digestion. Bile salts are synthesized from cholesterol and, in the process, some cholesterol, as well as bile salts, is secreted into the bile. The bile salts and lecithin form a soluble micelle (colloidal particle) with the cholesterol, thereby preventing cholesterol precipitation and gallstone formation. The solubility, however, depends on an alkaline solution, which is provided by HCO_3^-.

Bile is secreted continuously in all species and can be transported to the gallbladder and stored for later use or transported directly to the intestine. While in the gallbladder, bile can be concentrated by absorption of NaCl or of $NaHCO_3$ and water. The degree of concentration depends on the length of storage. In animals that eat once or twice per day, bile is highest in concentration, but its concentration is low in ruminants and the pig because they eat frequently and bile is therefore discharged from the gallbladder frequently. The horse does not have a gallbladder, and a large flow of hepatic bile continuously enters the duodenum; it is the only domestic animal without a gallbladder. The opening of the common bile duct into the duodenum is controlled by the **sphincter of Oddi**. Contraction of the gallbladder and relaxation of the sphincter are controlled by CCK, which is released in response to the presence of lipids and amino acids in the small intestine.

Bile secretion by the liver is primarily stimulated by the amount of bile salts being recirculated. On reaching the liver, the bile salts are absorbed from the hepatic sinusoids (portal circulation) into the hepatic cells and are then resecreted into the bile canaliculi by active transport (*Fig. 12-34*). Cations and water diffuse passively, so that the newly formed bile is iso-osmotic with plasma. Therefore, the larger the amount of bile salts recirculated, the higher is the rate of secretion of bile. Bicarbon-

ate and other electrolytes are secreted by the bile duct epithelium as well (biliary secretion), and their secretion is increased by CCK, secretin, and gastrin. The secretion of biliary bicarbonate is an important source of buffer for the intestine in some species. In the sheep, the rate of biliary secretion of HCO_3^- is much higher than that of the pancreatic secretion, and the liver plays a greater role than the pancreas in neutralizing the H^+ in the duodenum.

Fat in the intestine is **emulsified** (breakdown of fat globules into smaller globules) by the bile salts and by the lecithin present in the bile. This provides a greater surface area for digestion by the luminal lipases (lipid enzymes). Another important function of the bile salts is the removal of the products of lipid digestion (free fatty acids and monoglycerides) from the area of digestion so that digestion can continue without recombination to triglycerides. The bile salts accomplish this transport function by forming soluble micelles. In this form the digestion products are moved easily by diffusion to the intestinal epithelium for absorption.

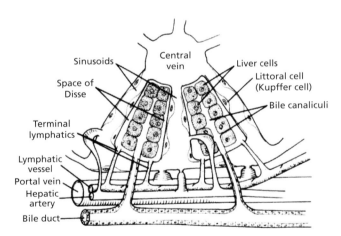

■ **FIGURE 12-34** Schematic representation of the microstructure of a liver lobule and its association with bile secretion. Most of the bile salts are reabsorbed from the intestine by active transport (others lost in feces), enter the portal vein, and pass to the liver (enterohepatic circulation). They are quickly absorbed from the sinusoids into the liver cells and are then resecreted into the bile canaliculi by active transport. The bile salts then enter the bile duct from the canaliculi. Small amounts of bile salts are secreted continuously by the liver cells, and this accounts for that which is lost in the feces. The secretion of bile by the liver is stimulated by the amount of bile salts being recirculated. Therefore, the larger the amount recirculated, the higher the rate of bile secretion. (From Guyton AC, Taylor AE, Granger HJ. Dynamics and Control of the Body Fluids. Philadelphia: WB Saunders, 1975.)

A summary of the major gastrointestinal hormones and their association with gastric, pancreatic, and biliary secretions is presented in *Figure 12-35.*

■ DIGESTION AND ABSORPTION

1. Are disaccharides absorbed from the intestine?
2. How are glucose, galactose, and fructose absorbed?
3. What is the limit of peptide size for its absorption? What electrolyte is involved?
4. What are the products of triglyceride digestion? How are they absorbed?
5. What are chylomicrons? Where are they formed? How do they get to the blood?
6. Is there enzymatic digestion in the large intestine of mammals? What accounts for the digestion that does occur in the large intestine?
7. What are the end products of microbial digestion?
8. What happens to the microorganisms associated with large intestine digestion?
9. What is the importance of large intestine microbial digestion in dogs and cats?

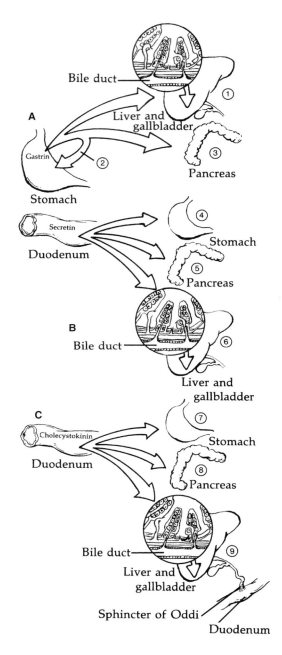

■ **FIGURE 12-35** The major mammalian gastrointestinal hormones and their association with gastric, pancreatic, and biliary secretions. **A)** Gastrin: 1, stimulates secretion of HCO_3^- and H_2O from bile duct epithelium; 2, stimulates HCl and pepsinogen secretion; 3, stimulates secretion of pancreatic enzymes. **B)** Secretin: 4, inhibits HCl secretion and stimulates pepsinogen secretion; 5, stimulates secretion of HCO_3^- and H_2O from pancreas; 6, stimulates secretion of HCO_3^- and H_2O from bile duct epithelium. **C)** Cholecystokinin: 7, inhibits HCl secretion; 8, stimulates secretion of pancreatic enzymes; 9, stimulates contraction of gallbladder and relaxation of sphincter of Oddi, and stimulates secretion of HCO_3^- and H_2O by bile duct epithelium.

Most of the digestion and absorption of the soluble carbohydrates, proteins, and fats occurs in the small intestine (except in ruminants). Only minimal hydrolysis of starches is thought to occur in the stomach (in pigs from salivary amylase), where the digestion of protein begins through the activity of pepsin. The intestinal phases of digestion for the nonruminant consist of those processes that occur in the lumen and on the brush border of the epithelial cells.

Carbohydrates

The only carbohydrate enzyme secreted by the pancreas that is present in the lumen of the intestine is amylase. Amylase hydrolyzes starch to maltose. Further degradation of starch occurs at the brush border surface under the influence of maltase, and the resulting glucose is absorbed by active transport into the epithelial cells. Sucrose and lactose (disaccharides) do not have a luminal phase of digestion, and their hydrolysis occurs at the brush border under the influence of sucrase and lactase. Glucose and fructose from sucrose, and glucose and galactose from lactose, are then absorbed, glucose and galactose by active transport and fructose by facilitated diffusion. Fructose is converted to glucose inside the epithelial cell and enters the portal vein blood in that form. Because the intracellular concentration of fructose is kept low, nearly all of the fructose in the intestine can be absorbed by facilitated diffusion. Glucose and galactose require the presence of Na^+ for their active transport (cotransport) into the cell. This is similar to the process in which glucose and amino acids are transported from the tubular lumen of the kidney nephron into the tubular epithelial cell (see Chapter 11).

Proteins

The pancreatic proteases are commonly categorized as exopeptidases (carboxypeptidases A and B) and endopeptidases (trypsin, chymotrypsin, and elastase). The **exopeptidases** hydrolyze proteins into smaller units, and the **endopeptidases** hydrolyze the smaller units into **oligopeptides** (fewer than 10 amino acids) and amino acids. Many oligopeptides must be degraded further because peptides with more than three amino acids cannot be absorbed. Further hydrolysis occurs at the brush border under the influence of oligopeptidases. The amino acids, dipeptides, and tripeptides are absorbed by active transport. Further degradation of dipeptides and tripeptides occurs within the cytoplasm of the epithelial cells.

The active transport of amino acids and peptides requires the presence of Na^+, as for glucose and galactose.

Fats

Dietary triglycerides are coarsely emulsified in the stomach as a result of stomach motility, whereby they are mixed with phospholipids and other chyme (a mixture of food with gastric secretions) components. Further emulsification occurs on entering the small intestine because of the presence of bile salts and lecithin. Further mixing with pancreatic lipase results in the formation of free fatty acids, monoglycerides, and glycerol. **Micellar solutions** (**microemulsions**) are formed with bile salts to provide for their ready transport to the brush border. Glycerol, fatty acids, and monoglycerides are absorbed by simple diffusion.

The fatty acids and monoglycerides are resynthesized to triglycerides inside the epithelial cell. The triglycerides are grouped with cholesterol and phospholipids and given a protein covering to form a chylomicron. **Chylomicrons** are similar to micelles in that they are water soluble and thus facilitate the transport of the water-insoluble triglycerides. The water solubility conferred by the protein coat permits exit from the cell so that the chylomicron can enter the central lacteal (lymphatic capillary) of the villus (see Fig. 12-13) for delivery to the blood.

Microbial Digestion in the Large Intestine

No enzymatic digestion occurs in the large intestine of mammals. The digestion that occurs results from microbial digestion, which is significant for the nonruminant herbivores and omnivores. The end products of digestion are **volatile fatty acids** (VFAs), mainly **acetic, propionic,** and **butyric acids** (*Fig. 12-36*). VFAs are important energy sources after absorption. The microorganisms associated with ruminant digestion are subsequently digested to provide amino acids, but the microorganisms involved with large intestine digestion in mammals are not digested and are voided with the feces. Some species, such as the rabbit, practice coprophagy (eating their feces) so that the microorganism protein is then subjected to small intestine enzymatic degradation.

An animal such as the horse obtains as much as 75% of its energy requirement from large intestinal absorption of VFAs. Although dogs and cats have little need for microbial fermentation as a source of energy from VFAs, it is an important mechanism from a water conservation standpoint. Any nutrients that escape enzymatic degradation or absorption contribute to an effective osmotic pressure (because the nutrients would not be absorbed) and retain water. Thus, large intestine fermentation salvages otherwise lost calories in the form of VFAs and decreases the effective osmotic pressure of large intestine contents so that water can be reabsorbed.

■ THE RUMINANT STOMACH

1. How do the camel and llama stomach differ from that of sheep and cattle?
2. What kind of epithelium lines the forestomachs of the ruminant?
3. Which side of the cow would be used to detect rumen motility or observe rumen distention from tympanites?
4. Why is bloat a hazard to breathing?
5. Which stomach compartment is largest in newborn calves? In adult ruminants?
6. At what age do calves begin ruminating (assuming they have access to roughage)?
7. Where are boluses first deposited when they enter the rumen? Why are ingested, pointed, hardware items a hazard?
8. What is the function of the reticular groove?
9. How many contractions of the rumen ought to be observed each minute? Where can the contractions be felt?
10. What was the name of the Jersey steer that made the rumen fistula famous?
11. What are functions of the ruminant stomach compartments?

Animals that regurgitate and remasticate their food are called ruminants. There are two suborders of ruminant animals: 1) Ruminantia, which includes the deer, moose, elk,

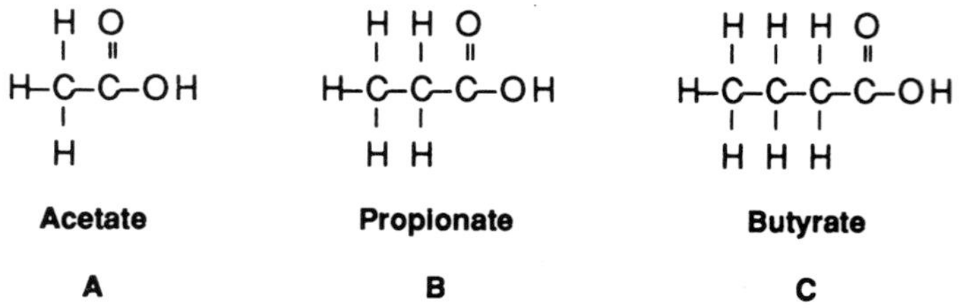

■ FIGURE 12-36 Chemical structure of principal volatile fatty acids derived from fermentation in the rumen and large intestine. **A)** Two carbon atoms. **B)** Three carbon atoms. **C)** Four carbon atoms.

reindeer, caribou, antelope, giraffe, musk ox, bison, cow, sheep, and goat; and 2) Tylopoda, which includes the camel, llama, alpaca, and vicuna. The principal difference between the two suborders is that Tylopoda do not have an omasum. Another difference is that Tylopoda have areas of cardiac glands that open into ventral sacculated surfaces of the reticulum and rumen. These small sacs have given rise to the myth that the camel stores water in its rumen, but no evidence has been found to support the idea that more water is present in the camel rumen than in the rumen of other ruminants.

The ruminant stomach is adapted for fermentation of ingested food by bacterial and protozoan microorganisms. Energy is obtained through fermentation that would not otherwise be made available. In their natural environment, the diet of ruminants includes mostly growing, mature, or dried grass, and the mammalian digestive enzymes cannot digest the cellulose in these materials. Microbial enzymes, however, can digest the plant cells through the fermentation process. Fermentation requires controlled conditions for a maximum rate of degradation; these are provided through appropriate secretions, motility, and temperature. Regurgitation and remastication (associated with rumination) assist fermentation by providing more finely divided material and thus a greater surface area for microbial digestion. Foraging ruminants often seize and swallow food over a prolonged period, with only a relatively short time given to mastication. Remastication is done during times of relative quiescence. Resalivation is also accomplished during remastication, and the additional saliva is also beneficial to the fermentation process.

Structure and Function

The ruminant stomach is composed of four compartments: 1) rumen (paunch), 2) reticulum (honeycomb), 3) omasum (many plies), and 4) abomasum (true stomach). The rela-

tionship of the compartments to each other is shown in *Figures 12-37* and *12-38*. The first three compartments are also known as the forestomach, because they precede the so-called true stomach. The forestomach is lined with stratified squamous epithelium and constitutes the esophageal region of the stomach (see Fig. 12-7). The rumen occupies a prominent portion of the viscera on the left side of the animal; its relationship to the thoracic viscera is shown in Figure 12-37. Note the proximity of the reticulum to the heart. The viscera, as seen from the right side, is shown in Figure 12-38. The abomasum is mostly on the right side. When the rumen and reticulum are distended with gas (tympanites, or bloat), pressure is applied in all directions, but becomes serious when pressure on the diaphragm prevents thoracic enlargement (needed for inspiration) and pulmonary ventilation is severely impaired. Tripe, a food product, is made from the rumen and reticulum after cattle are slaughtered. The rumen and reticulum are condemned for human food if they are ulcerated. The feeding of high-concentrate rations is associated with ulceration and condemnation.

The abomasum is the largest compartment of the newborn ruminant's stomach (*Fig. 12-39*). Forestomach development is associated with roughage intake and is lacking in calves that are fed only milk. Young ruminants usually begin ingesting limited roughage when they are 1 to 2 weeks old, and brief periods of rumination begin soon thereafter.

In the adult ruminant, the rumen is the largest forestomach compartment. It is separated from the much smaller reticulum by the ruminoreticular fold (see Fig. 12-37). Food enters the rumen through the cardiac opening of the esophagus and is deposited in the cranial sac (atrium) of the rumen (see Fig. 12-37). The next contraction of the cranial sac transfers the contents into the reticulum, from which they can be "pumped" by contractions of the reticulum to: 1) the cardiac opening for regurgitation, 2) the omasum through the reticulo-

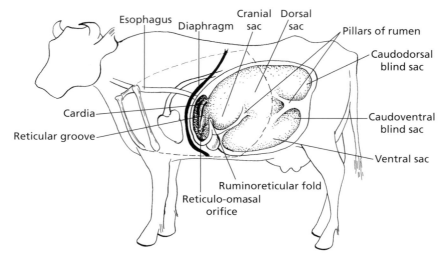

■ **FIGURE 12-37** The stomach of cattle (left view). The rumen and reticulum (shown) are two of the three compartments of the forestomach that precede the true stomach (abomasum). The reticulo-omasal orifice is the passageway to the third compartment known as the omasum. The rumen is divided into a number of sacs by muscular pillars. Pillar contraction is essential for movement of rumen content. The dashed line illustrates the extent of the rib cage.

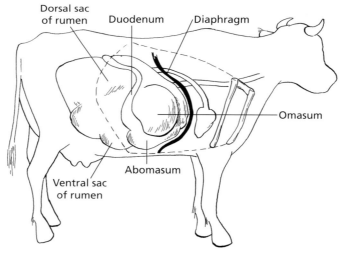

■ **FIGURE 12-38** The stomach of cattle (right view). The omasum is the third compartment of the forestomach, which has a short omasal canal that connects the reticulo-omasal orifice with the omaso-abomasal orifice. The dashed line illustrates the extent of the rib cage.

omasal orifice for transfer to the abomasum or for further digestion and absorption by the many plies of the omasum, or 3) more caudal parts of the rumen. Dense metal objects are often retained in the reticulum. If they are pointed objects, reticular contractions can result in their penetrating thoracic viscera (the heart or lungs), causing inflammation. This condition is known as traumatic pericarditis (heart involvement) or, more commonly, hardware disease.

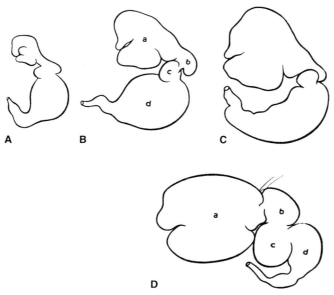

■ FIGURE 12-39 Relative sizes of the bovine stomach compartments at various ages. **A)** Three days old. **B)** Four weeks old. **C)** Three months old. **D)** Adult. a, Rumen; b, reticulum; c, omasum; d, abomasum. (From Nickel R, Schummer A, Seiferle E. The Viscera of the Domestic Mammals. 2nd Ed. Berlin: Verlag Paul Parey, 1979.)

The reticular groove (see Fig. 12-37) functions as a conduit for milk from the cardiac opening to the reticulo-omasal opening, from which it is conveyed to the abomasum through the omasal canal. Closure of the reticular groove (formerly called the esophageal groove) is a reflex initiated when receptors in the mouth and pharynx are stimulated. The reflex loses its responsiveness with age. Although certain chemicals have been shown to bring about closure of the reticular groove in adult ruminants, no function has been described for it in the adult.

The various pillars of the rumen (see Fig. 12-37) are muscular folds, which, when contracted, can move and mix large volumes of rumen content. One to two cycles of rumen contraction occur each minute. These can be felt when the hand is placed into the left paralumbar fossa (depression cranial to the pelvic hooks or tuber coxae, caudal to the ribs and ventral to the lumbar vertebrae). Assessment of rumen function is often made

by this technique. Recall that there is a reflex inhibition of gastrointestinal motility in the presence of peritonitis, gas distention, and pain.

A permanent opening into the rumen at the paralumbar location is known as a **rumen fistula**. These surgical interventions have been used for obtaining samples and for making various physiologic measurements for many years. The fistula openings are plugged during times of nonuse. A classic example of a rumen fistula is shown in *Figure 12-40*.

The functions of the ruminant stomach compartments can be summarized as follows:

1. The rumen allows for soaking and fermentation of bulk fibrous food and, because of its motility, the contents are continually mixed.
2. The reticulum serves as a pump that causes liquid to flow into and out of the rumen. The flow of liquid directs ingesta into the rumen, regulates its passage from the rumen

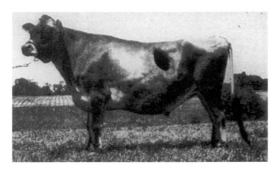

■ **FIGURE 12-40** "Bill," a Jersey steer with a large rumen fistula. The animal was born in May 1942, the fistula was made in March 1943 and, after a leg injury, the steer was euthanized in January 1955. This photograph was taken in June 1954. When not in use, the fistula was kept closed with a pneumatic plug. (From Dukes HH. The Physiology of Domestic Animals. 7th Ed. Ithaca, NY: Cornell University Press, 1955.)

to omasum, supplies moisture to rumen contents, and floods the cardia before regurgitation.

3. The omasum provides for continued fermentation and absorption (absorption enhanced by large luminal surface related to the plies or leaves), and regulation of onward propulsion between the reticulum and abomasum.

4. The abomasum provides true stomach functions. Digestion of degraded roughages and concentrates begins for fermentation residues that have not been already absorbed. Also, the microbes of fermentation are prepared for their own digestion. Using microbes for nutrition of their host is an advantage ruminants have over non-ruminant herbivores.

■ **CHARACTERISTICS OF RUMINANT DIGESTION**

1. What are the four phases of the rumination cycle?
2. How is regurgitation accomplished?
3. How many chews might be associated with remastication of a roughage bolus?

4. How does diet influence rumination time?
5. What are the two principal gases produced during ruminant fermentation? Which one predominates? What is the rate of gas production?
6. What is the stimulus for eructation, and where are the receptors located for its detection?
7. How are the eructation receptors related to the condition known as bloat?
8. Is all of the eructated gas expelled into the environment? If not, how is it directed elsewhere?
9. How do off-flavors occur in milk?

In addition to the mechanical activities of the ruminant stomach described above, fermentation and the digestive process are facilitated by rumination and eructation.

Rumination

The process of bringing food material back from the ruminant stomach to the mouth for further mastication is known as **rumination**. Rumination is a cycle of activity composed of four phases: 1) regurgitation, 2) remastication, 3) resalivation, and 4) redeglutition. It is a reflex initiated by mechanical stimulation of receptors in the mucosa of the reticulum and rumen in the area of the cardia.

The rumination cycle begins with regurgitation of a food mass bolus. **Regurgitation** is accomplished by taking a breath (inspiration) with a closed glottis (opening to the trachea). The thoracic cavity enlarges without lung inflation, and the intrapleural pressure decreases. The lowered intrapleural pressure is accompanied by a similar lowering of pressure in the mediastinal space and in the organs located within it (e.g., the esophagus, as it relates to regurgitation). The cardia (submerged in mixed rumen content) opens and, because of the lower pressure within the esophagus, the rumen content is aspirated into the esophagus. Reverse peristalsis is initiated in the esophagus, and the food mass bolus is quickly carried to the mouth. The passage of the food bolus can be observed on the left side of the neck. The reticulum contracts just before regurgitation to ensure a rumen mixture in the region of the cardia. It also aids in clearing the cardia of recently swallowed boluses.

Immediately after the regurgitated bolus arrives in the mouth, the liquid is squeezed from it and swallowed. **Remastication** and **resalivation** occur simultaneously, and remastication is thorough and deliberate. The number of chews given to each bolus varies depending on diet. For example, an all-roughage diet is remasticated more thoroughly and can be chewed 100 or more times before swallowing. A cow can secrete from 100 to 200 L (25 to 50 gal.) of saliva per 24 hours. During remastication, saliva might be swallowed two or three times. **Redeglutition** (reswallowing of a bolus) occurs at an appropriate time, and the next cycle of rumination begins in about 5 seconds. Actual tracings showing the sequence of several regurgitation events are shown in *Figure 12-41*.

The time spent in rumination each day varies with species and diet. Generally, the coarseness of the ration influences the time for rumination—cattle on a hay diet average about 8 hr/day. All of the rumination is not done at one time, but is spread out into periods (e.g., up to 14 periods/24 hr), with the periods being distributed rather evenly. Rumination time in sheep can be reduced from 9 to 5 hr/day by changing the ration from long or chopped dried grass to ground dried grass. When only concentrates are fed, rumination time can be reduced to about 2-1/2 hr/day.

Gas Production and Eructation

The gases produced in the rumen as a result of fermentation are mainly carbon dioxide and methane. Nitrogen, oxygen, and hydrogen

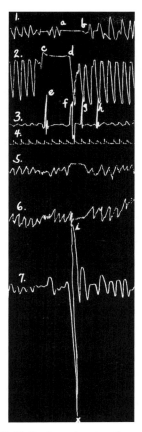

FIGURE 12-41 Tracings showing the mechanism of regurgitation in rumination. The writing points were vertically placed. The cow regurgitated at X. **1)** Movements of air in the nostrils. Note closure of the glottis from a to b. **2)** Movements of the jaw in mastication. Note the pause from c to d. **3)** Movements of boluses in the cervical part of the esophagus: e, the masticated bolus; f, the regurgitated bolus; g, h, the swallowed liquid pressed out of the regurgitated bolus. **4)** Time tracing showing 1-second intervals. **5)** Movements of the thoracic wall. **6)** Rectal pressure. It is not elevated during regurgitation. **7)** Pressure changes in the trachea. A sharp decrease coincident with regurgitation is seen. The increase of pressure as it is caused by the momentum of the liquid (bromoform) used in the recording manometer. (From Bergman HD, Dukes HH. An experimental study of the mechanism of regurgitation in rumination. J Am Vet Med Assoc 1926;69:600.)

might be present in trace amounts, but only briefly, because they are intermediaries for other reactions. Carbon dioxide is produced during the fermentation of carbohydrates and the deamination of amino acids. Carbon dioxide also can be produced from salivary bicarbonate when it neutralizes the fatty acids produced from microbial fermentation of lipids. Methane is formed by the reduction of carbon dioxide by methane-producing bacteria. In cattle, carbon dioxide composes about 60% to 70% of the rumen gas, and methane composes about 30% to 40%. The volume of gas produced in the ruminoreticulum of a dairy cow is about 0.5 to 1 L/min. It is not known how much gas is absorbed into the blood and lymph across the wall of the rumen and reticulum, but it is thought that most of the carbon dioxide and methane produced in the stomach is eliminated by eructation.

Eructation is the process by which gas from the forestomach is removed by way of the esophagus to the pharynx. Eructation occurs about once each minute. An eructation center exists in the medulla that receives afferent fibers from mechanoreceptors located in the dorsal sac of the rumen and around the cardia. The primary stimulus for eructation is the presence of gas in the dorsal sac. If gas is artificially placed into the dorsal rumen, the frequency and volume of eructation increases. A condition of **tympanism or bloating** occurs when the eructation mechanism fails. Two general types of bloat are recognized: 1) **feedlot or grain bloat**, which occurs in cattle as the result of feeding a high-concentrate diet, and 2) **legume bloat**, which can occur when cattle feed on lush, rapidly growing alfalfa or clover pastures. It is believed that these dietary bloats occur because the gas becomes trapped in tiny bubbles (frothy bloat) and the normal free gas bubble cannot accumulate on top of the ingesta in the dorsal sac of the rumen. The mechanoreceptors are effectively covered, and the presence of gas is thus not detectable, which ordinarily would initiate the eructation reflex. Tiny bubbles are formed because the surface tension of the rumen fluid has been increased. Surface-active agents (surfactants) can be used to lower the surface tension effectively and cause the bubbles to coalesce.

The normal occurrence of eructation requires that the cardia be clear of any ingesta. The cardia is reflexively closed when in contact with liquid rumen contents. Conditions that clear the cardia occur when the dorsally located gas bubble is moved cranially and ventrally toward the cardia by simultaneous contractions in the rumen of the dorsal sac, cranial pillar, and caudal pillar. At the same time, the reticulum relaxes to accommodate the forward-moving rumen content (see Fig. 12-37).

A similar expulsion of gas from the stomach in humans produces a sound; the process is characteristically referred to as a belch. Such a sound does not accompany eructation in ruminants. This might have evolved as a protective measure for ruminants in their natural environment so that their whereabouts would be less readily discovered by predators. The force of evacuation is lessened because a nasopharyngeal sphincter (in the pharynx) contracts, which assists in directing part of the eructated gas into the trachea. Subsequent inspiration moves eructated gas into the lungs. It is thought that over half of the eructated gas is directed into the lungs rather than being expelled through the nose to the outside. The inhaled carbon dioxide and methane provide a source of carbon to be reused in biochemical reactions. Labeled carbon in the form of $^{14}CO_2$ that was inhaled in this manner has been found to appear in plasma and other body fluids (*Fig. 12-42*).

Flavors that appear in milk from certain foods (e.g., wild onion, beet tops) are sometimes called **off-flavors**. They arise as volatile substances from rumen fermentation and become part of the eructated gas. The characteristic flavors get into the milk only if they are inhaled when eructated. When the eructated gas containing the off-flavor is experimentally directed away from the pharynx by a tracheal

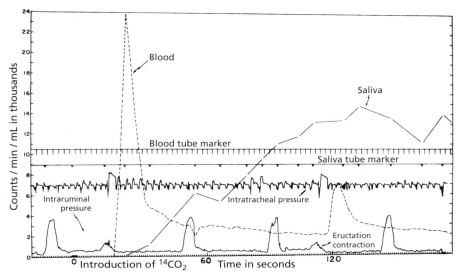

■ **FIGURE 12-42** Radioactivity in blood and saliva of the goat after intraruminal insufflation with CO_2. (From Dougherty RW, Mullinax CH, Allison MJ. Physiological disposition of ^{14}C-labeled rumen gas in sheep and goats. Am J Physiol 1964;207:1185.)

fistula, its inhalation is prevented, and the off-flavor in milk does not occur.

■ CHEMISTRY AND MICROBIOLOGY OF THE RUMEN

1. What composes the microbial population in the rumen?
2. What are the VFAs produced by microbial fermentation, and where are they absorbed?
3. What happens to glucose in the rumen?
4. What happens to protein in the rumen?
5. What happens to lipids in the rumen?
6. What vitamins are synthesized in the rumen? Which vitamin requires cobalt?
7. Note advantages of "up front" fermentation.

Fermentation that occurs in the rumen and reticulum of ruminants is accomplished by the action of **bacterial** and **protozoan microorgan-**

isms. Bacteria account for about 80% of the rumen metabolism (about 10^{11} bacteria/mL of content). Protozoa account for about 20% of the rumen metabolism (about 10^6 protozoa/mL of rumen content). These microorganisms are **anaerobic**, meaning that they thrive in the absence of oxygen.

Both bacteria and protozoa produce short-chain VFAs, carbon dioxide, and methane from their fermentation of foodstuffs. The principal VFAs are acetic, propionic, and butyric acids (see Fig. 12-36). These are mostly absorbed from the rumen before the ingesta reaches the duodenum. The usual proportions of VFAs in the rumen are about 60% to 70% acetic acid, 15% to 20% propionic acid, and 10% to 15% butyric acid. The concentration of propionic acid increases when the diet contains large quantities of soluble sugars or starch and decreases when animals are fed poor-quality hay. The acetic acid concentration varies in an inverse direction. The propionate-to-acetate ratio is increased by the presence of certain substances. For example, monensin, an ionophore antibiotic, inhibits certain organisms (H_2 producers) and favors others (succinate producers) and the propionate to acetate ratio increases.

The products of the fermentation of most carbohydrates are simple mixtures of VFAs with carbon dioxide. The rumen epithelium can absorb glucose as well as VFAs so that some ingested glucose or intermediary might be absorbed before fermentation. It seems likely, however, that most of the glucose yields VFAs.

The microorganisms of the rumen are also involved in the hydrolysis of protein. Hydrolysis occurs through the breakdown of peptides of decreasing chain length to free amino acids, which are largely destroyed by fermentative deamination with the production of carbon dioxide, ammonia, and VFAs. Some peptides and amino acids pass directly into bacterial cells, but it seems that many of the rumen bacteria can synthesize their nitrogenous cell constituents using ammonia as a principal source of nitrogen. **Ammonia** is the principal soluble nitrogenous constituent of rumen fluid. The ammonia can be derived from dietary protein, urea from saliva, and urea that diffuses through the rumen wall. Rumen fluid has urease activity, so that urea entering rapidly hydrolyzes to ammonia and carbon dioxide.

Triglycerides undergo hydrolysis in the rumen to **glycerol** and **fatty acids**. The hydrolysis is caused by rumen microorganisms and the glycerol is fermented further, mostly to propionic acid. The fatty acids continue into the duodenum for further digestion. Some of the unsaturated fatty acids might be hydrogenated in the rumen to saturated fatty acids.

Rumen bacteria can synthesize the **B complex vitamins**. B vitamin deficiencies are not observed in adult ruminants, except for vitamin B_{12}. **Vitamin B_{12}** requires **cobalt** (a trace mineral) for its synthesis—thus, a cobalt deficiency can result in vitamin B_{12} deficiency.

The types of digestion accomplished by microorganisms for ruminants are also carried out in the large intestine of nonruminant herbivores (see previous section, Microbial Digestion in the Large Intestine). Its occurrence in the forestomach of ruminants instead of the large intestine has certain advantages:

1. Microbial products of value to the host (VFAs and B vitamins) are presented to efficient absorptive sites, both in the rumen and in the small intestine.
2. Ammonia and substances metabolized to ammonia are used by microbes to synthesize high-quality microbial protein, which is subsequently subjected to abomasal and small intestine digestion and absorption.
3. Selective retention of particles at the reticulo-omasal orifice and the added opportunity for mechanical breakdown of fibers during rumination enhance digestion of coarse foods.
4. The large quantities of gas that are produced can be readily released from the system by eructation.
5. The large input of saliva provides a buffered fluid that permits effective mixing by rumen contractions.
6. Some toxic dietary substances can be rendered nontoxic by fermentation in the rumen, and small intestine absorption of toxin is thereby prevented.

■ RUMINANT METABOLISM

1.   What are the principal nonhexose sources of glucose for ruminants? Why do they need nonhexose sources? Why do they need glucose?
2.   Study energy production, entry routes of the VFAs into the tricarboxylic acid cycle, ketone production, and treatment rationale for ketosis.
3.   What is a summary statement for why bloat occurs?

Several indispensable uses for glucose in the body include its function as the principal

(usually within 6 weeks after calving), in which it is called **acetonemia**, and in late-gestation pregnant ewes, in which it is called **pregnancy toxemia**. In cows, there is a sudden or gradual loss of appetite, a rapid decrease in condition, and usually a marked decrease in milk flow. Although the onset is usually sudden, there may be a history of unthriftiness or a gradual loss in condition or milk production over a period of 1 to 4 weeks.

The treatment of ketosis in cattle is directed toward increasing the blood concentration of glucose. This can be done by intravenous infusion of glucose. The feeding of sucrose (table sugar) is usually ineffective because it is quickly fermented (first to glucose and fructose and then to VFAs). Some benefit might be obtained from absorbed glucose before its further fermentation and from propionate, a VFA obtained from its fermentation. Acetate and butyrate, however, would aggravate ketosis because they are ketogenic. The rationale for administering glucocorticoid (as injections) is that it stimulates **gluconeogenesis (production of new glucose)** from protein sources. The glucose formed or infused is degraded to pyruvate and then carboxylated to oxaloacetate, so that more acetyl CoA can enter the citric acid cycle and reduce the excess concentrations of ketone bodies (see Fig. 12-43). Feeding of sodium propionate might be of some value, but it seems to be unpalatable.

As long as the gas produced in the rumen and reticulum is permitted to collect in the dorsal part of the rumen without frothing, and as long as the eructation mechanism is functioning, no problem arises from gas production, even at high rates. Problems occur when gas cannot be eliminated and a condition known as **acute tympany**, or **bloat**, ensues. Bloat does not occur because of any change in the gas composition or because of any increase in the rate of gas production, but because of a failure of the eructation mechanism (see previous section, Energy Production).

Bloat has been variously described as being caused by the highly soluble protein content of the rumen, mucin in saliva, insufficient amount of saliva, bacterial slime, the high saponin content of ingested plants, and specific eructation inhibitors. It seems that bloat might have several causes. Eating alfalfa or clover pastures (legumes) often causes bloat. Birdsfoot trefoil, however, a leguminous plant, does not cause bloat.

■ AVIAN DIGESTION

1. What structures in birds provide for the mechanical breakdown of their ingested food?
2. Do birds have salivary glands and taste buds?
3. Where is the crop located, and what is its function?
4. What are the secretions of the proventriculus?
5. What is the function of the gizzard?
6. Do the common domestic birds have gallbladders?
7. What is the most noticeable function of the ceca?
8. What is the most striking feature of colonic motility?
9. What prevents colonic material from entering the ileum during anti-peristalsis?
10. What is the function of the bursa of Fabricius?
11. What part of the digestive tract accounts for most of the end products of digestion?
12. How does heat stress interfere with absorption?

Differences in the anatomy of the digestive tract were noted among the domestic mammalian species, and although there are general similarities between the domestic avian digestive tracts and those of mammals, there are major differences. The digestive tract of a turkey is shown in *Figure 12-45*, and it is similar to that of a chicken.

Inasmuch as birds do not have teeth, the mechanical breakdown of their ingested food is accomplished by their beak and by their muscular gizzard. Salivary glands are present in birds and are well developed in those that eat dry foods. Taste buds are located on the tongue and other parts of the mouth as in mammals.

The **esophagus** is divided into precrop and postcrop segments. It is comparatively larger in diameter than in mammals to accommodate the swallowing of large food items that would have been divided in mammals by teeth. Mucous glands are abundant in the esophagus to provide lubrication for food being swallowed. The crop is a dilatation of the esophagus and has a food storage function.

The **proventriculus** is located between the postcrop esophagus and the gizzard. The gastric secretions HCl and pepsinogen and the mucus are secreted by the proventriculus. Food does not stay in the proventriculus but rather continues into the gizzard, where gastric secretion activity (proteolysis) occurs.

The gizzard is the muscular stomach and is adapted for the mechanical reduction of food that has been ingested.

The small intestine has a well-defined duodenum, with the pancreas located between its loops (as in mammals), but distinction between jejunum and ileum is not apparent. The yolk sac vestige (**Meckel's diverticulum**) is noticeable and is located about midway on the small intestine. One of the liver hepatic ducts proceeds directly to the duodenum; another goes directly to the gallbladder. Gallbladders are present in chickens, turkeys, ducks, and geese. The mucosa of the small intestine is similar to that of mammals, except the villi have well-defined blood capillaries but no central lacteal.

The **ceca**, which are paired structures, are located at the junction of the small and large intestine. Not all of the food eaten by chickens and turkeys enters the ceca, and the ceca seem

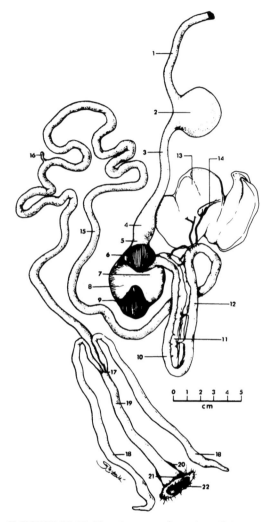

■ **FIGURE 12-45** Digestive tract of a turkey. **1)** Precrop esophagus; **2)** crop; **3)** postcrop esophagus; **4)** glandular stomach (proventriculus); **5)** isthmus; **6–9)** muscular stomach (gizzard); **10)** proximal duodenum; **11)** pancreas; **12)** distal duodenum; **13)** liver; **14)** gallbladder; **15)** jejunum; **16)** Meckel diverticulum (remnant of yolk sac); **17)** ileoc cocolic junction; **18)** ceca; **19)** colon; **20)** bursa of Fabricius; **21)** cloaca; **22)** vent. See text for description of the various parts. (From Duke G. Avian digestion. In: Swenson MJ, Reece WO, eds. Dukes' Physiology of Domestic Animals. 11th Ed. Ithaca, NY: Cornell University Press, 1993.)

to have lesser importance in domestic fowl as compared with wild fowl. The most noticeable function of the ceca is related to the microbial digestion of cellulose. This is of greater importance for the energy needs of some wild species. Urine that has entered the colon from the cloaca may pass into the ceca via antiperistalsis (oral direction). Antiperistalsis is the most striking feature of colonic motility and is believed to occur almost continuously. Because of antiperistalsis, the ceca are filled. A circular muscular ring of the ileum projects into the colon, and its contraction (sphincter-like action) effectively prevents reflux of colonic material into the ileum. In the ceca, the uric acid present in the urine becomes a nitrogen source for the microflora associated with cellulose digestion. Also, water reabsorption from the refluxed urine is another important function of the ceca.

The digestive tract ends with the **cloaca**, the site that is common to the digestive, reproductive, and urinary systems. The caudal opening to the exterior is known as the vent. The **bursa of Fabricius** is a dorsal diverticulum of the cloaca and is associated with the development of humoral immunity (see Chapter 3). It is an important site for the preprocessing of B lymphocytes.

The upper ileum is the most important site for absorption of the end products of digested fats, carbohydrates, and proteins. Heat stress and cold stress can be factors affecting absorption. This may be caused by altered mesenteric blood flow (to the intestines), which is decreased about 50% in chickens when the ambient temperature is 37°C (heat stress).

■ SUGGESTED READING

Allison MJ. Microbiology of fermentative digestion in the rumen and large intestines. In: Reece WO, ed. Dukes' Physiology of Domestic Animals. 12th Ed. Ithaca, NY: Cornell University Press, 2004.

Argenzio RA. General functions of the gastrointestinal tract and their control. In: Reece WO, ed. Dukes' Physiology of Domestic Animals. 12th Ed. Ithaca, NY: Cornell University Press, 2004.

Frandson RD, Wilke WL, Fails AD. Anatomy and Physiology of Farm Animals. 6th Ed. Baltimore: Lippincott Williams & Wilkins, 2003.

Goff JP. Disorders of carbohydrate and fat metabolism. In: Reece WO, ed. Dukes' Physiology of Domestic Animals. 12th Ed. Ithaca, NY: Cornell University Press, 2004.

Goff JP. Minerals. In: Reece WO, ed. Dukes' Physiology of Domestic Animals. 12th Ed. Ithaca, NY: Cornell University Press, 2004.

Goff JP. Vitamins. In: Reece WO, ed. Dukes' Physiology of Domestic Animals. 12th Ed. Ithaca, NY: Cornell University Press, 2004.

Guyton AC, Hall JE. Textbook of Medical Physiology. 10th Ed. Philadelphia: WB Saunders, 2000.

Leek BF. Digestion in the ruminant stomach. In: Reece WO, ed. Dukes' Physiology of Domestic Animals. 12th Ed. Ithaca, NY: Cornell University Press, 2004.

Trampel DW, Duke GE. Avian digestion. In: Reece WO, ed. Dukes' Physiology of Domestic Animals. 12th Ed. Ithaca, NY: Cornell University Press, 2004.

 SELF EVALUATION—CHAPTER 12

INTRODUCTORY CONSIDERATIONS

1. The reactions and conversions necessary to provide energy, build tissues, and synthesize secretions are collectively known as:
   a. digestion.
   b. absorption.
   c. intermediary metabolism.

THE ORAL CAVITY AND PHARYNX

2. For the sheep, the dental formula 2(0/4-0/0-3/3-3/3) would indicate that:
   a. the sheep has eight incisors in the lower jaw of its mouth.
   b. the sheep has 16 teeth in its mouth.
   c. there are four canine teeth on each half of the lower jaw.

3. A "smooth mouth" in a horse:
   a. indicates that it is about 5 years old.
   b. is represented by two complete enamel rings.
   c. is seen when the inner enamel ring disappears in all of the lower incisors and is replaced by the dental star (occurs at 11 to 13 year of age).
   d. has nothing to do with wear characteristics.

4. Mobility of the tongue of domestic animals is facilitated by:
   a. three-directional muscle fibers.
   b. greater innervation.
   c. the taste buds.
   d. greater mental concentration.

5. Which one of the following age brackets is characterized by equine incisors being "in wear"?
   a. 3 to 5 years
   b. 6 to 8 years
   c. 13 to 15 years

6. The filiform and conical papillae of the tongue:
   a. render it more mobile.
   b. serve as a plunger for transport of food from the mouth to the esophagus.
   c. provide traction for movement of food in the mouth and for grooming hair.
   d. discriminate between harmful and proper foods.

7. Which one of the following structures is elevated during deglutition to prevent food entrance into the nasal cavity?
   a. Soft palate
   b. Epiglottis
   c. Glottis
   d. Larynx

THE SIMPLE STOMACH

8. There are anatomically distinct esophageal sphincters, not only at the pharyngeal opening, but also where it enters the stomach.

a. True
b. False

9. Mucus is secreted by all of the stomach gland regions.
   a. True
   b. False

INTESTINES

10. Replacement of intestinal epithelium:
    a. does not occur (they are there for life).
    b. originates from the crypts and migrates to the tip of the villi.
    c. originates from the tips of the villi and migrates to the crypts.
    d. occurs in cycles.

11. Which one of the following does not characterize the small intestine?
    a. It contains two smooth muscle layers, one arranged circularly and the other longitudinally.
    b. The presence of villi, crypts, brush borders on cells, and folds combine to increase surface area.
    c. Digestion is accomplished by microbial enzymes rather than by mammalian enzymes.
    d. It is composed of the duodenum, jejunum, and ileum, in that order from cranial to caudal.

12. For those animals not requiring extensive fermentation of their food, where does most of the digestion and absorption take place?
    a. Cecum
    b. Small intestine
    c. Colon
    d. Stomach

13. Which one of the following is the smallest division of intestinal surface amplification?
    a. Microvilli (brush border)
    b. Intestinal folds (plications)
    c. Villus

14. Reabsorption of electrolytes and water and microbial digestion are characteristic of the:
    a. stomach.
    b. small intestine.
    c. large intestine.

ACCESSORY ORGANS

15. Which one of the domestic animals has the liver lobules surrounded by visible connective tissue septa?
    a. Horse
    b. Pig
    c. Cow
    d. Dog

16. Which one of the following organs has both endocrine and exocrine functions?
    a. Pancreas
    b. Salivary glands
    c. Liver
    d. Spleen

COMPOSITION OF FOODSTUFFS

17. Amino acids can be coupled by peptide linkages to form:
    a. glycogen.
    b. triglycerides.
    c. cellulose.
    d. proteins.

18. Cellulose, starch, and glycogen are classified according to which one of the following?
    a. Protein, polypeptide
    b. Lipid, triglycerides
    c. Carbohydrate, polysaccharides
    d. Carbohydrate, disaccharides

19. Foods containing a high percentage of cellulose with low digestibility are classified as:
    a. concentrates.
    b. roughages.
    c. junk foods.
    d. fast foods.

PREGASTRIC MECHANICAL FUNCTIONS

20. Seizing and conveying food to the mouth is known as:
    a. apprehension.
    b. tension.
    c. prehension.
    d. pension.

21. When a bolus of food is swallowed:
    a. the soft palate is folded over the glottis.
    b. the epiglottis is elevated, closing the nasal cavity from the pharynx.
    c. respiration is inhibited.

22. Which one of the following best describes prehension?
    a. Movement of food through the intestines
    b. Seizing and conveying food to the mouth
    c. Fear
    d. Emptying of the stomach

23. The tongue is more important as a prehensile organ in the:
    a. cow.
    b. pig.
    c. horse.
    d. dog.

GASTROINTESTINAL MOTILITY

24. Segmental contractions are noted for their ability to:
    a. mix intestinal contents.
    b. propel intestinal contents toward the anus.

25. Parasympathetic stimulation to the intestine:
    a. decreases the resting membrane potential (more negative), thus decreasing motility.
    b. increases the resting membrane potential (less negative), thus decreasing motility.
    c. decreases the resting membrane potential, thus increasing motility.

d. increases the resting membrane potential, thus increasing motility.

26. Intestinal contractions initiated by distention, which stimulates activity cranial to and inhibits activity caudal to the distention, thus moving contents and propagating the reflex, are called:
    a. twitches.
    b. spasms.
    c. segmentation.
    d. peristalsis.

27. Which one of the autonomic divisions depolarizes gastrointestinal smooth muscle, increases spiking, and results in more vigorous gastrointestinal activity?
    a. Parasympathetic
    b. Sympathetic

MECHANICAL FUNCTIONS OF THE STOMACH AND SMALL INTESTINE

28. Vomiting is often observed in horses and cattle.
    a. True
    b. False

MECHANICAL FUNCTIONS OF THE LARGE INTESTINE

29. Where does most of the water and electrolyte reabsorption occur?
    a. Stomach
    b. Duodenum
    c. Ileum
    d. Large intestine

30. Which one of the following is not characteristic of large intestine function?
    a. Water conservation occurs because incompletely digested foodstuffs are further digested and absorbed.
    b. Microbial digestion does occur.
    c. There is considerable digestion by mammalian enzymes.
    d. The large intestine is a major site for water reabsorption.

31. A defecation frequency of 10 times per day would be considered as diarrhea in:
    a. the horse.
    b. the cow.
    c. the dog.
    d. all of the above.

DIGESTIVE SECRETIONS

32. Among the domestic animals, bicarbonate for the gastrointestinal tract is secreted:
    a. only by the salivary glands.
    b. only by the bile ducts.
    c. only by the exocrine pancreas.
    d. by salivary glands, exocrine pancreas, and bile ducts.

33. Which one of the following hormones is best known for its association with stimulation of pancreatic enzyme secretions and contraction of the gallbladder?
    a. Cholecystokinin
    b. Secretin

34. Which one of the following is best associated with the milk-coagulating enzyme of calves?
    a. Bile, formed in liver
    b. Renin, formed in kidney
    c. Rennin, formed in abomasum
    d. Enterokinase, formed in intestine

35. Which one of the following statements is not a characteristic of bile?
    a. Released from gallbladder under the influence of cholecystokinin
    b. Important for digestion because of presence of bile salts
    c. Contains digestive enzymes
    d. Emulsifies fat and assists transport of monoglycerides and free fatty acids to epithelial cells for absorption

36. Protein digestion begins in the stomach because of the enzymatic action of:
    a. HCl.
    b. pepsinogen.
    c. rennin.
    d. pepsin.

37. Which one of the following salivary functions is either nonexistent or insignificant in ruminants?
    a. Enzymes for digestion
    b. Chemical buffers for rumen
    c. Bacterial growth media enhancement
    d. Prevention of froth

38. Which hormone is responsible for the secretion of the pancreatic digestive enzymes and precursors of enzymes?
    a. Secretin
    b. Cholecystokinin
    c. Oxytocin
    d. Antidiuretic hormone

39. Which one of the following best describes trypsinogen and chymotrypsinogen?
    a. Precursors of proteolytic enzymes secreted by the intestinal epithelium
    b. Precursors of lipolytic enzymes secreted by the intestinal epithelium
    c. Proteolytic enzymes secreted by the intestinal epithelium
    d. Precursors of proteolytic enzymes secreted by the pancreas

40. Which one of the following is not a function of HCl in the stomach?
    a. Lowers pH
    b. Kills bacteria
    c. Converts trypsinogen to trypsin
    d. Converts pepsinogen to pepsin

41. The hepatic portal circulation:
    a. receives blood from the kidneys.
    b. is that which perfuses the hypothalamus.
    c. receives blood that arises from the capillaries of the stomach, spleen, and small and large intestine; and this blood then perfuses the liver sinusoids before entering the hepatic vein.
    d. has to do with concentrating the urine.

42. A hyperosmotic solution in the stomach becomes isotonic before it is evacuated into the duodenum.
    a. True
    b. False

43. Which salivary function is most important for ruminants?
    a. Provision of evaporative water for cooling
    b. Provision of amylase (conversion of starch to maltose)
    c. Provision of bicarbonates and phosphates for buffering

44. Pancreatic fluid flow is continuous in the:
    a. horse.
    b. dog.
    c. both horse and dog.

45. Which one of the following is activated by enterokinase in the intestine so that the active form can then activate the other proteolytic proenzymes?
    a. Trypsinogen
    b. Chymotrypsinogen
    c. Elastase
    d. Carboxypeptidase A

46. Contraction of the gallbladder and relaxation of the sphincter of Oddi are initiated by:
    a. CCK.
    b. secretin.
    c. gastrin.

DIGESTION AND ABSORPTION

47. Fermentation in the gastrointestinal tract of the cat and dog:
    a. never occurs.
    b. takes place in the stomach.
    c. would occur in the large intestine.
    d. causes gas formation only.

48. The microbes of fermentation are digested in both ruminant and nonruminant herbivores.
    a. True
    b. False

49. No further digestion is required for the absorption of (select the response in which all are correct):
    a. glucose, sucrose, galactose.
    b. glycerol, fatty acids, monoglycerides.

    c. amino acids, polypeptides.

    d. glycerol, fatty acids, triglycerides.

50. Which one of the following best describes the digestion of carbohydrates in the small intestine?
    a. It is accomplished in the intestinal lumen by carboxypeptidase A and B, trypsin, chymotrypsin, and elastase.
    b. Conversion to glucose, galactose, and fructose occurs in the lumen.
    c. Pancreatic amylase is produced by the intestinal epithelium.
    d. Sucrose, maltose, and lactose are degraded to monosaccharides by enzymes in the brush border of the intestinal epithelium.

51. Which one of the following is most likely to be resynthesized to its beginning form and to enter the central lacteals of the intestinal villi for its entry to the circulation?
    a. Monoglycerides and fatty acids
    b. Amino acids
    c. Monosaccharide
    d. Fruitcake

52. Where would one find chylomicrons?
    a. Gallbladder
    b. Pancreas
    c. Central lacteal
    d. Intestinal lumen

53. Complete protein hydrolysis yields:
    a. monosaccharides.
    b. amino acids.
    c. glycerol and fatty acids.
    d. peptides.

THE RUMINANT STOMACH

54. Rumen contractions can be observed in the left paralumbar fossa and should approximate:
    a. 1 to 2 each minute.
    b. 5 to 10 each minute.
    c. 5 to 10 each hour.
    d. TNTC.

CHARACTERISTICS OF RUMINANT DIGESTION

55. Which one of the following is associated with the sequence of flooding of the cardia, opening of the cardia, inspiration with a closed glottis, entrance of rumen content into the esophagus, and reverse peristalsis of the esophagus?
    a. Redeglutition
    b. Eructation
    c. Regurgitation
    d. Rumen contractions

56. A good estimate for the volume of saliva produced by an adult cow in 24 hours is:
    a. 30 gallons.
    b. 30 pints.
    c. 30 quarts.
    d. 30 cups.

57. Which one of the following is a component of rumination?
    a. Defecation
    b. Vomiting
    c. Eructation
    d. Regurgitation

58. Deglutition, regurgitation, and eructation (assuming distention of the esophagus) could all be observed on the left side of the neck of a cow.
    a. True
    b. False

59. The presence of gas stimulates receptors in the region of the cardia and initiates:
    a. regurgitation.
    b. eructation.
    c. defecation.
    d. flatulence.

60. Regurgitation is facilitated by:
    a. inspiration with a closed glottis (decreases mediastinal pressure).
    b. expiration (mediastinal pressure increased).
    c. salivation.
    d. thorough mastication.

CHEMISTRY AND MICROBIOLOGY OF THE RUMEN

61. The principal end product(s) of dietary carbohydrates in ruminants is(are):
    a. volatile fatty acids.
    b. triglycerides.
    c. glucose.
    d. amino acids.

62. Which vitamin synthesized in the rumen requires cobalt for its structure?
    a. Vitamin B_{12}
    b. Vitamin K
    c. Vitamin A
    d. Vitamin C

RUMINANT METABOLISM

63. Bloat in cattle is caused by:
    a. an increase in the volume of gas produced.
    b. a failure of the eructation mechanism.

64. Bloat in ruminants is caused by a change in the composition of the gas produced.
    a. True
    b. False

65. Ketosis occurs in ruminants because there is not enough acetyl CoA to direct acetic and butyric acid (two of the VFAs) into the Krebs cycle.
    a. True
    b. False

66. Which one of the following VFAs is the least likely to be productive of ketosis in ruminants?
    a. Acetic acid
    b. Propionic acid
    c. Butyric acid

AVIAN DIGESTION

67. Which one of the avian digestive tract structures secretes HCl and pepsinogen?
    a. Crop
    b. Proventriculus
    c. Gizzard
    d. Ceca

68. Which one of the avian digestive tract structures is very muscular and serves to grind or break down food?
    a. Crop
    b. Proventriculus
    c. Gizzard
    d. Ceca

69. Which avian digestive tract structure provides for the microbial digestion of cellulose?
    a. Gizzard
    b. Ileum
    c. Ceca
    d. Cloaca

70. It is possible for uric acid to go from the cloaca to the ceca.
    a. True
    b. False

71. The avian vent:
    a. ventilates the cloaca.
    b. serves as an opening for the passage of feces, feces mixed with urine, and eggs.

72. The bursa of Fabricius:
    a. is a part of the small intestine.
    b. is associated with humoral immunity.
    c. produces erythrocytes.
    d. is a site for water reabsorption from the cloaca.

73. Heat stress associated with ambient temperatures of 37°C:
    a. has no affect on absorption from the ileum.
    b. decreases mesenteric blood flow and thereby reduces absorption.
    c. increases turkey intelligence.

ANSWERS TO SELF EVALUATION—CHAPTER 12

1.	c	20.	c	39.	d	58.	a
2.	a	21.	c	40.	c	59.	b
3.	c	22.	b	41.	c	60.	a
4.	a	23.	a	42.	b	61.	a
5.	b	24.	a	43.	c	62.	a
6.	c	25.	d	44.	a	63.	b
7.	a	26.	d	45.	a	64.	b
8.	b	27.	a	46.	a	65.	b
9.	a	28.	b	47.	c	66.	b
10.	b	29.	d	48.	b	67.	b
11.	c	30.	c	49.	b	68.	c
12.	b	31.	c	50.	d	69.	c
13.	a	32.	d	51.	a	70.	a
14.	c	33.	a	52.	c	71.	b
15.	b	34.	c	53.	b	72.	b
16.	a	35.	c	54.	a	73.	b
17.	d	36.	d	55.	c		
18.	c	37.	a	56.	a		
19.	b	38.	b	57.	d		

CHAPTER 13

Body Heat and Temperature Regulation

CHAPTER OUTLINE

- **BODY TEMPERATURE**
  Gradients of Temperature
  Diurnal Temperature
- **PHYSIOLOGIC RESPONSES TO HEAT**
  Circulatory Adjustments
  Evaporative Heat Loss
  Responses to Extremes of Heat
- **PHYSIOLOGIC RESPONSES TO COLD**
  Reduction of Heat Loss
  Increase of Heat Production

- **HIBERNATION**
  Awakening from Hibernation
  Brown Fat versus White Fat
- **HYPOTHERMIA AND HYPERTHERMIA**
  Hypothermia
  Fever
  Heat Stroke and Impaired Evaporation

The chemical reactions of the body—and therefore the body functions—depend on body temperature. An elevation of temperature accelerates the reactions, and a lowering of temperature depresses the reactions. To avoid fluctuations of function caused by temperature, mammals and birds have developed a means whereby body temperature is maintained at a relatively constant level regardless of the temperature of the surroundings. Mammals and birds are classified as homeotherm, or warm-blooded animals. Poikilotherm (cold-blooded) animals have a body temperature that varies with the temperature of the environment.

■ BODY TEMPERATURE

1. What factors can influence body temperature?
2. What is meant by core temperature?
3. Does a rectal temperature reading represent the temperature throughout the body?
4. What is meant by diurnal temperature?
5. Give an example of heat storage in an animal. What advantage is served by heat storage?
6. What is an approximate value for rectal temperature in common domestic animals?

An average body temperature is associated with each domestic animal species. These temperatures are shown in *Table 13-1*, along with their commonly observed ranges. The temperatures were obtained by rectal insertion of a thermometer in resting animals. A number of conditions can influence body temperature, including exercise, time of day, environmental temperature, digestion, and drinking of water.

Gradients of Temperature

Different parts of the body can differ in temperature because of differences in metabolic

TABLE 13-1 AVERAGE RECTAL TEMPERATURES OF VARIOUS SPECIES

	AVERAGE		RANGE	
ANIMAL	°C	°F	°C	°F
Stallion	37.6	99.7	37.2–38.1	99.0–100.6
Mare	37.8	100	37.3–38.2	99.1–100.8
Donkey	37.4	99.3	36.4–38.4	97.5–101.1
Camel	37.5	99.5	34.2–40.7	93.6–105.3
Beef cow	38.3	101	36.7–39.1	98.0–102.4
Dairy cow	38.6	101.5	38.0–39.3	100.4–102.8
Sheep	39.1	102.3	38.3–39.9	100.9–103.8
Goat	39.1	102.3	38.5–39.7	101.3–103.5
Pig	39.2	102.5	38.7–39.8	101.6–103.6
Dog	38.9	102	37.9–39.9	100.2–103.8
Cat	38.6	101.5	38.1–39.2	100.5–102.5
Rabbit	39.5	103.1	38.6–40.1	101.5–104.2
Chicken (daylight)	41.7	107.1	40.6–43.0	105.0–109.4

From Andersson BE, Jonasson H. Temperature regulation and environmental physiology. In: Swenson MJ, Reece WO, eds. Dukes' Physiology of Domestic Animals. 11th Ed. Ithaca, NY: Cornell University Press, 1993.

rate, blood flow, or distance from the surface. For example, the liver and the brain can have a temperature that is higher than that of the blood, and they are therefore cooled by blood circulation. The deep body temperature, or core temperature, is higher than the temperature of the limbs or even higher than the temperature observed rectally. **Rectal temperature** represents a true steady state of temperature, however, because it reaches equilibrium more slowly.

Diurnal Temperature

Variations in temperature related to the time of day are designated as **diurnal temperatures**. Animals that are active during the day and sleep at night have body temperatures that are lower in the morning than in the afternoon. The opposite is true for nocturnal (night-active) animals. Also, as a water conservation

measure, the body temperature of the camel is permitted to increase during the day so that the excess heat can be dissipated at night when the desert air is cool; this is known as heat storage. The temperature of a normal camel, watered every day and fully hydrated, varies by less than 2°C, between about 36°C and 38°C (more water available for evaporation and less need for heat storage). When the camel is deprived of drinking water, however, its morning temperature can be as low as 34°C and its highest temperature, in the late afternoon, can be nearly 41°C (Fig. 13-1).

■ PHYSIOLOGIC RESPONSES TO HEAT

1. How can the diversion of blood to the skin result in loss of body heat? How can heat loss by this means be regulated?

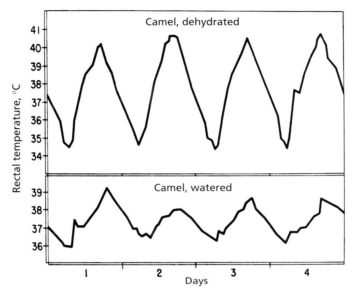

■ FIGURE 13-1 Diurnal temperatures in the watered and dehydrated camel. The rectal temperature elevations (heat storage) occur during the day, and the reductions occur at night. (From Schmidt-Nielsen K. Osmotic regulation in higher vertebrates. In: The Harvey Lectures, 1962–1963, Series 58. London: Academic Press, 1963.)

2. What is the stimulus for allowing heat to be lost via the skin?
3. Where are thermosensitive cells located in the brain?
4. Are there any reflexes associated with heat gain or heat loss?
5. What percent of the heat produced in the body is normally lost by insensible means?
6. What type of sweat glands predominate in animals?
7. What is the principal function of the apocrine sweat glands?
8. Is sweating an important mechanism for heat loss among domestic animals? Which one of the domestic animals represents the greatest use of this means? The least?
9. What function is accomplished by panting? What is panting? How is hyperventilation prevented while panting? Is panting only observed in the dog?
10. Which domestic animals are most able to withstand extremes of heat?
11. What are factors associated with the pig's intolerance to heat?
12. How does the cat increase evaporative heat loss?
13. What is an approximate body temperature of birds? Why is pulmonary ventilation more likely to cool the body of birds than that of mammals?

Heat is produced constantly in the body as a result of metabolism. If there were not provisions for losing heat, the temperature of the body would increase to intolerable levels. Two principal means for losing heat are: 1) radiation, conduction, and convection, and 2) evaporation of water from the skin and respiratory passageways. A third way considers the excretion of feces and urine that leave the animal at body temperature. Heat lost by excretion of feces and urine is small and is considered negligible. Under ordinary conditions, about 75% of ▓▓▓▓▓▓ from the body is dissipated ▓▓▓▓▓ conduction, and convection a▓▓▓▓▓▓d mostly by vasomotor activity.

Circulatory Adjustments

Inasmuch as circulating blood is a distributor of body heat, heat can be lost from the blood if blood is brought to the skin surface and exposed to a gradient for loss to the environment.

A schematic section of the skin of the dog (Fig. 13-2) illustrates the extensive network of blood vessels to the skin. The amount of blood circulating to the skin is controlled by sympathetic vasoconstrictor fibers to the blood vessels. An increase in tone results in constriction of blood vessels and diversion of blood from the surface, thereby conserving heat. A decrease in tone lets more blood go to the surface. A stimulus for a decrease in tone so that more heat can be lost from the body, is the temperature of the blood circulated to the brain. Thermosensitive cells in the rostral hypothalamus respond to warming by activating physiologic and behavioral heat loss mechanisms (Fig. 13-3). Similarly, cooling of the same region stimulates other thermosensitive cells to evoke thermoregulatory responses for heat gain. Reflexes to inhibit vasoconstrictor tone also arise from thermoreceptors in the skin and other parts of the body.

Evaporative Heat Loss

Evaporation of water results in cooling. Loss of water by evaporation is referred to as **insensible water loss**; this includes water lost from the skin surfaces and water lost in the heated exhaled air. Normally about 25% of the heat produced in an animal at rest is lost when water is lost by insensible means.

Evaporative heat losses are increased by sweating and panting. The relative importance of sweating as a heat loss mechanism varies among species. Generally, the function of sweat glands as dissipaters of body heat is less effective in domestic animals than in humans.

There are two types of sweat glands: **apocrine** and **eccrine**. Eccrine sweat glands are those typically found in humans, but are sparse among domestic animals. In the dog and cat they occupy only the foot pad location. This area does not subserve thermoregulation, it provides for a moist surface and subsequent improved traction. Horses, cattle, sheep, dogs, and cats have apocrine sweat glands disseminated over the body surface (Fig. 13-4). The composition, volume, stimulus for secretion, and function of apocrine sweat varies among

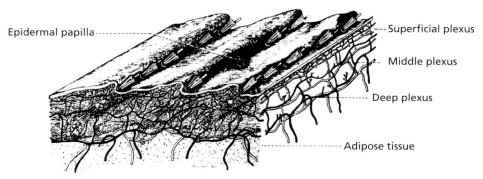

■ **FIGURE 13-2** Schematic section of dog skin showing the extensive network of blood vessels and the location of insulating adipose tissue. (From Evans HE. Miller's Anatomy of the Dog. 3rd Ed. Philadelphia: WB Saunders Company, 1993.)

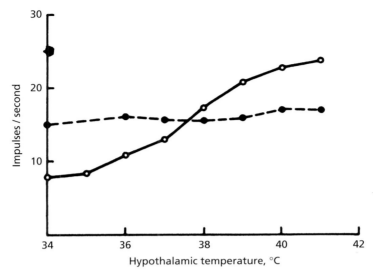

■ **FIGURE 13-3** Response of warmth-sensitive neurons (solid line) in the rostral hypothalamus of the cat to increasing hypothalamic temperature. Neurons insensitive to warmth (dashed line) do not increase their activity. (From Nakayama T, Hammel HT, Hardy JD, Eisenman JS. Thermal stimulation of electrical activity of single units of the preoptic region. Am J Physiol 1963;204:1122.)

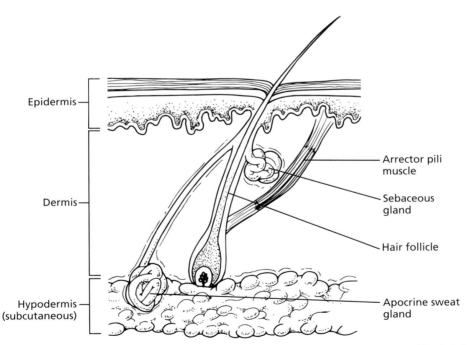

■ **FIGURE 13-4** Schematic representation of apocrine and sebaceous glands and their association with a hair follicle. The secretory parts of the apocrine glands are located in the dermal and subcutaneous layers of the skin. The excretory ducts pass upward through the dermis and empty into the hair follicles above the ducts of the sebaceous glands.

species. In the dog, and perhaps in other species, apocrine sweat is a proteinaceous, white, odorless, milky fluid that is formed slowly and continuously. On the skin surface, it mixes with sebum from the sebaceous glands to form a protective emulsion that acts as a physical and chemical barrier. Characteristic animal odors arise from bacterial flora action on apocrine secretions. Heat loss from sweating (thermo regulatory function) is probably greatest in the horse, followed (in order) by cattle, sheep, dogs, cats, and swine.

The panting mechanism is effective in dissipating the heat load because greater amounts of air are made to go over moist surfaces. Panting is most effective in the dog, but it is also observed in the other domestic animals. Essentially, panting is an increase in dead space ventilation without change in respiratory alveolar ventilation. A decreased tidal volume is associated with the increased respiratory frequency of panting; in this way, hyperventilation of the alveoli is prevented.

In cattle, panting is accompanied by increased salivation, and the salivary secretion promotes cooling by evaporation. Salivary secretion loss by evaporation and drooling (physical loss to the exterior of the body) can result in metabolic acidosis because of loss of bicarbonate and phosphate buffers contained in ruminant saliva.

Increases in sweating and panting are brought about by increased blood temperature, subsequent adjustments by the hypothalamus, and reflexes produced by local heating of the skin.

Responses to Extremes of Heat

Different animal species differ in their ability to withstand heat. The humidity of the air becomes a factor—as humidity increases, evaporation from insensible losses is reduced and less cooling occurs.

Of all domestic animals, cattle and sheep seem to be the most able to withstand extremes of heat. Open-mouth panting and sweating

occur as the temperature increases, and these animals can withstand temperatures as high as 43°C (109°F) with humidity above 65%.

The pig cannot tolerate a temperature above 35°C (95°F) with humidity above 65%. The intolerance of pigs to heat is recognized by transporters of livestock. During periods of heat, the transport of pigs is usually delayed until night, and they often are hosed with water. Pigs do not sweat copiously, and their small mouth makes them ineffective at panting. In addition, they often have substantial subcutaneous fat.

When the relative humidity is above 65%, the cat cannot withstand prolonged exposure to an environmental temperature of 40°C (104°F) or higher. In addition to panting, the cat can increase evaporative losses by spreading saliva over its hair coat.

Because the dog is effective at panting, it can withstand extreme environmental temperatures better than the cat, but it is in danger of collapse when its rectal temperature reaches 41°C (106°F).

In birds, the air sacs are extensions of the lungs, which extend into the body cavities. The body temperature of birds is about 41°C (106°F). Pulmonary ventilation air is more likely to cool the body of birds than that of mammals because of the larger gradient and because of the closeness of the air to the body organs (via air sacs, see Chapter 10). It seems that prolonged exposure of a hen to an air temperature of 38°C (100°F) is unsafe if the relative humidity is above 75%. A rectal temperature of 45°C (113°F) is the upper limit of safety in the chicken.

■ PHYSIOLOGIC RESPONSES TO COLD

1. How are responses to cold activated?
2. What is accomplished by the countercurrent flow of blood in the limbs of animals?
3. What are some behavioral responses for reducing heat loss?

4.   What is piloerection?
5.   Which farm animals have the lowest critical temperature?
6.   What is accomplished by shivering?
7.   What is the role of thyroid hormone in adaptation to cold?

Cold activates body heating mechanisms, just as excess heat activates body cooling mechanisms. With excess cooling, heat is either conserved by reducing heat loss or is generated to compensate for that which is lost. The physiologic responses to cold are activated by blood temperature and local reflexes, as are the responses to heat.

Reduction of Heat Loss

In an attempt to reduce heat loss, animals instinctively curl up when they lie down. This behavioral response reduces the surface area exposed to the cold. To increase the insulation value of their hair or fur, **piloerection** occurs. In this process the hair is made to become more erect by the arrector pili muscle of the hair follicle (see Fig. 13-4). With sustained exposure to cold, the hair coat thickens and the amount of subcutaneous fat increases.

In contrast to vasodilation, which occurs to accommodate heat loss, the peripheral vessels are constricted by an increase in vasoconstrictor tone.

Heat is also conserved by the arrangement of the deep blood vessels that supply the legs of animals. Blood returning in the veins from the colder legs is close to the warmer blood in the arteries going to the legs. Because of the temperature differences, heat is transferred from the arteries to the veins; this decreases the gradient for heat loss from the arterial blood to the environment. This arrangement of blood vessels is known as a **countercurrent system**.

Increase of Heat Production

When the ability to reduce heat loss is not adequate to maintain a normal body tempera-

ture, heat must be produced. The temperature to which body temperature decreases before heat generation begins is known as the **critical temperature**. Among farm animals, cattle and sheep have the lowest critical temperature, which means that they are better suited to withstand cold.

Shivering is one means by which heat is generated for withstanding cold. Shivering is a generalized rhythmic contraction of muscles. Because 30% to 50% of the energy of muscle contraction is converted to heat, the seemingly spasmodic contraction of muscle serves a useful purpose.

Other methods are used to generate heat in addition to shivering. **Epinephrine** and **norepinephrine** (see Chapter 6) are both released in increased amounts in the cold. **Brown fat** is an important source of thermogenesis (see Brown Fat versus White Fat later in this chapter). Epinephrine and norepinephrine are the stimuli for increased metabolism of brown fat. In addition to hibernating animals, brown fat is also found in newborn mammals. Epinephrine and norepinephrine have calorigenic effects with other cells as well, and the calorigenic effects are potentiated by the thyroid hormone. **Thyroid hormone** (see Chapter 6) is secreted in increased amounts during periods of cold.

■ HIBERNATION

1.   What is the favored definition of hibernation? Is a greatly reduced core temperature a necessary component of hibernation?
2.   Is the bear considered to be a true hibernant?
3.   Is hibernation characteristic of homeotherms or of poikilotherms?
4.   What prevents hibernants from freezing? Is there periodic awakening from hibernation?
5.   What is brown fat?

Hibernation is the act of resting in a dormant state in a protected burrow. This definition has recently returned to favor. Formerly, it was proposed that "Hibernation is the assumption of a state of greatly reduced core temperature by a mammal or a bird which has its active body temperature near 37°C, meanwhile retaining the capability of spontaneously rewarming back to the normal homeothermic level without absorbing heat from its environment" (Menaker M. Hibernation-hypothermia: An annual cycle of response to low temperature in the bat *Myotis lucifugus*. J Cell Comp Physiol 1962;59:16–174). According to the former definition, bears were not considered to be true hibernators because their core body temperature was not greatly reduced. The core body temperature of bears is reduced by only 6.8°C during their dormancy, as opposed to a reduction of 20°C to 30°C by animals that were considered to be true hibernators. The lesser reduction in body temperature of the bear is now believed to be a biologic protection for hibernating bears; accordingly, they are considered true hibernants. Because of their large body mass, it is thought that too much time would be involved in their revival to activity if their body temperature were lowered by 20°C to 30°C. The longer revival time would make them easy victims to another cannibalistic bear that had revived.

The characteristics of hibernation are as follows:

1. Hibernation is a process of warm-blooded animals.
2. The process is autonomous—the animal induces and reverses it by some self-contained mechanism.
3. The process is radical—changes involve not only overt physiologic functioning, but also cellular and subcellular changes.
4. All physiologic functions continue, but at a reduced rate.
5. During the process, body temperature is lowered significantly to a level compatible with survival for the species.

Awakening from Hibernation

Hibernating animals awake from their dormant state periodically. For example, the kidneys continue to form urine and the animal has a need to urinate. A protective mechanism against profound cooling also exists in winter hibernants. If the body temperature declines to levels near freezing, the animal awakes and rapidly rewarms.

Brown Fat versus White Fat

Brown fat is a connective tissue with a color that results from cytochrome pigments and a high density of mitochondria. It is typically found in hibernating animals and in smaller species. It is also present in the newborn of many species and disappears within the first few months of life. Its usual location is in the subcutaneous region between the scapulae (shoulder blades) and in the region of the kidneys as well as within the myocardium. The ability of hibernators to elevate their body temperature from reduced levels to the temperature necessary for arousal (nonshivering thermogenesis) is facilitated by their depots of brown fat. Brown fat differs from white fat not only in color, but also in metabolic characteristics. When brown fat cells are stimulated, they consume oxygen and produce heat at a high rate.

■ HYPOTHERMIA AND HYPERTHERMIA

1. What is hypothermia?
2. How can hypothermia occur in anesthetized animals?
3. What is fever? What are its beneficial effects?
4. Where is the need for fever sensed?
5. What are characteristics of heat stroke? How can its associated hyperthermia be relieved?

Reduction of the deep body temperature below normal in nonhibernating homeotherms is known as **hypothermia**; **hyperthermia** is the reverse.

Hypothermia

Hypothermia can readily occur during central nervous system anesthesia because the hypothalamic response to cold blood is depressed. It normally occurs as a result of prolonged exposure to cold, coupled with an inability of the heat-conserving and heat-generating mechanisms to keep pace. Tolerance to lowered body temperatures varies among species. In dogs, death can occur when the rectal temperature approximates 25°C (77°F). Hypothermia in any animal can become life threatening unless environmental conditions improve or external heat is provided.

It is important to monitor body temperature during and after procedures requiring anesthesia because of the depressed hypothalamic response. External heat sources are often fitted to surgical tables for the maintenance of body temperature. When these are used, there must be assurance that local injury to skin does not occur. When animals do not recover quickly after anesthesia (e.g., pentobarbital anesthesia), monitoring body temperature and provision of external heat is extremely important.

Fever

Fever is an elevation of deep body temperature that is brought on by microorganism-caused disease. Fever is usually beneficial because immunologic mechanisms are accelerated and the high temperature induced is detrimental to the microorganisms, but it can be damaging if allowed to go too high. In fever, the set point of the hypothalamus is elevated and the body senses that the blood is too cold, so heat-conserving and heat-generating mechanisms are recruited. Shivering and a feeling of coolness are characteristics of beginning fever. Fever is generally self-limiting; maximum temperatures of 41°C (106°F) can be approached.

Heat Stroke and Impaired Evaporation

Hyperthermia exclusive of fever can be associated with **heat stroke**. In this condition, heat production exceeds the evaporative capacity of the environment and occurs when the humidity is high. Hyperthermia can also develop when the evaporative mechanisms become impaired as a result of loss of body fluid or reduced blood volume. Antipyretic drugs (effective against fever) are ineffective in reducing the body temperature in heat stroke and impaired evaporation conditions, and relief is obtained only by whole-body cooling.

■ SUGGESTED READING

Andersson BE, Jonasson H. Temperature regulation and environmental physiology. In: Swenson MJ, Reece WO, eds. Dukes' Physiology of Domestic Animals. 11th Ed. Ithaca, NY: Cornell University Press, 1993.

Folk GE, Jr, Larson A, Folk MA. Physiology of hibernating bears. Proceedings of the third international conference on bear research and management, June 1974. In: Pelton MR, Lentfer JW, Folk GE, eds. Bears—Their Biology and Management. Morges, Switzerland: International Union for Conservation of Nature and Natural Resources, 1976:373–380.

Robertshaw D. Temperature regulation and the thermal environment. In: Reece WO, ed. Dukes' Physiology of Domestic Animals. 12th Ed. Ithaca, NY: Cornell University Press, 2004.

SELF EVALUATION—CHAPTER 13

BODY TEMPERATURE

1. The average rectal temperature in a healthy cow should be about:
   a. 98.6°F.
   b. 101.5°F.
   c. 104.0°F.
   d. 106.5°F.

2. Variations in temperature related to the time of day are known as:
   a. diurnal temperatures.
   b. core temperatures.
   c. poikilotherms.
   d. ambient temperatures.

3. Nocturnal animals have body temperatures that are lower in the morning than in the afternoon.
   a. True
   b. False

PHYSIOLOGIC RESPONSES TO HEAT

4. What part of the brain has a temperature regulating center?
   a. Medulla
   b. Thalamus
   c. Hypothalamus
   d. Cerebral cortex

5. Which sweat gland type predominates among the domestic animals?
   a. Eccrine
   b. Apocrine

6. Which one of the following animals has the greatest heat loss from sweating?
   a. Sheep
   b. Cats
   c. Dogs
   d. Horses
   e. Pigs

7. Increased blood flow to the skin would increase heat loss.
   a. True
   b. False

8. Which domestic animal(s) is(are) best able to withstand extremes of heat?
   a. Horse
   b. Dog
   c. Pig
   d. Cattle and sheep

PHYSIOLOGIC RESPONSES TO COLD

9. The countercurrent flow of blood to the limbs of animals assists in warming the limbs.
   a. True
   b. False

10. Which domestic animal(s) is(are) best able to withstand cold?
    a. Horse
    b. Dog
    c. Pig
    d. Cattle and sheep

11. Piloerection is a response to:
    a. heat.
    b. cold.
    c. watching television.

HIBERNATION

12. A true hibernant:
    a. is not represented by the bear.
    b. abandons homeothermy in cold weather but will awaken if body temperature approaches freezing or some other higher set point.
    c. abandons homeothermy in the cold and may freeze if body temperature becomes lower than freezing.
    d. maintains a constant body temperature even while it sleeps through cold weather.

13. White fat is more productive of heat production than brown fat.
    a. True
    b. False

HYPOTHERMIA AND HYPERTHERMIA

14. Which one of the following is characterized by greater heat production than the capacity for heat dissipation?

a. Fever
b. Heat stroke

15. Fever has no beneficial effects.
    a. True
    b. False

ANSWERS TO SELF EVALUATION—CHAPTER 13

1. b	5. b	9. b	13. b
2. a	6. d	10. d	14. b
3. b	7. a	11. b	15. b
4. c	8. d	12. b	

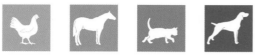

CHAPTER 14

Male Reproduction

CHAPTER OUTLINE

- **TESTES AND ASSOCIATED STRUCTURES**
  Epididymis
  Ductus Deferens
  Scrotum
- **DESCENT OF THE TESTES**
- **ACCESSORY SEX GLANDS AND SEMEN**
- **PENIS AND PREPUCE**
- **MUSCLES OF MALE GENITALIA**
- **BLOOD AND NERVE SUPPLY**
- **SPERMATOGENESIS**

Epididymal Transport
Spermatogenic Wave
Hormonal Control
Other Functions of Testosterone
- **ERECTION**
- **MOUNTING AND INTROMISSION**
- **EMISSION AND EJACULATION**
- **FACTORS AFFECTING TESTICULAR FUNCTION**
- **REPRODUCTION IN THE AVIAN MALE**

The reproductive functions of the male involve the formation of sperm and the deposition of the sperm into the female. Sperm are produced in the seminiferous tubules of the testes and are then transported through the rete testes to the epididymides, where they are stored and matured. The production of sperm is a continuous process once it has been initiated. However, it can change in rate at times in some species, depending on the amount of daylight (photoperiod). The introduction of semen into the female is preceded by erection of the penis so that it can enter the tubular genitalia of the female. Entrance is followed by emission of sperm into the penile urethra, along with stored secretions of the accessory glands. Actual transport of semen through the penile urethra to the region of the cervix or into the uterus of the female is accomplished by ejaculation. The process of male reproduction is assisted by hormones and the autonomic nervous system.

■ TESTES AND ASSOCIATED STRUCTURES

1. What are the seminiferous tubules?

2. Know the relative location of the Sertoli cells. Are they within the seminiferous tubules?

3. Know the relative location of the Leydig cells. Are they within the seminiferous tubules?

4. Which compartment of the seminiferous tubule provides a home for the spermatogonium? What must it move through to get into the other compartment? What is the name of the compartment where spermatozoa are finally formed?

5. What are the parts of the epididymis?

6. What is accomplished by storage of spermatozoa in the epididymis?

The two testes produce spermatozoa. Although they vary somewhat in size, shape, and location among species, they share a similar structure. The bull testicle and its associated genitalia are shown in *Figures 14-1* and *14-2*. The **seminiferous tubules** are convoluted and occupy the greatest portion of each testicle. The spermatozoa are produced within

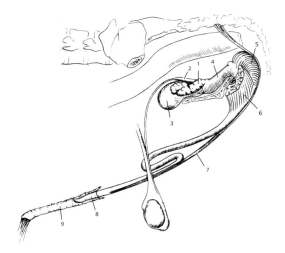

■ **FIGURE 14-1** Genital organs of the bull. **1)** Seminal vesicle; **2)** ampulla of vas deferens; **3)** bladder; **4)** urethral muscle surrounding pelvic urethra; **5)** bulbospongiosus muscle; **6)** ischiocavernosus muscle; **7)** retractor penis muscle; **8)** glans penis; **9)** preputial membrane and cavity. (From Roberts SJ. Veterinary Obstetrics and Genital Diseases [Theriogenology]. 3rd Ed. Woodstock, VT: Stephen J. Roberts, 1986.)

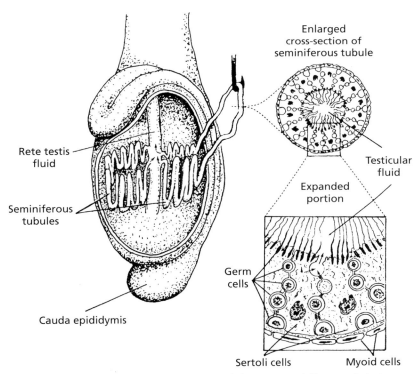

■ **FIGURE 14-2** Detailed structure of the testicle. Only two of the many seminiferous tubule loops are shown. Testicular fluid is secreted by Sertoli cells into the lumen of the seminiferous tubules. Myoid cells are contractile cells contained within the basement membrane. (From Hafez ESE, Hafez B. Reproduction in Farm Animals. 7th Ed. Baltimore: Lippincott Williams & Wilkins, 2000.)

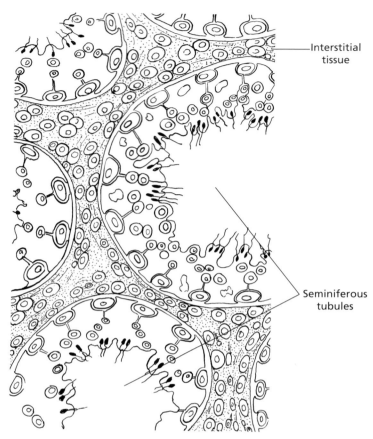

Interstitial
tissue

Seminiferous
tubules

■ **FIGURE 14-3** Relationship of the seminiferous tubules to each other and to the interstitial tissue. The interstitial tissue is occupied not only by the usual blood vascular network but also by Leydig cells (interstitial cells) and by connective tissue septa (provides support for seminiferous tubules) from the connective tissue capsule (tunica albuginea) of the testis.

them. The testicle is surrounded by a connective tissue capsule called the **tunica albuginea**. Support of the seminiferous tubules is provided by connective tissue extensions (**septa** or **trabeculae**) into the testis from the tunica albuginea. A cross section of the testicle (*Fig. 14-3*) shows the relationship of the seminiferous tubules to each other and to their connective tissue support (interstitial tissue).

In addition to spermatozoa in various stages of development, two other important cell types are the **Sertoli cell** (sustentacular cell) and the **Leydig cell** (interstitial cell). The Sertoli cell provides a "nurse" function for developing spermatozoa. Processes from Sertoli cells sur-

round spermatids and spermatocytes and provide intimate contact with all stages of spermatozoa production; in this respect they are known as sustentacular (supporting) cells. The arrangement of Sertoli cells and the details of seminiferous tubule compartments are shown in *Figure 14-4*. The Sertoli cells have their base at the periphery of the seminiferous tubules and extend toward the center. The basal junction (tight junction) with adjacent Sertoli cells forms a blood-testis barrier that permits control of the environment within the tubule and also prevents spermatozoa from entering the interstitium. The Sertoli cells divide the seminiferous tubules into two com-

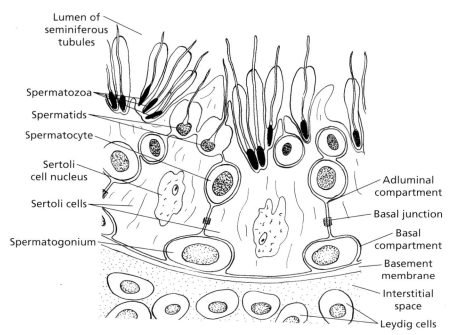

Lumen of
seminiferous
tubules

Spermatozoa

Spermatids

Spermatocyte

Sertoli
cell nucleus

Sertoli cells

Spermatogonium

Adluminal
compartment

Basal junction

Basal
compartment

Basement
membrane

Interstitial
space

Leydig cells

■ **FIGURE 14-4** Schematic representation of the periphery of a seminiferous tubule. The Sertoli cells divide the seminiferous tubule into adluminal and basal compartments at their basal junction (tight junction). Leydig cells are in the interstitial space. The basal junction forms a blood-testis barrier whereby the tubule environment is controlled and spermatozoa are prevented from entering the interstitium.

partments: 1) the **basal compartment**, which communicates with interstitial fluid and provides space for germinal epithelial cells; and 2) the **adluminal compartment**, which is the space between Sertoli cells that communicates centrally with the lumen of the tubule. Division of a germinal epithelial cell (spermatogonium) in the basal compartment provides a replacement cell and another cell, which must move through the Sertoli cell junction to enter the adluminal compartment. Here, further divisions occur and spermatozoa are finally formed. The Sertoli cells secrete a fluid into the adluminal compartment; its composition favors the developing spermatozoa.

Epididymis

The **epididymis** is a collection and storage tubule for the testis (*Fig. 14-5*). It begins at the pole of the testis in which blood vessels and nerves enter; this is known as the **head of the epididymis**. The head continues along one side of the testis as the **body of the epididymis**, which terminates before making a turn upward as the **tail of the epididymis**. The head of the epididymis receives sperm and adluminal fluid through efferent ducts from the rete testis (the intratesticular network of straight tubules that receives content from the convoluted seminiferous tubules). Spermatozoa move to the epididymis by the flow of fluid into the lumen of the seminiferous tubules from the adluminal spaces. Storage in the epididymis allows the spermatozoa to reach maturity and become motile. Reabsorption of much of the seminiferous tubular fluid occurs in the head of the epididymis.

Ductus Deferens

The **ductus deferens** (see Fig. 14-1), sometimes called the **vas deferens**, is the continuation of the duct system from the tail of the

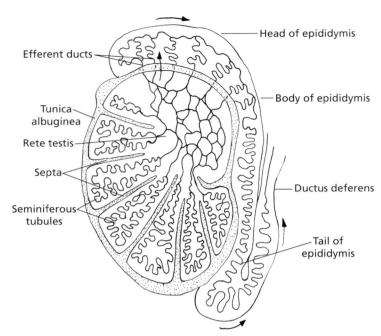

Head of epididymis

Efferent ducts

Body of epididymis

Tunica albuginea

Rete testis

Ductus deferens

Septa

Seminiferous tubules

Tail of epididymis

■ **FIGURE 14-5** Relationship of the seminiferous tubules to the rete testis, efferent ducts, epididymis, and ductus deferens. The rete testis is a network of straight tubules connecting convoluted seminiferous tubules with the highly convoluted epididymal tubule via efferent ducts (extratesticular). The flow of spermatozoa with their fluids is shown by the arrows.

epididymis to the pelvic urethra. As the ductus deferens leaves the testis, toward the abdomen, it is enclosed along with the testicular artery, vein, and nerve, and lymphatic vessels within the **visceral layer** of the **vaginal tunic**. This combination of structures is known as the **spermatic cord** (*Fig. 14-6*). The visceral layer of the vaginal tunic also envelops the testis and epididymis. It is derived from abdominal peritoneum of embryonic origin when the testes descended to the scrotum via the inguinal canal. The **inguinal canal** is an oblique passage from the abdominal cavity to the exterior of the body that extends from the **deep (interior) inguinal ring** to the **superficial (exterior) inguinal ring**. The inguinal rings are slits in the tendinous attachments of the two flat abdominal muscles to the pelvis. After the spermatic cord passes through the inguinal rings, the ductus deferens separates from the

spermatic cord to proceed to the pelvic urethra (see Fig. 14-1). The ductus deferens terminates with an enlarged, glandular area (variable size among species), known as the **ampulla of the ductus deferens** (absent in the boar). The relationship of the terminal ductus deferens to the urinary bladder, accessory glands, and pelvic urethra is also shown in Figure 14-1.

Scrotum

The **scrotum** is a cutaneous sac containing the testes. The scrotum contains a subcutaneous layer of smooth muscle fibers, the **tunica dartos**, which contracts in cold weather and holds the testes closer to the abdominal wall. The scrotum is lined with the **parietal layer** of the **vaginal tunic**, which is a continuation of parietal peritoneum into the scrotum.

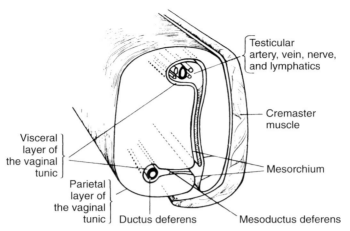

■ **FIGURE 14-6** Cross section of spermatic cord of mammals. (From Frandson RD, Wilke WL, Fails AD. Anatomy and Physiology of Farm Animals. 6th Ed. Baltimore: Lippincott Williams & Wilkins, 2003.)

■ DESCENT OF THE TESTES

1. What structures compose the spermatic cord?
2. Read and understand the relationship of scrotal hernias to the visceral and parietal vaginal tunics.
3. What are cryptorchid testes?

It is helpful to describe the lining of the scrotum and covering of the testis in more detail because it explains the origin of scrotal or inguinal hernias frequently encountered in pigs. During embryonic development the testes are intraabdominal but outside the peritoneum. They have not yet entered the scrotum, but each has a fibrous connection to the scrotum known as the **gubernaculum testis**. As development and growth progress, the gubernaculum testis pulls the testes through the inguinal canal into the scrotum that creates a double-walled tube of peritoneum. The testis, epididymis, ductus deferens, and testicular vessels, nerves, and lymphatics are enveloped by the inner tube of peritoneum known as the visceral vaginal tunic. The vessels, nerves, lymphatics, and ductus deferens are the components of the spermatic cord (see Fig. 14-6).

The **cremaster muscle** (an extension of the external abdominal oblique muscle) lies on the spermatic cord and assists with drawing the testes closer to the abdominal wall. The outer tube of peritoneum is known as the parietal vaginal tunic, and it lines the scrotum (*Fig. 14-7*). The testis and epididymis that are enveloped within the visceral vaginal tunic completely fill the scrotal cavity lined by the parietal vaginal tunic so that only a narrow space remains between the two tunics (the **vaginal cavity**). The vaginal cavity is continuous with the abdominal cavity at the deep vaginal ring (location where the parietal vaginal tunic of the scrotum is continuous with the parietal peritoneum of the abdominal cavity). The spermatic cord passes through the superficial and deep vaginal rings into the abdominal cavity. If the vaginal rings are too large, loops of intestine may enter the vaginal cavity to constitute what is known as an **inguinal hernia**. An inguinal hernia that has passed into the scrotum is known as a **scrotal hernia**. The herniated intestinal loops have the potential for **strangulation** (cut-off blood supply) or for **evisceration** (removal from the abdominal cavity) at the time of castration.

Cryptorchid testes are those that fail to descend. This condition seems to be most

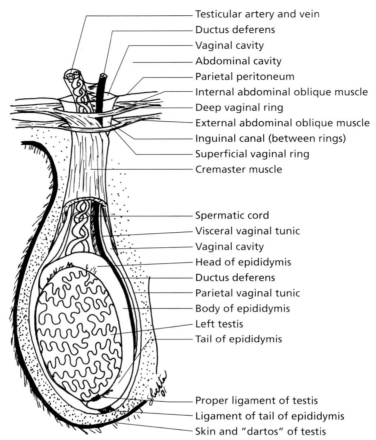

Testicular artery and vein
Ductus deferens
Vaginal cavity
Abdominal cavity
Parietal peritoneum
Internal abdominal oblique muscle
Deep vaginal ring
External abdominal oblique muscle
Inguinal canal (between rings)
Superficial vaginal ring
Cremaster muscle

Spermatic cord
Visceral vaginal tunic
Vaginal cavity
Head of epididymis
Ductus deferens
Parietal vaginal tunic
Body of epididymis
Left testis
Tail of epididymis

Proper ligament of testis
Ligament of tail of epididymis
Skin and "dartos" of testis

■ **FIGURE 14-7** The descended adult testis featuring its relationship to the enveloping visceral vaginal tunic, spermatic cord, the inguinal canal, deep and superficial vaginal rings, vaginal cavity, and abdominal cavity. The deep vaginal ring is the location where the parietal vaginal tunic of the scrotum is continuous with the parietal peritoneum of the abdominal cavity. The proper ligament of testis and ligament of tail of epididymis are remnants of gubernaculum testis.

prevalent in pigs and horses. When the testis is in the inguinal canal, but not in the scrotum, the horse is referred to as a **high flanker**. Often the testis or testes are retained entirely within the abdominal cavity.

■ ACCESSORY SEX GLANDS AND SEMEN

1. What composes the accessory sex glands? Which one is present in all of the domestic animals? What is the relationship of the accessory sex glands to the pelvic urethra?

2. What is the collective name of the accessory gland secretions? What is the difference between seminal plasma and semen?

3. What function is served by seminal plasma?

4. What function may be served by the prostaglandins present in seminal plasma?

5. Are we talking about big numbers when describing the number of sperm present for each artificial insemination? Give an example.

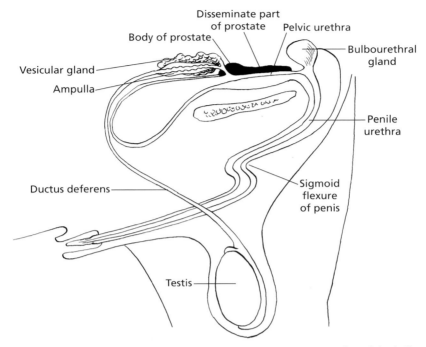

Disseminate part
of prostate   Pelvic urethra
Body of prostate
Vesicular gland
Ampulla
Bulbourethral
gland
Penile
urethra
Ductus deferens
Sigmoid
flexure
of penis
Testis

■ **FIGURE 14-8** Disposition of the accessory glands that discharge into the pelvic urethra of the bull.

The **accessory sex glands** provide secretions that empty into the pelvic urethra near their origin (*Fig. 14-8*). They vary in size and shape among species and can be absent in some. The accessory sex glands are composed of the **ampullae of the ductus deferentes**, the **vesicular glands** (sometimes called seminal vesicles), the **prostate gland**, and the **bulbourethral glands** (sometimes called the Cowper glands). The ampullae (absent in the boar and dog) are enlargements of the terminal part of the ductus deferentes, and their secretion empties into the lumens of the ductus deferentes. The vesicular glands (absent in the dog) are paired glands that empty into the pelvic urethra along with the ductus deferentes. The prostate gland is present in all domestic animals. It is prominent in the dog; it encircles the urethra. Enlargement can be a cause for obstruction of urine flow through the urethra; this condition is more common in

older dogs. Multiple ducts from this gland empty directly into the urethra. The paired bulbourethral glands (absent in the dog) are the most caudal of the accessory glands. At the time of ejaculation, the accessory sex gland secretions (collectively known as **seminal plasma**) are mixed with sperm and fluid from the epididymides to form **semen**.

The seminal plasma provides an environment conducive to the survival of sperm within the female reproductive tract. It is rich in electrolytes, fructose, ascorbic acid, and other vitamins. Whereas fertilization can occur with sperm unaided by seminal plasma, the greatest fertilization potential is achieved with it. Species differ in the composition of seminal plasma, but it seems that each species has solved the same fundamental problems in a different way. One unvarying component among all species, however, is fructose. The advantage of fructose as an energy source might be that it does not require metabolic energy for entrance into the spermatozoa.

Several **prostaglandins** (see Chapter 6) are present in seminal plasma. It is thought that they aid in fertilization in two ways: 1) prostaglandins react with cervical mucus and make it more receptive to sperm; and 2) some of the prostaglandins cause smooth muscle contraction, so it is believed that reverse peristalsis is initiated in the uterus and oviducts to facilitate transport of sperm toward the ovaries.

Most of the sperm in an ejaculate never reach the oviduct. In fact, only a few dozen might reach the vicinity of the oocyte, where only one is required for fertilization. Semen collected for artificial insemination is often diluted and mixed with extenders to obtain the greatest number of insemination units. The number of sperm intended for each artificial insemination varies among species, but approximates 10 and 125 million, respectively, for cattle and sheep, and 2 billion each for pigs and horses.

■ PENIS AND PREPUCE

1. Why is greater enlargement of the penis possible in the stallion than it is in the bull?
2. What is the urethral process of the ram penis?
3. How does the bulbus glandis of the dog penis participate in the "tie" associated with canine coitus?
4. Which domestic species have a sigmoid flexure of their penis?
5. Note the preputial diverticulum (pouch) in the boar and the double-folded prepuce in the stallion shown in Figure 14-9.

The **penis** is the male organ of copulation through which urine and semen pass by way of the penile urethra. The appearance of the penis of several farm animals and its associa-

tion with other structures is shown in *Figure 14-9*. The **roots (crura)** of the penis begin at the caudal border of the pelvic ischial arch. The forward extension from the roots is known as the **body**, and the free extremity is known as the **glans**. The internal structure (*Fig. 14-10*) is occupied mostly by **cavernous tissue** (commonly known as **erectile tissue**). Cavernous tissue is a collection of blood sinusoids separated by sheets of connective tissue. The stallion has a large amount of erectile tissue relative to connective tissue (see Fig. 14-10B), and greater enlargement is possible during erection than in the bull (see Fig. 14-10A), in which the ratio of erectile tissue to connective tissue is lower. The urethra is on the ventral aspect of the body of the penis (see Fig. 14-10).

The ram has a highly visible **urethral process** (see Fig. 14-9B), and sometimes, urethral calculi become lodged in its narrowed extremity. This can be corrected by amputation of the process. It is speculated that the function of the urethral process in the ram is to spray the cervical area with semen during ejaculation. The free end of such an extension would move in a circular pattern with the emission of fluid under pressure.

The dog has a **bulbus glandis** at the caudal part of the glans. The enlargement of the bulbus glandis is responsible for prolonged retention of the penis during coitus. Contraction of muscles in the vestibule of the female vagina caudal to the bulbus glandis assists this retention, commonly known as the **tie** (*Fig. 14-11*).

The bull, ram, and boar have a **sigmoid flexure** of their penis, resulting in an S shape when not erect (see Figs. 14-8 and 14-9). Erection causes extension of the flexure as shown for the bull in *Figure 14-12*.

The **prepuce** is an invaginated fold of skin that surrounds the free extremity of the penis (see Fig. 14-9). The stallion has a double-folded prepuce. Waxy accumulations known as **beans** sometimes form in the outer fold and must be removed manually. The boar has a

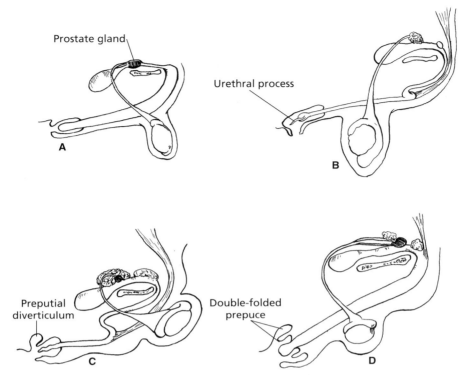

■ **FIGURE 14-9** Comparative anatomy of the male reproductive organs of various domestic animals. **A)** Dog. **B)** Ram. **C)** Boar. **D)** Stallion. Note the encirclement of the pelvic urethra by the prostate in the dog, urethral process in the ram, preputial diverticulum in the boar, and double-folded prepuce in the stallion.

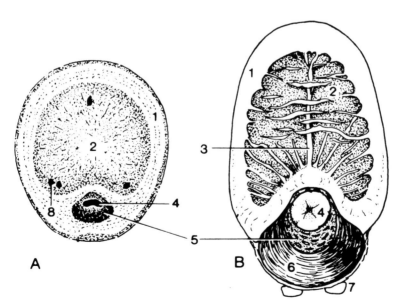

■ **FIGURE 14-10** Transverse sections of the fibroelastic penis of a bull **(A)** and the musculocavernous penis of a stallion **(B).** **1)** Tunica albuginea; **2)** corpus cavernosum; **3)** septum; **4)** urethra; **5)** corpus spongiosum; **6)** bulbospongiosus; **7)** retractor penis; **8)** large, thick-walled veins. (From Dyce KM, Sack WO, Wensing CJG. Textbook of Veterinary Anatomy. 3rd Ed. Philadelphia: WB Saunders, 2002.)

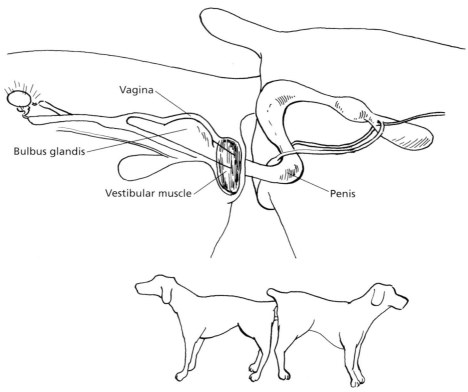

■ **FIGURE 14-11** "Locking" phase, or "tie" of canine coitus (lateral view). In the dog, erection involves primarily the glans penis. Enlargement of the bulbus glandis and contraction of vestibular muscles during intromission "lock" the dog's penis in the bitch's vagina.

preputial diverticulum (pouch) on the dorsal wall, which often contains decomposing urine and macerated epithelium. The fluid in the diverticulum also contains a pheromone (see Chapter 5) that causes sows to assume the immobile mating stance.

■ MUSCLES OF MALE GENITALIA

1. Note the functions for the external cremaster muscle, the internal cremaster muscle, the urethralis and bulbospongiosus muscle, the ischiocavernosus muscles, and the retractor penis muscles.

The cremaster muscle is formed from the caudal fibers of the internal abdominal oblique muscle. It passes through the inguinal canal and attaches to the outer aspect of the parietal vaginal tunic (see Figs. 14-6 and 14-7). This muscle pulls the testis up against the superficial vaginal ring, particularly in cold weather. The cremaster muscles are responsible for the testes being drawn into the abdominal cavity of the elephant, deer, and rabbit during times other than the breeding season.

A skeletal muscle, the urethralis (see Fig. 14-1), is the pelvic continuation from the smooth muscle wall of the urinary bladder. Peristaltic action of this muscle assists in the transport of urine or semen through the pelvic urethra.

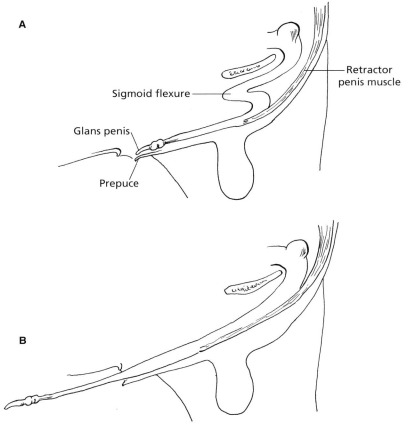

■ FIGURE 14-12 Penis of the bull. **A)** Nonerect position with its characteristic sigmoid flexure. **B)** Erect position with elimination of the sigmoid flexure and extension beyond the prepuce. The retractor penis muscle assists return of the penis to its nonerect position.

The **bulbospongiosus muscle** (Fig. 14-1 and *Fig. 14-13*) is a striated muscle continuation of the urethralis. It continues throughout the length of the penis in the horse, but only proceeds for a short distance along the penile urethra in other animals. The bulbospongiosus muscle continues the action of the urethralis in emptying the urethra.

The **ischiocavernosus muscles** are paired, striated muscles that converge on the body of the penis from their origins on the lateral sides of the ischial arch (see Figs. 14-1 and 14-13). When these muscles contract, they pull the penis upward against the floor of the pelvis. Much of the venous drainage from the penis is obstructed because of the location of the veins on the dorsal surface of the penis, and erection is thereby assisted.

The **retractor penis muscles** are paired striated muscles that originate from the suspensory ligaments of the anus. They continue forward and converge caudal to the body of the penis (see Figs. 14-12 and 14-13). After they join on the underside of the penis, they continue forward to the glans penis. The retractor penis muscles pull the flaccid penis back into the prepuce.

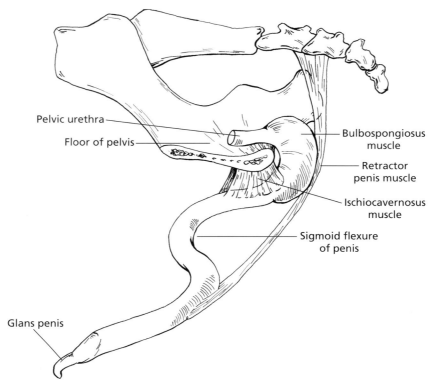

Pelvic urethra

Floor of pelvis

Bulbospongiosus
muscle

Retractor
penis muscle

Ischiocavernosus
muscle

Sigmoid flexure
of penis

Glans penis

■ **FIGURE 14-13** Penis of the bull and some of its associated muscles. The bulbospongiosus muscle assists in empty-ing the urethra. The ischiocavernosus muscle assists in the erection process, and the retractor penis muscle assists in the return of the penis to the prepuce after intromission.

■ BLOOD AND NERVE SUPPLY

1. **What is the function of the pampini-form plexus?**
2. **Where does stimulation occur to provide for the afferent side of the reflexes associated with erection and ejaculation?**

Blood to the testicles is supplied by the testicular arteries. The testicular veins parallel the testicular arteries. Both artery and vein are enclosed within the spermatic cord (see Fig. 14-6). A short distance above the testicle, the testicular vein is convoluted (the **pampiniform plexus**) and is in close association with the convoluted part of the testicular artery (*Fig. 14-14*). Their closeness, and because they are convoluted and are therefore longer, provides a means whereby blood entering the testis is cooled by the venous blood leaving the testis. The arteries and veins are also close to the surface of the testes, and so direct loss of heat from the testes is favored. Spermatogenesis requires a cooler temperature than normal body temperature. Arterial blood to the penis provides for filling of the cavernous tissue and provides nutrition to the tissues. The exclusive supply is the artery of the penis, a terminal branch of the internal pudendal arteries. The blood supply to the penis of the horse is slightly different than that of other species and is more extensive.

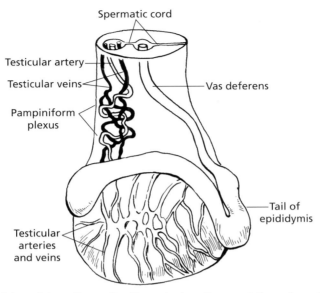

■ **FIGURE 14-14** Lateral view of the stallion testis with emphasis on the pampiniform plexus. The pampiniform plexus is illustrated by the intertwining of the testicular artery and vein. This allows for the cooler venous blood to cool the warmer arterial blood going to the testis.

In addition to autonomic nerve fibers to the testes, penis, and accessory sex glands, the penis is supplied by a spinal nerve, the pudendal nerve. Terminations of the pudendal nerve are located in the glans penis. Sensory stimulation of the glans provides the afferent side for reflexes associated with erection and ejaculation. Reflex centers for erection and ejaculation are located in the lumbar region of the spinal cord.

■ **SPERMATOGENESIS**

1. Define spermatogenesis.
2. Spermatids undergo nuclear and cytoplasmic changes and develop a tail. What is this maturation phase called?
3. What is spermiation?
4. Where is the fertilizing ability of spermatozoa attained? Where are they stored? What happens to spermatozoa that are not ejaculated?
5. What function is served by the spermatogenic wave?

6. Describe the negative feedback system that relates to the production of testosterone by Leydig cells. Why is luteinizing hormone called interstitial cell stimulating hormone (ICSH)?
7. What is the role of testosterone in spermatogenesis?
8. What are the assumed roles of FSH in the male?
9. Aside from spermatogenesis, what are other functions of testosterone in the male?
10. What embryonic structures stimulated by testosterone become tubular portions of the male reproductive system?
11. What metabolic function is served by testosterone?
12. What are C-16 unsaturated androgens that are secreted by boar testes?

The term **spermatogenesis** refers to the entire process involved in the transformation of germinal epithelial cells (stem cells) to spermatozoa and can be divided into two phases: 1) spermatocytogenesis and 2) spermiogenesis. **Spermatocytogenesis** is the proliferative phase whereby spermatogonial cells multiply by a series of mitotic divisions followed by the meiotic divisions which produce the haploid (n) number of chromosomes (*Fig. 14-15*).

The **stem cells (spermatogonia)** are located in the basal compartment of the seminiferous tubules (see Fig. 14-4). The mitotic division of a spermatogonium results in one cell being a replacement for the cell that has just divided (it stays in the basal compartment). The other cell becomes a **type A spermatogonium**, which migrates through the Sertoli cell barrier to the adluminal compartment. Type A spermatogonia undergo mitotic division (sometimes involving several generations) until large numbers (variable among species) of **type B spermatogonia** have been produced. Type B spermatogonia undergo the last of the mitotic divisions, which results in the formation of primary spermatocytes with 2n chromosome numbers. Primary spermatocytes undergo meiotic division (described previously) to form secondary spermatocytes, which in turn undergo meiotic division to form spermatids (n chromosome numbers). In the bull, 64 spermatids are formed from one type A spermatogonium.

The second phase of spermatogenesis, **spermiogenesis**, involves maturation of the spermatids while they are still in the adluminal compartment. Spermiogenesis is composed of a series of nuclear and cytoplasmic changes and a transformation from a nonmotile cell (not able to move) to a potentially motile cell in which a flagellum (tail) has formed. The mature spermatids produced during the final phase of spermio-genesis are released into the lumen of the seminiferous tubules as **spermatozoa**.

The release of matured spermatids into the lumen of the seminiferous tubules is known as **spermiation**. Spermatozoa from several animal species are compared in *Figure 14-16*.

Epididymal Transport

The newly formed spermatozoa are essentially immotile. They are transported to the epididymis by fluid secretions into the seminiferous tubules and rete testis and by activity of contractile elements in the testis that direct fluid flow to the head of the epididymis.

The fertilizing ability of an animal is attained progressively during the transit of spermatozoa through the epididymis. Changes include development of unidirectional (as opposed to circular) motility, changes in nuclear chromatin (DNA protein complex), and changes in the nature of the surface of the plasma membrane.

The major site of sperm storage within the male reproductive tract is the tail (last portion) of the epididymis. About 70% of the total number of spermatozoa in the ducts outside the rete testis (**excurrent duct system**) are found in the tail of the epididymis.

Many of the spermatozoa formed in the testes are either phagocytized in the excurrent duct system or lost into the urine. About 85% of the daily sperm production in sexually inactive rams are voided in the urine.

Spermatogenic Wave

If all segments of the seminiferous tubules were involved in the same activity at the same time, a continuous supply of spermatozoa would not be produced because about 64 days (in the bull) are required while in the adluminal compartment for spermalocytogenesis (development from spermatogonia to spermatozoa). While this development is proceeding, a new type A spermatogonium migrates through the Sertoli cell barrier into the adluminal compartment to begin its development behind the developing type A spermatogonium that preceded it. In the bull, this occurs every 14 days. Since 64 days are required for development to spermatozoa, there will be 4.6 cycles (64 ÷ 14) of beginning development

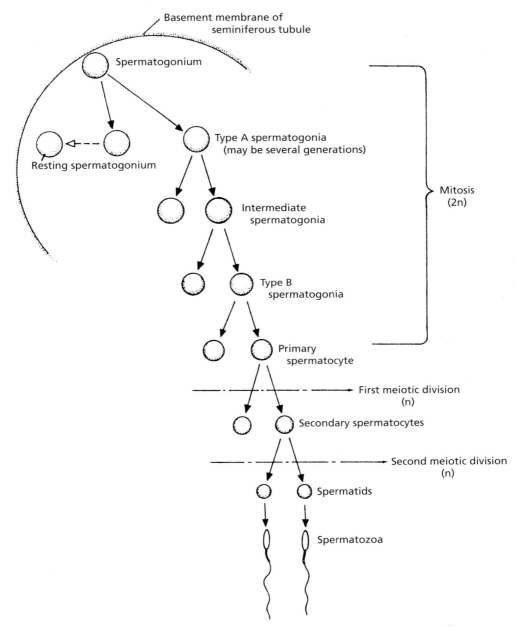

Basement membrane of
seminiferous tubule

Spermatogonium

Type A spermatogonia
(may be several generations)

Resting spermatogonium

Intermediate
spermatogonia

Type B
spermatogonia

Primary
spermatocyte

First meiotic division
(n)

Secondary spermatocytes

Second meiotic division
(n)

Spermatids

Spermatozoa

Mitosis
(2n)

■ **FIGURE 14-15** Diagrammatic representation of the stages of spermatogenesis in mammals. The chromosome number (2n, diploid; n, haploid) is also shown for each stage. (From Pineda MH. The biology of sex. In: Pineda MH, Dooley MP, eds. Veterinary Endocrinology and Reproduction. 5th Ed. Ames, IA: Iowa State Press, 2003.)

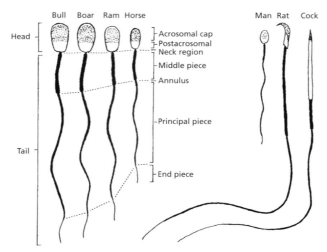

■ **FIGURE 14-16** Comparison of the spermatozoa of farm animals and other vertebrates. The major structural features are given. Note the differences in the relative size and shape. (From Hafez ESE, Hafez B. Reproduction in Farm Animals. 7th Ed. Baltimore: Lippincott Williams & Wilkins, 2000.)

before the first cycle from a given area of seminiferous epithelium begins to arrive at the rete testis. A cycle is defined as a series of changes in a given area of seminiferous epithelium between two appearances of developmental stages. A portion of tubule at one stage is usually adjacent to portions of tubule in stages just preceding it or following it in time. This sequential change in stage of cycle along the length of the tubule is known as the **spermatogenic wave**. A spermatogenic wave that involves a 12-day cycle is illustrated in *Figure 14-17*. The wave involves a sequence of stages beginning with the less advanced stages in the middle of the loop to progressively more advanced stages nearer the rete testis. The stages proceed in opposite directions from the **site of reversal** at the middle of the loop towards the rete testis.

A large number of spermatozoa are produced daily in the normal male animal, about 6.0×10^9 spermatozoa in the bull and about 16.5×10^9 in the boar. In the bull, daily sperm production increases with age, reaching a maximum at about 7 years.

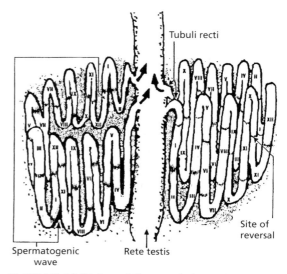

■ **FIGURE 14-17** A seminiferous tubule in which the wave of the seminiferous epithelium is schematically represented along the length of the tubule. The succession of stages I to XII (a 12-day cycle), the site of reversal in the middle of the tubule, and the relationship of the wave to the rete testis are shown. The more advanced stages of each wave are located nearer the rete testis. Any one tubule may have as many as 15 spermatogenic waves. (From Hafez ESE, Hafez B. Reproduction in Farm Animals. 7th Ed. Baltimore: Lippincott Williams & Wilkins, 2000.)

Hormonal Control

Leydig and Sertoli cells are responsible for hormone production within the testes. The production of **testosterone** by Leydig cells is controlled by the gonadotropin known as **luteinizing hormone (LH)** (sometimes called **interstitial cell stimulating hormone**, or **ICSH**). Low levels of testosterone cause an increase in LH secretion by the anterior pituitary. The increase in LH secretion causes the Leydig cells in the testes to secrete testosterone; when increased, testosterone inhibits the further secretion of LH and testosterone levels are thus stabilized. A subsequent decline in testosterone again stimulates LH secretion, and the cycle is repeated; this is known as a negative feedback system.

The influence of testosterone on spermatogenesis requires that it diffuse from the interstitial tissues into the seminiferous tubules. Within the seminiferous tubules, it seems that testosterone maintains spermatogenesis by supporting the meiotic process.

Another gonadotropic hormone, **follicle stimulating hormone (FSH)** from the anterior pituitary, stimulates production of an **androgen-binding protein** by the Sertoli cells. Androgen-binding protein is secreted into the lumen of the seminiferous tubules and binds with testosterone and other androgens to stabilize their concentrations and ensure appropriate amounts for spermatogenesis. It is also believed that FSH stimulates the secretion of estrogens by the Sertoli cells. The actual secretion of estrogen might arise from the intracellular conversion of testosterone (originating from Leydig cells) by the Sertoli cells. The Sertoli cells are also the source of a hormone known as **inhibin**, which inhibits secretion of FSH by the anterior pituitary.

Whereas LH is required continuously for spermatogenesis (testosterone-supported meiosis), FSH is not essential for the maintenance of spermatogenesis once it has been initiated. Initiation of spermatogenesis at puberty and after physiologic or pathologic interruptions requires FSH.

Other Functions of Testosterone

In addition to its spermatogenic activity, testosterone fulfills other functions in the peripheral circulation. After secretion of testosterone by Leydig cells into the interstitial space of the testes, a greater amount diffuses into the blood and lymphatic capillaries than that which diffuses into the seminiferous tubules. After entrance into the blood, testosterone is bound loosely with a plasma protein for its transport. Within 15 to 30 minutes, the testosterone is released from the protein to be fixed to target tissues or to be degraded, mainly by the liver, into inactive products that are subsequently excreted.

Other functions of testosterone include the development and maintenance of **libido**, secretory activity of the accessory sex glands, and general body features associated with the male.

Libido refers to sexual drive. It can be effectively eliminated by **castration** (removal of the testes). Castrated animals usually, but not invariably, lack libido. Small amounts of testosterone from other sources such as the adrenal gland (interconversion potential) might be sufficient to provide libido in some animals.

The structural development and physiologic functioning (production of secretions) of the accessory sex glands are influenced by testosterone. In this regard, hyperactive prostate glands (enlargement) can be treated effectively by estrogen administration. The estrogen inhibits the secretion of LH, and testosterone production by the Leydig cells is suppressed. A reduced concentration of testosterone causes the hyperactive prostate gland to reduce its activity, and its size decreases.

General body features associated with the male (**secondary sexual characteristics**) are influenced by testosterone. These features include increased bone growth (heavier bones), greater muscling, thicker skin, and deeper voice (in the bull). During fetal growth, testosterone directs the descent of the testes. The presence or absence of testosterone determines the respective development of a penis and scrotum or a clitoris and vagina. Before sexual differentiation in the embryo, the structures needed for the development of either sex are present. With normal male hormonal stimulation, the **wolffian ducts** become tubular portions of the male reproductive system, and the **müllerian ducts** regress. In the female the müllerian ducts become tubular portions of the reproductive system, and the wolffian ducts regress.

Metabolically, testosterone has protein anabolic functions that affect the greater muscling potential of males. Probably the thicker skin and laryngeal changes of the male are also related to this function of testosterone. Because of the desirability for more muscle and less fat in meat producing animals, the current trend is to use noncastrated males for meat production. The protein anabolic effect obtained from testicular testosterone is thereby retained.

Other Androgens

Testosterone is one of several steroid hormones classified as androgens. In addition to testosterone, the boar testes secrete large amounts of compounds known as **C-16 unsaturated androgens**. These androgens act as pheromones when they are excreted in boar saliva, and they cause the sow in heat to adopt the mating posture. When the C-16 unsaturated androgens are excreted in urine, they contribute to the characteristic odor of boar urine. These compounds are also responsible for the undesirable flavor of boar meat, which is known as **boar taint**.

■ ERECTION

1. **How is erection of the penis accomplished?**
2. **Does erection accomplish straightening of the sigmoid flexure?**
3. **What is an approximate blood pressure within the corpus cavernosum penis of the bull during coitus? What is hematoma of the penis?**

An increase in the turgidity of the penis is known as **erection**. It is caused by an increase of blood pressure within the cavernous sinuses of the penis as a result of greater blood inflow than outflow. The inflow of blood increases through vasodilation of the arteries caused by parasympathetic stimulation. The outflow of blood decreases through compression of the dorsal veins of the penis against the pelvis when the ischiocavernosus muscles contract. Contraction of the ischiocavernosus muscles also compresses the blood in the cavernous sinuses (now a closed system), which also assists erection by increasing blood pressure in the cavernous sinuses (see Fig. 14-13).

Complete erection of the glans penis of the horse is delayed until after introduction of the penis into the vagina of the mare. Mounting of the mare compresses the prepuce against the vulva, and venous drainage from the prepuce is impaired. Complete erection of the glans is then possible because venous drainage from the glans is directed to the prepuce, which is blocked.

In animals with a sigmoid flexure, the filling of the cavernous sinuses, coupled with relaxation of the retractor penis muscles, causes the flexure to be eliminated and the penis to be straightened. Although animals with a sigmoid flexure have a higher ratio of connective tissue to cavernous tissue (see Fig. 14-10), the length and diameter of the penis increase somewhat as a result of erection, in addition to penis straightening. As compared with the bull, ram, and boar, the penis of the horse has a lower ratio of connective tissue to cavernous tissue, and a relatively greater increase in the length and diameter of its penis occurs during erection.

Blood pressure within the corpus cavernosum penis of the bull has been measured during coitus. A pressure of approximately 14,000 mm Hg was associated with peak activity, and peak activity was correlated with an increased intensity of ischiocavernosus muscle contraction that furthered compression of blood in the cavernous tissue. Higher pressures have been recorded. It is believed that these high pressures, coupled with cavernous tissue capsule weakness, might be the cause of rupture of the corpus cavernosum penis (**hematoma of the penis**) in some bulls. The usual rupture site is on the dorsal surface of the distal curve of the sigmoid flexure (see Fig. 14-12).

■ MOUNTING AND INTROMISSION

1. **What are some causes for mounting failures?**
2. **Define intromission. Which domestic species has the longest and which has the shortest duration of intromission? What are causes for intromission failures?**

Mounting is the stance assumed by the male by which the penis is brought into apposition with the vulva of the female. Successful mounting must be preceded by a receptive stance on the part of the female. Failures in mounting are encountered when there are injuries, weakness, or soreness in the hindlimbs of the male.

Introduction of the penis into the vagina and its maintenance within the vagina during coitus is known as **intromission**. Pelvic thrusts assisted by the abdominal muscles assist penetration of the penis into the vagina. The duration of intromission varies among species—it is shortest for the bull and ram and longest for the boar. Failures of intromission occur in some animals; causes include **phimosis** (constriction of the preputial orifice), hematoma of the penis (as in the bull), and congenital deformities. Final distention of the penis does not occur in the dog until after intromission.

It is presumed that intromission is facilitated in the dog by the presence of the **os penis** (penis bone in the dog).

■ EMISSION AND EJACULATION

1. **Differentiate between emission and ejaculation.**

As sexual stimulation increases, a point is reached at which reflex centers in the spinal cord bring about **emission** and **ejaculation**. Emission precedes ejaculation. It results from sympathetic innervation whereby sperm and fluids in the vasa deferentia and ampullae are emptied into the urethra along with fluids from the other accessory glands (**seminal plasma**). The sympathetic innervation provides peristaltic movement for transport to the urethra and constricts the neck of the bladder to minimize reflux (backward flow) of sperm and fluids into the urinary bladder. Once emission has been accomplished, reflex peristalsis of the urethral muscles propels the urethral contents toward the external urethral orifice. The latter phase, peristalsis of the urethra, is assisted by contraction of the bulbospongiosus muscle, which in turn compresses the urethra. The combination of pressure and peristalsis forces the semen (mixture of seminal plasma and sperm and fluid from the epididymides) from the urethra to the exterior, the process of ejaculation. Stimulation for emission and ejaculation is derived from sensory nerves located in the glans penis.

Sperm and fluids are ejaculated near the opening of the cervix in cattle and sheep, directly into the uterus in swine, and partially into the uterus in the horse.

■ FACTORS AFFECTING TESTICULAR FUNCTION

1. **When does testicular function become manifest?**

2. How does puberty begin in the male?
3. What is the purpose of photoperiod influence on testicular function?
4. How does increasing photoperiod affect sheep and goats? Is this different in the stallion? Are cattle and swine influenced by photoperiod?
5. What gland mediates the photoperiod response?

Testicular function becomes manifest at the onset of **puberty**. It is believed that puberty is correlated with a decreased sensitivity of the hypothalamus to testosterone so that LH is secreted in greater amounts. An increased LH concentration stimulates the Leydig cells to secrete testosterone in greater quantities, and all aspects of testosterone function begin to appear. FSH is essential for the initiation of spermatogenesis at puberty.

In some species, **photoperiod (length of daylight)** changes have a marked influence on testicular function. Photoperiod is also related to ovarian activity in the female of these same species. The purpose of photo-period influence is the coordination of birth with favorable weather conditions. Sheep and goats have major periods of testicular regression during increasing photoperiods, which is restored by decreasing photoperiods. In the stallion a decreasing photoperiod reduces testicular function. The pineal gland (also known as the pineal body) is an endocrine gland attached by a stalk to the dorsal wall of the third ventricle of the cerebrum. The pineal gland is inhibitory to the gonads and is the principal mechanism in the known affect of photoperiod on testicular and ovarian function. The pineal gland mediates the photoperiod response in the ram and ewe and is probably involved in the response of the other species. Testicular function and photoperiod in cattle and swine are related only to a minor degree. When spermatogenesis is stopped during photoperiod inhibition, FSH is again required for its initiation.

■ REPRODUCTION IN THE AVIAN MALE

1. Contrast the location of avian testes with that of mammals.
2. Is there a pampiniform plexus for cooling of the testes in birds, as there is for most mammalian species?
3. How does the avian epididymis differ from that of mammals?
4. What are the storage sites for avian spermatozoa?
5. What structures provide for seminal plasma?
6. What name is given to the penis of birds?
7. Describe the route of ejaculated sperm from the vasa deferentia to the exterior in the cock and tom.
8. Which ones of the domestic birds accomplish intromission at the time of mating?
9. Where is maturation of spermatozoa accomplished in birds?
10. Is there a long life for spermatozoa once they are deposited into the female vagina?

The paired testes of the male bird are located within the body cavity, in contrast to those of most mammals (*Fig. 14-18*). In this location they are able to function at body temperature (about 41°C to 42°C for domestic species). The internal structure is composed of seminiferous tubules, Sertoli cells, stem cells, and Leydig cells, similar to that of mammals. The blood supply to the testes does not provide for a pampiniform plexus, which in mammals is present to assist in cooling the testes. Instead of an epididymis as arranged in mammals, there are tubules (vasa efferentia) conducting sperm from the testis to a short epididymal duct that is continued as the vas deferens. The vas deferens terminates as an enlargement before its opening into the cloaca at a papilla. The vas deferens and the enlargement serve as

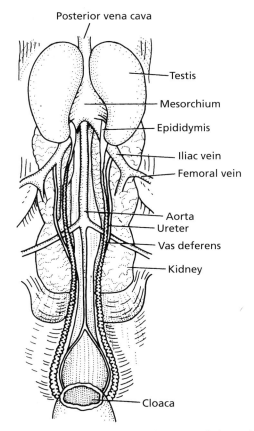

Posterior vena cava

Testis

Mesorchium

Epididymis

Iliac vein

Femoral vein

Aorta
Ureter

Vas deferens

Kidney

Cloaca

■ **FIGURE 14-18** The urogenital system of the male chicken (ventral view). The testes are located within the body cavity and the vasa deferentia conduct spermatozoa to the cloaca. (From Sturkie PD, Opel H. Reproduction in the male, fertilization, and early embryonic development. In: Sturkie PD, ed. Avian Physiology. 3rd Ed. New York: Springer-Verlag, 1976.)

storage sites for spermatozoa. The accessory organs of the male include the vasa efferentia, epididymides, vasa deferentia, ejaculatory groove, and phallus (penis). Seminal plasma is derived from the seminiferous tubules and vasa efferentia inasmuch as birds do not have a prostate gland, bulbourethral gland, and seminal vesicle. The ejaculatory groove of the erected phallus (*Fig. 14-19*) is formed at the time of sexual excitation when several folds in the ventral cloaca become engorged

with lymph. The engorged folds direct semen through the groove of the erect phallus. The phallus of the male chicken (cock or rooster) and turkey (tom) do not perform intromission, but rather transfer semen to the female by touching their phallus to the female vagina, that part of the female reproductive tract terminating at the cloaca. Ducks and geese have sizable penises, and intromission is accomplished at mating.

In the cock, protrusion of the genitalia and forceful expulsion of semen follows external stroking of the base of the tail. Phallic eversion follows similar stimulation in the tom, but semen is generally released only after pressure is applied to the terminal storage depots (terminal enlargements of the vasa deferentia).

The gonadotropic influence of LH and FSH on testicular function is similar to that of mammals, wherein LH acts on Leydig cells to promote their development and testosterone production, and FSH acts on Sertoli cells. Full testicular function results from the combined action of FSH and testosterone.

The collection of semen from cocks and toms is practiced widely. The average volume of cock ejaculate is about 0.5 mL, and that of the tom is about 0.3 mL. Sperm concentration of the cock is about 4 billion/mL, and it is about 10 billion/mL for the tom. The chemical composition of seminal plasma varies among birds as well as in mammals. See Figure 14-16 for the comparison of a spermatozoon of the cock with several mammalian species. Spermatozoa of toms are similar to those of cocks. It seems that cock sperm are functionally mature before they leave the testes. Much of the maturation of mammalian spermatozoa occurs in the epididymides.

After mating or artificial insemination, sperm are found in sperm storage glands of the female that are located in the vagina, near its junction with the uterus. They persist at this location for the fertile period of the female. It is likely that sperm are nourished by the uterovaginal sperm storage glands and/or are placed into reversible quiescence (quiet period).

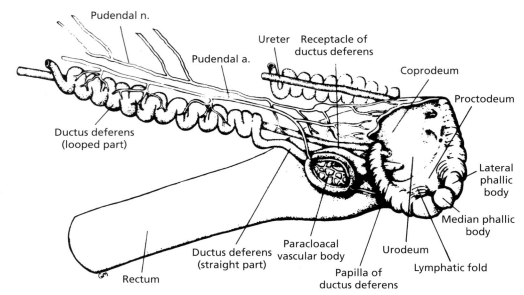

■ **FIGURE 14-19** Lateral view of the cloaca and the terminal part of the vas deferens (ductus deferens) of the domestic fowl. The ejaculatory groove (not shown) is formed at the time of sexual excitation when the lymphatic folds become engorged with lymph, forming a troughlike structure to direct the flow of semen. The paracloacal vascular body is the source of the lymph. The receptacle of the ductus deferens serves as a storage site for spermatozoa. (From Lake PE. Male genital organs. In: King AS, McClelland J, eds. Form and Function in Birds, Vol. 2. San Diego: Academic Press, 1981.)

■ SUGGESTED READING

Brackett BG. Male reproduction in mammals. In: Reece WO, ed. Dukes' Physiology of Domestic Animals. 12th Ed. Ithaca, NY: Cornell University Press, 2004.

Dyce KM, Sack WO, Wensing CJG. Textbook of Veterinary Anatomy. 2nd Ed. Philadelphia: WB Saunders, 1996.

Frandson RD, Wilke WL, Fails AD. Anatomy and Physiology of Farm Animals. 6th Ed. Baltimore: Lippincott Williams & Wilkins, 2003.

Hafez ESE, Hafez B. Reproduction in Farm Animals. 7th Ed. Baltimore: Lippincott Williams & Wilkins, 2000.

Kirby JD, Froman DP. Reproduction in male birds. In: Whittow GC, Ed. Sturkie's Avian Physiology. 5th Ed. San Diego: Academic Press, 2000.

Pineda MH. Male reproductive system. In: Pineda MH, Dooley MP, eds. Veterinary Endocrinology and Reproduction. 5th Ed. Ames, IA: Iowa State Press, 2003.

 S E L F   E V A L U A T I O N — C H A P T E R   1 4

TESTES AND ASSOCIATED STRUCTURES

1. Which one of the following cells lines the periphery of the seminiferous tubules, and provides a "nurse" function for developing spermatozoa?

   a. Leydig cells
   b. Spermatid
   c. Sertoli cells
   d. MPS cells

2. The ductus deferens (vas deferens):
   a. is not included in the spermatic cord.

b. is the same as the epididymis.

c. is a continuation of the duct system from the tail of the epididymis to the pelvic urethra.

d. is not present in all domestic males.

3. The scrotum is lined with:
   a. the visceral layer of the vaginal tunic.
   b. the parietal layer of the vaginal tunic.

DESCENT OF THE TESTES

4. A scrotal hernia exists when a loop of intestine:
   a. descends to the scrotum within the spermatic cord.
   b. descends to the scrotum in the vaginal cavity.
   c. is in the peritoneal cavity.
   d. occupies the pleural cavity.

5. The gubernaculum testis plays a role in:
   a. spermatogenesis.
   b. erection.
   c. descent of the testicles during fetal development.
   d. elevation of testicles to inguinal ring.

ACCESSORY SEX GLANDS AND SEMEN

6. Which one of the following hormones is found in seminal plasma, and is thought to assist fertilization by making cervical mucus more receptive to sperm and to facilitate sperm transport by contracting uterine smooth muscle?
   a. Prostaglandins
   b. Testosterone
   c. Estrogen
   d. FSH

7. Seminal plasma is:
   a. the same as semen.
   b. a component of blood.
   c. a collective name for accessory sex gland secretions.
   d. the fluid from the epididymides.

8. Which one of the following accessory sex glands would obstruct urine flow when it becomes enlarged?
   a. Bulbourethral glands
   b. Ampullae of the ducti deferentes
   c. Vesicular glands
   d. Prostate gland

PENIS AND PREPUCE

9. The bull has a large amount of erectile tissue relative to connective tissue, and greater enlargement is possible during erection than in the stallion, in which the ratio of erectile tissue to connective tissue is less.
   a. True
   b. False

10. A sigmoid flexure in the bull, ram, and boar is a characteristic of the erected penis.
    a. True
    b. False

11. A preputial diverticulum is present in the:
    a. boar.
    b. stallion.
    c. ram.
    d. dog.

MUSCLES OF MALE GENITALIA

12. The muscles that pull the testes up against the external inguinal ring, particularly in cold weather, are the:
    a. cremaster muscles.
    b. ischiocavernosus muscles.
    c. retractor penis muscles.

BLOOD AND NERVE SUPPLY

13. The pampiniform plexus:
    a. pampers the testicles.
    b. assists warming of the testicles.
    c. assists cooling of the testicles.
    d. is a nerve network to the testicles.

SPERMATOGENESIS

14. The maturation phase, whereby spermatids undergo nuclear and cytoplasmic changes and develop a tail, is known as:
    a. spermatidosis.
    b. spermiation.
    c. spermatogenesis.
    d. spermiogenesis.

15. Testosterone is produced by:
    a. Leydig cells in response to stimulation by LH.
    b. Sertoli cells in response to stimulation by FSH.
    c. Leydig cells in response to stimulation by FSH.
    d. Sertoli cells in response to stimulation by LH.

16. Which one of the following is an androgen?
    a. Testosterone
    b. Estrogen
    c. LH
    d. FSH

17. The spermatogenic wave:
    a. is a spectator performance at athletic events.
    b. ensures a continuous supply of spermatozoa.
    c. is an activity of the epididymis.
    d. is a friendly acknowledgement.

18. Maturation and storage of spermatozoa occurs in the:
    a. epididymis.
    b. seminiferous tubules.
    c. prostate gland.
    d. urethra.

19. Which one of the following is the principal androgen in the male?
    a. Interstitial cell stimulating hormone
    b. Testosterone
    c. Follicle stimulating hormone
    d. Cholesterol

20. The function of luteinizing hormone in the male animal is to:
    a. stimulate the production of estrogen by Sertoli cells.
    b. stimulate spermatogenesis.
    c. stimulate the production of testosterone by the interstitial cells (Leydig cells).
    d. cool the testicle.

ERECTION

21. An approximate blood pressure within the corpus cavernosum penis of the bull during coitus is:
    a. 140 mm Hg.
    b. THTM (too high to measure).
    c. 1400 mm Hg.
    d. about the same in mm Hg as Pike's Peak in Colorado is high in feet (14,000) above sea level.

22. Contraction of the ischiocavernosus muscle in the bull:
    a. pulls the testis up against the external inguinal ring.
    b. assists in emptying the urethra.
    c. pulls the penis upward against the floor of the pelvis, which obstructs venous outflow, thereby assisting erection.
    d. pulls the flaccid penis back into the prepuce.

MOUNTING AND INTROMISSION

23. Intromission is defined as:
    a. emptying of sperm and fluids from the vasa deferentia and ampullae into the urethra along with seminal plasma.
    b. a time-out between mounting and ejaculation.
    c. introduction of the penis into the vagina and its maintenance therein during coitus.
    d. the movement of urethral content toward the external urethral orifice.

EMISSION AND EJACULATION

24. Emission follows ejaculation.
    a. True
    b. False

FACTORS AFFECTING TESTICULAR FUNCTION

25. The degree of influence of photoperiod on testicular regression is the same in all animals.
    a. True
    b. False

REPRODUCTION IN THE AVIAN MALE

26. An intraabdominal location for avian testes is abnormal.
    a. True
    b. False

27. Cooling of avian testes below body temperature is:
    a. accomplished by their close proximity to the air sacs.
    b. accomplished by a vascular arrangement similar to the pampiniform plexus.
    c. not necessary for their functional integrity.

28. The avian penis is also known as the:
    a. malleus.
    b. phallus.
    c. incus.
    d. organ.

29. Intromission is a reproductive component for:
    a. all avian species.
    b. cocks (male chickens) and toms (male turkeys).
    c. drakes (male ducks) and ganders (male geese).
    d. cocks, toms, drakes, and ganders.

30. When avian semen is inseminated, the spermatozoa:
    a. are short lived (minutes).
    b. perish after a one-time fertilization.
    c. have a prolonged life in sperm storage glands of the female and persist at this location for the fertile period of the female.

ANSWERS TO SELF EVALUATION—CHAPTER 14

1. c	9. b	17. b	25. b
2. c	10. b	18. a	26. b
3. b	11. a	19. b	27. c
4. b	12. a	20. c	28. b
5. c	13. c	21. d	29. c
6. a	14. d	22. c	30. c
7. c	15. a	23. c	
8. d	16. a	24. b	

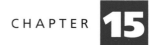
Female Reproduction

CHAPTER OUTLINE

- **FUNCTIONAL ANATOMY OF THE FEMALE REPRODUCTIVE SYSTEM**
  Ovaries
  Ovarian Follicles
  Tubular Genital Tract
  External Genitalia
  Blood Supply of Female Genitalia
- **HORMONES OF FEMALE REPRODUCTION**
  Estrogens
  Progesterone
  Gonadotropins
- **OVARIAN FOLLICLE ACTIVITY**
  Follicular Growth
  Ovulation
  Corpus Luteum Formation and
    Regression
  Summary of Ovarian Cycle Events
- **SEXUAL RECEPTIVITY**
- **ESTROUS CYCLE AND RELATED FACTORS**

Stages of Estrous Cycle
Photoperiod
Nutrition
Species Characteristics
- **PREGNANCY**
Transport of Oocyte and Spermatozoa
Fertilization
Implantation and Placentation
Hormones
Diagnosis
- **PARTURITION**
Signs of Approaching Parturition
Hormone Changes
Stages
- **INVOLUTION OF THE UTERUS**
Cow
Mare, Ewe, and Sow
Bitch
- **REPRODUCTION IN THE AVIAN FEMALE**

The reproductive functions of the female are production of oocytes and provision of an environment for growth and nutrition of the fetus that develops after fertilization of a mature oocyte by a spermatozoon. Terminal conditions of the latter function are to give birth at an appropriate time and to continue the nutritional function through lactation.

The complex relationships of hormones and tissue changes are coordinated for the female's role of perpetuating the species.

■ FUNCTIONAL ANATOMY OF THE FEMALE REPRODUCTIVE SYSTEM

1. When conducting a rectal palpation on a cow for the components of the female reproductive system, would one search dorsally (above) or ven-

trally (below)? What is the relative location of the urinary bladder?

2. Do all domestic animals (intact females) ovulate over the entire surface of the ovary?

3. Compare numbers of spermatozoa and oocytes that develop from one primary spermatocyte and one primary oocyte, respectively.

4. What is the process of oocyte formation known as?

5. What are primordial follicles? Does their number at birth, aside from those called to become mature oocytes, continue throughout the reproductive life of the female?

6. What function is served by the uterine tubes?

7. What are fimbria?

8. What is the serous covering of the uterine tubes known as?
9. What function is served by the uterus?
10. Is the endometrium glandular throughout in all domestic animals (intact females)?
11. What function is served by the glandular secretion of the endometrium?
12. Is the cervix open at all times?
13. What composes the myometrium, and what is its function?
14. What is the major support for the gravid uterus?
15. What is the landmark junction between vagina and vulva? What is the vestibule of the vagina?
16. What is the fornix?
17. What is the major blood supply to the uterus? What is fremitus?
18. What function is served by the intertwining of the uterine artery and vein?

The female reproductive system consists of two ovaries and the tubular genital tract composed of two uterine tubes, uterus, vagina, and the external genitalia (*Fig. 15-1*). The mammary glands are an important part of the reproductive system as well, and they are described separately. The location of the reproductive system relative to the rectum and bladder is shown in *Figure 15-2*.

Ovaries

The **ovaries** are paired glands that provide for the development of oocytes and for the production of hormones. Each ovary is located caudal to its respective right or left kidney and is suspended from the dorsal wall of the abdomen by a reflection of the peritoneum, the **mesovarium**. The mesovarium is part of the **broad ligament** (*Fig. 15-3*), an inclusive term that also refers to the suspensions of the uterine tubes (**mesosalpinx**) and uterus (**mesometrium**). The rather pendulous suspension

of the ovaries provides for easy manipulation by rectal palpation in the cow and horse. The ovaries are described as almond shaped in most species and as bean shaped (kidney shaped) in the mare (*Fig. 15-4*). In the sow the ovary resembles a cluster of grapes (berry shaped) because of the larger number of protruding follicles. Ovulation (release of mature oocytes) occurs throughout the entire surface of the ovary in most species but is confined to an **ovulation fossa** (an indentation) in the mare; this gives the latter its bean shape.

The ovary has a surface or superficial layer of epithelium that is underlain by the **tunica albuginea**, a connective tissue covering of the entire ovary. Beneath the tunica albuginea is the **cortex**, which contains a large mass of follicles in various stages of development. The **medulla** is centrally located and contains loose connective tissue, blood vessels, lymphatics, and nerves.

Ovarian Follicles

The follicles within the cortex are classified as: 1) primordial (sometimes called primary) follicles, 2) growing follicles, and 3) graafian follicles (*Fig. 15-5*). The **primordial follicles** contain a single oocyte that is surrounded by a single layer of granulosa cells. The granulosa cells are derived from the superficial epithelium, and the oocytes are derived from mitosis of oogonia in the embryonic genital ridge that then migrate to the ovary. **Growing follicles** are follicles that have begun growth from the resting stage as primordial follicles but have not developed a thecal layer or antrum (fluid-filled cavity; see Fig. 15-5). They have two or more layers of granulosa cells surrounding the oocyte. Additional layers are added with continued growth. A zona pellucida that surrounds the oocyte may also be present. The zona pellucida provides pores through which processes of granulosa cells can interact with the oocyte surface. Also, sperm must first recognize and then contact and traverse the zona pellucida to reach the oocyte plasma mem-

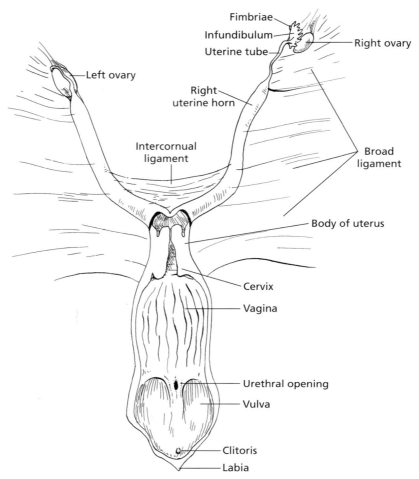

■ **FIGURE 15-1** Reproductive tract of the cow (dorsal aspect). The body of the uterus, vagina, and vulva (vestibule of the vagina) have been laid open and the right ovary withdrawn from the infundibulum. The broad ligament (a downward reflection of the peritoneum) suspends the reproductive tract from the dorsolateral abdominal wall.

brane. **Graafian follicles** are those in which an antrum is clearly visible. Two layers of thecal cells, theca interna and theca externa, are also present (see Fig. 15-5).

Follicle Regression

Considerable **atresia (regression)** of the many primordial follicles occurs by birth and throughout the reproductive life of the female. At the end of the female's reproductive life, only a few primordial follicles remain, and

even these undergo atresia soon thereafter. Growth of some number of primordial follicles does occur after birth and before puberty, but these never reach the graafian follicle stage and regress. The growth that occurs before puberty is not hormone related and is probably controlled by an unknown intraovarian factor. The formation of graafian follicles is hormone dependent and begins at puberty when tonic levels of LH and FSH begin to rise and fall with each estrous cycle. Many of the follicles that undergo growth and maturation with each

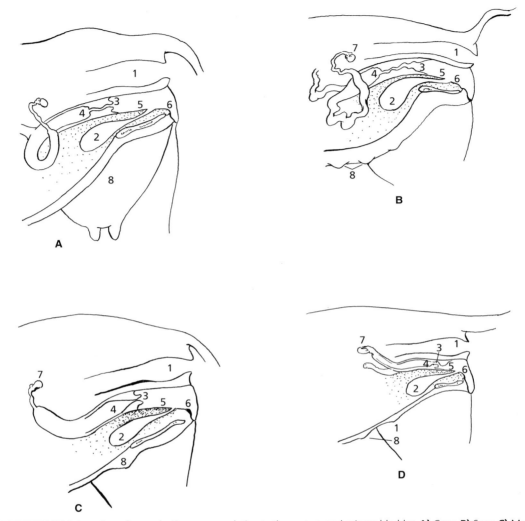

■ **FIGURE 15-2** Location of reproductive organs relative to the rectum and urinary bladder. **A)** Cow. **B)** Sow. **C)** Mare. **D)** Bitch. Note species differences in anatomy of the cervix and mammary gland(s). **1**, rectum; **2**, urinary bladder; **3**, cervix; **4**, uterus; **5**, vagina; **6**, vulva; **7**, ovary; **8**, mammary gland(s).

cycle never ovulate. Therefore, the number of primordial follicles that reach the graafian follicle stage and proceed to ovulation is a very small fraction of the birth number.

Oogenesis

The process by which oocytes are formed is known as **oogenesis**. The oocyte of the pri-

mordial follicle is a primary oocyte that is in a quiescent (arrested) stage of meiosis. Meiosis resumes at the time of ovulation. Whereas four spermatozoa arise from one primary spermatocyte, only one oocyte develops from the reduction division of a primary oocyte. A polar body, which lacks sufficient cytoplasmic material for viability, develops when a primary oocyte divides to form a secondary oocyte.

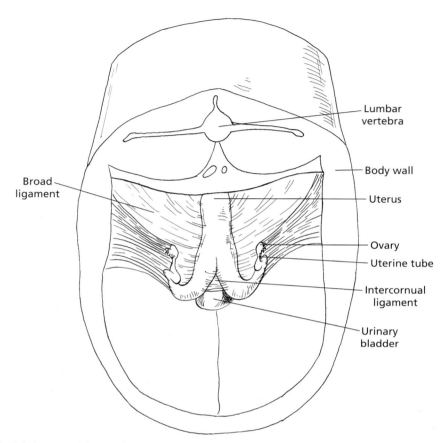

■ **FIGURE 15-3** Dorsocranial view of bovine female reproductive organs. The broad ligament is the inclusive term for the mesovarium, mesosalpinx, and mesometrium, which suspend the ovary, uterine tubes, and uterus, respectively, from the dorsolateral wall of the sublumbar region. The broad ligament is a reflection from the peritoneum.

Another polar body is formed by the division of the secondary oocyte at the time of ovulation. The surviving oocyte has a haploid (n) number of chromosomes (similar to a spermatozoon) so that the union of a spermatozoon with an oocyte produces a cell with a diploid (2n) number of chromosomes.

Tubular Genital Tract

The tubular genital tract is the location for transport of spermatozoa to the oocyte. If fertilization occurs, the tract becomes the site for development of the fetus.

Uterine Tubes

The **uterine tubes** are also called the oviducts and, less frequently, fallopian tubes. They are paired, convoluted tubes that conduct oocytes from the ovaries to the respective horn of the uterus. The uterine tubes serve as the site for fertilization of released oocytes by spermatozoa in domestic species. The portion of each tube adjacent to its respective ovary expands to form the **infundibulum** (see Fig. 15-1), and **fimbria** project from its free edge. The fimbria assist in directing the oocyte into the infundibulum at the time of ovulation.

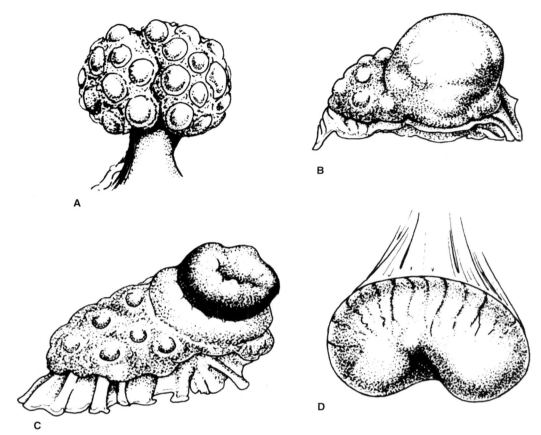

■ FIGURE 15-4 Ovarian differences resulting from species morphology and functional changes. **A)** Sow ovary (berry shaped). **B)** Cow ovary (almond shaped) with ripening follicle. **C)** Cow ovary with fully developed corpus luteum. **D)** Mare ovary (kidney shaped) with ovulation fossa (indentation on the lesser curvature). (From Dyce KM, Sack WO, Wensing CJG. Textbook of Veterinary Anatomy. 3rd Ed. Philadelphia: WB Saunders, 2002.)

The lumen of the uterine tubes are lined with secretory cells and ciliated cells. These cells provide an environment for the oocytes and transport the spermatozoa. Both longitudinal and circular smooth muscles are located within the walls of the uterine tubes, which assist in the transport of oocytes and spermatozoa by their contractions. The serous covering of the uterine tubes (see Fig. 15-3) is known as the mesosalpinx, which is a continuation of the mesovarium and a part of the broad ligament (providing the serous support system for the internal genitalia).

Uterus

The uterus provides a place for development of the fetus if fertilization has occurred. The **uterus** consists of a **corpus (body)**, a **cervix (neck)**, and two **cornua (horns)**. The relative proportions of corpus, cornua, and cervix vary among species. The corpus is largest in the mare, less extensive in the cow and sheep, and small in the sow and bitch (*Fig. 15-6*).

The mucous membrane lining the interior of the uterus (**endometrium**) is highly glandular. The glands are scattered throughout the

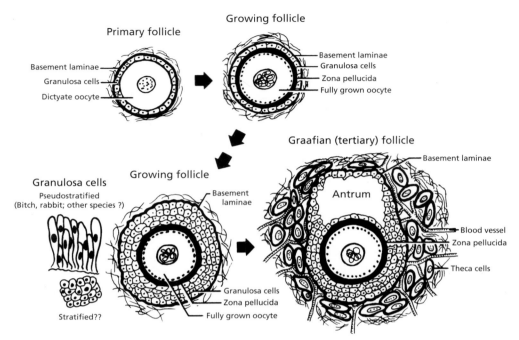

FIGURE 15-5 Development of an ovarian follicle from its primordial (primary) form to a graafian follicle. Growing follicles are those that have begun growth from the resting stage as primordial follicles but have not developed thecal layers or an antrum. (From Pineda MH. Female reproductive system. In: Pineda MH, Dooley MP, eds. Veterinary Endocrinology and Reproduction. 5th ed. Ames, IA: Iowa State Press, 2003.)

entire endometrium of the uterus except in ruminants, in which the **caruncles** (mushroom-like projections from the inner surface that provide attachment for the fetal membranes) are nonglandular (*Fig. 15-7*). The endometrium varies in thickness and vascularity with hormonal changes in the ovary and with pregnancy. The glandular secretion of the endometrium provides nutrients for the embryo before **placentation** (development of placental membranes), after which nutrition is provided by the mother's blood.

The **cervix** projects caudally into the vagina (see Fig. 15-2). This heavy, smooth muscle sphincter is tightly closed, except during estrus and at parturition (birth of young). The mucus seen at estrus is the secretion of cervical goblet cells. Goblet cell secretion of mucus during pregnancy and its outward flow pre-

vents infective material from entering from the vagina.

The **myometrium** is the muscular portion of the uterus, composed of smooth muscle cells. The myometrium hypertrophies during pregnancy, increasing both in cell number and cell size. The principal function of the myometrium is aiding in the expulsion of the fetus at parturition.

The serous covering of the uterus is continuous with the mesosalpinx; in the uterus it is known as the mesometrium. The mesometrium provides a suspensory support, particularly for the nongravid uterus. It should be noted (see Fig. 15-3) that there are two broad ligaments, each extending from the right or left sublumbar region and lateral pelvic wall to their respective ovary, uterine tube, and uterine horn and extending caudally onto the body of

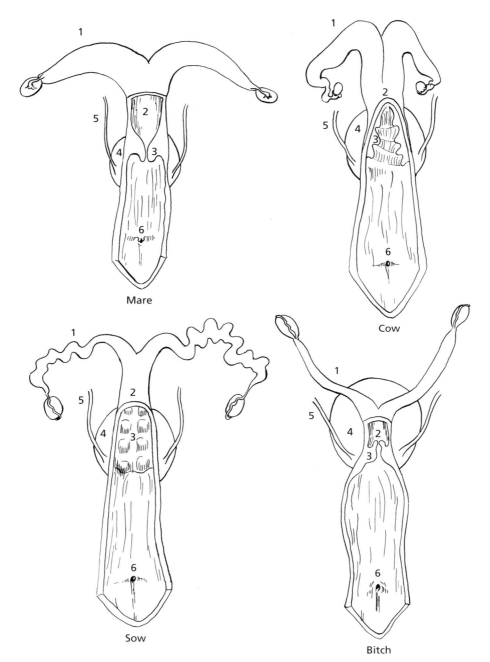

■ FIGURE 15-6 Genital tract comparisons among some domestic animals. **1**, Uterine horn; **2**, uterine body; **3**, cervix; **4**, urinary bladder; **5**, ureter; **6**, urethral opening. The genital tracts are opened dorsally near the body of the uterus, and the opening is extended caudally to the labia to show the cervix and urethral opening. Note that the relative proportions of uterine horns, uterine body, and cervix vary among species. The illustrations are not drawn to scale and do not compare size.

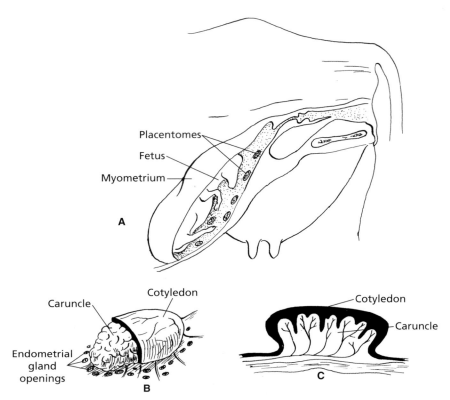

■ **FIGURE 15-7** Relationship of the bovine fetal placenta to the maternal endometrium. **A)** View of fetus within the uterus showing multiple placentomes. **B)** Magnification of a placentome that is surrounded by a number of endometrial gland openings. Only a part of the fetal cotyledon is shown so that the underlying maternal caruncle and endometrial gland openings can be visualized. **C)** Cross section of a placentome. The contribution by the fetal placenta is known as the cotyledon, and the maternal contribution is known as the caruncle.

the uterus. The **gravid (pregnant) uterus** enlarges, and major support is provided by the abdominal wall (*Fig. 15-8*).

Vagina

The **vagina** is the portion of the birth canal located within the pelvis, between the uterus cranially and the vulva caudally (see Figs. 15-1 and 15-2). The vagina serves as a sheath for the male penis during copulation. It is lined with stratified squamous epithelium, which is glandless. The **fornix** is the space formed cranial to the projection of the cervix

into the vagina. In some animals the fornix is only visible dorsally, whereas in others it can completely encircle the cervix or be entirely absent (as in the pig).

External Genitalia

The **external genitalia** consists of the **vulva, labia,** and **clitoris.** The vulva is the caudal portion of the female genitalia that extends from the vagina to the exterior. The external urethral orifice (opening) is the landmark junction of vagina and vulva. The **vestibule of**

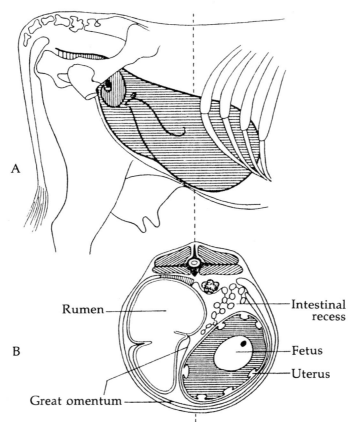

Rumen

Intestinal recess

Fetus

Uterus

Great omentum

■ **FIGURE 15-8** Position of the cow's uterus. **A)** The nongravid uterus (vertical striping) compared with the 6-month gravid uterus (horizontal striping). **B)** Location of the 6-month gravid uterus in transverse section (rumen on left and uterus on right side of abdomen). (From Dyce KM, Wensing CJG. Essentials of Bovine Anatomy. Philadelphia: Lea & Febiger, 1971.)

the **vagina** (*Fig. 15-9*) is another name for the vulva. It is the part of the external genitalia between the vagina and the labia (lips of the vulva). The clitoris (female vestigial counterpart of the penis) is concealed by the lowest part of the vulva. The clitoris is supplied with erectile tissue and sensory nerve endings. The external part of the vulva is its vertical opening, the labia (see Fig. 15-1).

Blood Supply of Female Genitalia

The ovary and oviduct receive their blood supply from the **ovarian artery**, and the vagina receives its blood supply from the **vaginal artery** (*Fig. 15-10*). The major blood supply to the uterus comes from the **uterine artery** (formerly called the middle uterine artery). The cranial part of the uterus is also supplied with blood from the ovarian artery, and the caudal part of the uterus receives blood from the vaginal artery. During pregnancy, the blood supply to the uterus increases dramatically. When the uterine artery is palpated, a vibration of the blood within it can be felt. This is called **fremitus** and is considered to be a good indicator of pregnancy. The ovarian artery is coiled and adheres closely to the uterine vein

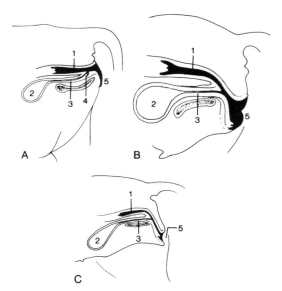

■ **FIGURE 15-9** Species variations in position of the vestibule of the vagina. **A)** Cow. **B)** Mare. **C)** Bitch. The vulva, and hence the vestibule of the vagina, extends caudally from the external urethral orifice. **1**, vagina; **2**, bladder; **3**, urethra; **4**, suburethral diverticulum (not present in mare and bitch); **5**, vulva. (From Dyce KM, Sack WO, Wensing CJG. Textbook of Veterinary Anatomy. 3rd Ed. Philadelphia: WB Saunders, 2002.)

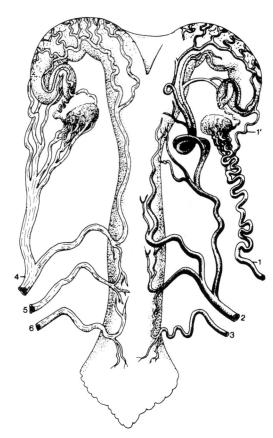

■ **FIGURE 15-10** Ventral view of blood supply to the reproductive tract of the cow. The arteries are shown on the right side and the veins on the left. **1**, ovarian artery; **1'**, uterine branch; **2**, uterine artery; **3**, vaginal artery; **4**, ovarian vein; **5**, uterine vein; **6**, vaginal vein. (From Dyce KM, Sack WO, Wensing CJG. Textbook of Veterinary Anatomy. 3rd Ed. Philadelphia: WB Saunders, 2002.)

(*Fig. 15-11*). Such an arrangement is important for the diffusion of the hormone **prostaglandin $F_{2\alpha}$ ($PGF_{2\alpha}$)** (see Chapter 6) from the uterine vein to the ovarian artery in some species (e.g., cow and ewe, perhaps others). Early transport by this arrangement avoids the general circulation, where much of it would be inactivated by vascular endothelial cells in the lungs. Production requirements are lower because most of the $PGF_{2\alpha}$ produced goes only to the target organ (ovary) and avoids general circulation (and subsequent inactivation) to all body parts. $PGF_{2\alpha}$ at the ovarian site initiates **luteolysis** (termination of the corpus luteum).

■ HORMONES OF FEMALE REPRODUCTION

1. Are diethylstilbestrol and estradiol-17β both estrogens? Are they both steroids?

2. Which female steroid hormone has activities that are performed in concert with estrogens and usually requires previous estrogen priming?

3. Which female steroid hormone prevents contractility of the uterus during pregnancy?

4. What are the main functions of the gonadotropins in the female?

5. Are tonic levels of the gonadotropins in the female increased or decreased by estrogens?

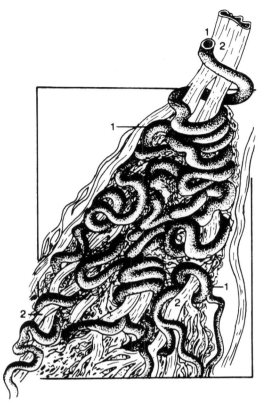

■ FIGURE 15-11 Relationship of the ovarian artery of a ruminant and its branches **(1)** with those of the uterine vein **(2)**. The intertwining ensures a large area of contact. (From Dyce KM, Sack WO, Wensing CJG. Textbook of Veterinary Anatomy. 3rd Ed. Philadelphia: WB Saunders, 2002.)

6. What is the role of the hypophysiopor-tal system in the release of FSH and LH?
7. What is the significance of gradually increasing concentrations of estrogen over a period of time on LH release?

The principal hormones associated with ovarian cycling, pregnancy, and parturition are estrogens, progesterone, and gonadotropins.

Estrogens

Estrogens occur naturally and synthetically. The important estrogens in mammals are ste-roids, produced by the ovary (granulosa cells of follicles), placenta, and adrenal cortex. A common synthetic estrogen is **diethylstilbes-trol**, which is not a steroid, but a complex alcohol with estrogenic properties. The chemical structures of diethylstilbestrol and estradiol-17β (a steroid) are compared in *Figure 15-12*. Regardless of production site, steroids share a common biosynthetic pathway (*Fig. 15-13*).

Estradiol-17β and estrone are estrogens that predominate in domestic nonpregnant and pregnant animals, respectively. Generally, the principal function of the estrogens is to cause cellular proliferation and growth of the tissues related to reproduction. Tissue responses caused by estrogens include: 1) stimulation of endometrial gland growth, 2) stimulation of duct growth in the mammary gland, 3) increase in secretory activity of uterine ducts, 4) initiation of sexual receptiv-ity, 5) regulation of secretion of luteinizing hormone (LH) by the anterior pituitary gland, 6) possible regulation of $PGF_{2\alpha}$ release from the nongravid and gravid uterus, 7) early union of the epiphysis with the shafts of long bones, whereby growth of long bones ceases, 8) protein anabolism, and 9) epitheliotropic activity. The protein anabolic effect of estro-gens is less pronounced than that associated with testosterone. Its effect is probably associ-ated more specifically with the sex organs rather than with a generalized effect. The epi-theliotropic function manifests at estrus when the epithelium in the vagina proliferates and cornification is more prevalent.

Progesterone

Progesterone, like the estrogens, is a steroid sex hormone produced by the corpus luteum (CL) of the ovary, placenta, and adrenal cortex. Its place in the common biosynthetic pathway scheme is shown in Figure 15-13. It is the principal progestational hormone. Certain synthetic and natural progestational agents are called **progestins**.

The activities associated with progesterone are often performed in concert with estrogens,

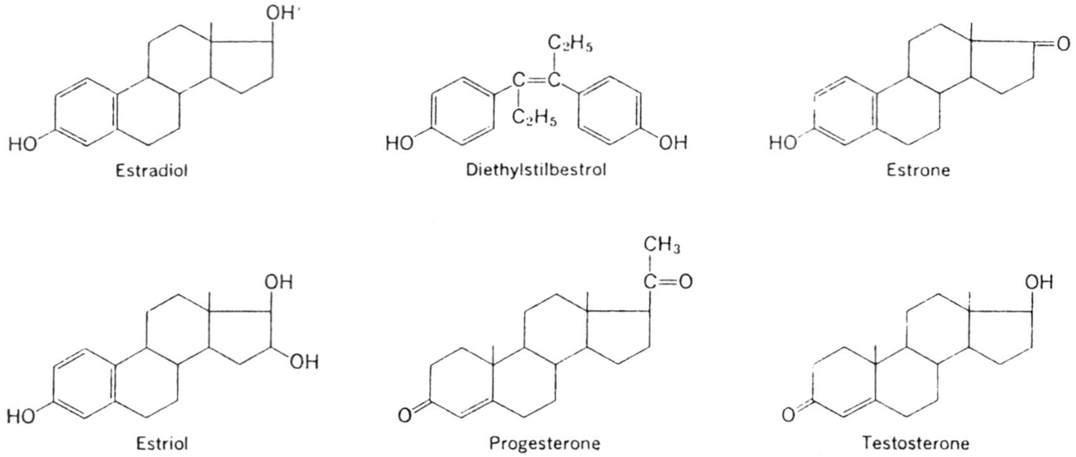

■ **FIGURE 15-12** Chemical structure of some steroid hormones, and diethylstilbestrol. (From Pineda MH. Female reproduction system. In: Pineda MH, Dooley MP, eds. McDonald's Veterinary Endocrinology and Reproduction. 5th Ed. Ames, IA: Iowa State Press, 2003.)

and usually require previous estrogen priming. The functions of progesterone include: 1) promotion of endometrial gland growth, 2) stimulation of secretory activity of the oviduct and endometrial glands to provide nutrients for the developing embryo before implantation, 3) promotion of lobuloalveolar growth in the mammary gland, 4) prevention of contractility of the uterus during pregnancy, and 5) regulation of secretion of gonadotropins.

The interrelationships of the estrogens, progesterone, and gonadotropins are described later in the discussions of the estrous cycle and pregnancy.

Gonadotropins

Follicle-stimulating hormone (FSH) and **luteinizing hormone (LH)** are collectively referred to as the gonadotropins because of their role in stimulating cells within the ovary and testis (the gonads). FSH and LH are hormones secreted by cells within the anterior pituitary. Both are classified chemically as **glycoproteins**. A glycoprotein is a conjugated protein in which the nonprotein group is a carbohydrate.

The main function of FSH in the female is promotion of the growth of follicles. LH is important for the ovulatory process and the luteinization of the granulosa, an essential aspect of CL formation.

Apparently, FSH and LH concentrations exist in the plasma at a tonic or basal level. These levels are controlled by negative feedback from the gonads. Tonic levels are increased by estrogen and decreased by progesterone.

The release of FSH and LH from the anterior pituitary is controlled by a releasing hormone from the hypothalamus. The circulatory system involved is known as the **hypophysioportal system** (*Fig. 15-14*). A portal system begins with capillaries and terminates with capillaries. The hypothalamic capillaries receive a secretion from sensing cells in the hypothalamus known as **gonadotropin releasing hormone (GnRH)**. GnRH is secreted in response to low levels of LH or FSH and is then followed by secretion of LH or FSH.

The concentrations of estrogens and progesterone also influence the amount of LH or FSH secretion. Generally, an increasing concentration of estrogen causes an increase in

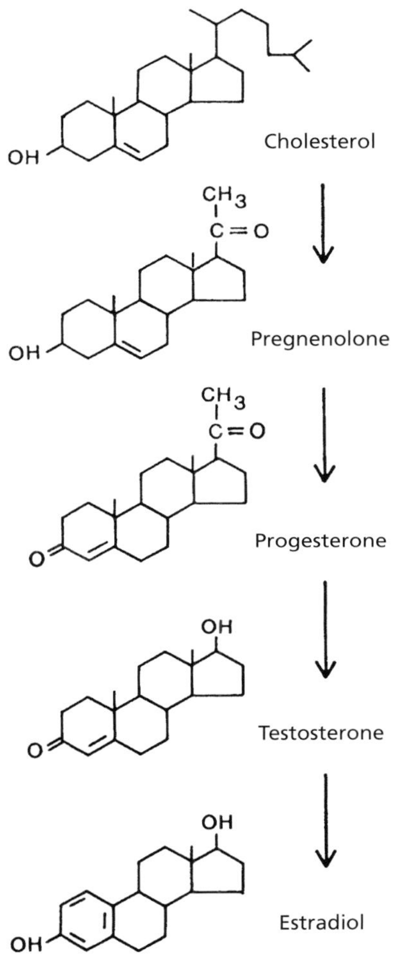

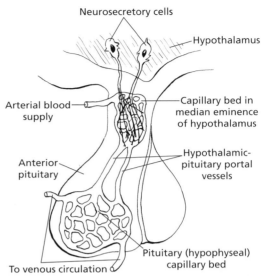

■ FIGURE 15-13 Biosynthesis of steroid hormones from cholesterol. (From Hafez ESE, Hafez B. Reproduction in Farm Animals. 7th Ed. Baltimore: Lippincott Williams & Wilkins, 2000.)

■ FIGURE 15-14 The hypophysioportal circulation involved with the secretion of anterior pituitary hormones. Cell bodies in the hypothalamus sense the need for a hormone and secrete a releasing hormone into the hypothalamic capillary bed. The releasing hormone enters the hypophyseal capillary bed and diffuses to specific cells, causing them to secrete their specific hormone.

sensitivity of the anterior pituitary to GnRH, and results in an increased release of gonadotropins. Progesterone decreases sensitivity of the anterior pituitary to GnRH, and LH and FSH concentrations decrease. These influences, particularly that of estrogen, depend on gradually increasing concentrations of estrogen over a period of time, which results in the preovulatory surge of LH release. Conversely, when estrogen concentration is basal and of short duration, LH and FSH secretions are suppressed.

■ OVARIAN FOLLICLE ACTIVITY

1. How do growing follicles become graafian follicles?
2. What part of the graafian follicle secretes androgens? Do androgens persist as androgens?
3. What hormones cause the formation of a fluid-filled space called an antrum?
4. What functions are served by the preovulatory (24 hours) surge of LH?
5. Do all animals ovulate before the end of estrus? What is the difference between spontaneous and reflex ovulation?
6. Does ovulation occur in all developing follicles? Do follicles continue to grow

and develop during all phases of the ovarian cycle? What must be a characteristic of follicles for them to ovulate?

7. What changes are involved in the formation of the corpus luteum? How is the corpus luteum maintained?

8. What is the natural luteolytic substance that causes regression of the corpus luteum? Does acute regression of the corpus luteum occur in the bitch and queen?

9. Note the unique delivery system of the natural luteolytic substance.

10. What is a persistent corpus luteum, and what is its most probable cause?

When reproductive cycling begins, select follicles within the ovary are influenced by hormones and proceed through growth and maturity, followed by ovulation, corpus luteum development, and its regression. These changes reoccur for other follicles at intervals characteristic for a species.

Follicular Growth

Puberty is defined as the beginning of reproductive life, which in the female is usually marked by the beginning of ovarian activity. The formation of graafian follicles from growing follicles is hormone dependent and begins at puberty when tonic levels of LH and FSH begin to rise and fall with each estrous cycle. Interstitial cells begin to surround the basement membrane of the granulosa cells to form the **theca**, which differentiates into a **theca interna** and **externa**. As the thecal cells are formed around the follicle, a capillary bed develops among them. These **thecal capillaries** increase in size and are concentrated in the theca interna close to the basement membrane that separates the theca interna cells from the granulosa cells (*Fig. 15-15*). LH receptors form on the cells of the theca interna, and receptors for FSH and estrogen form on the granulosa cells.

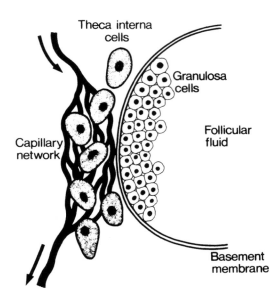

■ **FIGURE 15-15** Formation of a graafian follicle from a growing follicle. Wall structure. The theca interna cells are well supplied with blood. The basement membrane deprives granulosa cells of blood supply. (From Baird DT. Reproductive hormones. In: Austin CR, Short RV, eds. Reproduction in Mammals, Book 3. Cambridge, England: Cambridge University Press, 1972.)

During the hormone-dependent stage, under the influence of LH, **androgens** are produced by cells of the theca interna. The androgens diffuse from the theca interna to the granulosa cells. Under the influence of FSH, the granulosa cells convert the androgens to estrogens. The estrogens produced cause growth and division of the granulosa cells and, together with FSH, cause the granulosa cells to produce secretions that effect separation of the granulosa cells and formation of a space filled with **fluid (liquor folliculi)**, called an **antrum** (see Fig. 15-15). Also, FSH stimulates the formation of LH receptors on the granulosa cells. A **surge of LH output (preovulatory surge)** occurs about 24 hours before ovulation. In addition to its role in ovulation and formation of a corpus luteum, the LH surge causes a reduction in the number of FSH receptors on granulosa cells so that the output of estrogen by the granulosa cells decreases.

Ovulation

When the oocyte is released into the abdomen from its protruding follicle, it is covered by those granulosa cells that immediately surrounded it just before ovulation; these are known as the **corona radiata**. The oocyte and granulosa cells are evacuated with an enveloping viscous (gelatinous) follicular fluid. At ovulation, the oocyte, together with its surrounding cells and gelatinous mass, is swept into the uterine tubes by motility of the fimbriae. The relationship of ovulation to estrus for domestic animals and other factors involved in female reproduction are given in *Table 15-1*.

Ovulation is spontaneous (no stimulation needed) in all of the domestic species except the cat. The cat and other nonspontaneous ovulators (e.g., mink, rabbit, ferret) are **reflex ovulators**, in that coitus is required for ovulation to occur. Coital contact apparently brings forth an LH surge.

The selection of follicles for ovulation seems to occur primarily by chance. It is usually associated with the largest actively growing follicles present when the previous CL regressed (i.e., when progesterone decreased and FSH and LH output began to increase). Follicles continue to grow and develop during all phases of the ovarian cycle, with some impairment during the luteal phase; and the LH surge is necessary for ovulation to occur. Follicles close to full development, but without adequate LH receptors, do not ovulate in response to the LH surge and become atretic.

Corpus Luteum Formation and Regression

Formation of the CL involves **luteinization of the granulosa,** by which the granulosa is converted from estrogen secretion to progesterone secretion (LH receptors on the granulosa cells were previously induced by FSH). The process is initiated by the preovulatory LH surge. The cavity of the ruptured follicle and the fibrin clot within serve as the framework on which the granulosa cells develop. Blood vessels from the theca externa invade the developing CL, and it becomes vascularized. Maintenance of the CL is provided for by LH derived from the LH surge and by the basal circulating levels of LH. In the sheep, prolactin, a gonadotropin hormone for some species, is required to maintain the CL, in addition to LH.

The uterus (endometrium) plays a major role in controlling the life span of the CL in nonpregnant mares, cows, sows, ewes, and does (goats) but is not active in CL regression in the bitch (dog) and queen (cat). $PGF_{2\alpha}$ is released by the nonpregnant uterus about 14 days after ovulation and is considered to be the natural luteolytic substance (causes regression of the CL). The venous return of uterine blood to the right heart and from there to the lung before transport of arterial blood to the ovary results in inactivation by the vascular endothelium of about 90% of $PGF_{2\alpha}$. To ensure that enough $PGF_{2\alpha}$ is delivered directly to the ovary for luteolysis, the anatomic arrangement of the uterine vein and ovarian artery is such that $PGF_{2\alpha}$ can diffuse from the vein to the artery and ovarian perfusion of $PGF_{2\alpha}$ can occur before circulation through the lungs (*Fig. 15-16*). For $PGF_{2\alpha}$ to be effective when it enters the general circulation, it must either be secreted by the uterus in larger amounts, or be more resistant to degradation in the lungs, or both. Survival of $PGF_{2\alpha}$ for the general circulation is more important in the sow and mare.

The reason for final regression of the CL in the bitch and queen (bitch, 75 days; queen, 35 days) is not known. An acute lytic process does not occur.

Persistent Corpus Luteum

Prolongation of the luteal phase beyond 14 days to perhaps 1 to 5 months is known as **persistent corpus luteum**. The presence of a persistent CL prevents a return to the follicular phase and its next ovulation. The immediate reason for persistent CL is the

TABLE 15-1 FACTORS RELATED TO FEMALE REPRODUCTION

ANIMAL	ONSET OF PUBERTY (MO)	AGE FIRST SERVICE (AVERAGE)	LENGTH OF EXTROUS CYCLE (D)	LENGTH OF EXTROUS	GESTATION PERIOD (D)
Mare	18 (10–24)	2–3 yr	21 (19–21)	5 d (4.5–7.5 d)	336 (323–341)
Cow	4–24	14–22 mo	21 (18–24)	18 h (12–28 h)	282 (274–291)
Ewe	4–12 (first fall)	12–18 mo	16-1/2 (14–20)	24–48 h	150 (140–160)
Sow	3–7	8–10 mo	21 (18–24)	2 d (1–5 d)	114 (110–116)
Bitch	6–24	12–18 mo	6–12 mo	9 d (5–19 d)	63 (60–65)

ANIMAL	TIME OF OVULATION	OPTIMUM TIME FOR SERVICE	ADVISABLE TIME TO BREED AFTER PARTURITION
Mare	1–2 d before end of estrous	3–4 d before end of estrous; or 2nd or 3rd d of estrous	About 25–35 d or second estrous; about 9 d or first estrous only if normal in every way
Cow	10–15 h after end of estrous	Just before middle of estrous to end of estrous	60–90 d
Ewe	12–24 h before end of estrous	18–24 h after onset of estrous	Usually the next fall
Sow	30–36 h after onset of estrous	12–30 h after onset of estrous	First estrous 3–9 d after weaning pigs
Bitch	1–2 d after onset of true estrous	2–3 d after onset of estrous; or 10–14 d after onset of proestrous bleeding	Usually first estrous or 2–3 mo after weaning pups

From Frandson RD, Spurgeon TL. Anatomy and Physiology of Farm Animals. 5th Ed. Philadelphia: Lea & Febiger, 1992.

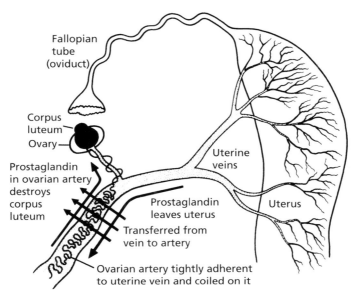

■ FIGURE 15-16 Postulated route by which prostaglandin secreted by the progesterone-primed uterus can enter the ovarian artery and destroy the corpus luteum in the ewe, and possibly other species. (From Short RV. Role of hormones in sex cycles. In: Austin CR, Short RV, eds. Reproduction in Mammals, Book 3. Cambridge, England: Cambridge University Press, 1972.)

failure of the endometrium to synthesize $PGF_{2\alpha}$. Often the failure is caused by an acute or chronic endometrial inflammation.

Summary of Ovarian Cycle Events

Events in the ovary associated with a cycle of hormone changes can be summarized as follows:

1. After regression of the CL (luteolysis caused by $PGF_{2\alpha}$), FSH and LH secretion increases (because of a decrease in the concentration of progesterone).
2. LH stimulates secretion of androgens by the theca interna cells, which diffuse into the granulosa cells.
3. FSH stimulates conversion of androgen to estrogen by the granulosa cells, and the estrogen concentration gradually increases.
4. FSH stimulates the formation of LH receptors on the granulosa cells.
5. Estrogen-rich fluid formed by the granulosa cells separates the granulosa cells and forms a pocket known as an antrum.
6. The gradually increasing estrogen concentration causes a preovulatory surge of LH release.
7. The LH surge promotes the maturation of oocytes by resuming meiosis through the first polar body stage.
8. The LH surge promotes the intrafollicular production of prostaglandins A and E (PGA and PGE), associated with rupture of the follicle.
9. Concomitant with PGA and PGE production is the formation of multivesicular bodies (MVB), which form as out-pockets of the exposed theca externa.
10. MVBs seem to secrete proteolytic enzymes that digest ground substance cementing the theca externa fibroblasts, allowing for the escape of the oocyte (ovulation).

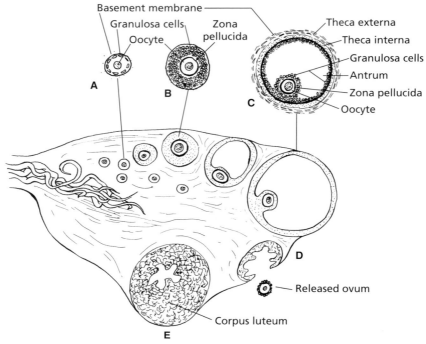

■ **FIGURE 15-17** Sagittal section of an ovary. **A)** Primary follicle. **B)** Growing follicle. **C)** Graafian follicle. **D)** Ruptured follicle. **E)** Corpus luteum. This schematic representation shows in sequence the origin, growth, and rupture of a graafian follicle and a corpus luteum that develops from the remains of the ruptured follicle.

11. The LH surge causes reduction in the number of FSH receptors on the granulosa cells, so the rate of conversion of androgen to estrogen diminishes.
12. LH attaches to granulosa cell LH receptors and begins the conversion of the granulosa from estrogen secretion in the follicular phase to progesterone secretion in the luteal phase.
13. At some point in the latter stages of these events, ovulation occurs, and the cavity previously occupied by the mature follicle becomes a corpus luteum.
14. The corpus luteum secretes progesterone, which causes a decrease in the output of FSH and LH by the anterior pituitary.
15. The corpus luteum regresses, and the output of progesterone begins to decrease.
16. A decrease in the level of progesterone causes FSH and LH secretion to increase, and the cycle is repeated.

The ovarian events are illustrated in *Figure 15-17*.

■ **SEXUAL RECEPTIVITY**

1. **What hormone is required for the initiation of sexual receptivity in all animals?**
2. **How does progesterone enhance receptivity in some domestic animal species?**
3. **What domestic animal species require estrogen synergism with progesterone?**

If copulation is to occur near ovulation, the female must be receptive to the male. Initiation of sexual receptivity in all animals requires estrogen derived from the antral follicles. Also, in some species (e.g., bitch, ewe, sow, cow), progesterone acts synergistically with estrogen for manifestation of receptivity. Neurons associated with a "**sex center**" are located diffusely in the hypothalamus and are critical in initiating the mechanisms of sexual behavior as a response to hormones. It seems that progesterone (tonic levels) acts as a primer for the hypothalamic sexual centers so that estrogen becomes effective. During the postpartum (after parturition) period in some cows and sows, the low progesterone concentration fails to prime the sexual centers of the hypothalamus, and the animals are not sexually receptive at the time of the first postpartum ovulation. In sheep, the priming of the hypothalamus with progesterone is essential, after their seasonal anestrus, before sexual receptivity is manifested. Accordingly, ewes do not show sexual receptivity in conjunction with the first ovulation of the breeding season.

During **proestrus** in the bitch, when estrogen levels increase, sexual receptivity is absent although they might be sexually attractive. It is only when the LH surge occurs near ovulation that sexual receptivity occurs. Preovulatory progesterone from the LH surge (luteinized granulosa cells) can be sufficient to prime the hypothalamus. Before proestrus, a long period of sexual inactivity (**anestrus**) occurs, during which progesterone levels are either low or nonexistent.

Some evidence has shown that GnRH has a role in the manifestation of sexual receptivity. Injection of GnRH without estrogen has been found to cause sexual posturing in some animals. Also, the onset of sexual receptivity is correlated closely with the preovulatory LH surge as caused by GnRH release.

Progesterone is not synergistic with estrogen in manifesting sexual receptivity in the doe, queen, and mare.

■ ESTROUS CYCLE AND RELATED FACTORS

1. How is an estrous cycle interval defined?
2. Know the stages of the estrous cycle and their relationships to ovarian activity.

3. Which steroid hormone predominates during the follicular periods?
4. Which stage of the estrous cycle is characterized by sexual receptivity?
5. Review photoperiod influence on the cat, horse, sheep, and goat. What does "turn-on" and "turn-off" time relate to?
6. How is nutrition related to puberty and postparturient resumption of ovarian activity?
7. Note species characteristics associated with their estrous cycles: cow—postestrus ovulation; ewe—short estrous cycle interval; bitch—vaginal cytologic changes and classical pseudopregnancy; queen—reflex ovulation, signs of estrus, coital behavior.

The term **estrous cycle** refers to the rhythmic phenomenon observed in all mammals involving regular but limited periods of sexual receptivity (estrus) that occur at intervals characteristic of a species. **One cycle interval** is defined as the time from the onset of one period of sexual receptivity to the next (the ovulatory interval).

Animals are usually classified as **monestrous** or **polyestrous**. Monestrous animals are characterized by experiencing estrus once each year. Most wild carnivorous mammals are monestrous and, with some variation, the bitch is usually considered to be monestrous. Polyestrous animals, including most domestic species, have more than one period of estrus in a year. A seasonally polyestrous animal is one that has repeated estrous cycles within a physiologic breeding season (some part of a year), followed by a period of anestrus until the next breeding season.

Stages of Estrous Cycle

The estrous cycle can be divided into several stages according to behavioral or ovarian changes:

1. **Estrus**—the time of sexual receptivity, sometimes referred to as "heat." Ovulation usually, but not always, occurs at the end of estrus.
2. **Metestrus**—the early postovulatory period, during which the CL begins development.
3. **Diestrus**—the period of mature luteal activity, which begins about 4 days after ovulation and ends with regression of the CL.
4. **Proestrus**—the period beginning after CL regression and ending at the onset of estrus. During proestrus, rapid follicle development leads to ovulation and to the onset of sexual receptivity.

The **follicular periods (proestrus and estrus)** are characterized by estrogen dominance. From the behavioral standpoint, the estrus—sexually receptive period encompasses estrus and the diestrus—sexually nonreceptive period includes metestrus, diestrus, and proestrus.

Photoperiod

Among the domestic animals, the seasonal breeders are considered to be the queen, doe, ewe, and mare. These animals are sexually inactive during certain times of the year. The resumption of sexual activity is correlated with conception, so that birth occurs when environmental conditions are more conducive to survival of the young.

The most important factor associated with seasonal breeding is **photoperiod** (relative lengths of alternating periods of lightness and darkness). Both the queen and mare become **anestrous (without estrous cycles)** late in the fall (turn-off time) because of decreasing light, and ovarian cycles are resumed in late winter or early spring (turn-on time) by increasing light. The phenomenon in the ewe and doe is opposite to that of the queen and mare, in that the ovarian cycle has a turn-on time associated with a decrease in daylight and a turn-off time associated with an increase in daylight. Not only do differences in photoperiod response

among species exist, but so do those within species as a result of genetic (breed) differences. Intraspecies difference is most apparent among sheep breeds and probably relates to their origin and related environmental differences. A representation of photoperiod influence on ovarian activity is shown for the queen, mare, ewe, and doe in *Figure 15-18*. Approximate dates of turn-on and turnoff vary according to distance from the equator and associated differences in photoperiods.

Nutrition

The influence of nutrition on the estrous cycle is most apparent at puberty and on reestablishment of the estrous cycle after parturition. Animals ingesting sound nutritional regimens reach puberty at an earlier age than nutritionally deprived animals. Consequently, breeding seasons can be delayed if calves are deprived of adequate nutrition. After parturition and during early lactation, cows can have a negative metabolic balance, which can result in an increased interval between parturition and resumption of ovarian activity.

Species Characteristics

Whereas the general pattern of the estrous cycle is similar among the domestic species, differences are noted in duration, not only for the cycle, but also for stages within the cycle. Duration of the cycle and for estrus is shown in Table 15-1 for domestic animals. The age of puberty onset also varies, and for some species it is affected by the breeding season for that species.

Cow

Smaller breeds of cows usually reach puberty at an earlier age than larger breeds (Jersey, 8 months; Holstein, 11 months). Behavioral changes associated with estrus include restlessness, mounting activity, standing to be mounted, being more alert to other animals,

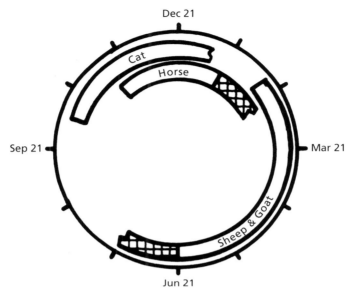

■ FIGURE 15-18 Effects of photoperiod on ovarian activity in the cat, horse, sheep, and goat at a latitude of 38.5° north (California). The open bars represent periods of ovarian inactivity (anestrus). The transition from anestrus to estrus (often erratic) is shown by the cross-hatched portion of the bars for the horse, sheep, and goat. (From Stabenfeldt GH, Edqvist L. Female reproductive processes. In: Swenson MJ, Reece WO, eds. Dukes' Physiology of Domestic Animals. 11th Ed. Ithaca, NY: Cornell University Press, 1993.)

and decreased appetite. At the same time decreased milk production, mucus discharge from the vulva, and redness and relaxation of the vulva are noted. It is important to detect estrus so that the correct time for artificial insemination can be determined.

Most domestic animals ovulate toward the end of estrus, but the cow ovulates 12 to 14 hours after estrus. The most successful artificial insemination occurs when it is performed about 12 hours after the beginning of estrus. In the cow, therefore, insemination precedes ovulation, and optimum fertilization is coupled with expected spermatozoon and oocyte life and with capacitation. Capacitation refers to a modification of ejaculated or inseminated spermatozoa within the female reproductive tract, enabling the spermatozoa to fertilize oocytes. The fertile life for bovine spermatozoa (time in female genitalia) is 30 to 48 hours and for bovine oocytes (after ovulation) is 20 to 24 hours. The effect of time of insemination on

conception rate in cattle is shown in *Figure 15-19.*

Mare

The onset of puberty in the mare occurs during the breeding season after birth. If the interval between birth and the next breeding season is short (e.g., summer birth), puberty can be delayed for 12 months. A wide range of age for puberty is seen in the mare, from 12 to 18 months.

The transition from winter anestrus to estrus in late winter or early spring is often erratic, in that follicles might be grown but not ovulated. This results in prolonged estrous periods. After the first ovulation, the length of the estrous cycle stabilizes, and the duration of estrus is 5 to 6 days.

Ovulation occurs about 24 hours before the end of estrus and causes the end of estrus, which is a good indication that ovulation has

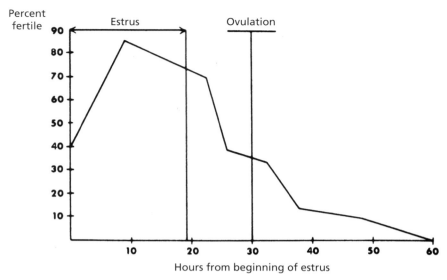

■ **FIGURE 15-19** The effect of time of insemination on conception rate in cattle. Conception rate is best when inseminated about 10 hours from beginning of estrus. (From Stabenfeldt GH, Edqvist L. Female reproductive processes. In: Swenson MJ, Reece WO, eds. Dukes' Physiology of Domestic Animals. 11th Ed. Ithaca, NY: Cornell University Press, 1993.)

occurred. Signs of estrus in the mare are elevation of the tail, standing with the hind legs apart, squatting and urinating, and rhythmically erecting the clitoris.

Ewe

Where lambs are normally born between December and March (in the northern hemisphere), puberty onset occurs the next fall, at about 8 to 9 months of age.

The estrous cycle in sheep is shorter than in the other domestic species because the antral phase of follicle growth is 3 to 4 days shorter. The physiologic breeding season lasts 6 to 7 months, during which repeated estrous cycles are observed in the absence of pregnancy.

A prominent sign of estrus is fluttering of the tail. Also, females separated from males by a barrier often assume a close proximity to the barrier.

Sow

Pigs born at any time of the year reach puberty at 6 to 7 months of age. Ovulation rates are

more pronounced at the third estrus after puberty.

Signs of estrus include swelling of the vulva, restlessness, and decreased appetite. Application of pressure on the sow's back during estrus brings forth the rigidity reflex that occurs during natural mating with a boar.

Ovulation occurs from both ovaries, and 14 to 16 oocytes can be released. Because of the large number of follicles or corpora lutea at any one time, the sow ovaries often appear to be lobulated (see Fig. 15-4).

Doe

The breeding season and gestation periods are similar for goats and sheep, and puberty is reached at about the same age (8 to 9 months). Breeding is often delayed, however, until the next breeding season.

Signs of estrus in the doe are similar to those in the ewe. When mating occurs, intromission and ejaculation are accomplished rapidly, usually within several seconds.

Pseudopregnancy is a condition in which a female has most signs of pregnancy but is not pregnant. Enlargement of the uterus occurs as a result of fluid accumulation. This phenomenon occurs in the goat and is believed to be caused by prolongation of the CL (see previous section, Persistent Corpus Luteum). The injection of $PGF_{2\alpha}$ results in CL regression and discharge of the accumulated uterine fluid.

Bitch

The onset of puberty in the bitch occurs 2 to 3 months after she reaches adult size. Among breeds it ranges from 6 to 12 months of age.

The bitch has an unusually long period of ovarian inactivity (anestrus) that is unrelated to photoperiod or nutrition. Because of this she is sometimes considered to be monestrous. Estrous cycles are common at all times of the year. The stages of the estrous cycle are different from those of the other species in that each is longer. Proestrus and estrus are each 7 to 10 days long, and diestrus is prolonged, lasting 70 to 80 days.

The LH surge occurs at the end of proestrus, followed by ovulation in 24 to 48 hours. The bitch might be sexually attractive during proestrus but is not sexually receptive until after the LH surge. Progesterone secretion thereafter is essential for receptivity and, although the estrogen level declines, sexual receptivity is maintained for 7 to 10 days.

Vaginal cytologic changes seem to be more pronounced in bitches than in other domestic species and have been correlated with each estrous cycle stage. Vaginal smears are useful for assessing the stage of estrus and for predicting the most suitable time for breeding. The principal cytologic changes are: 1) thickening and cornification of the vaginal epithelium, 2) loss of leukocytes because of the thickened epithelium, and 3) appearance of erythrocytes from the developing vascular system of the endometrium.

Among those animals that show pseudopregnancy, it is most often seen in the bitch. In the absence of pregnancy the corpus luteum persists, and during the exaggerated diestrus, progesterone continues to be produced for 50 to 80 days. This is a normal phenomenon in bitches because the uterus is not active in CL regression (production of $PGF_{2\alpha}$). The endometrium hypertrophies and endometrial glands develop, although no fetus is present. Some bitches have no other signs of the prolonged elevation of progesterone concentration, but others have mammary gland enlargement and relaxation of the pelvis. Occasionally, a maternal attitude develops that leads to nest building. Rarely, lactation begins and the bitch shows signs of labor.

The long period of progesterone dominance (long diestrus), coupled with the relatively long period of regression of the endometrium after luteolysis of the CL, predisposes the endometrium to pyometra (pus in the uterus). Pyometra is common in older bitches.

Queen

Cats born in the spring and summer months reach puberty in the next breeding season, at about 6 to 8 months of age. Cats born in the fall and early winter have their puberty delayed for 1 year, until the next breeding season. The breeding season is considered to be January to October in the northern hemisphere.

If the queen does not have coitus, ovulation does not occur, and no luteal phase intervenes until the next cycle. The 8-day follicular phase is followed, however, by an 8-day period of ovarian inactivity. If queens have coital contact but fail to conceive, a luteal phase prolongs the onset of the next proestrus, with a minimum time of 42 days between estrus. Pseudopregnancy occurs in queens if a luteal phase occurs without pregnancy. Development of the uterus, mammary glands, and abdomen is not as marked as in the bitch; and nest building and lactation seldom occur.

Signs of estrus in queens include an increase in affection, which can be shown to almost any object—humans, table legs, or other pieces of furniture. They also crawl with their thorax against the floor, roll about, and vocalize for prolonged periods.

Several coital contacts might be made, with intromission and ejaculation occupying only 10 to 15 seconds each time. A refractory period or lack of sexual receptivity occurs for 10 to 15 minutes after each intromission. During the first hour of contact, four or five intromissions and ejaculations might occur.

■ PREGNANCY

1. Know the length of gestation for each of the domestic species (see Table 15-1).
2. What is a sperm reservoir? Where are important ones located?
3. What is capacitation? Name one capacitation change.
4. What is the zona reaction associated with fertilization? Where does fertilization normally occur?
5. What is uterine milk?
6. What is implied by implantation?
7. What is placentation? What membranes compose the fetal placenta?
8. Know the relationship of the placental membranes to each other and to the fetus and mother. Where are the branches of the umbilical arteries and veins located?
9. What is a persistent urachus?
10. Which animals have a cotyledonary placenta? What composes a placentome?
11. Which steroid hormone predominates during pregnancy? Where is it produced? Do the sources and duration of their production vary among species? When is the corpus luteum source needed by all species?
12. What function is served by pregnant mare serum gonadotropin (PMSG)?
13. What are some signs of pregnancy in the cow as observed by rectal palpation?

Pregnancy is the condition of the female in which unborn young are contained within the body. Pregnancy is also called **gestation**, and its length is frequently known as the **gestation period**, extending from fertilization through birth. Its length for various domestic animals is shown in Table 15-1. Pregnancy begins with fertilization, ends with parturition, and includes the essential aspects of implantation and placentation. Before fertilization, the oocyte and sperm are transported to appropriate sites in the uterine tubes.

Transport of Oocyte and Spermatozoa

At ovulation, the fimbriae of the uterine tubes (see Fig. 15-1) are in close contact with the ovaries. The contractile activity of the fimbriae directs the shed oocyte into the funnel-shaped opening of the uterine tube. Within the uterine tube the oocyte is directed toward the uterus by cilia and by uterine tube motility.

The ejaculated spermatozoa are transported to the uterine tubes by increased motility within the uterus caused by the release of oxytocin at the time of coitus and by the presence of prostaglandins in semen. The oxytocin is effective because of the uterus being primed by estrogen. Another factor that assists in transport is thought to be the presence of a negative pressure (vacuum) in the uterus. Many spermatozoa are rapidly transported to the uterine tubes after ejaculation, but it is believed that these are not the ones destined for fertilization. Their presence might be coincidental with the spread of accessory fluids throughout the tubular genitalia. The spermatozoa destined for fertilization are transported more slowly from their sites of deposition (cervical canal, uterus, vagina) to **spermatozoa reservoirs**. The cervix of ruminants has prominent ridges and mucosal crypts that provide an extensive secretory surface (*Fig. 15-20*). The cervical crypts and their mucous covering aid in the physical entrapment of spermatozoa and serve as spermatozoa

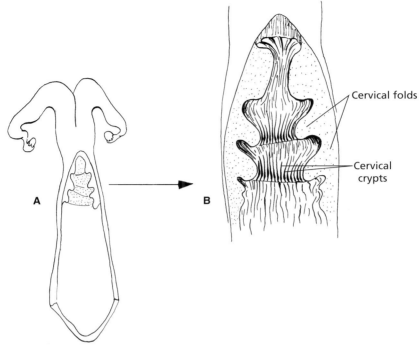

■ FIGURE 15-20 Dorsal view of the ruminant cervix. **A)** The cervix has been cut open and its lateral walls reflected to show the folds and crypts. **B)** Magnified view of the cervix. A mucous covering assists physical entrapment of spermatozoa destined for fertilization. The folds and crypts serve as sperm reservoirs and allow for capacitation of spermatozoa.

reservoirs. Another important spermatozoa reservoir is located at the junction of the uterine horns with the uterine tubes.

Within the spermatozoa reservoirs, the spermatozoa undergo changes necessary for later penetration of the zona pellucida and fertilization of the oocyte. These changes, known as **capacitation**, require several hours. One important change involves the **acrosome**, in which channels are established for the escape of hyaluronidase and a proteolytic enzyme; these substances are essential for penetration of the ovum. Capacitated spermatozoa are released slowly from the spermatozoa reservoirs and proceed to the ampulla of the oviduct (dilated portion near the infundibulum) for fertilization. Ovulation occurs after the onset of estrus so that insemination is accomplished before ovulation. This allows enough capacita-

tion time and, because the fertilizing life span is twice as long in spermatozoa as in oocytes, large numbers of spermatozoa are usually ready for fertilization at the time of ovulation. Oocytes retain viability for about 12 to 18 hours after ovulation in most domestic animals, and spermatozoa retain their fertilizing ability for 24 to 48 hours in the cow, ewe, and sow, for up to 90 hours in the bitch, and for 120 hours (5 days) in the mare.

Fertilization

Fertilization is the fusion of male and female gametes to form one single cell, the zygote. The first step in fertilization is penetration of the zona pellucida by the spermatozoon. This involves not only the enzymes **hyaluronidase** and **acrosin** (proteolytic enzyme from acrosome), but also spermatozoon motility. Motility ceases once contact with the oocyte has been made. In most domestic species, the second maturation division (meiosis) occurs when a spermatozoon penetrates the zona pellucida, whereas the first meiosis occurred a few hours before ovulation. The zona reaction occurs after penetration of the zona pellucida and protects the oocyte from further penetration by other spermatozoa. Penetration by more than one spermatozoon (**polyspermy**) is deleterious to normal development of the zygote.

Pronuclei develop from the nuclei of the spermatozoon and oocyte, which is followed by fusion of respective pronuclei to form a zygote with the diploid number of chromosomes (see Chapter 1). Fertilization is complete after the fused pronuclei have disappeared and are replaced by chromosome groups united in prophase of the first mitotic division.

Zygotes usually remain in the uterine tube for 3 to 4 days before being transferred to the uterus. Uterine motility is unfavorable for zygote survival, and estrogen dominance at estrus must be changed to progesterone dominance, which occurs with the formation of the corpus luteum. Progesterone has a quieting influence on the uterus and promotes development of a glandular endometrium that can secrete **uterine milk**, a nutrient medium for the embryo preceding its implantation. Cell division produces a 16- to 32-cell structure known as the morula. A cavity forms within the morula by 6 to 8 days of age, and the cell mass is called a blastocyst.

The period of the oocyte ends when the blastocyst attaches to the endometrium. This is the beginning of the embryonic period. The **embryonic period** is characterized by rapid growth; major tissues, organs, and systems develop, and the major features of external body form become recognizable. The **fetal period** extends from this time until birth, and begins at about day 45 of gestation in the cow.

Implantation and Placentation

The nutritive requirements of the developing blastocyst are satisfied by diffusion from yolk in the oocyte and by secretions of the uterine tube and uterus (uterine milk), until it becomes fixed in position in the uterus. **Implantation** of the embryo occurs when it becomes fixed in position and forms a physical and functional contact with the uterus. It occurs 2 to 5 weeks after fertilization. The interval is shortest for the cat (2 weeks) and longest for cattle and horses (5 weeks).

Because the embryo continues to grow, the central mass of cells becomes further removed from the surface. Diffusion of nutrients is no longer adequate, and membranes develop concurrent with a circulatory system that provide for receiving nutrients from the dam. The development of extraembryonic membranes is known as **placentation**, and the collective name for the membranes is the **fetal placenta**, which consists of the **chorion**, **allantois**, and **amnion**. The relationship of the fetal membranes to the fetus is shown in *Figure 15-21*. The chorion is the outermost membrane and is the one most intimately associated with the endometrium. The amnion envelops the fetus and contains **amniotic fluid** in the amniotic cavity. The amniotic fluid is derived from fetal urine from the urethra, from secretions from the respiratory tract and oral cavity, and from the maternal circulation. The amniotic fluid protects the fetus from external shock, prevents adhesion of fetal skin with amniotic membrane, and assists in dilating the cervix and lubricating the birth passage at parturition. The allantois outer layer is fused to the chorion, and the inner layer of allantois is fused to the amnion. The space between the two layers of allantois is called the allantoic cavity. It is continuous with the cranial extremity of the urinary bladder by way of the urachus, which passes through the umbilical cord. When the urachus fails to close at birth, a continuous drip of urine is observed from the navel, a condition known as persistent

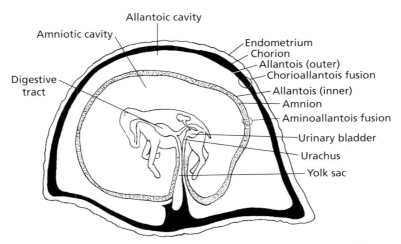

■ FIGURE 15-21 Fetus of horse within the placenta. The chorioallantois is the combination of the outer allantois with the chorion. Umbilical arteries and veins (not shown) occupy the space (blackened) between the outer allantois and chorion. The chorion is intimately associated with the endometrium. Attachment to endometrium not shown, and its extent varies with placental type. The inner allantois is fused with the amnion (stippled for contrast).

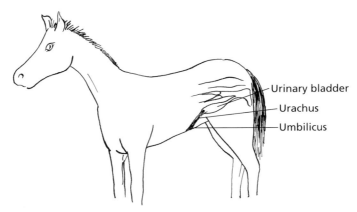

■ FIGURE 15-22 Diagrammatic view of persistent urachus in a foal. Failure of urachus closure at birth results in a continuous drip of urine at its umbilical exit.

urachus (*Fig. 15-22*). Allantoic fluid originates from fetal urine and from secretory activity of the allantoic membrane. The fluid brings the chorioallantoic membrane into close apposition with the endometrium during early attachment and stores fetal excretory products. Branches of umbilical arteries and veins are distributed between the outer layer of allantois and the chorion.

The yolk sac is connected to the fetal intestine (the remnant after birth is known as Meckel's diverticulum). It serves as a nutrition source early in development.

When the attachment (extension of chorionic villi) of fetal membranes to the endometrium is continuous throughout the entire surface of the fetal membranes, it is known as a **diffuse placenta**. A diffuse type of placenta

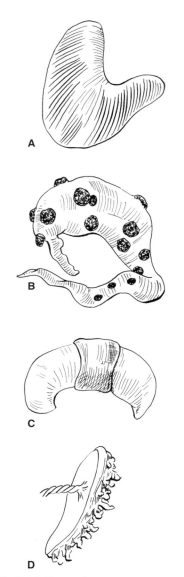

■ **FIGURE 15-23** Placental types according to the distribution of chorionic projections (villi) on the endometrium. **A)** Diffuse placenta of the horse and pig. **B)** Cotyledonary placenta of ruminants. **C)** Zonary placenta of the dog and cat. **D)** Discoid placenta of the human and monkey.

is found in the horse and pig (*Fig. 15-23A*). Ruminants have a **cotyledonary placenta**, in which attachment occurs only at the many mushroom-like projections from the endome-

trium (*Fig. 15-23B*). The fetal cotyledons are attached to the maternal caruncles, a combination known as a **placentome**. The fetal placentas of the dog and cat are attached by a girdle-like band that encircles the placenta, called a **zonary placenta** (*Fig. 15-23C*). The human placenta attachment is confined to a disk-shaped area and is called a **discoidal placenta** (*Fig. 15-23D*).

A sterile heifer born twin to a normal bull calf is called a **freemartin**. This occurs when the female calf develops in the uterus with a normal male twin and they share the same blood supply (anastomosis of the placental blood vessels). When this occurs, the sex hormones from the earlier developing male twin pass across to the female twin, causing sexual differentiation of both male and female to proceed under control of male hormones. About 90% of heifer calves born twin to a bull calf are freemartins and can usually be detected clinically because of the shortened vagina (short advancement of a blunt instrument) and an enlarged clitoris.

Hormones

Pregnancy is maintained as a result of the predominance of progesterone. During gestation, progesterone is produced by the placenta and CL. The contribution from placental and luteal sources and the duration of their contribution varies among species. The CL source is needed by all species during early pregnancy, but is not needed by the mare and ewe after about 100 and 60 days, respectively. A CL is needed for most of pregnancy in the cow, bitch, and queen and for the entire pregnancy in the sow and doe. Although progesterone from the CL is not needed by the ewe, regression of the CL does not occur and luteal production continues, but placental production is dominant. Regression of the CL occurs in the mare about midway, and the placenta is the sole source of progesterone for the maintenance of pregnancy.

In the mare, **endometrial cups** begin to be formed at about day 35 of gestation within the endometrium from cells migrating from the placenta. The cups begin to secrete a hormone known as **pregnant mare serum gonadotropin (PMSG)** at about 35 days, which continues until about 130 days of gestation. PMSG helps to form new follicles, which ovulate and provide for additional corpora lutea. A greater supply of luteal progesterone is thereby ensured until the endometrial supply of progesterone is adequate for maintenance. All corpora lutea regress by about 150 days. Early pregnancy in the mare can be diagnosed by analyzing for the presence of PMSG.

Diagnosis

It is often of economic importance to determine whether an animal is actually pregnant. Pregnancy is obvious during the late stages when the size of the fetus, uterus, and fetal fluids have increased to the point at which the abdomen has enlarged and definite dropping of the abdominal wall has occurred (known as **bellying down**). Rectal palpation is a useful procedure for detecting earlier signs of pregnancy, particularly in the cow. The hand is inserted into the rectum and structures located outside of the rectal wall can be felt.

Early pregnancy by rectal palpation in the cow is suggested if a corpus luteum is present and if one horn of the uterus is larger than the other. This condition can be apparent at 30 to 45 days. At about 3 months, the fetal membranes can be felt to slip away from the grasp when the uterus is lifted, and small caruncles in the uterine wall are palpable. Also at 3 months, a vibration or "buzzing" of blood in the uterine artery is palpable, known as fremitus. At 5 to 7 months the weight of the fetus causes the uterus to slip over the brim of the pelvis, and the cervix becomes taut. The ovaries and fetus are difficult to palpate when this occurs because of their distance from the palpator, but definite caruncles are palpable.

After the fetus has descended over the brim of the pelvis in the cow, it may be possible to detect pregnancy by an external technique known as **ballottement**. Pressure is exerted on the lower right abdominal wall (see Fig. 15-8) with the fist or knee in an inward and upward direction and then is released, causing the fetus to rise and fall in its suspending fluids. The fall should be felt by the manipulator.

The use of radiography for the diagnosis of pregnancy has had limited application in veterinary medicine. Penetration of the rays is restricted in large animals, and exposure of the film is difficult. In small animals, such as the dog, exposure is adequate, but differentiation of a fetus is not possible until calcification of bones is adequate for contrast. This does not occur until about 45 days in the dog, and other means, such as palpation and observation, are often more useful for earlier diagnosis of pregnancy.

A biologic test for the detection of pregnancy can be performed in the mare based on the production of PMSG by the endometrial cups (see previous text). Injection of serum taken from a mare at 40 to 130 days of pregnancy into a female rabbit that has been isolated from male rabbits for at least 30 days brings forth ovarian follicles that rupture and form reddened corpora hemorrhagica about 48 hours after injection. The corpora hemorrhagica can be seen when the rabbit is butchered or observed by other procedures when placed under anesthesia. Because the rabbit does not ovulate and form corpora hemorrhagica unless coitus occurs, only the injected PMSG could have caused the ovulation.

Human chorionic gonadotropin (HCG) is excreted in the urine of pregnant women. It is detectable about 8 days after ovulation, which is 1 day after implantation. Early detection of pregnancy in women is possible by diagnostic tests that use the presence of HCG in urine. Functionally, HCG is the signal for the corpus luteum to be maintained and thus sustain pregnancy.

■ PARTURITION

1. **What are some signs of approaching parturition?**

2. How is respiratory rate in the sow associated with closeness of farrowing? What happens to body temperature in the bitch just before parturition?
3. What functions are served by estrogen increase just before parturition?
4. What functions are served by $PGF_{2\alpha}$ at the time of parturition?
5. How do oxytocin and the presence of feet in the pelvic canal assist parturition?
6. What are the stages of labor?
7. What is meant by presentation of the fetus? How is it initiated?
8. What is the difference between an anterior and a posterior presentation? What is an example of an abnormal presentation?
9. What term is applied to difficulty encountered in expulsion of the fetus?

Parturition, sometimes called labor, is the physiologic process by which the pregnant uterus delivers the fetus and fetal membranes from the mother.

Signs of Approaching Parturition

Throughout pregnancy the abdomen continues to enlarge, and its maximum size is reached just before parturition. The mammary glands also continue to enlarge and, within a few days of parturition, begin to secrete a milky material. Other signs include swelling of the vulva and a discharge of mucus from the vulva. The abdominal muscles relax, which causes the belly to drop and the rump to sink on both sides of the tail head. It is believed that the hormone relaxin, in association with the increasing level of estrogen of late pregnancy, causes the relaxation of ligaments to enable the birth canal to enlarge. Also, it is thought that $PGF_{2\alpha}$ helps to relax the cervix. In addition to these physical signs,

certain behavioral signs are characteristic, such as restlessness, frequent lying down and getting up, and frequent urination. The bitch and sow often attempt to build elaborate nests.

Respiratory rates are better indicators than milk letdown that sows are close to farrowing. Respiratory rates increase steadily and peak 6 hours before farrowing in almost all sows. In contrast, some sows produce colostrum as long as 3 to 4 days before farrowing. An example of the respiratory rate index can be obtained from the following data:

1. Respiratory rates average 54 breaths/min during the 24- to 12-hour period before farrowing.
2. From 12 to 4 hours before farrowing, respiratory rates are the highest, averaging 91 breaths/min.
3. The lowest respiratory rates are recorded between 6 and 18 hours after birth of the last piglet, averaging 25 breaths/min.

Rectal temperature changes have also been studied as indicators of impending parturition under the assumption that certain hormones influence body temperature. For example, progesterone increases the basal body temperature because it causes an increase in the basal metabolic rate. The temperature index is most dramatic and reliable in the bitch, in which a decrease (loss of progesterone) of 28°C to 38°C (48°F or 58°F) might be observed 6 or 8 hours before parturition. Temperature index has not been found to be a reliable indicator in other species.

Hormone Changes

An important hormone change that occurs just before parturition is an increase in the production of estrogen. Estrone is produced by the fetoplacental unit as maturity of the fetus increases (approximately 3 to 4 weeks prepartum in the cow). The increase in production of cortisol by fetal adrenal cortices, concurrent with maturity of the fetus, initiates the prepartum increase in estrogen production. The secretion of estrogen assists in the production of uterine muscle contractile proteins before parturition. Estrogen might also be the signal for the secretion of $PGF_{2\alpha}$ that occurs in the immediate prepartum period (24 to 36 hours prepartum in the cow). $PGF_{2\alpha}$ initiates regression of the corpus luteum (if present) and subsequent lowering of progesterone levels. The increase in estrogen and decrease in progesterone levels convert the uterus from a state of quiescence to a state of potential contractility. The increase in estrogen level varies among domestic animals regarding time of occurrence before parturition (*Fig. 15-24*). The length of increase is longest for the cow and shortest for the ewe.

Changes in maternal hormonal levels do not seem to play a major role in parturition in the mare. At parturition the mare has relatively high levels of progestogens and low levels of estrogens. $PGF_{2\alpha}$ level increases, however, during foaling. The progesterone concentra-

tion does not decrease in the mare after $PGF_{2\alpha}$ secretion because no corpus luteum is present after about 150 days of pregnancy.

$PGF_{2\alpha}$ is also believed to increase the contractility of the uterus by permitting greater mobility of sarcoplasmic calcium. These early contraction increases might be important in positioning the fetus for delivery (presentation) through the pelvic canal. The presence of the fetus in the pelvic canal causes oxytocin to be released from the posterior pituitary. In the presence of an estrogen-primed uterus, the muscle contractions increase in intensity to assist in expelling the fetus. $PGF_{2\alpha}$ also increases the sensitivity of the uterus to oxytocin, which enhances the rhythmic contractions of the uterine musculature during delivery. The uterus can only assist in the expulsion of the fetus and must have the coordinated contraction of the abdominal muscles. The presence of the feet in the pelvic canal and the consequent stimulation of the vagina provides for reflex contraction of the abdominal muscles, similar to the straining that

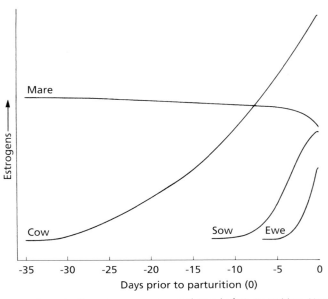

■ **FIGURE 15-24** Estrogen patterns in the mare, cow, sow, and ewe before parturition. Negative numbers refer to days before parturition (0). (From Edqvist LE, Stabenfeldt GA. Reproductive hormones. In: Kaneko JJ, ed. Clinical Biochemistry of Domestic Animals. 3rd Ed. New York: Academic Press, 1980.)

occurs when one attempts to replace a prolapsed uterus. The abdominal and uterine muscle contraction, coupled with relaxed pelvic ligaments, separation of the pelvic symphysis, and dilatation of the cervix, provide for expulsion of the fetus. A summary of the events associated with parturition, beginning with the prepartum secretion of fetal cortisol and ending with expulsion of the fetus, is shown in *Figure 15-25*.

Stages

The three stages of parturition are as follows:

1. Uterine contractions (contribute to dilatation of cervix and presentation of fetus)

2. Contractions associated with expulsion of fetus (involve abdominal muscle contraction)

3. Expulsion of fetal membrane

The stages of labor and related events are summarized in *Table 15-2*.

In monotocous (single birth) species, the fetus lies on its back during gestation. Just before birth, a position is assumed in the uterus that is characteristic for the species (presentation). Presentation can be initiated by early contractions of the uterus (see previous text). A proper presentation for the bovine fetus is shown in *Figure 15-26*. The front feet are pointed toward the cervix, the head is extended and tucked between the feet, and the

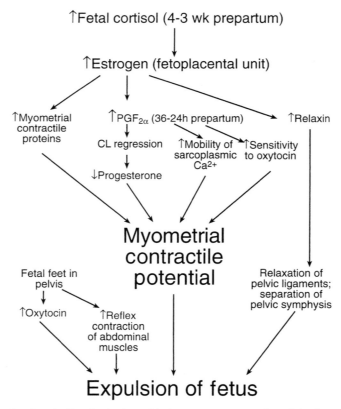

■ **FIGURE 15-25** Events of parturition beginning with the prepartum secretion of fetal cortisol and ending with expulsion of the fetus. PGF$_{2\alpha}$ (prostaglandin F$_{2\alpha}$); CL, corpus luteum.

TABLE 15-2 STAGES OF LABOR AND RELATED EVENTS IN FARM ANIMALS

STAGE OF LABOR	MECHANICAL FORCES	PERIOD	RELATED EVENTS
I. Dilation of cervix	Regular uterine contractions	Beginning of uterine contractions until cervix is fully dilated and continuous with vagina	Maternal restlessness, elevated pulse and respiratory rates Changes in fetal position and posture
II. Expulsion of fetus[a]	Strong uterine and abdominal contractions	From complete cervical dilation to end of delivery of fetus	Maternal recumbency and straining Rupture of allantochorion and escape of fluid from vulva Appearance of amnion (water bag) at vulva Rupture of amnion and delivery of fetus
III. Expulsion of fetal membranes	Uterine contractions decrease in amplitude	After delivery of fetus to expulsion of fetal membranes	Maternal straining ceases Loosening of chorionic villi from maternal crypts Inversion of chorioallantois Straining and expulsion of fetal membranes

[a]In polytocous species (sow) and twin-bearing species (sheep and goat), this stage cannot be separated from the next stage (III).

From Hafez ESE, Hafez B. Reproduction in Farm Animals. 7th Ed. Baltimore: Lippincott Williams & Wilkins, 2000.

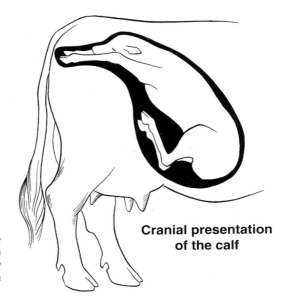

Cranial presentation of the calf

■ **FIGURE 15-26** Normal presentation for the bovine fetus, known as a cranial or anterior presentation. (From Frandson RD, Wilke WL, Fails AD. Anatomy and Physiology of Farm Animals. 6th Ed. Baltimore: Lippincott Williams & Wilkins, 2003.)

back of the calf is directed toward the sacral vertebrae. This is known as an **anterior or cranial presentation**. A **posterior or caudal presentation** with the hind feet extended into the pelvic canal is considered normal, but is less common. An example of an abnormal presentation is one in which there might be an anterior presentation, but with a deviation of the head and neck. Abnormal presentations usually require correction before the fetus can be expelled successfully.

Difficulties are often encountered during parturition, and delays are observed in what are considered normal durations of each stage. Undue delay in providing assistance often aggravates the condition and can injure the mother and cause death to the fetus. Rules of thumb for the average duration of the three stages of labor in the mare, cow, buffalo, ewe, and sow are given in *Table 15-3*. A difficulty encountered in expulsion of the fetus is referred to as a **dystocia**.

■ INVOLUTION OF THE UTERUS

1.   **What is meant by involution? What events characterize involution?**
2.   **What is "foal heat" in the mare?**
3.   **Is postfarrowing estrus (3 to 5 days after farrowing) in the sow fertile or nonfertile?**

The process by which the uterus returns to its nonpregnant size after parturition is known as **involution**. The points of attachment of the fetal placenta to the endometrium slough, and the exposed endometrium heals by forming new epithelium. In addition to new epithelial growth, the myometrium contracts and the cells shorten.

Cow

Within 6 to 7 days postpartum, the upper two-thirds of the maternal caruncle sloughs into the uterus, becoming part of the fluids discharged. The epithelial cells of the caruncle must be shed for the placenta to be expelled. Within 21 to 35 days, all cellular repair has occurred and endometrial gland function is restored. The caruncles have retracted and cannot be palpated. Normally, estrus is observed in 45 to 60 days postpartum. Suckling by the calf, low energy intake, infections, and heavy lactation delay estrus.

Mare, Ewe, and Sow

Involution in the mare is rapid, but not complete, by the time of "foal heat," which occurs within 6 to 13 days postpartum. Foal heat is usually accompanied by ovulation, and mares bred at this time can become pregnant. Conception rates are lower, however, when breeding occurs during the foal heat.

TABLE 15-3 AVERAGE DURATION OF THE THREE STAGES OF LABOR IN FARM ANIMALS (HOURS)

| | STAGE OF LABOR | | |
ANIMAL	I. DILATION OF CERVIX	II. EXPULSION OF FETUS(ES)	III. EXPULSION OF FETAL MEMBRANES
Mare	1–4	0.2–0.5	1
Cow, buffalo	2–6	0.5–1.0	6–12
Ewe	2–6	0.5–2.0	0.5–8
Sow	2–12	2.5–3.0	1–4

From Hafez ESE, Hafez B. Reproduction in Farm Animals. 7th Ed. Baltimore: Lippincott Williams & Wilkins, 2000.

In the ewe and sow, about 24 to 28 days are needed for complete involution. In the sow, a nonfertile (no ovulation) estrus occurs 3 to 5 days after farrowing. Estrus combined with ovulation is usually inhibited throughout lactation. Sows not nursing their litters during the first week after farrowing have estrus with ovulation within 2 weeks. Weaning of pigs at any time induces estrus with ovulation in 3 to 5 days.

Resumption of estrus in the ewe and mare is consistent with the photoperiod of estrous activity characteristic for these species.

Bitch

The interplacental areas return to normal within a few weeks, but the placental sites require about 12 weeks to involute and heal. Estrus usually does not occur until after the young are weaned.

■ REPRODUCTION IN THE AVIAN FEMALE

1. What is the oviduct in the avian female?
2. Is the avian reproductive tract bilateral? Which side persists?
3. What are the component parts of the oviduct?
4. What are the functions of the infundibulum?
5. What is the function of the magnum?
6. What is the function of the isthmus?
7. What are the functions of the uterus? What is the cuticle, and what is its function?
8. What is the function of the vagina?
9. What are sperm-host glands?
10. Where are the yolk proteins and lipids formed?
11. What is the function of the chalazia?
12. What is the immediate source of the calcium needed for hard shell formation?
13. What is the length of an ovulation cycle in the domestic hen? What is a clutch?
14. What is meant by "egg bound" in the avian female?
15. Describe oviposition in the avian female.

The term **oviduct** is the anatomic term used to describe the complete tubular genitalia of the avian female. It is highly coiled and extends from the ovary to the cloaca. In the sexually mature chicken, it can be straightened out to a length of 70 to 80 cm. With few exceptions, among the domestic species of birds, only the **left ovary and oviduct** reach functional development. The left ovary is cranial to the left kidney and is tightly attached to the dorsal body wall, caudal to the left lung, and adhered closely to the caudal vena cava.

The oviduct can be subdivided into five functional regions (*Fig. 15-27*). Beginning with the ovarian end and extending to the cloaca, they are the infundibulum, magnum, isthmus, uterus (shell gland), and vagina. As described in Chapters 10 and 11, the cloaca is a region through which digestive and kidney wastes and genital tract products pass. The function of the **infundibulum** is to envelop the ovulated oocyte with its yolk and begin its direction through the remaining portions of the oviduct. The infundibulum is also the location where fertilization would occur because it is assumed that spermatozoa would not be able to penetrate the oocyte after it begins to be covered by albumen (egg white). Secretion of albumen occurs in the **magnum**, and it is the longest segment of the oviduct. Albumen surrounds the central yolk mass and constitutes about two-thirds of the egg's weight. The **isthmus** secretes the fibrous inner and outer shell membranes that enclose the contents of the egg and provide support for deposition of the hard shell. The **uterus** adds fluid to the developing egg, secretes the hard shell, and adds the **cuticle** (a proteinaceous layer) to the

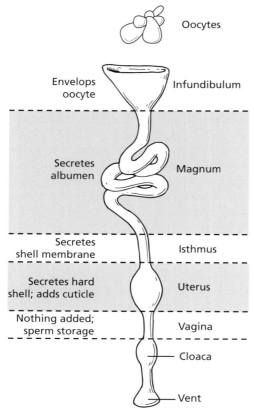

Oocytes

Envelops oocyte — Infundibulum

Secretes albumen — Magnum

Secretes shell membrane — Isthmus

Secretes hard shell; adds cuticle — Uterus

Nothing added; sperm storage — Vagina

Cloaca

Vent

■ **FIGURE 15-27** The five functional regions of the oviduct of the laying hen. The oviduct is the complete tubular genitalia of the avian female and consists of the infundibulum, magnum, isthmus, uterus, and vagina.

exterior of the hard shell. The cuticle functions as a blockade against the entrance of bacteria and reduces water loss. The uterus is also the location where pigment is added to the hard shell (e.g., brown eggs). The **utero-vaginal sphincter**, a constricting muscle, is the dividing point between the uterus and vagina. The oviduct terminates with the vagina that is attached to the cloaca. Nothing is added to the egg as it moves through the vagina; its function seems to be the prolonged storage of spermatozoa in its **sperm-host glands** (additional sperm-host glands of the chicken, but not turkey, are located in the infundibulum). Storage and maintenance of fertilizing capacity

for spermatozoa is possible in these glands for 7 to 14 days for chickens and 40 to 50 days for turkeys. A summary of the hen's egg formation is provided in *Table 15-4*.

As in mammals at the time of birth, only a small number of the ovarian follicles present at the time of hatching develop to the point of ovulation. The immature avian follicle consists of an oocyte surrounded by granulosa cells and proceeds to the mature follicle, which is quite large because of the addition of yolk material. The majority of yolk materials are deposited into the follicle during its rapid growth phase (final 7 to 11 days before ovulation). **Yolk protein** and **lipid formation** occur in the liver, and they are transported via the blood to the ovary. Deposition of yolk into the maturing follicle terminates about 24 hours before ovulation. Yellow egg yolk is a complex mixture of water, lipid, protein, and many components in very small amounts, including vitamins and minerals. Inasmuch as there will be no maternal source of nutrition, the yolk is the nutritional source for the developing embryo. Its counterpart in mammals is the yolk sac that exists in vestigial form after birth as Meckel's diverticulum (see previous text). The yellow color of egg yolk is caused by xanthophyll pigments in the diet. It is possible to have light yellow or white egg yolks when xanthophyll is low or lacking in the diet.

A cross section of a hen's egg is shown in *Figure 15-28*. There are four distinct **layers of albumen** in the laid egg: 1) the chalaziferous layer (thick), attached to the yolk; 2) the inner (liquid) layer; 3) the dense (thick) layer; and 4) the outer (thin) layer. Extending away from the yolk toward both ends of the egg are twisted strands of protein called the **chalazae**. They are extensions of the chalaziferous layer. It has been suggested that the function of the chalazae is to hold the yolk and developing embryo in the center of the egg so that adhesion of the embryo to the shell membranes does not occur. Most of the shell is secreted during the last 15 hours that the egg spends in the uterus. Its major composition is

TABLE 15-4 FORMATION OF THE HEN'S EGG

OVIDUCT SEGMENT	LENGTH[a] (CM)	FUNCTION	TIME SPENT
Infundibulum	8	Pick-up of ovulated ova	15 min
		Site of fertilization	
Magnum	33	Secretion of albumen	3 h
Isthmus	10	Secretion of shell membranes	1-1/2 h
Shell gland	12	Addition of fluid to egg (plumping)	20 h
		Stratification of albumen	
		Shell production	
		Secretion of shell pigments (if present)	
Vagina	12	Sperm storage	1 min
		Egg transport	

[a]Length of the segments differs with size of the hen and changes greatly depending on relaxation or contraction of the muscular walls.
From Burke WH. Avian reproduction. In: Swenson MJ, Reece WO, eds. Dukes' Physiology of Domestic Animals. 11th Ed. Ithaca, NY: Cornell University Press, 1993.

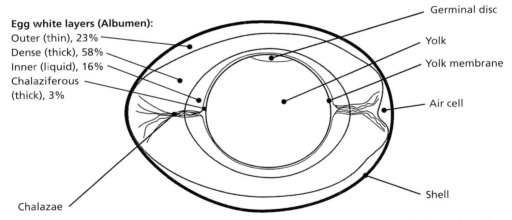

Egg white layers (Albumen):
Outer (thin), 23%
Dense (thick), 58%
Inner (liquid), 16%
Chalaziferous (thick), 3%

Chalazae

Germinal disc
Yolk
Yolk membrane
Air cell
Shell

■ **FIGURE 15-28** Midsagittal section of a hen's egg. The chalazae are extensions of the chalaziferous layer that hold the yolk and developing embryo in the center so that adhesions of the embryo to the shell membranes do not occur. The approximate percentage of the albumen for each layer is shown.

calcium carbonate. All of the calcium secreted into the uterus during shell formation comes from the blood. Because the amount of calcium in the shell exceeds the total amount of calcium in the blood, a dynamic interchange of skeletal calcium with blood calcium must occur. A sizeable amount of each shell's calcium is therefore derived from the bones. Blood and bone calcium is replaced by dietary calcium.

The **ovulatory cycle** in the domestic hen is about 24 to 26 hours long, and cycles may be repeated day after day without interruption. The period of time from one interruption to the next is called a **clutch**. In chickens, the clutches can range from one to 30 or more eggs. Oocytes not enveloped by the infundibulum are reabsorbed. Occasionally, an atypical large egg may become lodged in the lower end of the shell gland or in the cloaca. The condition is referred to as "**egg bound**" and if not relieved, it can lead to death of the bird.

The act of laying of the egg is known as **oviposition**. The muscles of the shell gland contract, and the sphincter separating the shell gland from the vagina relaxes. The shell gland contractions coordinate with abdominal muscle contractions (bearing-down reflex) to expel the egg.

Some commercial flocks of egg-laying hens begin to lay at about 22 weeks of age and continue for about 1 year. In this case an average production of about 260 eggs per hen per year is typical. Those breeds of chickens that are selected for meat production lay far fewer eggs.

Aside from those breeds selected for egg production, there is a tendency among turkeys and breeds of chickens selected for meat production to show **broodiness**, an incubation behavior in birds. After a few weeks of laying eggs, there is a desire to incubate them by setting on them in a nest. When hens become broody, the ovaries regress and egg production ceases. The hormone **prolactin** causes the ovarian and behavioral changes associated with broodiness.

■ SUGGESTED READING

Dyce KM, Sack WO, Wensing CJG. Textbook of Veterinary Anatomy. 3rd Ed. Philadelphia: Saunders, 2002.

Frandson RD, Wilke WL, Fails AD. Anatomy and Physiology of Farm Animals. 6th Ed. Baltimore: Lippincott Williams & Wilkins, 2003.

Hafez ESE, Hafez B. Reproduction in Farm Animals. 7th Ed. Baltimore: Lippincott Williams & Wilkins, 2000.

Johnson AL. Reproduction in the female. In: Whittow GC, ed. Sturkie's Avian Physiology. 5th Ed. San Diego: Academic Press, 2000.

Johnson PA. Avian reproduction. In: Reece WO, ed. Dukes' Physiology of Domestic Animals. 12th Ed. Ithaca, NY: Cornell University Press, 2004.

Pineda MH, Dooley MP. McDonald's Veterinary Endocrinology and Reproduction. 5th Ed. Ames, IA: Iowa State Press, 2003.

 SELF EVALUATION—CHAPTER 15

FUNCTIONAL ANATOMY OF THE FEMALE REPRODUCTIVE SYSTEM

1. The endometrium is:
   a. the muscle layer of the uterus, and it expels the fetus at the end of gestation.
   b. composed of skeletal muscle.
   c. the support system for the uterus.
   d. the lining of the uterus that secretes uterine milk.

2. Intertwining of the ovarian artery with the uterine vein serves to:
   a. cool the ovary.
   b. suspend the ovary.
   c. transport $PGF_{2\alpha}$ from the uterus to the ovary.
   d. transport spermatozoa from the uterus to the ovary.

3. The mare's ovary is described as:
   a. almond shaped.
   b. berry shaped.
   c. bean shaped.
   d. strawberry shaped.

4. An antrum (fluid-filled cavity) is clearly visible in:
   a. graafian follicles.
   b. primordial (primary) follicles.
   c. growing follicles.
   d. all follicles.

5. The reduction division of a primary oocyte will result in the formation of four oocytes.

a. True
b. False

6. Fertilization of oocytes released by the ovary occurs in the:
   a. abdominal cavity.
   b. uterine tubes.
   c. uterus.
   d. vagina.

7. The mesosalpinx is the serous covering of the:
   a. ovary.
   b. uterine tubes.
   c. uterus.
   d. vagina.

8. The cervix (the caudal projection of the uterus into the vagina):
   a. is a heavy smooth-muscle sphincter.
   b. is tightly closed except during estrus and at parturition.
   c. has a goblet cell secretion seen at estrus and during pregnancy.
   d. all of the above.

HORMONES OF FEMALE REPRODUCTION

9. Which one of the following best describes the action of progesterone?
   a. Increases libido
   b. Increases blood supply and motility of the uterus
   c. Increases endometrial development and glandular secretion of the endometrium, and decreases motility of the uterus
   d. Assists follicular rupture and subsequent development of the corpus luteum

10. Tonic levels of LH and FSH in the female are increased by increases in:
    a. estrogen.
    b. progesterone.
    c. androgen.

11. The female steroid hormone that prevents contraction of the uterus during pregnancy is:

a. estrogen.
b. progesterone.
c. LH.

OVARIAN FOLLICLE ACTIVITY

12. Which one of the following best describes the action of LH (luteinizing hormone) in the female?
    a. Causes lysis or reduction in size of the corpus luteum
    b. Increases the blood supply and motility of the uterus
    c. Assists in the maturing of an ovarian follicle, its rupture, and subsequent development and maintenance of a corpus luteum
    d. Stimulates the interstitial cells (Leydig cells) to secrete testosterone

13. The theca interna:
    a. is the outer cell layer of the primary and antral follicles.
    b. has LH receptors and secretes androgen.
    c. has FSH receptors and converts androgen to estrogen.
    d. secretes estrogen.

14. What hormone has its concentration increased greatly just before ovulation (preovulatory surge), which assists ovulation and conversion of a ruptured follicle to a corpus luteum?
    a. FSH
    b. Estrogen
    c. LH
    d. Progesterone

15. Which one of the following best describes the action of FSH (follicle-stimulating hormone) in the female?
    a. Causes lysis or reduction in size of the corpus luteum
    b. Causes granulosa cells to convert androgen to estrogens
    c. Assists in the maturing of an ovarian follicle, its rupture, and subsequent

development and maintenance of a corpus luteum

d. Stimulates the interstitial cells (Leydig cells) to secrete testosterone

SEXUAL RECEPTIVITY

16. Sexual receptivity in some species requires priming of the hypothalamic sexual center by progesterone so that estrogen then becomes effective.
    a. True
    b. False

17. During proestrus, the bitch is sexually attractive and sexually receptive without the requirement of priming by progesterone.
    a. True
    b. False

ESTROUS CYCLE AND RELATED FACTORS

18. Proestrus is characterized by:
    a. sexual receptivity.
    b. increasing amounts of relaxin.
    c. beginning after regression of the corpus luteum and ending at the onset of estrus.
    d. early corpus luteum development.

19. Which one of the following would not normally be expected in the sexual cycle of the cow and sow?
    a. Proestrus
    b. Estrus
    c. Metestrus
    d. Diestrus
    e. Anestrus (long periods of ovarian inactivity)

20. Which one of the following is the best example of a seasonally polyestrous animal?
    a. Cow
    b. Sow
    c. Bitch
    d. Ewe

21. An estrous cycle interval is:
    a. diestrus to proestrus.
    b. one period of sexual receptivity to the next.
    c. the same in all animals.
    d. puberty to the end of reproductive life.

22. Pseudopregnancy is most commonly observed in the:
    a. bitch.
    b. mare.
    c. doe.
    d. queen.

23. The estrous cycle stage that begins after corpus luteum regression and ends at the onset of estrus is:
    a. metestrus.
    b. diestrus.
    c. proestrus.

24. The most predominant steroid hormone at the time of estrus is:
    a. LH.
    b. FSH.
    c. progesterone.
    d. estradiol.
    e. LSMFT.

PREGNANCY

25. Which one of the following most closely approximates the gestation period for the sow?
    a. 21 days
    b. 150 days
    c. 16 days
    d. 114 days

26. Implantation is achieved when the uterus is dominated by:
    a. relaxin.
    b. progesterone.
    c. estradiol.
    d. diethylstilbestrol.

27. Which one of the following approximates the gestation period for the mare?

a. 21 days
b. 16 days
c. 282 days
d. 336 days

28. Which one of the following represents the most intimate attachment of the placenta with uterine tissue?
    a. Amnion–allantois
    b. Allantois–chorion
    c. Chorion–amnion
    d. Heart–lung preparation

29. A freemartin of the bovine species is:
    a. a sterile female calf that develops in same uterus with a normal male twin and shares a common blood supply with the male while in the uterus.
    b. same as answer a, except refers to the male as being sterile.
    c. infrequently sterile (reproductively).
    d. a calf with a free spirit.

30. The urachus is:
    a. an extension of the placental chorion.
    b. an extension of the fetal urinary bladder that empties into the allantoic cavity.
    c. an extension of the fetal urinary bladder that empties into the amniotic cavity.
    d. a musical instrument.

PARTURITION

31. Difficulty in giving birth to the young is called:
    a. fremitus.
    b. libido.
    c. dyspnea.
    d. dystocia.

32. Parturition refers to the:
    a. length of the estrous cycle.
    b. length of time for development of the fetus.
    c. act of giving birth to the young.
    d. return of the uterus to normal function and size.

INVOLUTION OF THE UTERUS

33. Involution refers to:
    a. the attachment of the embryo to the endometrium.
    b. increase in size of the uterus during gestation.
    c. a return of the uterus to its nonpregnant size after parturition.
    d. anestrus.

REPRODUCTION IN THE AVIAN FEMALE

34. The oviduct in the avian female:
    a. extends from the ovary to the horns of the uterus.
    b. extends from the ovary to the cloaca.
    c. does not include a component known as the uterus.
    d. serves only to transport the oocyte.

35. The reproductive tract of the avian female is characterized by:
    a. a single left ovary and its oviduct.
    b. a single right ovary and its oviduct.
    c. a right and left ovary connected to a single oviduct.
    d. right and left ovaries and oviducts, both terminating at the cloaca.

36. Envelopment of the ovulated oocyte in the avian oviduct is a function of the:
    a. magnum.
    b. isthmus.
    c. uterus.
    d. infundibulum.

37. Fertilization of the oocyte in the avian oviduct would occur in the:
    a. vagina.
    b. uterus.
    c. magnum.
    d. infundibulum.

38. Secretion of albumen in the avian oviduct takes place in the:
    a. infundibulum.
    b. magnum.

c. isthmus.
d. uterus.

39. Egg yolk proteins and lipids are formed in the:
    a. ovary.
    b. oviduct.
    c. liver.
    d. cloaca.

40. The cuticle for the egg functions to:
    a. add hardness to the shell.
    b. stabilize the albumen and yolk.
    c. reduce bacterial contamination and water loss.
    d. glamorize the egg.

41. Sperm-host glands in the avian female are present in the:
    a. cloaca.
    b. vagina.
    c. uterus.
    d. ceca.

42. "Egg bound" refers to:
    a. the ultimate location of the oocyte.
    b. eggs with shells that escape from the oviduct and are in the abdomen.
    c. oocytes and yolk not enveloped by the infundibulum.
    d. eggs stuck in either the lower shell gland or the cloaca.

43. Oviposition refers to:
    a. competition for an oocyte by spermatozoa.
    b. the act of laying the egg.
    c. the location of the oocyte within an egg.
    d. the position of the female during mating.

44. Which plasma cation has the greatest turnover during egg production?
    a. Na^+
    b. K^+
    c. $Ca2+$
    d. $Mg2+$

ANSWERS TO SELF EVALUATION—CHAPTER 15

1. d	12. c	23. c	34. b
2. c	13. b	24. d	35. a
3. c	14. c	25. d	36. d
4. a	15. b	26. b	37. d
5. b	16. a	27. d	38. b
6. b	17. b	28. b	39. c
7. b	18. c	29. a	40. c
8. d	19. e	30. b	41. b
9. c	20. d	31. d	42. d
10. a	21. b	32. c	43. b
11. b	22. a	33. c	44. c

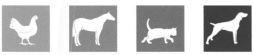

CHAPTER 16

Lactation

CHAPTER OUTLINE

- **FUNCTIONAL ANATOMY OF FEMALE MAMMARY GLANDS**
  Mammary Gland of Cows
  Mammary Glands of Other Animals
- **MAMMOGENESIS**
  Development in Cattle
  Development in Other Animals
- **LACTOGENESIS AND LACTATION**
  Hormones and Their Interactions
  Hormonal Maintenance of Lactation
- **COMPOSITION OF MILK**
  Proteins
  Carbohydrates

Lipids
Minerals
Vitamins
Other Substances
Species Variation in Composition
Colostrum
- **MILK REMOVAL AND OTHER CONSIDERATIONS**
  Milking Interval
  Regression of the Mammary Gland

Provision of food to the newborn is essential for its survival, so lactation is an important component of the reproductive process. Rapid development of the female mammary glands begins at puberty and functional development (prolactational) is reached during pregnancy. Lactation begins after parturition because of the hormonal changes that occur.

■ FUNCTIONAL ANATOMY OF FEMALE MAMMARY GLANDS

1. Note the relationship of alveoli, lobules, lobes, ducts, and lactiferous sinus (gland cistern, teat cistern).
2. What is the milk-secreting unit of the mammary gland? Is it part of the parenchyma or stroma?
3. Do teat canal, papillary duct, and streak canal refer to the same thing?
4. What seems to be the function of the rosette of Fürstenberg?
5. What seems to be the function of the venous plexus in the teat wall?
6. What function is served by inward folds of the empty teat wall?
7. What function is served by the sphincter muscle that encircles the streak canal?
8. What function is served by the suspensory apparatus?
9. What is the venous circle of the mammary gland, and where is it located? What is the milk vein? What is the milk well?
10. What is the function of the myoepithelial cells?

The physiology of lactation among the domestic animal species is similar; however, anatomic differences exist related to outward appearance, location, and numbers of glands, teats, and teat openings. Because of their widespread use in milk production, the bovine female will be presented as the lactation model.

Mammary Gland of Cows

The mammary gland (udder) of the cow has an inguinal location with distinct right and left halves, and each half has a front and hindquarter (*Fig. 16-1*). Each half is independent from its counterpart in regard to its blood and nerve supply, lymphatic drainage, and suspensory apparatus. A longitudinal furrow marks the ventral separation of the halves. The two quarters of each half are separate in regard to gland tissue and duct system. All of the milk from one teat is produced by the glandular tissue of that quarter. The **parenchyma** of the mammary gland refers to the epithelial or glandular tissues, as opposed to the **stroma**, which is the connective tissue framework of the mammary gland. The milk-secreting unit of the mammary gland is the **alveolus** (*Fig. 16-2*). A number of alveoli converge on **ducts** that convey milk to a cistern within the gland and finally to a **cistern** within the **teat**. Expulsion of milk from

the teat occurs through the **teat canal**, which is kept tightly closed by a muscular sphincter. A number of alveoli grouped together and surrounded by a layer of connective tissue is known as a **lobule**. A larger connective tissue division surrounds a number of lobules to form a **lobe**. The secreting units of the mammary gland are thus divided into lobules and lobes.

Duct System

The various ducts converge to form larger ducts that empty into a large basin known as the **lactiferous sinus**. The ducts are referred to as lobular or lobar, depending on whether they serve lobules or lobes, respectively. Accordingly, intralobular and interlobular refer to ducts within and between lobules, respectively. Interlobular ducts converge on a single intralobar duct; when it emerges from the lobe, it becomes an interlobar duct. Interlobar

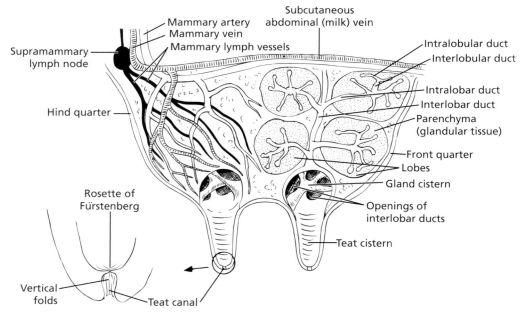

■ **FIGURE 16-1** Sagittal section of the cow udder through the left half. The four circular areas in the front quarter are schematically shown to illustrate the organization of the glandular tissue and also the various orders of ducts. The lobes are distributed throughout the parenchyma. The lobes are further divided into lobules (not shown). The gland cistern and teat cistern for each quarter are collectively known as the lactiferous sinus. The teat canal magnification shows the vertical folds of the teat canal, and also the rosette of Fürstenberg at the upper end.

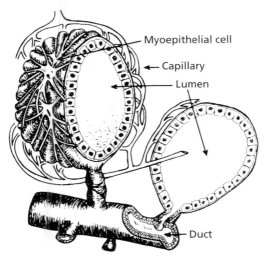

■ **FIGURE 16-2** Alveolus surrounded by blood vessels and myoepithelial (contractile) cells. Several alveoli in a group form a lobule. Each alveolus converges on an intralobular duct. (From Larson BL. Biosynthesis and cellular secretion of milk. In: Larson BL, ed. Lactation. Ames, IA: Iowa State University Press, 1985.)

ducts empty into the lactiferous sinus, which is composed of the **gland cistern** (within the gland) and the **teat cistern** (within the teat). Dilatations that occur along many of the ducts also store milk, in addition to the lactiferous sinus.

The Teat

The part of the mammary gland from which milk is extracted and suckled by the young is called the teat, with one teat for each quarter of the udder. A section of the cow's teat is shown in *Figure 16-3*. The duct extending from the teat cistern to the teat orifice is the **papillary duct** (**teat canal**). The teat canal has also been called the **streak canal**. It is normally closed by a **smooth muscle sphincter** (reinforced by elastic tissue) that encircles the teat canal (*Fig. 16-4*). Closure of the teat canal prevents leakage of the milk that accumulates within the lactiferous sinus. The mucosa of the teat canal is marked by vertical ridges that radiate upward from the internal opening, forming the **rosette of Fürstenberg** (see Fig.

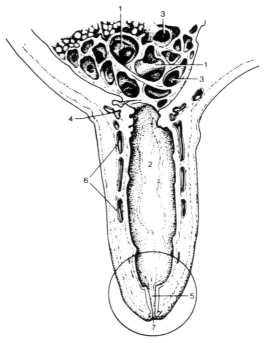

■ **FIGURE 16-3** Sagittal section through a cow's teat (circled area is shown in Figure 16-4). 1, Gland cistern; 2, teat cistern (gland cisterns and teat cisterns are collectively known as lactiferous sinuses); 3, openings of interlobar ducts; 4, submucosal venous ring; 5, teat canal; 6, venous plexus in teat wall; 7, teat orifice (opening). (From Dyce KM, Sack WO, Wensing CJG. Textbook of Veterinary Anatomy. 3rd Ed. Philadelphia: WB Saunders, 2002.)

16-1 and 16-4), which appears as folds of mucosa. The weight of milk in the lactiferous sinus exerts a downward thrust on the folds, thus covering the inner opening to the teat canal and assisting with retention of milk within the udder. External pressure and downward pull on the teat at milking causes the overlapping folds to be withdrawn so that milk can escape through the teat orifice. Inflammation or injury to the rosette can lead to excessive development, resulting in partial restriction or blockage of the teat canal. Epithelial cells associated with the Fürstenberg rosette are believed to secrete a bacteriostatic agent. The wall of the empty teat cistern is

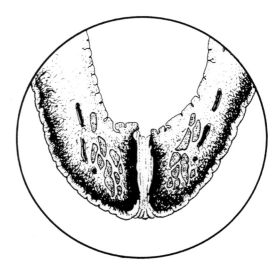

■ **FIGURE 16-4** Section of the teat (circled area is shown in Figure 16-3) showing the smooth muscle encircling the teat canal (papillary duct). The thickened area above the teat canal, which would encircle it, is the rosette of Fürstenberg. (From Dyce KM, Sack WO, Wensing CJG. Textbook of Veterinary Anatomy. 3rd Ed. Philadelphia: WB Saunders, 2002.)

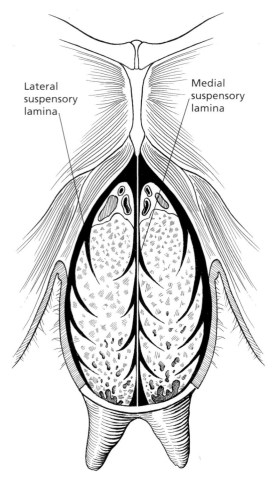

■ **FIGURE 16-5** Suspensory apparatus of the cow. Udder is shown in transverse section through hindquarters. (From Frandson RD, Wilke WL, Fails AD. Anatomy and Physiology of Farm Animals. 6th Ed. Baltimore: Lippincott Williams & Wilkins, 2003.)

characterized by numerous longitudinal and circular folds. When the teat is filled with milk, these folds are obliterated. The presence of the folds permits expansion of the teat wall without tension. The venous plexus of the teat wall (see Fig. 16-3) constitutes a form of erectile tissue and becomes congested when the teat is stimulated.

The ease with which milk can be withdrawn from the teat is often determined by the tightness of the sphincter that keeps the teat canal closed. A sphincter that is not tight enough can allow milk to leak from the teat in the interval between milkings. A loose sphincter also predisposes to mastitis (inflammation of the mammary gland usually resulting from infection by microorganisms).

Suspensory Apparatus

Support from the longitudinal axis of the body is provided to the udder by the **suspensory apparatus**, which is composed of medial and lateral suspensory ligaments (*Fig. 16-5*). The **medial suspensory ligament** is derived from the elastic fibers (connective tissue) that cover the abdominal wall. It passes down between the two halves of the udder and intimately covers the medial side of each half, passes around the front to about the middle of the cranial quarters, and passes around the back to about the middle of the caudal quarters. The **lateral suspensory ligaments** are composed of white, fibrous, connective tissue (with little elasticity) derived from the subpelvic tendon. The lateral ligaments cover the lateral side of each half and meet the medial suspensory ligament at the front and back of each half. A number of connective tissue extensions (**laminae**) are given off from both the medial and lateral suspensory ligaments to enter the mammary gland. The laminae divide each quarter into lobes and lobules. Collectively, the laminae form the stroma (framework) of the mammary gland.

The function of the elastic fibers in the suspensory apparatus becomes apparent when the cow is mature and in production. The fibers allow for absorption of the shock created when the cow walks and permit movement of the udder while the cow is lying down.

Blood Supply and Venous Drainage

The principal blood supply to each half of the mammary gland is the **external pudendal artery** (called the mammary artery in the cow)

(see Fig. 16-1). It passes through the inguinal canal and divides to supply the front and hindquarters on the same side as the artery. The **external pudendal vein** (mammary vein in the cow) collects blood from the cranial and caudal quarters of the respective side and returns blood through the inguinal ring to the caudal vena cava (*Fig. 16-6*). The mammary veins are continuous cranially with the subcutaneous abdominal milk veins and caudally with anastomosing (joining) ventral labial veins so that a **venous circle** is formed at the base of the udder. The milk veins are relatively large, tortuous (winding) veins on the ventrolateral wall that disappear suddenly at a forward location (**milk well**) to enter the internal thoracic vein. Some believe that blood can enter the venous circle from the milk veins (a reverse direction). As in other tissues, the interstitial fluid has auxiliary drainage by way of lymphatic vessels with lymph nodes along their length. The major lymph node on each side is the **superficial inguinal** (mammary or

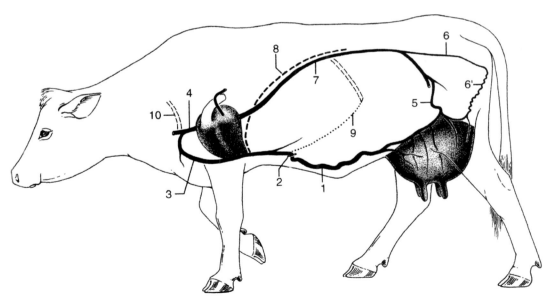

■ **FIGURE 16-6** Venous drainage of the udder. 1, Subcutaneous abdominal (milk) vein; 2, milk well; 3, internal thoracic vein; 4, cranial vena cava; 5, external pudendal vein (mammary vein); 6, internal pudendal vein; 6', ventral labial vein; 7, caudal vena cava; 8, diaphragm; 9, costal arch; 10, first rib. (From Dyce KM, Sack WO, Wensing CJG. Textbook of Veterinary Anatomy. 3rd Ed. Philadelphia: WB Saunders, 2002.)

supramammary) lymph node, located near the inguinal ring above the caudal part of the base of the udder (see Fig. 16-1). Capillary networks are present, as in other tissues, and for the udder these surround the alveoli and ducts much as capillaries surround alveoli in the lungs.

Myoepithelial Cells

The myoepithelial cells are contractile cells that surround the alveoli and ducts. Because of their location relative to the alveoli, they have been called basket cells (see Fig. 16-2). When contracted, they provide compression on the alveoli and ducts and hence cause milk to be directed toward the lactiferous sinus. They contract when the hormone oxytocin circulates and brings about milk letdown.

Mammary Glands of Other Animals

Pigs, Dogs, and Cats

The sow normally has seven pairs of mammary glands (range, four to nine). The teat of the sow has two teat canals, and each is continuous with its respective teat cistern, gland cistern, and associated ducts. In the bitch and queen, five pairs of mammary glands are most common, and each mammary gland has a mammary papilla, or nipple. The nipples have numerous fine openings (seven to 16) at their distal ends for the ducts of the glands. In the sow, bitch, and queen, the mammary glands are located in two rows parallel to the midline.

Sheep and Goats

The mammary gland has an inguinal location in both the ewe and doe. Each half has only one teat, one teat canal, one teat cistern, and one gland cistern. The sphincter muscles at the tips of the teats are poorly developed, and closure is assisted by elastic connective tissue.

Horse

The horse has an inguinal location for its mammary gland, and each half has only one

teat. Each teat has two teat canals and two teat cisterns; each teat cistern is continuous with a gland cistern that has its own system of ducts and alveoli.

■ MAMMOGENESIS

1. What is the state of mammary gland development in the female at birth?
2. How is mammogenesis affected with successive estrous cycles after puberty?
3. What are the mammary gland changes that occur during pregnancy?

Mammogenesis refers to the growth and development of the mammary gland. During embryologic development, a milk (or mammary) line appears on each side of the abdominal wall parallel to the midline (*Fig. 16-7*). In most animals, mammary glands develop only in the inguinal area of the milk line.

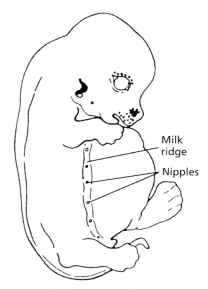

■ **FIGURE 16-7** A 20-mm pig embryo, showing the milk ridge (milk line) (original magnification, ×515). (From Frandson RD, Spurgeon TL. Anatomy and Physiology of Farm Animals. 5th Ed. Philadelphia: Lea & Febiger, 1992.)

Development in Cattle

At birth, the female calf has teat and gland cisterns that are already somewhat mature in form. The mammary ducts are short and are confined to the region of the gland cistern. The stroma is well organized and is interspersed with fat.

The rate of growth of the mammary gland from birth to puberty is the same as for the rest of the body. The mammary gland is a **skin gland** that responds to female sex hormones. These are present in low concentrations until puberty. At the beginning of puberty, follicle-stimulating hormone (FSH) and luteinizing hormone (LH) are released from the anterior pituitary at cyclic intervals that characterize the estrous cycles. FSH and LH activity cause the ovary to secrete the female sex steroid hormones, estrogens (primarily estradiol) and progesterone. Estradiol is secreted mostly during the follicular phase of the estrous cycle, and progesterone is secreted mostly during the luteal phase. An effective response of the mammary gland to estradiol and progesterone depends on the synergism (working with) provided by the two anterior pituitary hormones, prolactin and somatotropin (STH; growth hormone). During the first several cycles, the growth affected by the synergism of estradiol, progesterone, STH, and prolactin consists of duct lengthening, thickening, and branching. By the age of 18 months, heifers have a system of ducts in the mammary glands. Differentiation of the ducts into alveoli continues with each recurring estrous cycle. The maximum amount of lobule and alveolar growth produced by estrous cycles alone is thought to occur at about 30 to 36 months of age.

When pregnancy begins, the concentrations of estrogen, progesterone, STH, and prolactin increase to cause changes in the uterus that are essential for the survival of the fertilized oocyte. Most mammary gland growth occurs during pregnancy in response to the greater hormone concentrations. The adipose is slowly eroded and replaced by ducts, lobule alveoli, blood vessels, lymph vessels, and the connective tissue structures of the suspensory apparatus. Duct and alveolar growth continues throughout gestation.

The source of hormones varies with species. In cattle the placenta is a source of estrogen only. The corpus luteum continues as the major source of progesterone. A **placental lactogen** (hormone) that contributes to mammogenesis and is similar to STH and prolactin is secreted in several species and is directed from the fetal placenta to maternal blood. Placental lactogen secretion occurs at midpregnancy and continues until parturition. However, in contrast to other species, secretion of placental lactogen in cattle is directed to the fetal circulation, and its role in mammary gland development is unknown.

In addition to the pituitary, ovarian, and placental hormones already mentioned as contributors to mammogenesis, other hormones can have a peripheral role, such as adrenal steroids, thyroid hormone, insulin, and relaxin.

Development in Other Animals

In the dog, cat, and sow, mammary glands develop along the entire length of the milk line. In the elephant and primates, mammary glands develop only in the pectoral region.

The placenta becomes a source of both estrogens and progesterone in many species (but not in cattle; see previous text). In sheep and goats, the greatest secretion of placental lactogen coincides with the greatest lobule and alveolar growth of the mammary gland.

■ LACTOGENESIS AND LACTATION

1. What is meant by lactogenesis?
2. Why is progesterone withdrawal a prerequisite for lactogenesis?
3. How is the increase in estrogen concentration before parturition associated with lactogenesis?
4. What is the role of prolactin in lactogenesis?

5. What is accomplished by a growth hormone surge just before parturition?
6. What is the role of growth hormone in the maintenance of lactation in cattle?

Lactogenesis is the process by which mammary alveolar cells acquire the ability to secrete milk. The first stage includes increases in mammary enzymatic activity and differentiation of cellular organelles that coincide with limited secretion of milk before parturition. The second stage is associated with copious secretion of all milk components shortly before parturition in most species, continuing for several days after parturition.

Hormones and Their Interactions

The hormones involved in the second stage of lactogenesis (onset of copious milk secretion at parturition) include increased secretion of prolactin, adrenocorticotropic hormone (ACTH), and estrogen, and a decrease or virtual absence of progesterone. ACTH stimulates the secretion of glucocorticoids.

Prolactin concentration in cattle does not change appreciably during gestation, but a major increase occurs within 48 to 24 hours before parturition. Other hormones, glucocorticoids, growth hormone, prostaglandins, and estradiol also increase concurrently, and the progesterone level declines (*Fig. 16-8*).

These hormones interact in various ways:

1. Prolactin induces gene expression in mammary tissue for casein synthesis, and glucocorticoids are required for this process.
2. The presence of progesterone prevents the formation of prolactin binding sites in mammary tissue and also saturates the sites where glucocorticoids would bind. The withdrawal of progesterone is thus a prerequisite for lactogenesis.
3. Prostaglandin increase just before parturition causes lysis of the corpus luteum and

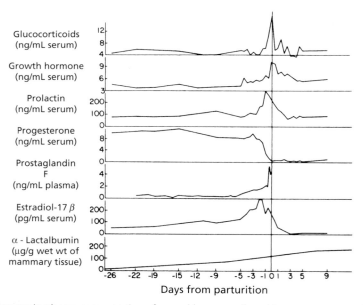

■ **FIGURE 16-8** Changes in plasma concentration of several hormones found in cows near parturition. (From Tucker HA. Endocrine and neural control of the mammary gland. In: Larson BL, ed. Lactation. Ames, IA: Iowa State University Press, 1985.)

a consequent decline in the progesterone level.

4. In cattle, the concentration of estrogens begins to increase about 1 month before parturition and reaches a maximum about 2 days before parturition. Lactogenesis is thus enhanced because estrogens stimulate the secretion of prolactin and possibly other hormones from the anterior pituitary.

5. A surge in growth hormone (from the anterior pituitary) occurs just before parturition, perhaps assuming its role of directing nutrients to the mammary gland for milk synthesis.

Hormonal Maintenance of Lactation

The increase in milk yield in cattle after parturition peaks in 2 to 8 weeks and gradually decreases thereafter. To continue with lactation, mammary alveolar cell numbers and alveolar cell activity must be maintained, and the milk produced must be removed regularly. Hormones required for milk synthesis include prolactin, growth hormone, insulin, parathyroid hormone, ACTH, and thyroid-stimulating hormone. The latter two hormones are required for their subsequent stimulation of glucocorticoid and thyroid hormone production, respectively.

Prolactin

In cows and goats, once lactation has been established, the concentration of basal circulating prolactin (see Chapter 6) and the release of prolactin at milking can be reduced to low levels without affecting milk yield. This situation contrasts markedly with that in nonruminants and even in other ruminants, particularly sheep. The increase in prolactin secretion during milking is brought about by stimulation of the udder and teats. No prolactin is released when the udder is denervated.

Growth Hormone

Whereas prolactin is important for milk secretion in nonruminants, growth hormone is more important in the maintenance of ruminant lactation. Growth hormone (see Chapter 6) is galactopoietic (increases milk yield) in cattle and is essential for the maintenance of lactation in the goat. Growth hormone does not directly stimulate the mammary gland but instead seems to direct nutrients from body tissues toward milk synthesis. It has been shown that plasma growth hormone concentration is significantly higher in high-yielding than in low-yielding cows and that a significant reduction occurs when high-yielding cows cease lactating.

Thyroid Hormone

Thyroid hormone is essential for the maintenance of lactation in cattle. Partial removal of the thyroid gland causes a decrease in milk production that can be restored by treatment with thyroactive compounds. Treatment of thyroid-intact cattle with thyroactive compounds can increase milk yields that are associated with increases in metabolism at the expense of body fat and protein.

Insulin

Glucose is required for lactose synthesis. Various adaptations favor mammary gland priority in glucose metabolism. In goats and cattle, insulin is not required for glucose transport into the mammary gland alveolar cells or for milk synthesis. Therefore, other tissues do not compete for the available glucose. Also, insulin concentrations are low during early lactation (when milk production is high) and increase as milk production declines. Low insulin concentrations reduce glucose uptake by those tissues that require its presence for transport and permit greater use by those cells that do not (e.g., alveolar epithelium). In cattle and goats, the pancreas releases less insulin in response to a glucose load. In animals other than cattle and goats, mammary uptake of insulin (associated with uptake of glucose) is maintained throughout lactation and is essential for maintenance of lactation.

Corticosteroids

Intact adrenal glands are essential for the maintenance of lactation in both ruminants and nonruminants. Mineralocorticoid and glucocorticoid components are needed. Plasma corticosteroid concentrations are higher in lactating than in nonlactating animals and are higher in high-yielding than in low-yielding cows. The exact role of the corticosteroids has not been established but might be correlated with metabolic rate.

Parathyroid Hormone

In view of the relatively high calcium content of milk, it is not surprising that parathyroid hormone is related to the maintenance of lactation. Parathyroid hormone stimulates bone resorption of calcium and the conversion of vitamin D to its active form, **1,25–dihydroxycholecalciferol [1,25 (OH)$_2$D$_3$]**, which is necessary for the absorption of calcium from the intestine. The concentration of 1,25 (OH)$_2$D$_3$ in plasma is markedly elevated during lactation.

■ COMPOSITION OF MILK

1.   **What composes the milk solids?**
2.   **What composes the major part of the milk protein?**
3.   **What is the difference between milk curd and whey?**
4.   **What is the principal carbohydrate in milk?**
5.   **What are the major lipids and minerals in milk?**
6.   **What vitamins are normally found in ruminant milk and are not associated with the diet?**
7.   **How do off-flavors get into ruminant milk?**
8.   **Why does milk from marine mammals have a high concentration of fat?**
9.   **What is colostrum, and what are its highlights?**

The gross composition of milk refers to the proportions of water, fat, carbohydrate, protein, and minerals it contains. Water content is determined by the loss of weight observed when milk is dried. Fat content is determined by extraction with defined methods. Carbohydrate in milk is usually expressed as lactose equivalent and can include other carbohydrates. Protein content represents all proteins, including enzymes. Milk minerals are usually expressed as ash, which represents the residue remaining after incineration. Tables that show the composition of milk often present only the percentages of fat, protein, lactose, and ash and delete water. The aggregate of fat, protein, lactose, and ash is referred to as dry matter, or milk solids.

Proteins

The **caseins** (alpha, beta, gamma, and kappa) constitute the major part of the milk proteins. These protein fractions are insoluble at a pH of 4.6 and make up what is known as the **curd**. The other proteins are alpha-lactalbumin, beta-lactoglobulin, blood serum albumin, immunoglobulins, and a proteose-peptone fraction. These other proteins are soluble at pH 4.6 and are referred to as the **whey proteins**. The **immunoglobulins** are present in very small amounts, except in colostrum. All of the proteins are synthesized in the mammary gland from amino acids except gamma-casein, blood serum albumin, and immunoglobulins (the immunoglobulin fraction of colostrum, however, is synthesized in the mammary gland). The minor proteins, including the enzymes, are present in milk in small amounts.

Carbohydrates

The principal carbohydrate in milk is lactose. It is synthesized in the mammary gland. Lactose is a disaccharide that contains glucose and galactose moieties. It is unique to the mammary gland, but small amounts are found in plasma during lactation. The principal precursor of lactose in the blood is glucose; propionate is also a precursor, by way of glucose. Propionate is important in ruminants because of its availability from fermentative processes in the rumen.

Lipids

Milk lipids consist primarily of triglycerides. Other lipids include small amounts of phospholipids, cholesterol, free fatty acids, monoglycerides, and fat-soluble vitamins. Milk fat synthesis in ruminants proceeds mostly from acetic and butyric acids. Acetic acid constitutes about 60% to 70% of the volatile fatty acids from rumen fermentation. A reduction in milk fat concentration occurs when fermentation changes cause a decrease in production of acetic acid.

Minerals

The major minerals in cow's milk are calcium (0.12%), phosphorus (0.10%), sodium (0.05%), potassium (0.15%), and chlorine (0.11%). Other minerals found in trace amounts include magnesium, sulfur, copper, cobalt, iron, iodine, and zinc.

Vitamins

The B vitamins and vitamin K are synthesized by ruminants, and their concentration in milk is not influenced by diet. Vitamin K is also synthesized by the intestine, so its presence in nonruminant milk does not depend on diet. Vitamins A, D, and E are not synthesized in the rumen, so their presence in milk does depend on the diet. The amount of vitamin C in milk is not greatly influenced by diet.

Other Substances

Many drugs pass readily into the milk from the blood. Milk must therefore be withdrawn from the market for a certain period when cows have been treated with specific drugs, particularly antibiotics.

Off-flavors are sometimes detected in milk when cows have eaten certain foods. Often fermentation is a prerequisite to its being detected. Inhalation of volatile components in eructated gas might be the entry route for these off-flavors. The off-flavor component is produced as a result of fermentation in the rumen and, because it is volatile, it becomes part of eructated gas (much of eructated gas is inhaled, see Chapter 12). The inhaled portion is readily absorbed from the lung, whereas it might not have been absorbed from the rumen.

Species Variation in Composition

The approximate gross composition of milk is presented in *Table 16-1* for several domestic animals, whales (marine mammal), and humans. The milk of marine mammals has a high fat content (33.2% in the whale as compared with 3.5% in the Holstein cow), which is a consequence of the concentration necessary to conserve isotonic water. The isotonic water intake of marine mammals is restricted and is limited to that obtained from the fish they eat, so conservation is required. Lactose composition is probably the most constant among species but still varies considerably. Some have thought that milk with a high protein content is characteristic of species with fast-growing offspring, but this is not a consistent finding. Variations are apparent among breeds within a species (e.g., fat and protein when comparing Holstein and Guernsey cows). Differences exist among individuals within a breed and within an individual, depending on the stage of lactation and on whether the milk drawn from the udder is first drawn or last drawn. Last-drawn milk in cows has a higher fat percentage. Also, the fat composition in cow's milk is higher during the first 2 weeks after parturition, decreases slightly for 3 to 4 months, and gradually decreases thereafter. Fat and protein content of milk is not affected by altering the fat and protein content in the diet.

TABLE 16-1 COMPOSITION OF MILK FROM VARIOUS SPECIES (%)

SPECIES	COMPONENT			
	FAT	PROTEIN	LACTOSE	ASH
Cat	7.1	10.1	4.2	0.5
Cattle				
Ayrshire	4.1	3.6	4.7	0.7
Brown Swiss	4.0	3.6	5.0	0.7
Guernsey	5.0	3.8	4.9	0.7
Holstein	3.5	3.1	4.9	0.7
Jersey	5.5	3.9	4.9	0.7
Shorthorn	3.6	3.3	4.5	0.8
Dog	9.5	9.3	3.1	1.2
Goat	3.5	3.1	4.6	0.8
Horse	1.6	2.4	6.1	0.5
Human	4.3	1.4	6.9	0.2
Mule	1.8	2.0	5.5	0.5
Sheep	10.4	6.8	3.7	0.9
Swine	7.9	5.9	4.9	0.9
Whale	33.2	12.2	1.4	1.4

Modified from Jacobson NL, McGilliard AD. The mammary gland and lactation. In: Swenson MJ. Dukes' Physiology of Domestic Animals. 10th Ed. Ithaca, NY: Cornell University Press, 1984.

Colostrum

Colostrum has been variously defined, but it is considered to be the initial mammary secretion after parturition. The composition of colostrum is decidedly different from milk composition that is considered normal for the species. The differences apparent in colostrum persist in descending magnitude for 4 to 6 days after parturition.

Colostrum is high in the whey proteins, particularly the immunoglobulins. Passive immunity is transferred to the offspring from the mother by immunoglobulins in colostrum. The period during which absorption occurs extends for 1 to 2 days after birth in the pig, horse, cow, and dog. Under normal circumstances, the period is estimated to be 4 days or less in sheep and goats. Beyond this time, the immunoglobulins are more subject to digestion by proteolytic enzymes. Other significant differences between colostrum and regular milk are its higher concentrations of vitamin A, vitamin E, carotene, and riboflavin. Generally, colostrum also contains more protein, ash, and fat and less lactose than regular milk.

■ MILK REMOVAL AND OTHER CONSIDERATIONS

1. What causes the intramammary gland pressure increase associated with milk letdown?
2. What is the usual recommendation for "drying off" of a pregnant cow that is lactating with regard to time before parturition?

It was formerly believed that milk secretion occurred during milk removal and that certain stimulating factors caused this to occur. The intramammary pressure of milk accumulation in the alveoli was thought to create the pressure difference by which milk could be withdrawn from the mammary gland.

It is now known that all of the milk removed at a single milking is present in the mammary gland at the time of milking. The pressure increase that directs the milk from the alveoli through the ducts, cisterns, and teat canal is provided by the myoepithelial cells that surround the alveoli and ducts.

Stimulation of the teats or udder results in a reflex secretion of **oxytocin** (see Chapter 6) from the posterior pituitary gland, which, on reaching the myoepithelial cells, causes them to contract. Often the presence of the calf or other conditioned reflexes can cause the release of oxytocin. The phenomenon associated with contraction of the myoepithelial cells is generally referred to as milk letdown (*Fig. 16-9*). The

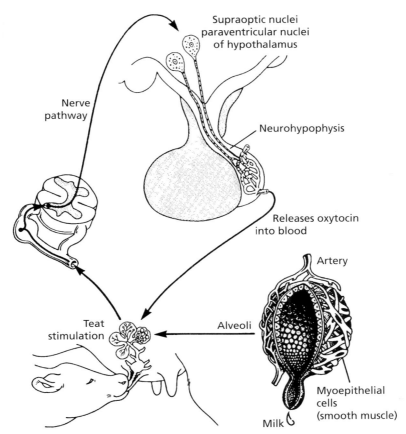

■ **FIGURE 16-9** Milk letdown. Stimulation of the teats or udder results in a neuroendocrine reflex secretion of oxytocin from the posterior pituitary gland that, on reaching the myoepithelial cells, causes them to contract. (From Hafez ESE, Hafez B. Reproduction in Farm Animals. 7th Ed. Baltimore: Lippincott Williams & Wilkins, 2000.)

milk letdown effect ends in 10 to 15 minutes because of dissipation of the oxytocin. Until milk letdown, the pressure within the mammary gland is relatively low (0 to 8 mm Hg), but it increases to 30 to 50 mm Hg at the beginning of myoepithelial cell contraction.

The secretion of oxytocin for milk letdown is usually associated with tranquil situations, and it can be inhibited by stressful situations. Milk is not let down by tormented or frightened animals.

Milking Interval

It was generally believed that the intervals between milking should be evenly spaced, whether milking occurred twice or three times daily. Although some slight decreases are noted, it is now accepted that significant reductions do not occur if the intervals are not evenly spaced. It would seem that regularity of intervals might be a more important factor.

Regression of the Mammary Gland

Lactation does not continue indefinitely, either because animals are "dried off" (milk secretion is not removed) or because the secretion is gradually diminished to an insignificant amount. Several drying-off techniques can be used, including the intermittent, incomplete, and abrupt methods. In the **intermittent**

method, the accumulated milk is removed at 2- or 3-day intervals and then stopped. In the **incomplete method**, milk is only removed partially at the usual regular intervals. The **abrupt method** is probably most widely used, and milk removal ceases completely. Milk secretion ceases when alveolar pressure increases to a certain point. The usual alveolar and duct accommodation is exceeded, and milk secretion ceases. The milk components are enzymatically digested, or reabsorbed, the alveolar cells break up, and the gland is infiltrated by phagocytic cells. In a nonpregnant cow that is dried off, insufficient hormones are present to stimulate or maintain mammary growth, and the lobules decrease in size, the alveoli collapse, and stromal tissue increases. These changes progress until ultimately the lobules are reduced to a few branching ducts.

In the lactating cow that is pregnant and is dried off 2 months before parturition, little regression occurs in the lobule and alveolar tissue. Unless 2 months are allowed for a dry period before the next parturition, milk yield in the subsequent lactation is depressed. Continued lactation apparently interferes with the normal renewal or regeneration of alveolar cells.

■ Suggested Reading

Dyce KM, Sack WO, Wensing CJG. Textbook of Veterinary Anatomy. 3rd Ed. Philadelphia: WB Saunders, 2002.

Frandson RD, Wilke WL, Fails AD. Anatomy and Physiology of Farm Animals. 6th Ed. Baltimore: Lippincott Williams & Wilkins, 2003.

Larson BL. Biosynthesis and cellular secretion of milk. In: Larson BL, ed. Lactation. Ames, IA: Iowa State University Press, 1985.

Park CS, Lindberg GL. The mammary gland and lactation. In: Reece WO, ed. Dukes' Physiology of Domestic Animals. 12th Ed. Ithaca, NY: Cornell University Press, 2004.

 SELF EVALUATION—CHAPTER 16

FUNCTIONAL ANATOMY OF FEMALE MAMMARY GLANDS

1. The milk well is the:
   a. location of milk storage.
   b. same as the external pudendal vein.
   c. location where the subcutaneous abdominal vein disappears and joins the internal thoracic vein.
   d. exit location of vessels through the inguinal ring.

2. The function of the mammary gland suspensory apparatus is to:
   a. provide upward support.
   b. absorb shock when a cow runs or walks and the udder is full.
   c. allow movement and stretch from the elastic element when the cow is lying down.
   d. all of the above.

3. The milk-secreting unit of the mammary gland is the:
   a. myoepithelial cell.
   b. alveolus.
   c. lactiferous sinus.
   d. interlobular duct.

4. Tissue with potential for assisting retention of milk within the udder between milkings coupled with their secretion of a bacteriostatic agent is known as the:
   a. teat canal.
   b. longitudinal and circular folds in the wall of the teat cistern.
   c. rosette of Fürstenberg.
   d. parenchyma.

MAMMOGENESIS

5. Growth and development of the mammary gland is known as:

a. mammogenesis.
b. lactogenesis.
c. mammary gland regression.
d. all of the above.

6. Most mammary gland growth occurs during:
   a. the follicular and luteal phases of the estrous cycles.
   b. pregnancy.
   c. lactation.

LACTOGENESIS AND LACTATION

7. Which one of the anterior pituitary hormones is essential for the initiation of milk secretion (lactogenesis)?
   a. Oxytocin
   b. Estradiol
   c. Prolactin
   d. Progesterone

8. Which one of the following hormones must be withdrawn at the time of parturition in the cow for the mammary gland alveolar cells to begin milk secretion?
   a. Progesterone
   b. Estrogen
   c. Prostaglandins
   d. Prolactin

9. Estrogen increases in the cow toward the end of gestation. What is the significance of the increase to lactogenesis?
   a. Causes lysis of corpus luteum
   b. Prevents the formation of prolactin
   c. Directs nutrients to the mammary gland for milk synthesis
   d. Stimulates the secretion of prolactin and some other hormones from the anterior pituitary

10. Which one of the following hormones is most important for maintenance of lactation in cows?
    a. Prolactin
    b. Growth hormone

11. What is the relationship of parathyroid hormone to the maintenance of lactation?

a. Increases metabolic rate
b. Assists transport of glucose into alveolar epithelium
c. Increases plasma concentration of calcium
d. Stimulates alveolar protein synthesis

COMPOSITION OF MILK

12. Which one of the following statements best describes colostrum?
    a. The secretions of the colon
    b. Food material mixed with stomach secretions
    c. The last-drawn milk at a particular milking, which is higher in fat content
    d. The first milk drawn after birth of the young, which is high in vitamin A and high in immunoglobulins

13. The major part of the milk proteins are the:
    a. lactalbumins.
    b. caseins.
    c. lactoglobulins.
    d. immunoglobulins.

MILK REMOVAL AND OTHER CONSIDERATIONS

14. Which one of the following hormones causes contraction of the alveolar myoepithelial cells resulting in milk letdown?
    a. ADH
    b. Relaxin
    c. Oxytocin
    d. Secretin

15. With continued milk secretion, alveolar pressure increases. What happens when alveolar, duct, and sinus accommodation is exceeded?
    a. Milk secretion ceases.
    b. Teat canal sphincter and rosette of Fürstenberg retention potential is overcome and milk leaks to ground.
    c. Milk is reabsorbed.
    d. Cows get mean.

ANSWERS TO SELF EVALUATION—CHAPTER 16

1. c	5. a	9. d	13. b
2. d	6. b	10. b	14. c
3. b	7. c	11. c	15. a
4. c	8. a	12. d	

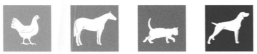

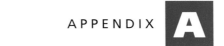

Normal Blood Values

TABLE 1 ARTERIAL BLOOD GAS VARIABLE RANGES FOR EQUINE, BOVINE, CANINE, AND FELINE SPECIES

	EQUINE	BOVINE	CANINE	FELINE
pH	7.32–7.44	7.35–7.50	7.31–7.42	7.24–7.40
P_{CO_2} (mm Hg)	38–46	35–44	29–42	29–42
P_{O_2} (mm Hg)	85–95	85–95	85–95	85–95
HCO_3^- (mEq/L)	24–30	20–30	17–24	17–24

Data from Clinical Pathology Laboratory, Department of Veterinary Pathology, College of Veterinary Medicine, Iowa State University.

TABLE 2 NORMAL BLOOD VALUES FOR THE DOG

	ERYTHROCYTIC SERIES			LEUKOCYTIC SERIES	
	RANGE	AVERAGE		RANGE	AVERAGE
Erythrocytes ($\times 10^6$/µL)	5.5–8.5	6.8	Leukocytes/µL	6,000–17,000	11,500
Hemoglobin (g/dL)	12.0–18.0	15.0	Neutrophil (band)	0–300	70
PCV (%)	37.0–55.0	45.0	Neutrophil (mature)	3,000–11,500	7,000
MCV (fl)	60.0–77.0	70.0	Lymphocyte	1,000–4,800	2,800
MCH (pg)	19.5–24.5	22.8	Monocyte	150–1,350	750
MCHC (%)	32.0–36.0	34.0	Eosinophil	100–1,250	550
Reticulocytes (%)	0.0–1.5	0.8	Basophil	Rare	0
RBC diameter (µm)	6.7–7.2	7.0	Percentage distribution		
RBC life span (days)	100–120		Neutrophil (band)	0–3	0.8
Resistance to hypotonic saline (%)			Neutrophil (mature)	60–77	70.0
Minimum	0.40–0.50	0.46	Lymphocyte	12–30	20.0
Maximum	0.32–0.42	0.33	Monocyte	3–10	5.2
Myeloid–erythroid ratio	0.75–2.5:1	1.2:1.0	Eosinophil	2–10	4.0
Other data			Basophil	Rare	0.0
Thrombocytes ($\times 10^5$/µL)	2–5	3.0			
Icterus index (units)	2–5				
Total plasma proteins (g/dL)	6.0–8.0				
Plasma fibrinogen (g/dL)	0.2–0.4				

From Jain NC. Essentials of Veterinary Hematology. Philadelphia: Lea & Febiger, 1993.

TABLE 3 HEMATOLOGIC REFERENCE RANGE FOR CATS[a]

DATA	RANGE	UC DAVIS VALUES[b]
Erythrogram		
Erythrocytes ($\times 10^6$/μL)	5.0–10.0	6.0–10.2
Hemoglobin (g/dL)	8.0–15.0	9.0–15.1
PCV (%)	24.0–45.0	29.0–48.0
MCV (fL)	39.0–55.0	41.5–52.5
MCHC (%)	31.0–35.0	30.0–33.5
Reticulocytes[c] (%)		
Aggregate	0–0.4	
Punctate	1.4–10.8	
RBC diameter (μm)	5.5–6.3	
Erythrocytes life span (d)	66–78	
Leukogram		
Leukocytes (μL)	5,500–19,500	5,000–15,000
Neutrophils (band)	0–300	Rare
Neutrophils (seg)	2,500–12,500	2,500–11,300
Lymphocyte	1,500–7,000	1,400–8,100
Monocyte	0–850	0–800
Eosinophil	0–1,500	0–1,500
Basophil	Rare	Rare
Other data		
Platelet count ($\times 10^5$/μL)	3–8	200,000–600,000
MPV (fL)	12–17[d]	
Plasma proteins (g/dL)	6.0–8.0	6.8–8.3
Fibrinogen (g/dL)	0.05–0.30	

[a]From Clinkenbeard KD, Meinkoth JH. Normal hematology of the cat. In: Feldman BF, Zinkl JG, Jain NC, eds. Schalm's veterinary hematology. 5th ed. Baltimore: Lippincott Williams & Wilkins, 2000:1064–1068.
[b]Recently determined values from the University of California, Davis, Veterinary Medical Teaching Hospital.
[c]Cramer DV, Lewis RM. Reticulocyte response in the cat. J Am Vet Med Assoc 1972;160:61–67.
[d]For nonaggregated platelets. Zelmanovic D, Hetherington EJ. Automated analysis of feline platelets in whole blood, including platelet count, mean platelet volume, and activation state. Vet Clin Pathol 1998;27:2–9.
Note: PCV, Packed cell volume; MCV, mean cell volume; MCHC, mean cell hemoglobin concentration; RBC, red blood cell; MPV, mean platelet volume.

TABLE 4 NORMAL BLOOD RANGES FOR THE HORSE

	HOT-BLOODED BREEDS (BASED ON 147 CLINICALLY NORMAL HORSES)	COLD-BLOODED BREEDS (COLLECTED FROM THE LITERATURE)
Erythrocytic series		
Erythrocytes ($\times 10^6$/µL)	6.8–12.9	5.5–9.5
Hemoglobin (g/dL)	11.0–19	8.0–14.0
PCV (%)	32–53	24.00–44.0
MCV (fL)	37.0–58.5 (37.0–58.0)[a]	–
MCH (%)	12.3–19.9 (10.0–20.0)[a]	–
MCHC (%)	31.0–38.6 (31.0–36.0)[a]	–
RBC diameter (µm)	5.0–6.0	–
RDW (%)	24–27	–
Leukocytic series		
Total leukocytes/µL	5,400–14,300	6,000–12,000
Neutrophil (band)	0–100 (0–100)	–
Neutrophil (seg)	2,260–8,580	–
Lymphocyte	1,500–7,700	–
Monocyte	0–1,000	–
Eosinophil	0–1,000	–
Basophil	0–290	–
Percentage distribution		
Neutrophil (band)	0–8	0–2
Neutrophil (seg)	22–72	35–75
Lymphocyte	17–68	2–10
Monocyte	0–14	2–12
Eosinophil	0–10	0–3
Basophil	0–4	–
Other data		
Plasma proteins (g/dL)	5.8–8.7	–
Fibrinogen (g/dL)	0.1–0.4	–
Thrombocytes ($\times 10^3$)	1.0–3.5	–
Erythrocyte life span (days)	140–150	–
Myeloid–erythroid ratio	0.5–1.5 : 1.0	–

From Kramer JW. Normal hematology of the horse. In: Feldman BF, Zinkl JG, Jain NC, eds. Schalm's veterinary hematology. 5th ed. Baltimore: Lippincott Williams & Wilkins, 2000:1069–1074.

[a]Parentheses contain recently determined values from the University of California, Davis, Veterinary Medical Teaching Hospital.

Note: PCV, Packed cell volume; MCV, mean cell volume; MCH, mean cell hemoglobin; MCHC, mean cell hemoglobin concentration; RBC, red blood cell; RDW, red cell distribution width.

TABLE 5 NORMAL BLOOD VALUES FOR CATTLE

	RANGE	MEAN
Erythrocytic series		
Erythrocytes ($\times 10^6$/µL)	5.0–10.0	7.0
Hemoglobin (g/dL)	8.0–15.0	11.0
PCV (%)	24–46	35
MCV (fL)	40–60	52
MCH (%)	11.0–17.0	14.0
MCHC (%)	30–36	32.7
RBC diameter (µm)	4.0–8.0	5.8
Leukocytic series		
Total leukocytes/µL	4,000–12,000	8,000
Neutrophil (band)	0–120	20
Neutrophil (seg)	600–4,000	2,000
Lymphocyte	2,500–7,500	4,500
Monocyte	25–840	400
Eosinophil	0–2,400	700
Basophil	0–200	50
Percentage distribution		
Neutrophil (band)	0–2	0.5
Neutrophil (seg)	15–45	28
Lymphocyte	45–75	58
Monocyte	2–7	4.0
Eosinophil	0–20	9.0
Basophil	0–2	0.5
Miscellaneous data		
Plasma proteins (g/dL)	7.0–8.5	
Fibrinogen (mg/dL)	300–700	
Thrombocytes ($\times 10^3$)	1,100–800	500
RBC life span (days)	160	
Myeloid–erythroid ratio	0.3–1.9	0.7–1.0

From Kramer JW. Normal hematology of cattle, sheep, and goats. In: Feldman BF, Zinkl JG, Jain NC, eds. Schalm's veterinary hematology. 5th ed. Baltimore: Lippincott Williams & Wilkins, 2000:1075–1084.
Note: PCV, Packed cell volume; MCV, mean cell volume; MCH, mean cell hemoglobin; MCHC, mean cell hemoglobin concentration; RBC, red blood cell.

TABLE 6 NORMAL BLOOD VALUES FOR SHEEP

	RANGE	MEAN
Erythrocytic series		
Erythrocytes (×10^6/μL)	9–15	12.0
Hemoglobin (g/dL)	9–15	11.5
PCV (%)	27–45	35
MCV (fL)	28–40	34
MCH (%)	8–12	10.0
MCHC (%)	31–34	32.5
RBC diameter (μm)	3.2–6.0	4.5
Leukocytic series		
Total leukocytes/μL	4,000–12,000	8,000
Neutrophil (band)	Rare	–
Neutrophil (seg)	700–6,000	2,400
Lymphocyte	2,000–9,000	5,000
Monocyte	0–750	200
Eosinophil	0–1,000	400
Basophil	0–300	50
Percentage distribution		
Neutrophil (band)	Rare	–
Neutrophil (seg)	10–50	30.0
Lymphocyte	40–75	62
Monocyte	0–6	2.5
Eosinophil	0–10	5.0
Basophil	0–3	0.5
Miscellaneous data		
Plasma proteins (g/dL)	6.0–7.5	
Fibrinogen (mg/dL)	100–500	
Thrombocytes (×10^3)	1,100–800	500
RBC life span (days)	140–150	
Myeloid–erythroid ratio	0.77–1.7	1.1

From Kramer JW. Normal hematology of cattle, sheep, and goats. In: Feldman BF, Zinkl JG, Jain NC, eds. Schalm's veterinary hematology. 5th ed. Baltimore: Lippincott Williams & Wilkins, 2000:1075–1084.

Note: PCV, Packed cell volume; MCV, mean cell volume; MCH, mean cell hemoglobin; MCHC, mean cell hemoglobin concentration; RBC, red blood cell.

TABLE 7 NORMAL BLOOD VALUES FOR GOATS

	RANGE	MEAN
Erythrocytic series		
Erythrocytes ($\times 10^6/\mu L$)	8.0–18.0	13.0
Hemoglobin (g/dL)	8.0–12.0	10.0
PCV (%)	22–38	28
MCV (fL)	16–25	19.5
MCH (%)	5.2–8.0	6.5
MCHC (%)	30–36	33
RBC diameter (μm)	2.5–3.9	3.2
Leukocytic series		
Total leukocytes/μL	4,000–13,000	9,000
Neutrophil (band)	Rare	
Neutrophil (seg)	1,200–7,200	3,250
Lymphocyte	2,000–9,000	5,000
Monocyte	0–550	250
Eosinophil	50–650	450
Basophil	0–120	50
Percentage distribution		
Neutrophil (band)	Rare	
Neutrophil (seg)	30–48	36.0
Lymphocyte	50–70	56.0
Monocyte	0–4	2.5
Eosinophil	1–8	5.0
Basophil	0–1	0.5
Miscellaneous data		
Plasma proteins (g/dL)	6.0–7.5	
Fibrinogen (mg/dL)	100–400	
Thrombocytes ($\times 10^3$)	300–600	450
RBC life span (days)	125	
Myeloid–erythroid ratio	0.7	

From Kramer JW. Normal hematology of cattle, sheep, and goats. In: Feldman BF, Zinkl JG, Jain NC, eds. Schalm's veterinary hematology. 5th ed. Baltimore: Lippincott Williams & Wilkins, 2000:1075–1084.

Note: PCV, Packed cell volume; MCV, mean cell volume; MCH, mean cell hemoglobin; MCHC, mean cell hemoglobin concentration; RBC, red blood cell.

TABLE 8 NORMAL BLOOD VALUES FOR THE PIG

	ERYTHROCYTIC SERIES			LEUKOCYTIC SERIES	
	RANGE	AVERAGE		RANGE	AVERAGE
Erythrocytes ($\times 10^6$/µL)	5.0–8.0	6.5	Leukocytes/µL	11,000–22,000	16,000
Hemoglobin (g/dL)	10.0–16.0	13.0	Percentage distribution		
PCV (%)	32–50	42.0	Neutrophil (band)	0–4	1.0
MCV (fL)	50–68	60	Neutrophil (mature)	28–47	37.0
MCH (%)	17.0–21	19.0	Lymphocyte	39–62	53.0
MCHC (%)	30.0–34.0	32.0	Monocyte	2–10	5.0
Reticulocytes (%)	0.0–1.0	0.4	Eosinophil	0.5–11	3.5
ESR (mm in 1 hr)	Variable		Basophil	0–2	0.5
RBC diameter (µm)	4.0–8.0	6.0			
RBC life span (d)	86 ± 11.5		Other Data		
Resistance to hypotonic saline (%)			Thrombocytes ($\times 10^5$/µL)	5.2 ± 1.95	
Minimum		0.70	Icterus index (units)	<5	
Maximum		0.45	Plasma protein (g/dL)	6.0–8.0	
Myeloid–erythroid ratio	1.77 ± 0.52:1		Fibrinogen (g/dL)	0.1–0.5	

From Thorn CE. Normal hematology of the pig. In: Feldman BF, Zinkl JG, Jain NC, eds. Schalm's veterinary hematology. 5th ed. Baltimore: Lippincott Williams & Wilkins, 2000:1089–1095.
Note: PCV, Packed cell volume; MCV, mean cell volume; MCH, mean cell hemoglobin; MCHC, mean cell hemoglobin concentration; ESR, erythrocyte sedimentation rate; RBC, red blood cell.

TABLE 9 HEMATOLOGIC VALUES FOR THE CHICKEN (GALLUS GALLUS DOMESTICUS)

PARAMETER	INTERVAL
Erythrocytes/µL	2,500,000–3,500,000
Hemoglobin (g/dL)	7–13
PCV %	22–35
MCV (fL)	90–140
MCH (%)	33–47
MCHC (%)	26–35
Reticulocytes (%)	0–0.6
Leukocytes/µL	12,000–30,000
Heterophil (band)	Rare
Heterophil	3,000–6,000
Lymphocyte	7,000–17,500
Monocyte	150–2,000
Eosinophil	0–1,000
Basophil	Rare

From Bounous DI, Stedman NL. Normal avian hematology: chicken and turkey. In: Feldman BF, Zinkl JG, Jain NC, eds. Schalm's veterinary hematology. 5th ed. Baltimore: Lippincott Williams & Wilkins, 2000:1147–1154.
Note: PCV, Packed cell volume; MCV, mean cell volume; MCH, mean cell hemoglobin; MCHC, mean cell hemoglobin concentration.

Index

Figures are indicated with italicized page numbers; tables are noted with a *t*.

A

A band, 211, *212*
Abdominal aorta, *238*
Abdominal breathing, 279
Abdominopelvic cavity, 22–23
Abducens nerve (VI), 100*t*
    in dog, *101*
Abnormal presentations (parturition), 492
Abomasum (true stomach), 367, 401, *402*, 403, 404
Abrupt method, of drying-off, 514
Abscess, 50
Absolute number of leukocytes, 54–55
Absolute polycythemia, 63–64
Accessory foods, 383–384
Accessory nerve (XI), 100*t*
    in dog, *101*
Accessory sex glands, 438–440, 449
Accommodation, lens and, 143–145
ACE. *See* Angiotensin converting enzyme
Acetabulum, 184
Acetate
    chemical structure of, *400*
    energy production and, 410
Acetic acids, 400, 407
Acetoacetate, 410
Acetone, 410
Acetonemia, 411
Acetylcholine, 108, *109*, 216, 394, 395
Acetyl coenzyme A, 6, 410
ACh. *See* Acetylcholine
Acid-base balance maintenance, 344–347
    chemical buffer systems, 345–347
        mechanisms of action for, 346
        relative merits of, 346–347
    mechanism of H+ secretion by kidneys, 345
    relationship of ph to H+, 345
    respiratory system and, 345
Acidemia, 344, 345
Acidosis, 344, 345
Acids, 344
Acrosin, 483
Acrosome, 483
ACTH. *See* Adrenocorticotropic hormone
Actin, 71, 210, 211
    muscle contraction and, 216–217
    myosin interacting with, sequence of, *219*
Actin filaments
    comparison of contraction among muscle types and, 222
    conformational changes of, after calcium binding, *218*
    smooth muscle contraction and, *223*
Action potentials, 108, 125
Activated B cells, 53
Activated factor IX, 69
Activated factor X (FXa), 69, *69*
Activated FIX (FIXa), 70
Active transport, 29–30
Acute tympany, 411
Adaptation, 125
Adductors, 209
Adenine, DNA replication and, *9*
Adenohypophysis, 162
Adenosine diphosphate, 7
    oxidative phosphorylation of, 7
    in platelets, 67
    skeletal muscle contraction and role of, 219, *219*, 220
Adenosine triphosphatase (ATPase), 217
Adenosine triphosphate, 7, 67
    skeletal muscle contraction and role of, 219, *219*, 220
    water gain and, 39
ADH. *See* Antidiuretic hormone
Adipose tissue, in dogs, *424*
Adluminal compartment, 435, *435*
ADP. *See* Adenosine diphosphate
Adrenal cortex, 164, 469
    aldosterone and, 338
    hormones of, 170
Adrenal glands, 169–170
    canine kidneys and, *314*
    diagrammatic representation of, *171*
Adrenaline, 173
    structural formula for, *173*
Adrenal medulla
    hormones of, 173–174
    nerve supply to, 170
Adrenal steroids, mammogenesis and, 507
Adrenergic system, 109
Adrenocortical hormones, structural formula of, *171*
Adrenocorticosteroid hormones, Cushing's disease and, 52

Adrenocorticotropic hormone, 164
   lactogenesis and, 508
   secretion of, 172
Adventitious sounds, 282
Aerobic stage, in catabolism, 6
Afferent arteriolar feedback mechanism, 326
Afferent arterioles, *318, 319, 320,* 322
   glomerular filtration rate and diameter of, 326
   kidney blood flow and, *321*
Afferent limb, 112
Afferent lymphatics, *243*
Afferent neuron, spinal cord of dog and, *95*
Agglutination, 53, *54*
Agonists, platelet activation and, 68
Agranular endoplasmic reticulum, *5*
Agranulocytes, 47, 48
Agricultural chemicals, inhalation of, 296
Air, as excellent radiographic contrast media, 275
Air capillaries, in birds, 302
Air flow, avian respiration and, 303–304, *305*
Air sacculitis, 303
Air sacs
   in birds, 302, *302*
      infection of, 306
Airways, to lungs, 270–275
Albumen, 493
   in hen's egg, *495*
   layers of, in laid yolk, 494
Albumin (plasma protein), 75
Alcohol consumption, inhibition of ADH secretion and, 335
Aldosterone, 164, 170, 327
   function of, 337–338
   secretion of, 172–173
Alkalemia, 296–297, 300, 344, 345
Alkaline tide, 394
Alkalosis, 344
Allantoic cavity, 484
Allantoic fluid, 485
Allantois, 484
Allergic reactions, basophils and, 52
All-or-none principle, 108
All-trans-retinal, 149
Alpacas, 401
Alpha cells (glucagon), 174, 378
Alpha globulins, 75
Alpha-glycerophosphate dehydrogenase, 167
Alpha granule, in platelet, *67*
Alpha-lactalbumin
   in milk, 510
   plasma concentration of, in cows near parturition, *508*

Alpha receptors, 174
Alveolar air pressure, atmospheric air pressure *vs.,* 283–284
Alveolar clearance, 297, 298, 300
Alveolar duct, 275
Alveolar membrane, *274*
Alveolar sac, 275
Alveolar ventilation, humoral control and, 294
Alveolus (alveoli), 273, 275
   blood vessels and myoepithelial cells around, *503*
   carbon dioxide loss at, 292
   of mammary gland, 502
Alzheimer's disease, 87
Ameboid movement, of neutrophils, 50
Amine chemical class, 173
Amine hormones, 161, 165
Amino acid nitrogen, values of, in blood from mature domestic animals, 76*t*
Amino acids
   proteins and, 381–382
   reabsorption of, 327–328
Ammonia, 408
   excretion of, 353
   uric acid formation and, 353
Amnion, 484
Amniotic cavity, 12
Amniotic fluid, 484
Amorphous ground substance, 19, 37, *38*
Ampulla, 136, *137*
   of ductus deferens, 436, 439
   of vas deferens in bull, *433*
Ampullary crista, structure of, in semicircular duct, *137*
Amylase, 393, 399
Anaerobic microorganisms, 407
Anaphase, 9, *10*
Anasarca, 265
Anatomy, 3
Androgen-binding protein, 449
Androgens, 450, 472
Anemia, 63–64, 338
Anestrus, 477
Angiotensinases, 327
Angiotensin converting enzyme, 326
Angiotensin I, 172
Angiotensin II, 40, 172, 327, 338
   conversion of angiotensinogen to, 326, *326*
   juxtaglomerular apparatus and, 321
Angiotensinogen, 172
   conversion of, to angiotensin II, 326, *326*

Annulus fibrosus, 181
Anosmatic sense of smell, 131
Anoxia, 301
ANS. *See* Autonomic nervous system
Ansa spiralis, 374, 375
  of cow, *376*
  of pig, *375*
Antebrachium, 187t, *188*
Antelope, 401
Anterior chamber, of eyeball, *142, 144,* 145, *146*
Anterior cornea, 142
Anterior epithelium, 143
Anterior lobe, 162, *162*
Anterior pituitary, 163
  adrenocorticotropic hormone and, 164
  beta-lipoprotein hormone and, 164
  gonadotropic hormones, prolactin and, 164
  growth hormone and, 163–164
  hypophysioportal circulation and secretion of
      hormones in, *471*
  thyroid-stimulating hormone and, 164
Anterior presentation, 492
Anterior semicircular canal, *135,* 136, *136*
Anthracosis, 298
Antibodies, 53, 239, 241
Anticoagulant protein C pathway, 73
Anticoagulants, 72
Antidiuretic hormone, 164–165, 333–335
Antigen-antibody agglutination and precipitation, *54*
Antigens, 239, 241
Antiperistalsis, colonic motility and, 413
Antipyretic drugs, 429
Antithrombin III, 71–73
Antithyroid compounds, thyroid deficiency and,
      167–168
Antrum, 388, 390, 472, 475, *476*
Anulus fibrosus, *184*
Anus, 375
  in dog, *374*
Anvil, 134
Aorta, 232, 235, 236
  in canine kidneys, *314*
  in horse, *278*
  in male chicken, *453*
  mean pressure and, *237*
Aortic arch, *254*
Aortic bodies, 293
Aortic semilunar valves, 231, *233*
Aortic sinuses, 253, 293
Apex, of heart, 229, *232*
Aplastic anemia, 63

Apnea, 280
Apneustic center, in respiratory center, 292, *292*
Apocrine glands, secretions of, 18
Apocrine sweat, characteristics of, 426
Apocrine sweat glands, 424, *425*
Aponeurosis, 209
Apotransferrin, 63
Appendicular skeleton, 56, 181–182, 184, 186–187
Apposition, bone growth by, *196*
Appositional mechanism, 195
Aqueous collecting veins, 145
Aqueous humor
  formation of, *146*
  pressure maintained by, 145
Aqueous scleral vein, *146*
Aqueous veins, in eyeball, *144*
Arachidonic acid, 175, *176*
Arachnoid, 114, 115, *134*
Arachnoid granulations, 115
Arachnoid villi, *114,* 115
Arcades, of teeth, 362
Arch, *183*
Arrector pili muscle, 425, 427
Arterial blood, pH of, 47
Arterial blood partial pressure, 282
Arterial pressure, 254
Arteries, 232, 234, 235
  major, decreasing pressures to major veins, *237*
  mammary, *502,* 505
  ovarian, 467
  pulmonary, 275
  renal, 313
  testicular, 444
  uterine, 467
  vaginal, 467
Arterioles, 234, *235, 236*
  mean pressure and, *237*
Arthritis, 199
Arthrology, 198
Articular cartilage, 190, *190,* 201–202
Artificial insemination, 438–440
Asbestosis, 298
Ascending aorta, *239*
Ascending colon, 374
  in cow, *376*
  in dog, *374*
Ash, milk minerals expressed as, 510
Asparagine, 341
Asphyxia, 301
Association fibers, 90
Asters, 9

Astrocytes, 86, 119
Atelectasis, 301
Atmospheric air pressure, alveolar air pressure *vs.*, 283–284
ATP. *See* Adenosine triphosphate
Atresia, of follicles, 460
Atria, *246*
    heart, *233, 235*
    muscle fibers of, 245
Atrial syncytium, 245
Atrioventricular (A-V) valves, 231, *233*
Atrium, *238*
    in canine heart, *232*
    of heart, 231
Atrophy, 224
Attitudinal reflexes, 113
Auditory area, of brain, 90
Auditory ossicles (bones), 133, 139
Auditory reflex center, *90*
Auditory tube, 133, *134*
Auerbach plexus, 369
    cells of, *370*
August, Marie, 275
Auricles, 231
    in canine heart, *232*
Auscultation, 281
Automatic adjustments, 92
Autonomic nerves, 95
Autonomic nervous system, 98–104
    autonomic reflexes and, 103–104
    central components of, 98–99
    heart rates and, 251, 253
    hypothalamus and, 94
    male reproduction and, 432
    parasympathetic efferent distribution in, 103
    peripheral components of, 100, 102
    role of, 98
    saliva and, 393
    subdivisions within, 98
    sympathetic efferent distribution and, 102–103
Autonomic reflexes, 103
Autonomic stimulation, actions of, 102*t*
Autoregulation
    of blood flow, 257
    of cardiac output, 253
    of glomerular filtration, 326–327
A-V bundle, 246, *246*
Avian digestion, 411–413
Avian lungs
    cross-current gas exchange system in, *306*
    impaired ventilation of, 306

Avian respiration, 301–306
    general considerations related to, 304, 306
    mechanics of respiration and air circulation in, 303–304
Avian respiratory morphology, general scheme of, 302–303
Avian urinary system, 347–353
    anatomic features of, 349–350
    concentration of avian urine in, 353
    modification of ureteral urine in, 353
    renal portal system and, 350–351
    uric acid formation and excretion in, 351–353
    urine characteristics and flow in, 353
Avuscular, 143
Axial skeleton, 56, 180–181
Axolemma, 85, *85*, 87
Axons, 85, *85*
Ayrshire cows, milk composition and, 512*t*
Azurophilic granules, 49

B
Bacterial infections, leukocytosis and, 54
Bacterial microorganisms, 407
Bainbridge reflex, 253
Ballottement, 487
Band cells, 48
Band neutrophil, *48*
Basal compartment, 435, *435*
Basal daily needs, for water, 39
Basal junction, *435*
Basal lamina (basement membrane), 234
Basal metabolism conditions, 39
Basal nuclei, 89, 90, *90*, 92
Base, of heart, 229
Basement membrane, *236*
    function of, 15
    in seminiferous tubule, *435, 447*
Bases, 344
Basilar membrane, 138, *139, 140, 141*
Basket cells, 506
Basophils, 48, *48*, 52
B cells, 52
    life span of, *49*
B complex vitamins, rumen bacteria and, 408
Beaks, food ingestion and, 412
Beans, 440
Bean-shaped kidneys, in sheep, *314*
Bears, hibernating, 428
Beats per minute, 251
Beef cows, average rectal temperature of, 422*t*
Belch, 406

Bellying down, 487

Beta cells, 174, 378

Beta globulins, 75

Beta-hydroxybutyrate, 410

Beta-lactoglobulin, 510

Beta-lipoprotein hormone, 164

Beta receptors, 174

Bicarbonate, carbon dioxide transport and, 290

Bicarbonate buffers, in saliva, 393

Bicarbonate buffer system, 345, *346*

    formula representation for, 346

    relative merits of, 346–347

Bicuspid valve, 231

Bile, 369, 378, 379, 396

Bile canaliculi, *397*

Bile duct, *240*, 369, *380*, *397*, *398*

Bile salts, 378, 396, *397*, *397*

Biliary bicarbonate, secretion of, 397

Biliary secretions, 396–398

Bilirubin, 46, 60, 61

    urine color and, 340

    values of, in blood from mature domestic animals, 76*t*

Bilirubin diglucuronide, *61*

Bilirubin glucuronide, 60

Biliverdin, 60, 61

Binocular area of vision, 150

Bipolar neurons, 85

Birds. *See also* Avian digestion; Avian respiration; Avian urinary system

    absent contact activation pathway in, 74

    air flow associated with inspiration and expiration in, *305*

    basophils in, 52

    domestic, retinas of, 146

    eosinophils in, 52

    extremes of heat and responses of, 426

    fundi of, *148*

    male reproduction in, 452–454

    monocytes in, 52

    respiration and utilization coefficient for, 306

    stomach of, 365–366

    uric acid in, 352–353

    urine formation and elimination in mammals *vs.* in, 349

    veins in renal portal system of, *353*

Birth, 458

Birth canal, 466

Bison, 401

Bitch. *See also* Dogs

    corpus in, 463

    estrous cycle in, 481

    factors related to female reproduction in, 474*t*

    genital tract in, *465*

    location of reproductive organs relative to rectum and urinary bladder in, *461*

    vestibule of the vagina in, *468*

Bitter taste, 130

Black-and-white vision, rods and, 142, 146

Bladder, *24*, 315

    in bull, *433*

    neck of, 316, *316*

Blastoceles, 12

Blastula, 12

    mitotic division from zygote to, *14*

Bloating

    causes of, 411

    in ruminants, 410–411

    types of, 406

Blood, 19

    cells of, 45

    color of, 46

    functions of, 45

    general characteristics of, 45–47

    hematocrit and, 46

    iron absorption from intestinal epithelium into, 63

    pH of, 47

    total leukocytes per microliter of, and percentage of each leukocyte, 50*t*

    values of some constituents of, from mature domestic animals, 76*t*

Blood-brain barrier, 119

Blood circulatory systems, 236–237

Blood clot, major stages in formation of, *65*

Blood coagulation

    clot growth, 71

    clot retraction, 71

    fibrin formation, 70–71

    pathways to thrombin formation, 69–70

    prevention of, 71–73

        in normal circulation, 72–73

        in withdrawn blood, 73

    species differences and, 74

    tests for, 73–74

Blood diversion, cardiac output and, 257

Blood flow, 256–260

    breathing and, 257, 259

    in dog, diversion of according to need, *258*

    intralobular, *353*

    through heart, 232, 234

Blood-gas analysis, 286

Blood loss, 63

Blood pressure, 254–256
    characteristic, in adult, resting animals, 257*t*
    measurement in dog, taken from carotid artery, 256
    measurements of, 256
    pressure generation and flow, 254–255
    reflexes for control of, *254*
    simultaneous recording of electrocardiogram, phonocardiogram, respiration and, *252*
    systolic and diastolic pressures, 255
Blood supply
    to female genitalia, 467–468
    to mammary glands, 505–506
    to nephrons, *320*
    in synovial joint, *201*
    to testicles, 444
Blood values
    for cattle, 520*t*
    for dogs, 517*t*
    for goats, 522*t*
    for pigs, 523*t*
    for sheep, 521*t*
Blood variables, average values for several, 57*t*
Blood vessels, 234–236. *See also* Arteries; Capillaries; Veins
    in dog, *424*
    heat conservation and, 427
Blood volume
    calculation of, 47
    defined, 46
Boar
    ampullae absent in, 439
    ampulla of the ductus deferens absent in, 436
    anatomy of male reproductive organs in, *441*
    preputial diverticulum in, *441*, 442
    sigmoid flexure of penis in, 440
    spermatozoa of, *448*
Boar taint, 450
Body
    of canine stomach, *366*
    of epididymis, 435, *436*
    of penis, 440
    of stomach, 366
    of uterus, 463
    of vertebrae, *183, 184*
Body cavities, 21–24
    abdominal, schematic sagittal plane of, *24*
    abdominopelvic, 22–23
    dorsal, 22
    peritoneum, 23
    thoracic, 22
    ventral, 22

Body sense area, 90
Body size, heart rate and, 251
Body systems, *14*
Body temperature, 421–422. *See also* Heat
    average rectal temperatures for various species, 422*t*
    diurnal temperature, 422
    gradients of, 421–422
    pulmonary ventilation and, 297
Body water distribution, 36–37
    intracellular and extracellular fluid, 37
    total body water and fluid compartments, 36–37
Bolus, 361
    intestinal peristalsis and movement of, *389*
    mastication process and, 385
    rumination and, 404–405
    swallowing and, *386*
    transport of, 366
Bone(s), 19, 179. *See also* Skeleton
    cells of, 192–193
    of chicken, *182*
    composition of, 190
    formation of, 193–196
    fractures of, 196–197
        repairing, *199*
    haversian systems and, 190–192
    of horse, *180*
    long
        growth of, 193–195
        shaft of, *191*
        structure of, *190*
    metacarpal and phalangeal, of horse, *189*
    of ox, *181*
    remodeling of, 193, 195–196
    repair of, 196–198
    structure of, 187–193
    of thoracic and pelvic limbs, comparison of, 187*t, 188, 189*
Bone varrow, 188
Boundary marking, pheromones and, 132
Bovine fetal placenta, relationship of, to maternal endometrium, *466*
Bovine fetus, proper presentation for, 490, *491*
Bovine ketosis, 171
Bovine reproductive organs, dorso-cranial view of, *462*
Bovine species, arterial blood gas variable ranges for, 517*t*
Bovine spermatozoa, fertile life for, 479
Bovine stomach compartments, relative sizes of, at various ages, *403*
Bovine tongue, dorsal surface of, *365*

Bowman capsule, *318, 320, 321, 322*
   glomerular filtration dynamics and, 319, 323, 325, *325*
Bowman gland, 131
Bowman membrane, 143, *143*
bpm. *See* Beats per minute
Brachial plexus, 97
   of horse, *99*
Brachiocephalic trunk, *238, 239*
Brachium, 187*t*
Bradykinin, in basophil granules, 52
Bradypnea, 280
Brain, 89–94
   cerebellum, 92–93
   cerebral hemispheres, 89–90, 92
   cooling blood supply to, 270
   gross divisions of, 89
   meninges of, 114–116
   subdivisions of, *90*
      according to development from primary embryonic vesicles, *91*
      in dog, *92*
      relative locations of, *91*
   ventricles of, 116–117
Brain stem, 89, *90*, 93–94
Braking effect, 296–297
Breathing, 279–282
   blood flow and, 257, 259
   illustration of mechanics of, 259, *260*
   lung sounds, 280–282
   main function of, 283
   pulmonary volumes and capacities, 280
   reflex inhibition of, 293–294
   respiratory cycles, 279
   respiratory frequency, 280
   states of, 279
   types of, 279
Breath sounds, 282
Bright quality, of pain, 127
Broad ligament, 459
   bovine, *462*
   in cow, *460*
Bronchi, 273
   in birds, 302, *303*
   in horse, 271
Bronchial tree, contributors to moving mucous blanket of, *299*
Bronchioles, 274, 275
   inertial deposition and, 298
   laminar, low-velocity flow in, 280–282
Broodiness, 496

Brown eggs, 494
Brown fat
   heat production and, 427
   white fat *vs.*, 428
Brownian motion, deposition by, 297
Brown Swiss cows, milk composition and, 512*t*
Buccal surface, of tooth, 362
Buffalo, average duration of three stages of labor in, 492*t*
Buffer systems, relative merits of, 346–347
Buffy coat, 46
Bulbar conjunctiva, 154
Bulbospongiosus muscle, 443, 451
   in bull, *444*
   in fibroelastic penis of bull and musculocavernous penis of stallion, *441*
Bulbo-urethral glands, 439
Bulbus glandis
   canine coitus and, *442*
   in dog, 440
Bulk flow
   diffusion and, 261–262
   mechanisms of, 262
Bulls
   disposition of accessory glands, discharging into pelvic urethra of, *439*
   erectile tissue in, 440
   erection in, 450–451
   genital organs of, *433*
   penis of, *443*
      hematoma of, 451
      sigmoid flexure of, 440
      some associated muscles and, *444*
   rupture of corpus cavernosum penis in, 451
   spermatogenic wave in, 446, 448
   spermatozoa of, *448*
   transverse sections of fibroelastic penis of, *441*
Burrows, hibernation in, 428
Bursa of Fabricius
   function of, 413
   of turkey, *412*
Butyrate
   chemical structure of, *400*
   energy production and, 410
Butyric acids, 400, 407
BV. *See* Blood volume
B vitamins, in milk, 511

C
Calcified matrix, 193, *194*
Calcitonin, 168
Calcitriol, 338

Calcium, 383
  in milk, 511
  values of, in blood from mature domestic animals, 76t
Calcium binding, conformational changes of actin
    filament after, 218
Calcium ions, 216
  homeostasis and, in cow, 339
  regulation of, parathyroid hormone and, 168–169
Callus, 197
Caloric expenditure, 39
Calorigenesis, 174
Calvaria (brain case), 114
Calveolae, 223
Calving process, lack of adduction and, 209
Camels, 401
  adapting to lack of water and, 41
  average rectal temperature of, 422t
  rumen of, 401
  watered and dehydrated, diurnal temperature of, 422,
    423
Canaliculi, 191, 380
Canal of Schlemm, 145
Canary, blood pressures in, 257t
Cancellous bone, 188, 190
Canine adrenal glands, 170
Canine brain ventricles, 117
Canine glottis, cranial view of, 273
Canine heart, 229
  sagittal section of, 232
Canine kidneys, ventral view of, 314
Canines. See also Dogs
  arterial blood gas variable ranges for, 517t
  dental formulas and eruption times for, 362t
Canine teeth, 361
Canine thorax, healthy, radiographs of, 277
Canine thyroid gland, 165
Cannon bone, 186
Capacitation, 479, 483
Capillaries, 234, 235, 235, 236, 237, 237, 274
  of central nervous system, 119
  imbalances in, 262–265
  joints and, 200
  physical factors associated with filtration at arterial
    end and reabsorption at venous end of, 263
  pressures determining fluid filtration and reabsorption
    in, 263t
  of pulmonary circulation, 274
Capillary bed, schematic representation of, 236, 261
Capillary dynamics, 260–265
  capillary imbalances, 262–265
  diffusion and bulk flow, 261–262

imbalances in, as causes for interstitial fluid
    accumulation, 264
  interstitial fluid colloidal osmotic pressure, 262
  venous side increases vs. arterial side increases, 264–
    265
Capillary endothelium, 274
  basement membrane, 322
  fenestrated, 322
Capillary hydrostatic pressure, increases in, 263
Capillary pericytes, 234–235
Capillary pressure (P_c), bulk flow and, 262
Capillary tube method, for blood coagulation test, 73
Capsular space, 322
Carbamino compounds, 291
Carbohydrates, 380–381, 396
  digestion and absorption of, 399
  in milk, 510–511
Carbon dioxide
  diffusion of, 286
    direction for, 288
    from tissues into erythrocytes, 291
  fermentation and production of, 405, 406
  humoral control and influence of, 294
  in plasma, 78
  respiration and, 269
Carbon dioxide receptors, in avian lungs, 306
Carbon dioxide transport, 290–291, 290
  carbamino compounds, 291
  hydration reaction, 290–291
  loss of carbon dioxide at the alveolus, 292
Carbonic anhydrase, 345
Carbon monoxide, hemoglobin and, 56
Carbon monoxide poisoning, ventilation and, 295
Carbonmonoxyhemoglobin, 56
Cardia
  of canine stomach, 366
  of stomach, 366
Cardiac auscultation, 251
Cardiac contractility, 245–247
  cardiac cycle, 247
  conduction of the impulse, 245–247
  origin of the heartbeat, 245
Cardiac cycle, 247, 248
Cardiac gland, 367
Cardiac muscles, 206–207, 209
  cells of, in their longitudinal and cross-sectional
    planes, 207
  changes in size of, 224
  contraction of, 222
  frequency of contraction in, 245
  hypertrophy in, 224

Cardiac output
  blood diversion and, 257
  for dog in normal state of hydration, 324t
Cardioinhibitory center, 253, 254
Cardiovascular system, 228–265. *See also* Heart
  blood flow, 256–260
  blood pressure, 254–256
  blood vessels, 234–237
  capillary dynamics, 260–265
  cardiac contractility, 245–247
  electrocardiogram, 247–250
  embryonic development of, 228
  heart and pericardium, 228–234
  heart rate and its control, 251–253
  heart sounds, 251
  lymphatic system, 237–242
  spleen, 242–245
Caribou, 401
Carnivorous (or flesh-eating) animals, 360
Carotid arteries, 239, 254
Carotid bodies, oxygen and, 293
Carotid sinuses, 253, 293
Carpus, 21, 187t
Cartilage, 19, 202
Cartilage cells, 193
Cartilage plate, four zones of, 194
Caruncles, 464, 466
Cascade phenomenon, 69
Caseins, in milk, 510
Castration, 437, 449
Catabolism
  aerobic stage of, 6
  of proteins, fats, and carbohydrates, 7
Catecholamines, 161, 173
  structural formulas for, 173
Cats
  accommodation in, 144–145
  apocrine sweat glands in, 424
  approximate number of nephrons in each kidney for, 317t
  average rectal temperature of, 422t
  blood pressure in, 257t
  extremes of heat and responses of, 426
  field vision of, 152
  fundi of, 148
  heart rates in, 253t
  heat loss from sweating in, 426
  hematologic reference range for, 518t
  lengths of intestinal parts in, 372t
  life span of erythrocytes in, 60
  mammary glands of, 506

  mammogenesis in, 507
  milk composition from, 512t
  ovarian activity in, 479
  percentage of long-looped nephrons in, 318
  polycythemia vera in, 64
  purring in, 300–301
  respiratory frequency for, under different conditions, 281t
  response of warmth-sensitive neurons in rostral hypothalamus of, 425
  total leukocytes per microliter of blood in and percentage of each leukocyte, 50t
  urine volumes and specific gravities for, 341t
  zonary placenta of, 486
Cattle. *See also* Cows
  apocrine sweat glands in, 424
  approximate number of nephrons in each kidney for, 317t
  bloating in, 406
  critical temperature in, 427
  effect of time of insemination on conception rate in, 480
  ejaculation of sperm in, 451
  extremes of heat and responses of, 426
  gastrointestinal tract in, 360
  heat loss from sweating in, 426
  ketosis treatment in, 411
  kidney's shape in, 313
  life span of erythrocytes in, 59–60
  mammogenesis in, 507
  milk composition from, 512t
  normal blood values for, 520t
  number of sperm intended for artificial insemination in, 440
  panting in, 426
  polycythemia vera in, 64
  rumination time and, 405
  stomach of, left and right views, 402
  stunning of, breathing and heart beat in, 284
  traumatic pericarditis in, 127
  urine volumes and specific gravities for, 341t
  wooden tongue in, 384
Cauda epididymis, 433
Cauda equina, 95
  caudal extremity of spinal cord showing, 96
Caudal (Cd) vertebrae, 181
Caudal direction, 20, 21
Caudal lobe, in avian kidney, 349
Caudal nerves, 95
Caudal presentation, 492
Caudal vena cava, 232, 233, 235, 238, 240, 246

in canine kidneys, *314*

in cow, *505*

in horse, *278*

Caudodorsal blind sac, *402*

Caudoventral blind sac, *402*

Cavernous tissue, 440

C cells, 168

CCK. *See* Cholecystokinin

Ceca

avian, 412

of turkey, *412*

Cecal contractions, large intestine and, 391

Cecum, 374

in cattle, *360, 376*

in dog, 360, *360, 374*

in horse, 360, *360, 376*

in pig, *375*

Cell-mediated immunity, 52

Cell membranes, 4

structure of, *29*

Cells

band, 48

blood, 45

bone, 192–193

cardiac muscle, *207*

crenated, 33

endothelial, 234, *236*

number of, in animals, 4

schematic drawing of, and its organelles seen in electron photomicrographs, *5*

segmented, 48

smooth muscle, *207*

Cellulose, 381

Celom, 12

Central canal of the spinal cord, 116

Central component, in autonomic nervous system, 99–100

Central incisors, 363

Central lacteals, 373

Central nervous system, 85, 89–95

blood-brain barrier and, 119

blood requirement for, 119

brain and, 89–94

of mammals, examples of neuron placement in, *111*

metabolism of, 119

spinal cord and, 94–95

Central neurotransmitters, 109

Central organ, reflexes and, 112

Central pattern generator, 292

Centrifugation, 46

Centrioles, 5, 6

Centrosomes, 9

Cerebellum, 89, *90*, 92–93

of dog, sources of input to, *93*

Cerebral aqueduct, 116

Cerebral cortex, *91*, 293

characteristics of, 89–90

neuron circuit from periphery to, *112*

Cerebral hemispheres, 89–90, *91*, 92

Cerebral meninges, *114*

Cerebral peduncles, *91*

Cerebral striata, *91*

Cerebrospinal fluid

circulation and function of, 117–119

normal pressure of, 117–119

pathway of flow from choroid plexus to arachnoid villi, *118*

principal function of, 118

Cerebrum, 89, *90*

Cervical (C) vertebrae, 181

Cervical nerves, 95

Cervical vertebrae, *183*

Cervix, 463, 464

in mare, cow, sow, and bitch, 461, *465*

ruminant, dorsal view of, *483*

Chalazae, 494, *495*

Cheek teeth, 361

Chelating agents, 72, 73

Chemical buffer systems

acid-base balance maintenance and, 344, 345–347

mechanisms of action for, 346

relative merits of, 346–347

Chemical synaptic transmission, 86

Chemoreceptors, pulmonary ventilation and, 297

Chemotactic products, 50

Chemotaxis, 53

"Cherry eye," 155

Chewing, uneven wear of tooth surfaces and, 362

Chickens

average rectal temperature of (daylight), 422*t*

blood pressures in, 257*t*

broodiness in, 496

extremes of heat and responses of, 426

heart rates in, 253*t*

hematologic values for, 523*t*

hydrated, urine flow for, 353

life span of erythrocytes in, 60

male, urogenital system of, *453*

skeleton of, *182*

stark white pectoralis muscle of, 208

temperature and drinking water by, 130

Chickens (*contd.*)
  total leukocytes per microliter of blood in and
    percentage of each leukocyte, 50*t*
  values of some constituents of blood from, 76*t*
  vertebral formulas for, 183*t*
Chlorine, 383
  in milk, 511
  values of, in blood from mature domestic animals,
    76*t*
Chlorpromazine, 168
Cholecystokinin, 175, 390, 391, 395, 396, *398*
Cholesterol, 161, 383, 396, 399
  biosynthesis of steroid hormones from, *471*
  values of, in blood from mature domestic animals,
    76*t*
Cholinergic system, 109
Chondrocytes, 193–194, *194, 195,* 202
Chordae tendineae, 231, *233*
  in canine heart, *232*
Chorion, 484
Choroid, 142, *142, 144*
Choroid plexus, 87, 116, 118
Chromatids, 8
Chromatin, 4, *5,* 8
Chromium, 383 ˇ
Chromosomes, 8, 9, 11, 12
Chronic renal failure, impaired concentrating ability
    and, 336
Chylomicrons, 399
Chyme, 367, *388*
Chymotrypsin, 399
Cilia, 17
Ciliary body, 142, *142,* 143, *144*
Ciliary muscles, 144, *144*
Ciliary processes, *144,* 145, *146*
Circularly arranged fibers, 145
Circulation time, 259–260
Circulatory adjustments, body temperature and,
    424
Circulatory system, 236–237. *See also* Arteries;
    Blood; Capillaries; Heart; Veins
  schematic representation of, *235*
Circumferential lamellae, 191
Cistern, within teat, 502, *502*
Cisternae, *5*
Citric acid cycle, 6, 410, *410*
CL. *See* Corpus luteum
Cl-, reabsorption of, 327–328
Clavicle, 182
Clitoris, 450, 466
  of cow, *460*

Cloaca, 349
  avian, 413, 453, 493
    lateral view of, *454*
  of male chicken, *453*
  of turkey, *412*
Clostridium tetani, 220
Clot formation, 68–72
  clot growth, 71
  clot retraction, 71
  fibrin formation, 70–71
  key reactions involved in, 69
  pathways to thrombin formation, 69–70
Clot growth, 71
Clot retraction, 71
Clutch, 496
CNS. *See* Central nervous system
CoA. *See* Acetyl coenzyme A
Coagulation defects, 74
Coagulation pathway, major components of, 66*t*
Coarse mesh, lymph node, *243*
Cobalt, 383
Cochlea
  pressure waves transmitted in, *140*
  structure and function of, 138–139
Cochlear aqueduct, 136, *136, 137*
Cochlear duct, *134, 137,* 138, *141*
Cochlear nerve, 134, *141*
  in dog, *101*
Cochlear portion, of inner ear, 134, *135*
Cochlear sac, 136
Cochlear window, 133
Cocks
  phallus of, 453
  spermatozoa of, *448*
Coffin bone, 186
Coffin joints, 186
Coiled colon, for ruminants, 375
Coitus, 451
  dog, "locking" phase or "tie" during, *442*
Cold
  physiologic responses to, 426–427
  sense of, 124
Cold-blooded animals, body temperature and, 421
Cold environments, inhibition of ADH release and, 335
Cold stress, avian digestion and, 413
Collagen, 19, *20,* 66, 143
Collagenase, 49
Collecting ducts, 315, 319, *321*
  nephron, *318*
Collecting tubules, 315, 319, *321*
Colloid, 165

Colloidal osmotic pressure, plasma proteins and, 75, 77–78
Colon, *240*, 374
  in cow, *376*
  descending, *24*
  divisions of, 374
  in dog, *374*
  in dog, horse, and cattle, *360*
  in horse, *376*
  peristaltic movements in, 391
  in pig, *375*
  transverse, *24*
  in turkey, *412*
Color vision, cones and, 142, 146
Colostrum, composition of, 512
Columnar epithelium, 16
Commissural fibers, 90
Common meatus, 271
  of horse, *271*
Compact bone, 188, *190*
Complementary relationships, 8
Complement system, 53
Concentrates, 380
Concentrating capacity, relationship of structure to, in mammalian kidneys, 336*t*
Concentration failure, 335–336
Conchae, 271
Conduction, heat loss and, 423
Cone protein, 149
Cones, 145, 146
  color vision and, 142, 147
  outer segments of, *147*
Conical papillae, *129*
Conjunctivae, 142, *142*, 154
Conjunctival membrane, 154
Conjunctival sac, 154
Connecting tubules, *320*
Connective tissues, 14
  functions of, 19
  ordinary, 19
Constipation, 392
Contact activation pathway (intrinsic system), 70
Contact surface, of tooth, 362
Contractile proteins, 71
Contraction
  contracture vs., 220
  increasing muscle strength by increasing frequency of, *221*
  microstructure of skeletal muscle and, 210–221
  of muscle fibers, 247
  of skeletal muscles, 209

Contraction strength, 220–221
  tetanus, 220
  treppe, 221
Contracture, contraction vs., 220
Contralateral side of body, cerebellum and, 92
Convection, heat loss and, 423
Converging circuit, 110, *111*
Convex lenses, 143
Copper, 383
Coprodeum, avian, *454*
Coprophagy, rabbits and, 400
Copulation, sexual receptivity and, 476–477
Coracoid, 182
Cornea, *142*, *144*, *146*
  anterior, 142
  histologic organization of, *143*
  hydration of, 143
  layers of, 143
Corneoscleral meshwork, 145
Corner incisors, 363
Cornified cells, 17
Cornua, 463
Corona radiata, 473
Coronary arteries, 233, 236, 239
Corpora hemorrhagica, 487
Corpora quadrigemina, *91*
Corpus
  of stomach, 388
  of uterus, 463
Corpus cavernosum, in fibroelastic penis of bull and musculocavernous penis of stallion, *441*
Corpus cavernosum penis, rupture of, in bulls, 451
Corpus luteum, 164, 469, 472, 476
  formation and regression of, 473
  persistent, 473, 475
  pregnancy and, 486–487, 507
Corpus spongiosum, in fibroelastic penis of bull and musculocavernous penis of stallion, *441*
Cortex, *90*
  of horse kidney, *315*
  of kidney, *319*
  of ovary, 459
Cortical collecting tubules, 319, *320*
Cortical nephron, *318*
Corticomedullary nephrons, 318
Corticosteroids, maintenance of lactation and, 510
Corticotrope, 164
Cortisol, 170
  eosinophil count and, 52
  parturition and, 488

Costal arch, in cow, *505*

Costal breathing, 274

Costal pleura, 22

  in horse, *278*

Cotyledon, *466*

Cotyledonary placenta, of ruminants, 486, *486*

Countercurrent exchanger system, 330, 332

Countercurrent mechanism, 329–330

Countercurrent multiplication, in loop of Henle and
  recirculation of urea, *331*

Countercurrent multiplier system, 330

Countercurrent system, heat loss reduction and, 427

Cowper glands, 439

Cows, 401. *See also* Cattle

  average duration of three stages of labor in, 492*t*

  average rectal temperature of, 422*t*

  blood pressure in, 257*t*

  blood supply to reproductive tract of, ventral view,
    468

  changes in plasma concentration of hormones in, near
    parturition, *508*

  circulation showing pulmonary system in, *238*

  corpus in, *463*

  dental formulas and eruption times for permanent
    teeth in, 362*t*

  estrous cycle in, 478–479

  factors related to female reproduction in, 474*t*

  fundi of, *148*

  gastrointestinal tract of, *376*

  genital tract in, *465*

  heart's location in, relative to reticulum, *230*

  involution of uterus in, 492

  location of reproductive organs relative to rectum and
    urinary bladder in, *461*

  mammary gland of, 502–506

    blood supply and venous drainage, 505–506

    duct system, 502–503

    myoepithelial cells, 506

    regression in, 514

    suspensory apparatus, 504–505

    teat, 503–504

  midsaggital section of head of, with nasal septum
    removed, *275*

  nostrils of, *270*

  ovaries in, *463*

  pelvic bones of, 186

  red blood cell number count in, 58

  relationship of parathyroid hormone, kidneys, and
    calcium ion homeostasis in, *339*

  reproductive tract of, *460*

  right kidney, ventral view in, *314*

    suspensory apparatus of, *504*

    total leukocytes per microliter of blood in and
      percentage of each leukocyte, 50*t*

    traumatic pericarditis in, 229

    urinary bladder and urethra relative to other organs
      in, *317*

    uterine position in, *467*

    values of some constituents of blood from, 76*t*

    vestibule of the vagina in, *468*

Coxofemoral (hip) joint, *189*

CP. *See* Creatine phosphate

Crackles, 282

Cranial cavity, 22

Cranial direction, 20, *21*

Cranial lobe, in avian kidney, 349

Cranial nerves, 94, 95, 97–98, 100*t*

  in dogs, origin and distribution of, *101*

  twelve pairs of, 97

Cranial presentation, 492

Cranial vena cava, 232, *232*, *233*, *235*, *238*, *246*

Cranioesophageal sphincter, 366

Craniosacral origin, of nerves, 100

Cranium, 180

Creamster muscle, 437

Creatine phosphate, 220

Creatinine, values of, in blood from mature domestic
  animals, 76*t*

Creatinine clearance, 343–344

Cremaster muscles, 437, *438*, 442

Crenated cells, 33

Crista, 136, 138

Critical temperature, 427

Crop

  in avian esophagus, 412

  of turkey, *412*

Cross bridges, 217

Cross-current flow, avian respiration and, 304

Crossed extensor response, 113

Crus (tibia and fibula), *189*

Cryptorchid testes, 437

Crypts of Lieberkün, 370

C-16 unsaturated androgens, 450

Cubical epithelium, 16

Cupula of cochlea, *136*, *137*

Curd, 510

Current flow, 105

Cushing's disease, eosinophils and, 52

Cutaneous pain afferent fiber, *128*

Cuticle, 493–494

Cyanosis, 301

Cytoplasm, 4

Cytosine, DNA replication and, *9*
Cytotoxic T cells, 53

D

Dairy calf, respiratory frequency for, under different
    conditions, 281*t*
Dairy cows
    average rectal temperature of, 422*t*
    heart rates in, 253*t*
    respiratory frequency for, under different conditions,
        281*t*
Dark adaptation, 149–150
Daughter chromosomes, 11
Dead space ventilation, 284, 300
Deep (interior) inguinal ring, 436
Deep surface, 21
Deer, 400
Defecation, frequency of, 392
Defibrillation, 247
Deglutition, 364, 385
Dehydration, 40
Delta cells (somatostatin), 174
Dendrites, 85, *85*
    of postsynaptic neuron, *86*
Denervation atrophy, 224
Dense body
    in platelet, *67*
    smooth muscle contraction and, 223
Dense connective tissues, 19
Dense irregular tissues, 19
Dense regular tissues, 19
Dense tubular system, in platelet, *67*
Dental formula, 361
    for permanent teeth, 362*t*
Dental pad, 361
Dental rasp, 362
Dental star, 363
Depolarization, 105, 107, *107*, 108
    of heart muscle, voltage changes and, 248–249
    of internodal pathways, 246
    mammalian intestinal smooth muscle and, 387,
        387
    of muscle fibers, 216
    recording of transmembrane potential during, *106*
Deposition, physical forces of, 297–298
Depraved appetite, 130
Depth perception, 150
Dermis, *425*
Descemet endothelium, 143, *143*
Descemet membrane, 143, *143*
Descending aorta, *239*

Descending colon, *24*, 374
    in cow, *360*, *376*
    in dog, *360*, *374*
    in horse, *360*
    in pig, *375*
Desert animals, urine-to-plasma osmolal ratio and,
    335
Detrusor muscle, 315
Diabetes insipidus, ADH and, 334, 335
Diabetes mellitus, transport maximum and, 329
Diapedesis, 50, 51
Diaphragm, *24*, 278, 285
    in cow, *230*, *505*
Diaphysis, 188, *190*, *194*
Diarrhea, 392
Diastole, 247
Diastolic blood pressure, 255
Dicoumarol, 74
Diencephalon, *91*
Diestrus, defined, 478
Diet. *See also* Foods
    basic foodstuffs in, 380
    rumination time and, 405
Diethylstilbestrol, 469
Differential white blood cell count, 54
Diffuse junctions, 223
Diffuse placenta, 485
    of horse and pig, *486*
Diffusion, 29–30
    barriers to, 29
    bulk flow and, 261–262
    of respiratory gases, 286
Diffusional flow, 261
Digestion and absorption, 359–413. *See also* Colon
    accessory organs, 376–377
    avian digestion, 411–413
    of carbohydrates, 399
    characteristics of ruminant digestion, 404–407
    chemistry and microbiology of the rumen, 407–408
    composition of foodstuffs, 379–384
    digestive secretions, 392–398
    of fats, 399
    gastrointestinal motility, 385–388
    intestines, 367–375
    mechanical functions of large intestine, 391–392
    mechanical functions of stomach and small intestine,
        388–391
    microbial digestion in large intestine, 400
    oral cavity and pharynx, 361–365
    pregastric mechanical functions, 384–385
    of proteins, 399

Digestion and absorption (*contd.*)
    ruminant metabolism, 408–411
    ruminant stomach, 400–404
    simple stomach, 365–367
Digestive secretions, 392–398
    biliary secretions, 396–398
    gastric secretions, 393–395
    pancreatic secretions, 395–396
    saliva, 393
Digestive tract
    filling of, respiratory frequency and, 280
    of turkey, *412*
Digit, *188*, *189*
Dipeptides, 382
Diphosphoglycerate mutase, 167
Diploid (2n) number of chromosomes, oocytes and, 12,
    462
Directional terms and planes, 19–21, *21*
Dirunal temperatures, in watered and dehydrated camel,
    422, *423*
Disaccharides, 380, 399
    chemical structure of, *381*
Discocytes, advantages of, 58
Discoid placenta, of humans and monkeys,
    486
Disease, respiratory frequency and, 280
Disseminated intravascular coagulation, 74
Distal direction, 21, *21*
Distal duodenum, of turkey, *412*
Distal tubule, *318*, *319*, *319*, *320*, *321*, 322
Disuse atrophy, 224
Diuresis, 164, 329
Diurnal animals, corneas of, 143
Diurnal temperature, 422
Diverging circuit, 110, *111*
Diving ducks, respiratory center sensitivity to postural
    changes in, 306
DNA
    replication of, 8, *9*
    two polynucleotide chains in double helix of, *8*
Does
    estrous cycle in, 480–481
    photoperiod response in, 478
Dogs. *See also* Bitch
    adrenal glands in, *170*
    ampullae absent in, 439
    anatomy of male reproductive organs in, *441*
    apocrine sweat glands in, 424
    approximate number of nephrons in each kidney for,
        317t
    average rectal temperature in, 422t

blood pressure measurement taken from carotid artery
    in, *256*
brain in, gross subdivisions of, *92*
brain ventricles in, *117*
bulbus glandis in, 440
cecum and colon in, dorsal view of, *374*
cecum in, 360
dental formulas and eruption times for permanent
    teeth in, 362t
diversion of blood flow in, *258*
dorsal view of stomach, duodenum, and pancreas in,
    369
efferent autonomic nervous system of, *103*
erythrocyte size in, 59
examples of different electrode placements and
    characteristic wave forms for, *249*
external ear of, *133*
extremes of heat and responses of, 426
extrinsic eye muscles of, *153*
female, side view of, showing general location of
    urinary system and vagina, *313*
final distention of penis in, 451
fundi of, *148*
gastrointestinal tract in, *360*
GFR determination by endogenous creatinine
    clearance method in, 244t
glottis in, cranial view of, *273*
heart in and its major vessels in the thorax, *229*
heart rates in, 253t
heat loss from sweating in, 426
iridocorneal angle region of, *147*
kidney function variables in, 324t
kidneys in, ventral view of, *314*
kidney size in, 317
lacrimal production and drainage system in eye of,
    154
latex cast of inner ear of, *136*
lengths of intestinal parts in, 372t
life span of erythrocytes in, 60
"locking" phase or "tie" during coitus in, *442*
mammary glands of, 506
mammogenesis in, 507
milk composition and, 512t
normal blood values for, 517t
normal lead II P-QRS-T complex, close-up of, *250*
nostrils of, *270*
olfactory region in, 130
olfactory region of, and cells associated with smell,
    132
origin and distribution of cranial nerves in, *101*
osmotic fragility of erythrocytes from, 34, 34t

polycythemia vera in, 64
prostate gland enlargement in, 439
prostate gland in, *441*
red blood cell number count in, 58
relationship of ciliary processes with ciliary body,
    zonular fibers, and posterior chamber in, *144*
respiratory frequency for, under different conditions,
    281*t*
salivary gland locations in, *377*
schematic of association of spinal nerves with
    vertebrae in, *97*
sound frequencies perceived by, 140
sources of input to cerebellum of, *93*
spinal cord of
    structure of, *94*
    transverse section of, *95*
spinal nerves in, 95
spleen, in relationship to other body organs in, *243*
splenic contraction in, 245
third eyelid in, *155*
thorax of, radiographs of, *277*
tongue of, taste buds associated with papillae on,
    129
total leukocytes per microliter of blood in and
    percentage of each leukocyte, 50*t*
urine volumes and specific gravities for, 341*t*
values of some constituents of blood from, 76*t*
vertebral formulas of, 183*t*
zonary placenta of, *486*
Dog skin, schematic section of, showing blood vessels
    and insulating adipose tissue, 424, *424*
Domestic mammals, retinas of, 146
Donkeys
    adapting to lack of water and, 42
    average rectal temperature of, 422*t*
Dopamine, structural formula for, *173*
Doppler effect, 256
Doppler flow method, of blood pressure measurement,
    256
Dorsal branch, 96–97
Dorsal cavity, 22
Dorsal colon, 375
Dorsal concha
    of cow, 272
    of horse, 271
Dorsal direction, 20, 21, *21*
Dorsal horn
    of gray matter, 95
    in spinal cord of dog, *95*
Dorsal meatus, 271
    of horse, *271*

Dorsal oblique muscle, in dog, *153*
Dorsal rectus muscle, in dog, *153*
Dorsal respiratory group, 292
    in respiratory center, 292
Dorsal root
    in spinal cord of dog, *95*
    in spinal nerve, 96
Dorsal root ganglion, 96
    in spinal cord of dog, *95*
Double-folded prepuce, in stallion, *441*
Double helix (DNA), 8, *8*
DRG. *See* Dorsal root ganglion
Dromedary, adapting to lack of water and, 41. *See also*
    Camels
Drying-off techniques, regression of mammary gland
    and, 513–514
Dry matter (milk solids), 510
Ducks, penises of, 453
Ductless glands, 17
Ducts, in mammary gland, 502
Duct system, in cow mammary glands, 502–503
Ductus deferens, 435–436, *436*, *438*
    avian, *454*
    spinal cord of mammals and, *437*
Duodenum, 367, 369, 377, 378, 388
    canine, dorsal view of, *369*
    of cow, *376*
    of pig, *375*
Dural sinuses, 117
Dura mater, 114, *114*, 115, *134*
Dyspnea, 279
Dystocia, 492
Dysuria, 340

E
Ear canal, in dog, *133*
Eardrum, 139
Ears
    of dog, *133*
    external, 133
    hearing, equilibrium and, 133
    inner, 134, 136
    middle, 133–134
    sound wave pathway into, *141*
Eat-or-sleep concept, 99
Eccrine sweat glands, 424
ECF. *See* Extracellular fluid
ECG. *See* Electrocardiogram
Ectoderm, 12
    formation of, *15*
Edema, 239, 265

Effective osmotic pressure, 32
  of the plasma, 75
Effector organ, 112
Efferent arteriolar feedback mechanism, 326
Efferent arterioles, *320, 321,* 322
  glomerular filtration rate and diameter of, 326
  mammalian nephrons and, *318,* 319
Efferent ducts, *436*
Efferent limb, 112
Efferent lymphatic vessels, *241, 243*
Efferent neurons, in spinal cord of dog, *95*
Efferent (outflowing) fibers, 94
Efferent renal sympathetic nerve activity, 336, *337*
Egg
  hen's, formation of, 493–495, 495*t*
  hen's, midsaggital section of, *495*
Egg bound, 496
Egg-laying hens, commercial flocks, production of, 496
Egg white, 493
Ejaculation, 432, 445, 451
Elastase, 399
Elastic fibers, 19, *20,* 284
  connective in large arteries, 255
  in suspensory apparatus, 505
Elbow joint, *188*
Electrocardiogram, 247–250
  isoelectric line, 249–250
  simultaneous recording of phonocardiogram,
    respiration, blood pressure and, *252*
  wave forms in, *249*
Electrocardiography, 247
Electrolytes
  intestinal transport of, 392
  values of, in blood from mature domestic animals,
    76*t*
Electron transfer chain, 7
11-*cis*-retinal, 149
Elk, 400
Embryo, implantation of, 484–486
Embryology, 12
Embryonic period, 484
Emesis (vomiting), 390–391
Emission, 451
Emphysema, 301
Enamel ring, 363
Endocarditis, 234
Endocardium, 234
Endochondral ossification, 193
Endocrine functions, of pancreatic gland, 377–378
Endocrine glands, 17
  development of, *18*

Endocrine system, 160–176. *See also* Hormones
  adrenal glands, 169–174
  hormones, 160–161
  pancreatic gland, 174–176
  parathyroid glands, 168–169
  pituitary gland, 161–165
  thyroid gland, 165–168
Endocrine transmission, 161
Endocytosis, 166
Endoderm, 12
  formation of, *15*
Endogenous creatinine clearance method, 343–344
Endolymph, 136
Endometrial cups, 486–487
Endometrium, 463–464
  bovine fetal placenta in relationship to, *466*
  placental types according to distribution of chorionic
    projections on, *486*
Endomysium, 209, *211*
Endopeptidases, 399
Endoplasmic reticulum, 4, *5*
Endosteum, *190,* 195, 197
Endothelial cells, *20,* 236
  classification of, 234
Endothelium, 16, 66, 234
Endotracheal tube
  placement of, 273
  in place relative to structures encountered,
    273
Energy production, 6–7
  ruminant metaboism and, 409–410
Enteric nervous system, 99
Enterogastric reflex, 390
Enterogastrone reflex, 390
Enterokinase, 396
Eosinophils, *48,* 52
Ependymal cells, 87, 116
Epiblasts, 12
Epicardium, 229, 234
Epicrine transmission, 161
Epidermal papilla, in dogs, *424*
Epidermis, *425*
Epididymal transport, of spermatazoa, 446
Epididymis, 435, 437
  in male chicken, *453*
Epiglottis, 272, *386*
  in cow, *272*
  endotracheal tube in place relative to, *273*
Epimysium, 209, *211*
Epinephrine, 161, 170, 173, 174, 427
Epiphyseal bone, *194*

Epiphyseal plates, 190, *190*, 193
  appearance presented by both longitudinal and cross
      sections of areas of, *195*
  growth hormone and, 163
Epiphysis, 188, *190*
Epithalamus, *90, 91*, 94
Epithelial membranes, kinds of, 18
Epithelium (epithelial tissue), 14, 234
  classification of, 15–17
  origination of, 15
  tissue classifications, *16*
EPO. *See* Erythropoietin
Equilibrium
  hearing and, 132–140
  inner ear and sense of, 134
Equine species, arterial blood gas variable ranges for,
      517*t. See also* Horses
Equine thorax
  cross section of, *259*
  schematic transverse plane of, 23
  transverse section of, *278*
Equivalents, 35
  pathways for interconversion of grams, osmoles and,
      35
ER. *See* Endoplasmic reticulum
Erectile tissue, 440
Erection, 432, 450–451
  reflex centers for, 445
  sigmoid flexure of penis and, 440
ERSNA. *See* Efferent renal sympathetic nerve activity
Eructation, 406, 411
Eructed gases, off-flavors and, 511
Eruption, of teeth, 361, 362*t*
Erythrocyte development, stages of, *58*
Erythrocyte indices, 58, 59
Erythrocytes (red blood cells), 45, *48*, 55–61
  canine, changes in volume of, attributable to tone of
      suspending NaCL solution, 34*t*
  effect of tone of solutions on, *32, 33*
  fate of, 60–61
  life span of, 59–60
  number of, 58
  osmotic fragility of, from normal dogs and normal
      goats, *34*, 34*t*
  processes occurring when carbon dioxide diffuses
      from tissues into, *291*
  shape of, 58–59
  size of, 59
Erythropoiesis, 56–58, 63
Erythropoietin, 58, 338
Esophageal region, 367

Esophagus, 272, 361, 364, 366, *386*
  avian, 412
  canine, *366*
  in cow, 272
  endotracheal tube in place relative to, *273*
  in horse, *278*
  swallowing and, *385*
Essential amino acids, 382
Esters, 382
Estradiol, *471*
  mammary gland response to, 507
  plasma concentration of, in cows near parturition, *508*
Estradiol-17-β, 469
Estrogen(s)
  functions of, 469
  parturition and increase in, 488, 489
  patterns in mare, cow, sow, and ewe before
      parturition, *489*
  sexual receptivity and, 476–477
Estrone, 469, 488
Estrous cycle, 477
  Graafian follicles and, 459
  nutrition and, 478
  species characteristics of, 478–482
    bitches, 481
    cows, 478–479
    does, 480–481
    ewes, 480
    mares, 479–480
    queens, 481–482
    sows, 480
  stages of, 477–478
Estrus
  cervix and, 464
  defined, 478
Eupnea, 279
  Hering-Breuer reflexes and, 293
  intrapulmonic pressure during, 284
Eustachian tubes, 271, 364
Evaporative heat loss, 42, 423, 424, 426
Ewes. *See also* Sheep
  average duration of three stages of labor in, 492*t*
  estrogen patterns in, before parturition, *489*
  estrous cycle in, 480
  factors related to female reproduction in, 474*t*
  involution of uterus in, 492–493
  photoperiod response in, 478
  prostaglandins, progesterone-primed uterus and
      destruction of corpus luteum in, *475*
Excitotoxicity, 87
Excurrent duct system, 446

Exocrine functions, of pancreatic gland, 377–378
Exocrine glands, 17
    development of, *18*
Exocrine transmission, 161
Exogenous creatinine clearance method, 343
Exopeptidases, 399
Expiration, 278
    in birds, air flow associated with, *305*
    intrapleural and intrapulmonic pressures associated
        with, *285*
    lung volume and, *281*
Expiratory reserve volume, 280, *281*
Extensors, 209
External abdominal oblique muscle, *438*
External acoustic meatus, 133, *134*
External callus, 197
External ear, 133
External pudendal vein, 505, *505*
External sphincter, 316, *316*
Exteroceptors, 124
Extracellular fluid, 37, *37*, 312, 336–337
Extracellular hydration, regulation of, *334*
Extraembryonic membranes, 12
Extraglomerular mesangium, 322
Extravascular hemolysis, 60
Extrinsic muscles, of dog's eyes, *153*
Eyeball, 142
    structure of, *142*
    tunics of, 142
Eyelids, 142
    lower, *144*
Eye(s), *141*
    cornea, 143
    external, *142*
    humors of, 145
    iris, 145
    lens, 143–145
    retina, 145–146
    structure and functions of, 142
Eyeshine, 150
Eye teeth, 361

F
Facial bones, 180
    of chicken, *182*
    of horse, *180*
    of ox, *181*
Facial nerve (VII), 100*t*
    in dog, *101*
Facilitated diffusion, 29
    postulated mechanism for, *30*

Factor IX
    activation of, and contact phase for, *70*
    clot formation and activation of, 69
Factor X, clot formation and activation of, 69, *69*
Factor XII, absence of, blood coagulation time and,
        74
FAD. *See* Flavin adenine dinucleotide
Fallopian tubes, 462
Fangs, 361
Farm animals
    spermatozoa of, compared with other vertebrates,
        448
    stages of labor and related events in, 491*t*
Farrowing, respiratory rates and, 488
Fascicles, 209
Fasciculus, 86
Fat cells, *20*
Fats, 396
    digestion and absorption of, 399
    emulsification of, in intestine, 397
    in milk, 510
Fat-soluble vitamins, 383
Fatty acids, 408
F cells (pancreatic polypeptide), 174
FDPs. *See* Fibrin degradation products
Feces, 392
Feedlot bloat, 406
Feline cerebellar hypoplasia, 92–93
Feline species, arterial blood gas variable ranges for,
        517*t*. *See also* Cats
Feline urologic syndrome, 340
Female genitalia
    blood supply to, 467–468
    external, 466–467
Female mammary glands, functional anatomy of,
        501–506
Female reproduction, 458–496
    avian, 493–496
    estrous cycle and related factors, 477–482
    factors related to, in various animals, 474*t*
    functional anatomy of, 458–468
    hormones of, 468–471
    involution of uterus, 492–493
    location of reproductive organs relative to rectum and
        urinary bladder, *461*
    ovarian follicle activity, 471–476
    parturition, 487–492
    pregnancy, 482–487
    sexual receptivity, 476–477
Femoral vein, in male chicken, *453*
Femur, 184, *189*

Fermentation
  in large intestine, 374, 391
  ruminant stomach and, 401
Ferric (Fe³⁺) oxidation state, 62
Ferritin, 60, 63
Ferrous (Fe²⁺) oxidation state, 62
Fertilization, 12, 482. *See also* Pregnancy
  defined, 483
  in infundibulum, 493
  prostaglandins and, 440
  schematic diagrams of, *13*
  seminal plasma and, 439
  uterus and, 463
Fetal period, 484
Fetal placenta, 12, 484
Fetlock, 186
Fetus, 458, *466*
  expulsion of, *490*
Fever, 429
FF. *See* Filtration fraction
Fibrillation, 247
Fibrin, *69*, *72*
  degradation of, 71
  formation and degradation of
    major components of coagulation pathway involved
      in, *66t*
  formation of, 68–69
    pathways to, 69, 70–71
Fibrinogen, *69*, 70, 75
Fibrinolysis, 65, 71, *72*
Fibroblasts, 19, *20*
Fibrocytes, 19
Fibrous tunic, 142
Field of vision, 150–152
  in cat, *152*
  in horse, 151–152, *153*
"Fight-fright-flight" reaction
  autonomic nervous system and, 99
  catecholamines and, 174
Filliform and conical papillae, on bovine tongue,
  365
Filtrate reabsorption, for dog in normal state of
  hydration, *324t*
Filtration, 262
Filtration fraction, 324
  for dog in normal state of hydration,
    324t
  renal clearance and, 341
Filtration slit diaphragm, 322
Fimbria, 462
  of cow, *460*

Final common pathway, 109, *110*
Fine mesh, of lymph node, *243*
First heart sound, 251
FIXa. *See* Activated FIX
Flavin adenine dinucleotide, 6
Fleshy attachment, 209
Flexors, 209
Fluid compartments, total body water distributed
  among, 36, *37*
Fluorine, 383
Foal, persistent urachus in, *485*
Foal heat, 492
Follicles, 165
  Graafian, 460, *476*
  growing, 459, *476*
  primary, *476*
  primordial, 459
  ruptured, *476*
Follicle-stimulating hormone, 163, 164, 449, 470,
  471
  avian male reproduction and, 453
  Graafian follicles and, 459
  mammogenesis and, 507
Follicular fluid, *472*
Follicular growth, *472*
Follicular period, 478
Follicular periods, 478
Food deprivation, death and, 359
Foods. *See also* Diet
  accessory, 383
  composition of, 379–383
  proper, 383
Foodstuff classification, 379–384
  carbohydrates, 380–381
  lipids, 382–383
  minerals, 383
  proteins, 381–382
  vitamins, 383–384
Foramen of magendie, 116
Foramen of Monro, 116
Foramina of Luschka, 116, 117
Forebrain, *91*
Forestomach, 374, 401
Fornix, 466
Four-footed animals, directional terms and planes
  applied to, 20–21, *21*
Fourth ventricle, 116
Fovea centralis, 145
Foveal region, 145
Fowl, lateral view of cloaca and terminal part of vas
  deferens in, *454. See also* Chickens

Fractures
  bone, 196–197
  pelvis, 184
  repair of, *199*
Free bilirubin, 60
Free iron, 61
Freemartin, 486
Free nerve endings, *126*
Fremitus, 467, 487
Frequencies, sound waves, 138–139
Fructose, 399, 439–440
FSH. *See* Follicle-stimulating hormone
Full mouth, in horse, 363, *364*
Functional residual capacity, 280, *281*
Fundic gland region, 367
Fundus (fundi), 388
  of canine stomach, *366*
  of seven domestic animals, as seen by
    ophthalmoscopy, *148*
  of stomach, 366
Fungiform papillae, 364
  on bovine tongue, *365*
Fur, pilorection and, 427
FVIIa complex, *69*

G
GABA. *See* Gamma-aminobutyric acid
Galactose, 399
  chemical structure of, *381*
Gallbladder, 369
  avian, 412
  horses and lack of, 397
  of turkey, *412*
Gametes, 12, 483
Gamma-aminobutyric acid, 109
Ganglion, 86
Gap junctions, 192
Gas distention, 388
Gas production, in rumen, 405–406
Gastric emptying
  delay of, 390
  inhibiting, 395
Gastric glands, 367
Gastric inhibitory polypeptide, 390, 395
Gastric juice, 366
Gastric mucosa, mechanism of hydrochloric acid
    secretion by parietal cells of, *394*
Gastric secretions, 393–395
Gastrin, 175, 391, 393, 394, 395, *398*
Gastrointestinal hormones, mammalian, *398*
Gastrointestinal motility, 385–388

Gastrointestinal tract
  comparison of, in dog, horse, and cattle, *360*
  of cow, *376*
  mammalian, schematic representation of, *370*
Geese, penises of, 453
Genetic code, 11
Genetic coding, role of, in protein synthesis and related
    cell functions, *11*
Genitalia
  female, external, 459, 466–467
  male, muscles of, 442–443
Germ cells, in testicles, *433*
Germ layers
  establishment of, 12
  formation of, *15*
Gestation period, 482, 486. *See also* Fertilization;
    Pregnancy
GFR. *See* Glomerular filtration rate
GIP. *See* Gastric inhibitory polypeptide
Giraffe, 401
  blood pressure in, 257*t*
Gizzards, 412
  food ingestion and, 412
  of turkey, *412*
Gland cisterns, of cattle, 507
Gland of von Ebner, 128, *129*
Glands, 17–18
  ANS innervation to, 99
  classification of, 17
  development of, 17–18
Glandular stomach, of turkey, *412*
Glans penis, 440, 445
  in bull, *433*, *443*, *444*
Glial cells (glia), 85, 86–87, 116
Globin, 5, 61
Globulins, 75
Glomerular capillaries, 322
Glomerular epithelium basement membrane,
    322
Glomerular epithelium foot process, 322
Glomerular filtrate, 323
Glomerular filtrate volume, for dog in normal state of
    hydration, 324*t*
Glomerular filtration, 323, *323*, 324–327
  autoregulation of, 326–327
  dynamics of, *325*, 325–326
  filtration factors and, 326
  rate of, 324
    arteriole diameters and, 326
    creatinine clearance as measurement of, 343
    for dog in normal state of hydration, 324*t*

endogenous creatinine clearance method and determination of, in healthy 14-kg dog, 244*t*

renal clearance and, 341

Glomerular membrane, 325

Glomerulus (glomeruli), 317, *318*, 319, *320*, *321*, 324

Glossopharyngeal nerve (IX), 100*t*, *254*

in dog, *101*

Glottis, 272, *273*, 364, 366

in cow, *272*

endotracheal tube in place relative to, *273*

Glucagon, 170, 174, *175–176*, 378

Glucocorticoids, 170

functions and regulation of, 170–172

gluconeogenic effect of, 171

plasma concentration of, in cows near parturition, *508*

secretion of, 172

Gluconeogenesis, 170, 174, 409, 411

Glucose, 381, 399, 409

chemical structure of, *381*

facilitated diffusion of, 30

reabsorption of, 327–328

renal clearance and, 341, 342

transport maximum and, 329

values of, in blood from mature domestic animals, 76*t*

Glutamate, 87

Glycerol, 408, 409

Glycine, 109

Glycogen, 381

Glycogen molecule, highly branched, *381*

Glycoproteins, 470

GnRH. *See* Gonadotropin releasing hormone

Goats, 401

average rectal temperature in, 422*t*

erythrocyte size in, 59

heart rates in, 253*t*

lengths of intestinal parts in, 372*t*

life span of erythrocytes in, 60

mammary glands of, 506

milk composition and, 512*t*

normal blood values for, 522*t*

osmotic fragility of erythrocytes from, 34, 34*t*

ovarian activity in, *479*

pancreatic duct in, 377–378

photoperiods and, 452

red blood cell number count in, 58

total leukocytes per microliter of blood in and percentage of each leukocyte, 50*t*

urine volumes and specific gravities for, 341*t*

vertebral formulas of, 183*t*

Goblet cells, 17, 155

Goblet cell secretion, 464

Goiter, 167–168

Goitrin, 168

Goitrogen, 168

Golgi apparatus, 5, 6

Golgi tendon organs, 125

Gonadotrope cells, 163

Gonadotropic hormones, 164

Gonadotropin releasing hormone, 470, 477

Gonadotropins, 470

Graafian follicles, 460, *476*

formation of, from a growing follicle, *472*

Graded responses, 125

Gradients of temperature, 421–422

Grain bloat, 406

Gram-atom measurements, 47

Grams, 35

pathways for interconversion of osmoles, equivalents and, *35*

Granular content, platelet release reaction and, 68

Granular endoplasmic reticulum, *5*

Granulocytes, 47

life span and numbers of, 48

types of, 48

Granulocytic system, 49

Granulosa, luteinization of, 473

Granulosa cells, 472, *476*

Gravid uterus, 466

Gravitational settling, 297

Gray matter, 94

in spinal cord of dog, *95*

Great omentum, uterine position in cow relative to, *467*

Grinding (table) surface, of tooth, 361–362

Gross anatomy, 3

Growing follicles, 459, *476*

formation of Graafian follicle from, *472*

Growth hormone, 163–164

maintenance of lactation and, 509

plasma concentration of, in cows near parturition, *508*

Guanine, DNA replication and, *9*

Gubernaculum testis, 437

Guernsey cows, milk from, 511, 512*t*

Guinea pigs, blood pressure in, 257*t*

Gustation, 128

Gustatory cells, 128, *129*

H

H+, secretion of, 329, 345

Hair, pilorection and, 427

Hair cells, 139

of cristae, 138

of inner ear, *139*

Hair follicles, apocrine and sebacous glands and association with, *425*

Hammer, 134

Haploid (n) number of chromosomes, oocytes and, 12, 462

Haptoglobin, 60

Hard palate, 271

Hardware disease, 402

Haustra, 375

Haustral contractions, large intestine and, 391

Haversian canals, 190–191, 197

Haversian system, 190–192, *192*, 194, *195*, 196

Hb. *See* Hemoglobin

HCG. *See* Human chorionic gonadotropin

HCl. *See* Hydrochloric acid

Head, of epididymis, 435, *436*, *438*

Hearing, 124, 132–140
    cochlear structure and function related to, 138–139
    external ear, 133
    inner ear, 134, 136
    middle ear, 133–134
    sound reception summary, 139–140
    vestibular structure and function related to, 136, 138

Heart, 181, 229–234, *239*, *254*. *See also* Cardiovascular system
    blood flow through, 232, 234
    blood pathway through, *233*
    description of, 229
    horse, cross-sectional view of, at ventricular level, *231*
    mammalian
        cardiac cycle of, *248*
        conduction system of, *246*
        cross-sectional schematic representation of, *230*
    myocardium, 229, 231
    valves of, 231, *233*

Heartbeat, origin of, 245

Heart chambers, 229, 231

Heart rate
    in adult, resting animals, 253*t*
    autonomic nervous system and, 251, 253
    autoregulation of, 253
    metabolic rate and, 251
    reflexes related to, 253–254

Heart-shaped kidney, in horse, 313, *314*

Heart sounds, 251

Heat. *See also* Body temperature
    circulatory adjustments to, 424
    evaporative loss of, 424–426
    extremes of, responses to, 426

physiologic responses to, 422–426
    production of
        in the body, 423
        increase in, 427
        reducing loss of, 427
    sense of, 124

Heat (estrus), 478

Heat stress, avian digestion and, 413

Heat stroke, 429

Helicotrema, 138

Helper T cells, 53

Hemacytometer, 54, 58

Hematocrit, 46

Hematopoietic stem cells, 52

Hematoxylin and eosin (H&E) stain, 48

Heme, 60, 61

Heme group, schematic representation of, and its associated polypeptide chain, *56*

Hemoglobinemia, 34, 60–61

Hemoglobin (Hb), 55
    as chemical buffer, 347
    degradation of, *61*
    forms of, 55–56
    oxygen saturation of, in birds, 306
    transport of oxygen and, 288

Hemoglobinuria, 34, 61

Hemolysis, 34

Hemolytic disease, 60

Hemosiderin, 60, 63

Hemostasis, prevention of blood loss and, 64–71

Hemostatic components, 65–67
    platelets, 67
    proteins, 65–66
    vascular endothelium, 66–67

Hen, ovulatory cycle in, 495–496

Hen's egg
    formation of, 493–494, 495*t*
    midsaggital section of, *495*

Heparin, 72, 73

Hepatic artery, *240*, *380*, *397*

Hepatic portal system, 237, *240*, 379

Hepatic veins, *240*, 379

Herbivores (plant eaters), 360
    diet of, 380
    field of vision in, 150

Hering-Breuer reflexes, receptors for, 293

Hernias, 437

Herniated intervertebral disk, 181

Heterophils, 50

Heteroplastic ossification, 193

Hexokinase, 167

Hibernation, 427–428
  awakening from, 428
  brown fat *vs.* white fat and, 428
  characteristics of, 428
High-frequency sound waves, 138
Hindbrain, *91*
Histamine, 52, 394, 395
Histones, 8
Hock, 21, *189*
Hog, vertebral formulas of, 183*t*. *See also* Pigs
Holocrine glands, 18
Holstein cows
  legume hay consumption and daily water balance of, 39*t*
  milk from, 511
    composition of, 512*t*
  puberty and, 478
Homeotherm (warm-blooded) animals, 422
Hook bones, 184
Hopping reaction, 114
Horizontal plane, 20, *21*
Hormones, 160–161
  of adrenal cortex, 170
  of adrenal medulla, 173–174
  adrenocorticotropic, 164
  amine classification of, 165
  of anterior pituitary, 163–164
  antidiuretic, 164–165
  beta-lipoprotein, 164
  biochemistry of, 161
  changes in plasma concentration of, in cows near
      parturition, *508*
  defined, 160
  of female reproduction, 468–471
    estrogens, 469
    gonadotropins, 470–471
    progesterone, 469–470
  gonadotropic, 164
  growth, 163–164
  lactogenesis and, 508–509
  of male reproduction, 432
    androgens, 450
    testosterone, 449–450
  modes of transmission for, 161
  oxytocin, 165
  pancreatic, 174–175
  parathyroid, 168–169
  parturition and changes in, 488–490
  of posterior pituitary, 164–165
  pregnancy and, 486–487
  prolactin, 164
  pulmonary ventilation and, *297*

spermatogenesis and, 449
  thyroid-stimulating, 164, 165–168
Horns, of uterus, 463
Horses
  accommodation in, 150
  apocrine sweat glands in, 424
  blood pressure in, 257*t*
  brachial plexus of, *99*
  bulbospongiosus muscle in penis of, 443
  cecum and colon of, 360, *376*
  dental formulas and eruption times for permanent
      teeth in, 362*t*
  diffuse placenta of, *486*
  ejaculation of sperm in, 451
  erection in, 450
  fetus of, within placenta, *485*
  field of vision in, 151–152, *153*
  full mouth in, 363
  fundi of, *148*
  gastrointestinal tract in, *360*
  heart rates in, 253*t*
  heat loss from sweating in, 426
  incisor exam and gauging age of, 362–363
  incisors of, wear characteristics on, *364*
  kidney of, midsagittal plane of, *315*
  kidney shape in, 313
  lengths of intestinal parts in, 372*t*
  life span of erythrocytes in, 59
  mammary glands of, 506
  metacarpal and phalangeal bones of thoracic limb of,
      189
  milk composition from, 512*t*
  normal blood ranges for, 519*t*
  nostrils of, 272
    dilatation of, 271
  number of sperm intended for artificial insemination
      in, 440
  ovarian activity in, *479*
  prehensile structures in, 384
  rate of enzyme secretion in, 395
  red blood cell number count in, 58
  respiratory frequency for, under different conditions,
      281*t*
  right kidney, ventral view in, *314*
  scapula of, lateral and medial views, *185*
  skeleton of, *180*
  spermatozoa of, *448*
  stomach in, inner regions of, *368*
  thorax of
    cross section view, *259*
    transverse section view, *278*

Horses (*contd.*)
    total leukocytes per microliter of blood in and
        percentage of each leukocyte, 50*t*
    transverse section of head of, showing division of
        nasal cavities, *271*
    upper and lower teeth in, *363*
    urine of, 341
    urine volumes and specific gravities for, 341*t*
    values of some constituents of blood from, 76*t*
    vertebral formula for, 181, 183*t*
    visual streak in, 151
    volatile fatty acids and, 400
    vomiting in, 390–391
HP. *See* Hydrostatic pressure
Human chorionic gonadotropin, 487
Humans
    amylase in saliva, amount of, 393
    approximate number of nephrons in each kidney for,
        317*t*
    blood pressure in, 257*t*
    discoid placenta of, *486*
    heart rates in, 253*t*
    knee joint in, *200*
    milk composition and, 512*t*
    percentage of long-looped nephrons in, 318
    sound frequencies perceived by, 140
    sweat glands as dissipaters of heat in, 424
    urine volumes and specific gravities for, 341*t*
    vertebral formulas for, 183*t*
Humerus, *188*
Humidity, 283, 426
Humoral control, 160, 294–297
    braking effect, 296–297
    importance of oxygen regulation, 294, 295–296
    influences of carbon dioxide and hydrogen ions,
        294
Humoral immunity, 53
Humors, of eye, 145
Hyaline cartilage, *184*, 190
Hyaluronic acid, 37, *38*, 201, 202
Hyaluronidase, 483
Hydration reaction, 290–291, 394
Hydrocephalus, 118
Hydrochloric acid, 367, 393
Hydrogen ion concentration (H+), 47, 345
Hydrogen ions, humoral control and influence of,
    294
Hydrolysis, 380, 382
    of simple lipid, *382*
Hydrostatic pressure, 324, 325
Hypercalcemia, 168

Hypercapnia, 301
Hyperglycemia, 174
Hyperkalemia, 172
Hypermagnesemia, 168
Hypermetria, 93
Hyperosmolality, 333
    relieving, cycle of events for, *335*
    thirst center and, 334
Hyperplasia, 224
Hyperpnea, 279
Hyperpolarization, mammalian intestinal smooth muscle
        and, 387, *387*
Hyperthermia, 429
Hyperthyroidism, 168
Hypertonic solutions, 32
    erythrocytes and, *33*
Hypertrophy, 193, *194*, 224, 250
Hyperventilation
    in birds, heat stress and, 306
    oxygen lack and, 295
Hypoblast, 12
Hypocapnia, 301
Hypodermis (subcutaneous), *425*
Hypoglossal nerve (XII), 100*t*
    in dog, *101*
Hypoglycemia, in ruminants, 410
Hypomagnesemia, 169
Hypoosmolality, 333
Hypophyseal vein, *162*
Hypophysioportal circulation, 162, *162*
Hypophysioportal system, 470
Hypophysis, 94
Hypophysis cerebri (pituitary gland), 162
Hypothalamic temperature, in cat, *425*
Hypothalamus, *90, 91,* 94, 162, 470
    cell bodies of neurosecretory neurons in,
        162
    extracellular hydration and role of, *334*
    fever and set point of, 429
    neurons associated with sex center in, 477
    osmoreceptor cells of, 333
Hypothermia, 429
Hypothyroidism, 168
Hypotonic solutions, 32
    erythrocytes and, *33*
Hypovolemia, 40, 336, *337*
Hypoxemia, 286
Hypoxia, 301
    age and tolerance levels to, 119
    S-T segment depression and, 250
H zone, *212*

I
I band, 210, *212*
ICF. *See* Intracellular fluid
ICSH. *See* Interstitial cell stimulating hormone
Icterus, 60
IgD, 75
IgE, 52, 75
IgG, 75
IgM, 75
Ileoc cocolic junction, of turkey, *412*
Ileocecal junction, 373
Ileum, 184, 367, 373
    in dog, *374*
    in pig, *375*
    upper, in birds, 413
Iliac vein, in male chicken, *453*
Ilium, 182
Immune response, lymphocytes and, 52
Immunity, humoral, 53
Immunoglobulins, 53, 75, 510
Impaired evaporation, 429
Implantation, 484–486
Impulse conduction, cardiac contractility and, 245–247
Incisors, 361
    age of horse and, 362–363
    dental formulas and eruption times for, *362t*
    of horse, wear characteristics on, *364*
Incomplete method, of drying-off, 514
Incontinence, urinary, 340
Incubation behavior, in birds, 496
Incus, 133, *134, 135, 140*
Indifferent taste response, 130
Inertia, deposition of particles and, 297–298
Inferior canaliculus, *154*
Inferior hypophyseal artery, *162*
Inflammatory reactions, monocytes and, 51
Infundibulum, 363, *364, 462,* 493
    in cow, *460*
    formation of hen's egg and, *495t*
Inguinal canal, 436, *438,* 442
Inguinal hernias, 437
Inguinal rings, 436
Inhaled particles, percentage of unit density deposited in
        lung according to their size, *298*
Inhibin, 449
Inhibitory agents, 175
Inner cavity, of mitochondria, 6
Inner ear, 134, *136*
    cochlear portion of, *139*
    of dog, latex cast of, *136*
    pathway of infections in, 136

right, *135*
schematic of, *134*
Inner medullary collecting duct, *320*
Inner membrane, of mitochondria, 6
Inner mucinoid layer, 155
Inorganic salts, 380
Insensible water losses, 39, 424
Insertion, of skeletal muscle, 209
Inspiration, 278
    in birds, air flow associated with, *305*
    intrapleural and intrapulmonic pressures associated
        with, *285*
    lung volume and, *281*
    schematic of thorax during, *279*
Inspiratory capacity, 280, *281*
Inspiratory reserve volume, 280, *281*
Insulin, 174, 378
    controlling secretion of, 175–176
    maintenance of lactation and, 509
    mammogenesis and, 507
Interbrain, *90,* 93
Intercalated disc, 207
Intercellular clefts, 235, *236,* 261
Intercellular substances, 37
Intercornual ligament
    bovine, *462*
    in cow, *460*
Intercostal muscles, 278, *279*
Interlobular artery, *318*
Interlobular ducts, in cow udder, 502, *502*
Interlobular vein, *318*
Intermediate incisors, 363
Intermediate skeletal muscle cells, 207
Intermittent method, of drying-off, 513–514
Internal abdominal oblique muscle, *438*
Internal callus, 197
Internal pudendal vein, *505*
Internal sphincter, 316
Internodal pathways, 245, 246, *246*
Interoceptors, 124
Interphase, 9
Interstitial cell stimulating hormone, 449
Interstitial fluid, 4, 37, *37,* 191, *241, 328*
    countercurrent exchanger system and, 330
    countercurrent multiplier system and, 330
    proteins and, 239
    tubular reabsorption and, 327
Interstitial fluid colloidal osmotic pressure, bulk flow
        and, 262
Interstitial fluid loss, reduced, plasma protein depletion
        and, 265

Interstitial fluid pressure (P_{if}), bulk flow and, 262
Interstitial lamellae, 191, 192
Interstitial space, 37
Interstitial tissue, seminiferous tubules in relationship to, 434
Interstitium, 37
Interventricular septum, 246
Intervertebral disk, 181, 184
Intervertebral foramina, 96, 97
Intestinal parts, lengths of, for several species, 372t
Intestinal peristalsis, movement of contents and, 389
Intestinal reflexes
    peristalsis, 387–388
    segmentation, 387
Intestinal smooth muscle, mammalian, membrane potentials in, 387
Intestinal tract, of pig, 375
Intestinal transport, of electrolytes and water, 392
Intestines, 367–375
    large, 373–375
    small, 367, 369–371, 373
Intracellular fluid, 37, 37
Intracellular hemolysis, 60
Intracellular messengers, platelet activation and, 68
Intralobular blood flow, 353
Intralobular ducts, in cow udder, 502, 502
Intramembranous bone formation, 193
Intraperitoneal pressure, 287
Intrapleural pressure, 284
    inspiration and expiration relative to, 285
Intrapleural space, 259, 275
    in horse, 278
Intrapulmonic pressure, 284
    inspiration and expiration relative to, 285
Intravascular fluid, 37
Intrinsic factor, 395
Intromission, failures of, 451
Involuntary nervous system, 98
Involution of uterus
    in bitch, 493
    in cow, 492
    in mare, ewe, and sow, 492–493
Iodine, 165, 383
Ipsilateral side of body, cerebellum and, 92
Iridocorneal angle, 145, 146
Iridocorneal angle region, of dog, 147
Iris, 142, 142, 144, 145
Iron, 383
    absorption of, 62, 62–63
    metabolism of, 61–63
    toxicity related to, 63

Ischiocavernosus muscles, 443
    of bull, 444
    erection and, 450
Ischium, 182, 184
ISF. See Interstitial fluid
Islets of Langerhans. See Pancreatic islets
Isoelectric line, in electrocardiogram, 249–250
Isohydric principal, buffer systems and, 347
Isotonic solution, 33
Isthmus, 493
    formation of hen's egg and, 495t
    of turkey, 412

J
Jaundice, 60
Jejunum, 367
    in pig, 375
    in turkey, 412
Jersey cows
    milk composition and, 512t
    puberty and, 478
Jersey steer ("Bill"), with large rumen fistula, 404
JG cells, 321
Joint capsule, 179, 199
Joint receptors, 125
Joints, 179, 198
    blood, lymph, and nerve supply of, 200–201
    in chicken, 182
    in horse, 180
    in ox, 181
Juxtaglomerular apparatus, 321, 322
Juxtaglomerular cells, 322
Juxtamedullary (long-looped) nephron, 318
    component parts of, 319
Juxtamedullary nephrons, 318

K
K+, secretion of, 329
Keratinized cells, 17
Ketone bodies, 410
Ketosis, in ruminants, 410–411
Kidney function
    aldosterone and, 337–338
    angiotensin II and, 326–327, 338
    antidiuretic hormone and, 333–335, 338
    erythropoietin and, 338
    parathyroid hormone and, 338
    prostaglandins and, 338–339
    renal clearance and, 341–344
Kidney function values, in dog in normal state of hydration, 324t

Kidneys. *See also* Glomerular filtration
 action of PTH on, 169
 assessing health status of, 343
 avian, 349, *349*
  anatomic features of, 349–350, *350*
  renal portal system and, 350–351
 awakening from hibernation and, 428
 blood flow to, for dog in normal state of hydration, 324*t*
 canine, ventral view of, *314*
 in cow, *317*
 in dog, *170*
 extracellular hydration and role of, *334*
 functions of, 312
 gross anatomy of, 312–317
 location of, 313, *313*
 in male chicken, *453*
 mammalian, relationship of structure to concentrating capacity in, 336*t*
 mechanism of H+ secretion by, 345
 nephron function and function of, 317
 relationship of parathyroid hormone, calcium homeostasis and, in cow, *339*
 shape of, in different animals, *314*
Killer cells (cytotoxic T cells), 53
Kinesthesia, nerve supply to joint and, 200
Knee jerk reflex, 112
Knee joint, *189*
 in human, *200*
Krause end bulbs, *126*
Krebs cycle, 6, 410, *410*
Krogh, August, 275
Küpffer cells, 52, 379, 397

L
Labia, 466
 of cow, *460*
Labial surface, of tooth, 362
Labor
 average duration of three stages of, in farm animals, 492*t*
 stages of, 490, 491*t*
Lacrimal apparatus, 142, 153–155
Lacrimal gland, 153, *154*, 155
Lacrimal production system, in dog's eye, *154*
Lacrimal sac, *154*
Lactate, 409
Lactation, 458, 501–514
 composition of milk, 510–512
 functional anatomy of female mammary glands, 501–506

 hormonal maintenance of, 509–510
  corticosteroids, 510
  insulin, 509
  parathyroid hormone, 510
  prolactin, 509
  thyroid hormone, 509
 lactogenesis and, 507–510
 mammogenesis and, 506–507
 milk removal and other considerations related to, 512–514
Lactic acid, values of, in blood from mature domestic animals, 76*t*
Lactiferous sinus, 502
Lactoferrin, 49, 75
Lactogenesis
 defined, 508
 lactation and, 507–510
Lactose, 399, 510–511
Lacunae, 191, *195*
Lamellae, 5, 191
Laminae, stroma of mammary gland and, 505
Lamina propria, *373*
Laplace's law, 236
Large colon, 375
Large intestines, 361, 373–375
 mechanical functions of, 391–392
 microbial digestion in, 400
Large lymphocytes, 52
Large phagocytic cells, 51
Larynx, 272, 364, *386*
 endotracheal tube in place relative to, *273*
 of horse, *271*
Lateral canthus, *142*
Lateral direction, 21
Lateral masses
 in spinal cord of dog, 95
 of ventral horns, 95
Lateral rectus muscle, in dog, *153*
Lateral semicircular canal, *135*, 136, *136*
Lateral spinothalamic tract, 94
Lateral suspensory ligaments, of udder, *504*, 504–505
Lateral ventricles, 116
Laying hen, five functional regions of oviduct in, *494*
Lecithin, 396
Left atrium, of heart, *274*
Left bundle branch, 246, *246*
Left cerebral hemisphere, 89
Left coronary artery, *239*
Left kidney, *314*

Left ventricle, of heart, 232, *233*, *234*, *235*, 236
  blood pressure and contraction of, 254–255
  pulmonary circulation and, *238*
Legume bloat, 406
Lens, *142*, 143–145, *144*
Lesser curvature, of stomach, 366
Leukemia, 54
Leukocytes (white blood cells), 45, 47–55
  basophils, 52
  classification and appearance of, 47–48
  diagnostic procedures related to, 54–55
  eosinophils, 52
  function, 49
  life span and numbers of, 48–49
  lymphoctes, 52–54
  monocytes, 50–52
  neutrophils, 49–50
  total per microliter of blood and percentage of each
    leukocyte, 50t
Leukocytosis, 54
Leukopenia, 54
Levator palpebrae muscle, in dog, *153*
Leydig cells, *434*, *435*, 449, 452
LH. *See* Luteinizing hormone
Libido, testosterone and maintenance of, 449
Ligaments, 23
Light adaptation, 149–150
Light-sensitive retina, 142
Limbus, *142*
Lingual surface, of tooth, 362
Lipid bilayers, 29
Lipid formation, 494
Lipids, 380, 382–383, 511
Lipolysis, 174
Lips, as prehensile organ, 384
Liquor folliculi, 472
Littoral cell, *397*
Liver, *24*, *240*, 361, 369, 377
  bile secretion by, 397
  functions of, 378–379
  hepatic portal system in, 237
  iron storage in, 63
  lobule of, *240*
    microstructure of, *397*
    portion of, *380*
  in pig, *379*
  ruminant, major metabolic pathways in,
    409
  of turkey, *412*
Llamas, 401
LMNs. *See* Lower motor neurons

Lobes
  in avian kidney, 349, *350*
  in mammary glands, 502, *502*
Lobular ducts, 502
Lobulated kidney, in cow, 313, *314*
Lobules
  of liver, *240*, 378, *397*
  in mammary glands, 502
Lockjaw, 220
Locomotion, nerve supply to joint and, 200
Long bones
  bone deposition and resorption sites in, lengthening
    and remodeling of, *197*
  growth of, 193–195
  shaft of, three-dimensional view, *191*
  structure of, *190*
Long pastern bone, 186
Loops of Henle, 315, 317, 318, 319, 320–321, *321*
  ascending and descending, *318*, *319*, *320*
  autoregulation of glomerular filtration and, 326
  countercurrent exchanger system and, 332
  countercurrent mechanism and, 330
  countercurrent multiplier system and, 330, *331*
  mammalian-type nephrons and, 349
  recirculation and, 333
Loose connective tissues, 19
  fibers and cells of, *20*
Lower motor neurons, 109, *110*
Low-frequency sound waves, 138
Lub-dub heart sounds, 251
Lubrication, of synovial joints, 202
Lubricin, 202
Lumbar nerves, 96
Lumbar vertebrae, *183*
Lumbosa cral plexus, 97
Lumen, 4, *370*, 503
  of seminiferous tubules, *435*
  of uterine tubes, 463
Lungs, 181, 274–278, *279*
  airways to, 270–273
  avian, schematic representation of, *302*
  in birds, 302
  in horse, *278*
  lobes of, *274*
  mast cells in, 72
  in mouse, electron micrograph of, *276*
  pulmonary circulation and, *238*
  subdivisions of, *274*
  surface area of inner aspects of, 296
  ventilation in, 283
Lung sounds, 280–282

Lung volume, 277
  subdivisions of, *281*
Luteinization of the granulosa, 473
Luteinizing hormone, 163, 164, 449, 452, 469, 470, 471
  avian male reproduction and, 453
  Graafian follicles and, 459
  mammogenesis and, 507
Luteolysis, 468
Lymph, 239, 242
Lymphatic capillaries, *241*
  special structure of, *242*
Lymphatic folds, avian, *454*
"Lymphatic" function, of cerebrospinal fluid, 118
Lymphatic obstruction, causes of, 265
Lymphatic system, 237, 239, 241–242
Lymph drainage, schematic representation of, *241*
Lymph nodes, *24*, 48, 241, 242
  enlarged, 242
  internal structure of, *243*
Lymphoblasts, 48, 52
Lymphocytes, 48, 241, *243*
  in birds, 54
  classification of, 52
  large and small, *48*
  population of, *49*
Lymph vessels, *241*
  joints and, 200
  liver lobule and, *397*
Lysis, 53
Lysosomes, *5*, 6, 166
Lysozyme, 52, 155

M
Macrominerals, 383
Macrophages, *20*, 51, 237, 242
Macrosmatic sense of smell, 131
Macula, 136
Macula densa, 321, 322, 326
Magnesium, 383
  values of, in blood from mature domestic animals, 76*t*
Magnum, 493
  formation of hen's egg and, 495*t*
Male genitalia, muscles of, 442–443
Male reproduction, 432–454
  accessory sex glands and semen, 438–440
  avian, 452–454
  blood and nerve supply related to, 444–445
  comparative anatomy of organs of various domestic
    animals, *441*
  descent of the testes, 437–438
  emission and ejaculation, 451

erection, 450–451
factors affecting testicular function, 451–452
mounting and intromission, 451
penis and prepuce, 440–442
spermatogenesis, 445–450
testes and associated structures, 432–436
Malleus, 133, *134*, *135*, *140*
Maltose, 381
  chemical structure of, *381*
Mammalian nephrons
  in avian kidneys, 349
  within lobule, *350*
Mammalian skeletal muscle fiber, cross section of, *213*
Mammalian-type nephrons, avian, location of, *351*
Mammals
  examples of neuron placement within central nervous
    system of, *111*
  summary of neurotransmission in, *107*
  urine formation and elimination in birds *vs.* in, 349
Mammary artery, *502*, 505
Mammary glands, 459
  in cats, 506
  in cow, sow, mare, and bitch, *461*
  in cows, 502–506
    blood supply and venous drainage, 505–506
    duct system, 502–503
    myoepithelial cells, 506
    suspensory apparatus, 504–505
    teat, 503–504
  in dogs, 506
  functional anatomy of, 501–506
  in goats, 506
  in horses, 506
  in pigs, 506
  pregnancy and enlargement of, 488
  regression of, 513–514
  in sheep, 506
Mammary lymph vessels, *502*
Mammary veins, *502*, 505
Mammogenesis, 506–507
  in cattle, 507
  in dog, cat, and sow, 507
Mammotrope cells, 163
Man, spermatozoa of, *448*. *See also* Humans
Mandible
  of cow, *272*
  of horse, *271*
Mandibular salivary glands, 377
  in dog, *377*
Manganese, 383
Mantle, in birds, 302

Mares
average duration of three stages of labor in, 492t
average rectal temperature of, 422t
corpus in, 463
estrogen patterns in, before parturition, 489
estrous cycle in, 479–480
factors related to female reproduction in, 474t
genital tract in, 465
involution of uterus in, 492–493
location of reproductive organs relative to rectum and
urinary bladder in, 461
mounting of, 450
ovarian shape in, 459
ovaries in, 463
ovulation fossa in, 459
parturition and hormonal levels in, 489
photoperiod response in, 478
vestibule of the vagina in, 468
Margination, 50, 51
Marine mammals, milk of, 511
Marrow (medullary) cavity, 188
Mast cells, 20, 52, 72
Mastication, 384–385
Mastitis, 504
Mating stance, 442
Matrix, of mitochondria, 6
Mean blood pressure, 255
Measured potential, 105
Measurement, interconverting units of, 35–36
Meatus, 271
Mechanoreceptors, pulmonary ventilation and, 297
Meckel's diverticulum, 412, 485, 494
in turkey, 412
Medial canthus, 142
Medial direction, 20
Medial rectus muscle, in dog, 153
Medial suspensory ligament, in udder, 504, 504–505
Median plane, 20, 21
Mediastinal pleurae, 22
in horse, 278
Mediastinal pressure, 285
Mediastinal space (mediastinum), 22, 257, 259, 275
Medulla
of horse kidney, 315
of kidney, 319
of ovary, 459
Medulla oblongata, 90, 91, 93, 94, 254
Medullary cavity, 179
in long bone, 190
Medullary cone, 349
in avian kidney, 351

Medullary substance, 89, 90
Medullary washout, 332
Meibomian glands, 154–155
Meiosis, 12, 13, 461
Meissner plexus, 369
Melanin, 142
Membrane nictitans, 142
Membranous labyrinth, 136, 137
Memory, central nervous system and, 89
Memory B cells, 53
Memory T cells, 53
Meninges
of brain, 114–115
of spinal cord, 115–116, 116
Meningitis, 136
Meniscus, 200
Merkel endings, 126
Merocrine glands, 18
Mesangial cells, 322, 338–339
Mesangial matrix, 322
Mesencephalon (midbrain), 91
Mesenchymal epithelium, 16
Mesenteric nodes, of cow, 376
Mesentery, 23, 24, 369, 370
Meshwork, eyeball, 144
Mesoderm, 12
formation of, 15
Mesoductus deferens, 437
Mesometrium, 459, 464
Mesorchium, 437
in male chicken, 453
Mesosalpinx, 459, 463, 464
Mesothelium, 16
Mesovarium, 459, 463
Messenger RNA, 11, 11
Messner corpuscles, 126
Metabolic rate, 251
Metabolic water, 38, 269
Metabolism, of central nervous system, 118–119
Metacarpal bones, 186
of horse, 189
Metacarpus, 187t, 188
Metaphase, 9, 10
Metaphysis, 188, 190
appearance presented by both longitudinal and cross
sections of areas of, 195
Metarteriole, 236
Metatarsus, 189
Metencephalon, 91
Metestrus, defined, 478
Methane, fermentation and production of, 405, 406

Methemoglobin, 56
Micellar solutions, 399
Microbial digestion, in large intestines, 400
Microglia, 87
Microhematocrit, 46, *46*
Microscopic anatomy, 3
Microtubular contraction, platelet release reaction and, 68
Microtubules, 9
    in platelet, 67
Microvilli, 370, *371*
Micturition, 339–340
    descriptive terms related to, 340
    reflexes and, 339–340
    transfer of urine to urinary bladder and, 339
Midbrain, 90, *91*, 93, 94
Middle ear, 133–134
    inside view of, *135*
    schematic of, *134*
Middle lobe, of avian kidney, 349
Middle meatus, 271
    of horse, *271*
Milk, withdrawal of, from teat, 502, 503–504
Milk composition, 510–512
    carbohydrates, 510–511
    colostrum, 512
    gross, 510
    lipids, 511
    minerals, 511
    other substances in, 511
    proteins, 510
    species variation relative to, 511
    from various species, 512*t*
    vitamins, 511
Milk fever, 216
Milking, milk removal at time of, 512
Milking interval, 513
Milk letdown, 488
    oxytocin and, 165, 506, 512–513, *513*
Milk line, 506, *506*
Milk removal, 512–514
Milk well, 505, *505*
Mineralocorticoids, 170, 172–173
Minerals, 383, 511
Mitochondria, 5, *6*
Mitosis, 12
    description of, 9, 11
    stages of, *10*
Mitotic division, from zygote to blastula, *14*
Mitotic spindle, 9
Mitral valve, 231, *233*

Mixed nerves, 96
Mixing time, 260
Modified symphysis, 181
Molars, 361
    dental formulas and eruption times for, 362*t*
Moles, 35
Molybdenum, 383
Monestrous animals, 477
Monkey, discoid placenta of, *486*
Monoblasts, 48
Monocular area of vision, 150
Monocytes, 48, *48*, 50–52
    enzyme systems of, 51
    life span and numbers of, 48–49
Monomolecular layer of protein, 72
Mononuclear phagocytic system, 51, 72, 192, 244–245
Monosaccharides, 380
    chemical structure of, *381*
Moose, 400
Morula, 12, *14*
Motor (efferent) cranial nerves, 97–98
Motor unit, 214
    distribution of terminal branches from nerve fiber to individual muscle fibers in, *215*
Mounting, failures of, 451
Mouse
    blood pressure in, 257*t*
    lungs in, electron micrograph of, *276*
Mouth, 271, 361, 385
"Mouthing," aging horses by, 363
Moving mucous blanket, 297, *299*
MPS. *See* Mononuclear phagocytic system
mRNA. *See* Messenger RNA
Mucous membranes (mucosae), 18, 369
Mucus, 377
Mules, milk composition and, 512*t*
Müllerian ducts, 450
Multipolar neurons, 85
Multivesicular bodies, 475
Murmurs, 251
Muscle capillary, cross section through endothelial wall of, *236*
Muscle fibers
    depolarization of, 216
    division of, 210–211, *211*
Muscle(s), 206–224
    ANS innervation to, 99
    arrangement of, 208–209
    cardiac, 206–207, 209
    classification of, 206–208
    comparison of contraction among types of, 222–223

Muscle(s) (*contd.*)
  of eyeball, 142, *142*
  function of, 209
  of male geintalia, 442–443
  skeletal, 207–208
  smooth, 206, 209
Muscle size, changes in, 223–224
Muscle spindles, 125
Muscle tissue, 14
Muscle tonus (tone), postural reflexes and, 113
Muscularis mucosae, 369, *370*, *371*, *373*
Muscular stomach, of turkey, *412*
Musculocavernous penis, of stallion, *441*
Musk ox, 401
MVB. *See* Multivesicular bodies
Myelencephalon (medulla oblongata), *91*
Myelinated nerve fibers, 90
Myelinated pain fibers, 127
Myelin sheath, 85, *85*, 87
Myeloblasts, 48, *49*
Myocardium, 229, 231
Myoepithelial cells, around alveoli and milk ducts, *503*, 506
Myofibrils, 210, *211*, 213, *213*
  division of, into sarcomeres, *212*
Myofilaments, 210
Myoglobin, 56
Myoid cells, in testicles, *433*
Myometrium, 464, *466*
Myosin, 71, 210, 211
  actin interacting with, sequence of, *219*
  comparison of contraction among muscle types and, 222
  filaments of
    muscle contraction and, 216–217
    smooth muscle contraction and, 223
Myotatic (stretch) spinal reflex, 112

N
Na+
  reabsorption of, 327–328
    aldosterone secretion and, 338
  transport of, from tubular lumen into tubular
    epithelial cell and its cotransport with glucose, 328
NaCL solution, suspending, changes in volume of
    canine erythrocytes attributable to tone of, 34*t*
NAD. *See* Nicotinamide adenine dinucleotide
Nasal cavities, *154*, 271, 364, *386*
  of cow, 272
  of horse, division of, *271*

Nasal septum, 271
  of horse, *271*
Nasolacrimal ducts, *154*
Navicular bone, 186
Navicular disease, 186
Neck of the bladder, 316, *316*
Neopulmonic parabronchi, 303
Nephron ducts, 319–320
Nephron(s), 317–322, *319*
  approximate number of, in each kidney for domestic
      animals and humans, 317*t*
  components of, 318–321
    juxtaglomerular apparatus, 321
    loop of Henle, 320–321
    nephron tubules and ducts, 319–320
  functional
    with blood supply, *320*
    urine formation and, 323
  mammalian, types of, *318*
  summary of kidney blood flow and tubular fluid flow
      in, *321*
  types of, 317–318
Nephron tubules, 319–320
Nerve fibers, 85
Nerve impulses, mechanisms of transmission to, 104–
    108
Nerves, 86
Nerve supply
  in joints, 200–201
  in synovial joint, *201*
Nerve tunic, 145
Nervous system, 84–119. *See also* Autonomic nervous
      system; Central nervous system; Peripheral
      nervous system, 160
  meninges and cerebrospinal fluid, 114–119
  nerve impulse and its transmission, 104–110
  organization of, 87–104
  reflexes and, 111–114
  structure of, 84–87
Nervous tissue, 14
Net diffusion, 31
Neural control, 160, 293–294
Neural retina, 145
Neurilemma, 85, *85*
Neurocranium (brain case), 180
Neurocrine transmission, 161
Neuroglia, 85
Neurohypophysis, 162
Neuromuscular junction, 214, *215*, 216
Neuron placement, schemes of, 110
Neurons, 85, *85*

polarity of, 85
  synapses and, 85–86
Neurotransmission, summary of, in mammals, *107*
Neurotransmitters, 108–109
  central, 109
  peripheral, 108–109
Neutral fats, 382
Neutralization, 53
Neutrophilic band, *49*
Neutrophilic metamyelocyte, *49*
Neutrophilic myelocyte, *49*
Neutrophilic segmented, *49*
Neutrophils, 48, 49–50
  life span of, 50
  mechanism of movement for, 50
NH₃, secretion of, 329
Nicotinamide adenine dinucleotide, 6
Night vision, vitamin A and, 149
Nitrate poisoning, methemoglobin and, 56
Nitrogen, in plasma, 78
Nitrogenous component, in urine, 341
Nociceptors, *126*
Nocturnal animals
  body temperature and, 422
  corneas of, 143
Nodes of Ranvier, 85, *85*, 87, *89*
Nonapeptides, 164
Nonkeratinized stratified squamous epithelium, 17
Nonmyelinated nerve fibers, 143
Nonperfused alveoli, 287
Nonprotein nitrogen, 78
  values of, in blood from mature domestic animals, 76*t*
Nonruminants, 365
Noradrenaline, 173
  structural formula for, *173*
Norepinephrine, *109*, 161, 173, 174, 427
Nostrils (nares), 270
  of several domestic animals, *270*
Nuclear membrane (nuclear envelope), 4, *5*
Nuclear pores, 4
Nuclear sap (nucleoplasm), 4
Nuclei and fiber tracts, of the brain, *90*
Nucleolus, 4, *5*
Nucleotides, 8
Nucleus, 4, *5*, 85
Nucleus pulposus, 181, *184*
Nutrition, estrous cycle and, 478. *See also* Diet; Foods

O
Obturator foramen, 184
Obturator nerves, 184

Ocular conjunctiva, 154
Ocular fundus, 146
Oculomotor nerve (III), 100*t*
  in dog, *101*
Odors
  animal, apocrine secretions and, 426
  perception of, 131
Off-flavors, in milk, 406, 511
Olfaction, 131
Olfactory area, of brain, 90
Olfactory epithelium, 272
Olfactory nerve (I), 100*t*
  in dog, *101*
Olfactory receptor, 131
Olfactory region, 130, 131
Oligodendrocytes, 86, 87, *88*
Oligopeptides, 382, 399
Omasal canal, 403
Omasum, 401, *402*, 404
Omentum, 23
Omnivorous animals, 360
Oncotic pressure, 75, 262
One atmosphere, total pressure of, 283
One cycle interval, estrous cycle, 477
1,25-dihydroxycholecalciferol, 169, 510
One-stage prothrombin time, 73
Oocytes, *13*, 440, 458, 459, 473, 476
  diploid (2n) of chromosomes and, 12
  formation of, 461
  haploid (n) of chromosomes and, 462
  pregnancy and transport of, 482–483
Oogenesis, 12, 461–462
Open canalicular system, platelet release reaction and, 68
Opsonization, 53
Opsonized forms, of eosinophils, 52
Optic disc, *142*, 146, *147*
Optic nerve (II), 100*t*, 142, *142*, 146, *147*
  in dog, *101*
Oral cavity, 361–365, *364*, *386*
  in horse, *271*
  pharynx, 364–365
  teeth, 361–363
  tongue, 363–364
Ordinary connective tissues, 19
Organelles, 4–6
  centrioles, 6
  endoplasmic reticulum, 4
  Golgi apparatus, 6
  lysosomes, 6
  mitochondria, 6
  nucleus, 4

Organic molecules, secretion of, 329
Organ of Corti, 138, 139, *139*, 140, *140*, *141*
Organs, 14
Orientation in space, 124
Origin, of skeletal muscle, 209
Oscillometer, 256
Osmoconcentration, 40
Osmolality, of several solutions as determined by vapor
    pressure lowering osmometry, *32t*
Osmolar concentrations, 31
Osmole (osm), 31, 35
    pathways for interconversion of grams, equivalents
        and, *35*
Osmometer, *32t*
Osmoreceptors, 333, 390
Osmoregulation, 336
    antidiuretic hormone and, 333–335
Osmosis, 30, *31*
    hypothetical example of tone of solutions on: before
        and during, *33*
Osmotic diuresis, 329
Osmotic fragility test, 34
Osmotic pressure, 31
    comparison of, for several solutions, *32t*
    effective, 32
Os penis, in dog, 451
Osseous labyrinth, 134, *139*
Ossification, 193
Osteoblasts, 169, 190, 192, 194, 196
Osteoclasts, 169, 192, 196
    bone remodeling and, *198*
Osteocytes, 191, 192, *194*
Osteolysis, 169
Osteon (haversian system), 191, *192*
Osteoprogenitor cells, 190, 192
Otoconia, 136
Otolithic membrane, 136
Otoliths, 136, 138
    in otolithic membrane, *138*
Outer medullary collecting duct, *320*
Oval window, *135*, *140*, *141*
Ovarian artery, 467
    relationship of a ruminant and its branches, *469*
Ovarian cycle events, summary of, 475–476
Ovarian follicle activity, 471–473, 475–476
    corpus luteum formation and regression, 473, 475
    follicular growth, 472
    ovulation, 473
Ovarian follicles, 459–462
    oogenesis, 461–462
    regression of, 460–461

Ovarian hormones, mammogenesis and, 507
Ovaries, 459
    bovine, *462*
    in cow, *460*
    in cow, sow, mare, and bitch, *461*, *463*
    left, functional development in birds, 493
    sagittal section of, *476*
    sperm transport toward, 440
Oviducts, 440, 462
    in avian female, 493
    in laying hen, five functional regions of, *494*
    left, functional development in birds, 493
Oviposition, 496
Ovulation, 164, 459, 473
    follicular growth and, 472
    sexual receptivity and, 476–477
Ovulation fossa, 459
Ovulatory cycle, in domestic hen, 495–496
Ox
    lengths of intestinal parts in, *372t*
    pelvis of, *185*
    skeleton of, *181*
    vertebral formulas of, *183t*
Ox coxae, 184
Oxidative phosphoryolation, 7
Oxygen
    consumption of, thyroid hormone and, 167
    diffusion of, 286–287
        direction for, *288*
    enrichment of, respiratory frequency and, *296*
    humoral control and influences of, 294–296
    in plasma, 78
    respiration and, 269
Oxygen-hemoglobin dissociation curve, 289–290,
    290
Oxygen transport, 287–290, *289*
    oxygen-hemoglobin dissociation curve, 289–290
    transport scheme, 288
Oxytocin
    milk letdown and, 506, 512–513, *513*
    release and function of, 165

P
Pacemakers, 222
Pacinian corpuscles, *126*
Packed cell volume, 46, 47
Pain, 125, 127
    referred, 127
    sense of, 124
    visceral, 127
Pain receptors, pulmonary ventilation and, 297

Pain reflex, joint disease and, 200
Paleopulmonic parabronchi, 303
Palmar direction, 21
Palpebral conjunctiva, 154
p-aminohippuric acid, 343
Pampiniform plexus, 44
   in stallion, *445*
Pancreas, *240*, 361, 377
   canine, dorsal view of, *369*
   left lobe of, *24*
   location and appearance of, *378*
   secretions of, 395–396
   in turkey, *412*
Pancreas hormones
   glucagon, 174–175
   insulin, 174
   pancreatic polypeptide, 175
   somatostatin, 175
Pancreatic amylase, 396
Pancreatic duct, 377
Pancreatic gland, 174–175
   functions of, 377–378
Pancreatic islets, 378
Pancreatic lipase, 396
Pancreatic polypeptide, 174, 175
Panting, 42, 424
   heat load dissipation and, 426
   patterns of, 300
Papillae, *129*, 364
   on dog's tongue, taste buds associated with, *129*
Papillary duct (teat canal), 503
Papillary muscles, 231
Parabronchi, in birds, 302
Paracrine transmission, 161
Parafollicular hormones, 168
Parallel circuit, 110, *111*
Paralumbar fossa, 403
Parasympathetic division, of autonomic nervous system, 145
Parasympathetic efferent distribution, 103
Parasympathetic nerves, micturition and, 340
Parasympathetic nervous system, 98
Parasympathetic stimulation, 253
Parathyroid glands, 168–169, 338
Parathyroid hormone
   calcium ion regulation and, 168–169
   homeostasis in cow and, *339*
   kidneys and, 169, 338
   lactation and, 510
   1,25-dihydroxycholecalciferol formation, 169
Paraventricular nuclei, 164

Parenchyma, 244
   of mammary glands, 502, *502*
Parietal layer, of vaginal tunic, 436
Parietal pericardium, 229, *230*
Parietal peritoneum, *438*
Parietal pleura, 22
Parietal vaginal tunic, *437*, *437*, *438*
Parkinson's disease, 87
Parotid salivary glands, 377
   in dog, *377*
Partial pressure, 282
Particles in a solution, osmotic pressure and, 31
Parturient paresis, 216
Parturition, 482, 487–492
   approaching, signs of, 488
   cervix and, 464
   changes in plasma concentration of hormones in cow
      in advance of, *508*
   estrogen patterns in mare, cow, sow, and ewe before,
      489
   events of, *490*
   hormone changes related to, 488–490
   lactation begins after, 501
   oxytocin and, 165
   stages of, 490, 492
Pastern, 186
Patella, 187, *189*
PCV. *See* Packed cell volume
Pectoral girdle (shoulder), 182
Pelvic bones, of cow, 186
Pelvic cavity, 22, 23
Pelvic floor, of bull, *444*
Pelvic girdle (pelvis), 182, 184
Pelvic limbs
   anatomy of bones, comparison of, *189*
   bones of thoracic limbs *vs.* bones of, 187*t*
Pelvic urethra, of bull, *444*
Pelvis, *189*
   in dog, *374*
   fractures to, standing ability and, 184
   of ox, lateral and dorsal views of, *185*
Penis, 440, 442, 450
   of avian male, 453
   of bull, *443*
      some associated muscles, *444*
   canine coitus and, 442
   fibroelastic, of bull, *441*
   penetration of, into vagina, 451
Pepsin, 393–394
Pepsinogen, 393, 395
Peptide bond, 382

Peptide class, 163
Peptide hormones, 161
Pericardial coelom, *230*
Pericardial sac, 229, *230*
 in horse, *278*
Pericardium, 229, 234
Pericytes, *20*, 234, *236*
Perilymph, 136, 140
Perimysium, 209, *211*
Periosteum, *134*, 190, *190*, 195, 197
Peripheral components, of autonomic nervous system, 100, 102
Peripheral nervous system, 85, 95–98
 cranial nerves, 97–98
 spinal nerves, 95–97
Peripheral neurotransmitters, 108–109
Peristalsis, 387–388
 large intestine and, 391
Peristaltic reflex, swallowing food bolus and, *386*
Peritoneum, 23, *24*
Peritonitis, 127, 279, 388
Peritubular capillaries, 319, *320*, *321*, *324*, *328*
 structures separating tubular fluid in tubular lumen from plasma in, *327*
Perivascular space, *115*
Permanent teeth, 361
Permolars, dental formulas and eruption times for, 362*t*
Persistent corpus luteum, 473, 475
Persistent urachus, 484–485
Petrous temporal bone, *134*
pH
 blood, 47
 relationship of, to H+ concentration, 345
Phagocytized particles, alveolar clearance and, 298
Phagocytosis, 49
Phalangeal bones, of horse, *189*
Phalanges, 187*t*, *188*, *189*
Phallic body, avian, *454*
Pharynx, 272, 361, 364–365
 of cow, *272*
 endotracheal tube in place relative to, *273*
 swallowing and, *385*, *386*
Phasic receptor organ, 125
Pheromones, 131–132, 161, 442, 450
Phimosis, 451
Phonocardiogram, 251
 simultaneous recording of respiration, blood pressure, electrocardiogram and, *252*
Phosphate, 382
Phosphate buffers, in saliva, 393
Phosphate buffer system, 345, 347

 formula representation for, 346
 relative merits of, 347
Phospholipids, 4, 69, *69*, 382
Phosphorus, 383
 in milk, 511
 values of, in blood from mature domestic animals, 76*t*
Photoperiod
 effects of, on ovarian activity in cat, horse, sheep, and goat, *479*
 intraspecies differences and, 478
 sperm production and, 432
 testicular and ovarian function related to, 452
Photopsin, 149
Photoreceptors, 145
Phrenico-abdominal artery and vein, in canine kidneys, *314*
pH symbol, 47
Physiologic contracture, 220
Physiologic dead space, 284
Physiology, 3
Pia mater, 114, *114*, 116
Pica, 130
Pig embryo, milk line shown on, *506*
Pigeons, crimson red pectoralis muscles of, 208
Pigs
 amylase in saliva of, amount of, 393
 approximate number of nephrons in each kidney for, 317*t*
 average rectal temperature of, 422*t*
 baby, anemia in, 63
 dental formulas and eruption times for permanent teeth in, 362*t*
 diffuse placenta of, *486*
 extremes of heat and responses of, 426
 fundi of, *148*
 heart rates in, 253*t*
 hernias in, 437
 intestinal tract of, schematic representation of, *375*
 lengths of intestinal parts in, 372*t*
 life span of erythrocytes in, 60
 liver in, relative to other organs, *379*
 mammary glands of, 506
 normal blood values for, 523*t*
 nostrils of, *270*
  dilatation in, 270
 number of sperm intended for artificial insemination in, 440
 percentage of long-looped nephrons in, 318
 red blood cell number count in, 58
 respiratory frequency for, under different conditions, 281*t*

rooting by, 384
schematic representation of outer part of skin from, *38*
stomach in, inner regions of, *368*
total leukocytes per microliter of blood in and percentage of each leukocyte, 50*t*
values of some constituents of blood from, 76*t*
variability of taste in, 130
Piloerection, 427
Pin bones, 184
Pineal gland (or pineal body), 94, 452
Pinna, 133, 139
    in dog, *133*
Pinocytotic vesicles, 235
Pituitary gland, *90*, 94, 161–165, 470
    anterior pituitary and its hormones, 162, 163–164
    posterior pituitary and its hormones, 164–165
Pituitary hormones, mammogenesis and, 507
Placenta, 12, 469
    diffuse type of, 485–486
    fetus of horse within, *485*
Placental lactogen, 507
Placentation, 464, 484–486
Placentomes, *466*, 486
Plantar direction, 21, *21*
Plasma, 37, 46, 74–75, 77–78, 239
    color of, 46
    defined, 75
    other constituents in, 78
    proteins in, 75, 77–78
        colloidal osmotic pressure and, 75, 77–78
        origin of, 75
Plasma amino acids, reversible equilibrium among plasma proteins, tissue proteins and, 77
Plasma cells, *20*, 53
Plasma colloidal osmotic pressure, bulk flow and, 262
Plasma membrane, 4
Plasma protein depletion, causes of, 265
Plasma proteins, reversible equilibrium among tissue proteins, plasma amino acids and, 77
Plasma volume, 46
Plasmin, 71, 72
Plasminogen, 71, 72
Plasticity, 59
Platelet adhesion, *65*, 67–68
Platelet plug, stabilized, 69
Platelets, 45, *48*, 67
    activation of, 68
        platelet aggregation, 68
        release reaction, 68
    cross-section of, *68*
    internal details of, 67

Pleasant taste response, 130
Pleura, 22, 275–278, *273*, *274*
Pleural cavity, 22
Pleural sac, *274*
Pleuritis
    abdominal breathing and, 279
    pain with, 127
PMSG. *See* Pregnant mare serum gonadotropin
Pneumatic bone, in birds, 302
Pneumonia, 280, 301
Pneumotaxic center, in respiratory center, 292, *292*
Pneumothorax
    description of, 285–287
    ventral view, *286*
PNS. *See* Peripheral nervous system
Poikilotherm (cold-blooded) animals, 422
Polar bodies, oogenesis and, 461–462
Polarity of a neuron, 85
Polarized membrane, 105
Polycythemia, 63–64
Polycythemia vera, 64
Polydipsia, 334, 335
Polyestrous animals, 477
Polynucleotide chains, 8
Polypeptide chain, *382*
Polypeptides, 161, 168, 382
Polypnea, 279
Polyribosomes, 57
Polysaccharides, 380
Polyspermy, 484
Polyuria, 334, 335, 340
Pons, *90*, *91*, *93*, 94
Portal systems, 236, 237
Portal vein, *240*, *380*, *397*
Position, inner ear and sense of, 134
Postccrop esophagus, of turkey, *412*
Posterior chamber, *144*, 145, *146*
    in dog, *144*
    of eyeball, *142*
Posterior endothelium, 143
Posterior limiting lamina, 143
Posterior lobe, 162, *162*
Posterior pituitary, 162
    ADH release and, 335
    antidiuretic hormone and, 164–165
    extracellular hydration and role of, *334*
    oxytocin and, 165
Posterior presentation, 492
Posterior sclera, 142
Posterior semicircular canal, *135*, 136, *136*
Postganglionic neurons, 102

Postmortem carcass examination, inspection for lymph node enlargement and, 242
Postpartum period, sexual receptivity and, 477
Postsynaptic neuron, *86*
Postural reflexes, 94, 113–114
Posture, nerve supply to joint and, 200
Potassium, 383
 in milk, 511
 values of, in blood from mature domestic animals, 76*t*
Potential, 104
Poultry production, temperature, taste and, 130
Precapillary sphincter, *236*
Precipitation, 53, *54*
Precorneal film, 154–155
Precrop avian esophagus, 412
Precrop esophagus, of turkey, *412*
Precursor of body cavities, 12
Predatory animals, field of vision in, 150
Preference test, 130
Preganglionic neuron, for sympathetic nerve, 102
Pregnancy, 482–487
 defined, 482
 diagnosis of, 487
 fertilization and, 483–484
 goblet cell secretion and, 464
 hormones and, 486–487
 implantation and placentation, 484–486
 mammary gland growth during, 507
 prolactional development during, 501
 respiratory frequency and, 280
 transport of oocyte and spermatozoa and, 482–483
 uterine blood supply during, 467
Pregnancy toxemia, 411
Pregnant mare serum gonadotropin, 487
Pregnant uterus, 466
Pregnenolone, *471*
Prehension, 384
Premolars, 361
 of horse, *271*
Preovulatory surge, 472
Prepuce, 440, 442
 of bull, *443*
 double-folded, in stallion, *441*
Prepuptial membrane and cavity, in bull, *433*
Preputial diverticulum, in boar, *441*, 442
Pressure, sense of, 124
Pressure receptors, pulmonary ventilation and, *297*
Pressure waves, transmission of, in cochlea, *140*
Presynaptic neuron, *86*
Presynaptic terminal bulb, 108
Prevertebral ganglia, 102

Primary follicles, *476*
Primordial follicles, 459
Procoagulants, 67, 72
Proctodeum, avian, *454*
Proenzymes, 396
Proestrus, 477
 defined, 478
Progesterone, 471, *471*
 fertilization and, 484
 functions of, 469–470
 mammary gland response to, 507
 parturition and decrease in, 489
 plasma concentration of, in cows near parturition, *508*
 pregnancy and, 486
 sexual receptivity and, 476–477
Progestins, 469
Projection fibers, 90
Prolactin, 163
 broodiness and, 496
 lactogenesis and, 508
 maintenance of lactation and, 509
 plasma concentration of, in cows near parturition, *508*
Prolapsed intervertebral disk, 181
Proliferation, 193, *194*
Promyelocyte, *49*
Prone position, 21
Pronuclei, 484
Proper foods, 383
Prophase, 9, *10*
Propionate, 409, 410
 chemical structure of, *400*
Propionic acids, 400, 407
Proprioceptive impulses, 94
Proprioceptors, 124–125
Prosencephalon (forebrain), *91*
Prostacyclin (PGI$_2$), 67, 176, *176*
Prostaglandins, 160–161
 corpus luteum formation and regression, 473, *475*
 female reproduction and, 468
 functions of, 175–176
 kidney function and, 338–339
 lactogenesis and, 508–509
 parturition and, 489
 plasma concentration of, in cows near parturition, *508*
 in seminal plasma, 440
 synthesis of, major pathways for, *176*
Prostate gland, 439
 in dog, 439, *441*

Protein buffer systems, 345

Protein channels, 29

Protein components, of blood coagulation pathway, 65–66

Protein molecules, 4

Proteins, 4, 380, 381–382, 396
androgen-binding, 449
as buffers, 346
digestion and absorption of, 399
gluconeogenesis and, 409
interstitial fluid and, 239
microorganisms of rumen and hydrolysis of, 408
in milk, 510
in plasma, 75, 77–78
quality of, 382
synthesis of
reduced, plasma protein depletion and, 265
RNA and, 11

Proteoglycans, 326

Prothrombin, 69
conversion of, to thrombin, 69

Prothrombinase complex, 69, 69

Protozoan microorganisms, 407

Proventriculus, 412

Proximal direction, 21, 21

Proximal duodenum, of turkey, 412

Proximal tubule, 318, 319, 319, 320, 321, 322

Pseudopods, 68

Pseudopregnancy, 481

Pseudostratified ciliated columnar epithelium, with goblet cells, 16, 17

Pseudounipolar neurons, 85

PSNS. See Parasympathetic nervous system

Psychic component, saliva and, 393

PTH. See Parathyroid hormone

Puberty
bitch and onset of, 481
defined, 472
mammogenesis and, 501, 507
mare and onset of, 479
testicular function and, 452

Pubis, 182, 184

Pudendal nerve, 445

Pulmonary alveoli, 275

Pulmonary arteries, 235, 275

Pulmonary arterioles, 274

Pulmonary circulation, lungs and, 238

Pulmonary interstitial edema, 286

Pulmonary semilunar valves, 231, 233

Pulmonary system, 236
mammalian circulation and, 238

Pulmonary trunk, 238

Pulmonary veins, 235, 274, 275

Pulmonary ventilation, 283–287
dead space ventilation, 284
factors related to, 297
mediastinal pressure, 285
pneumothorax, 285–287
pressures that accomplish ventilation, 284–286
regulation of, 292–297

Pulmonary venule, 274

Pulmonary volumes and capacities, 78–280

Pulp cavity, 363

Pulse pressure, 255

Pupil, 142, 145

Purine bases, 8

Purkinje fibers, 222, 246, 247

Purring, 300–301

Pus, 50

PV. See Plasma volume

P wave, in electrocardiogram, 249

Pyloric antrum, 366
canine, parts of, 366

Pyloric gland regions, 367

Pyloric sphincter, 388

Pylorus, in canine stomach, 366

Pyrimidine bases, 8

Q

QRS wave, in electrocardiogram, 249

Quadrupeds, directional terms and planes applied to, 20–21, 21

Queens
estrous cycle in, 481–482
photoperiod response in, 478

R

Rabbits
average rectal temperature of, 422t
blood pressure of, 257t
coprophagy practiced by, 400
lengths of intestinal parts in, 372t

Radially arranged fibers, 145

Radiation, heat loss and, 423

Radiography, pregnancy diagnosis with, 487

Radiopacity, lungs and, 275

Ramp-shaped retina, 150

Rams
anatomy of male reproductive organs in, 441
sigmoid flexure of penis in, 440
spermatozoa of, 448
urethral process in, 440, 441

Rarsus, *189*

Rats
  blood pressure in, *257t*
  spermatozoa of, *448*

RBCs. *See* Red blood cells

RBF. *See* Renal blood flow

Reabsorption, 262

Reaction threshold, to pain, 127

Receptor hair cells, 136

Receptors, 112

Recirculation, 332

Recoil tendency, 285

Rectal temperatures
  accuracy of, 422
  average, of various species, *422t*
  parturition and changes in, 488

Rectum, 375
  avian, *454*
  in cow, *317*
  in cow, sow, mare, and bitch, *461*
  in dog, *374*
  in pig, *375*

Red blood cells, 45
  fate of, 60–61
  hemoglobin and color of, 46
  life span of, 59–60
  numbers of, 58
  shape of, 58–59
  size of, 59
  spleen as important reservoir of, 245

Redeglutition, 404, 405

Red (or dark) skeletal muscle cells, 207, 208

Red pulp, of spleen, 244, *244*

Referred pain, 127

Reflex arc, 112

Reflex centers, 113

Reflexes, 111–114
  autonomic, 103–104
  for blood pressure control, *254*
  within cardiovascular system, 253
  defined, 112
  emesis and, 390
  gastric emptying and, 390
  intestinal, 387–388
  micturition, 339–340
  postural, and reactions, 113–114
  somatic and visceral, 113
  spinal, 112–113
  swallowing and sequence of, 385
  thermoreceptors and, 424

Reflex ovulators, 473

Reflex responses, joint disease and, 200

Refractory period, 108, 247

Regression, of follicles, 460–461

Regurgitation, 404
  tracings showing mechanism of, in rumination, *405*

Rehydration, 41

Reindeer, 401

Relative medullary thickness, derivation of, 335

Relative polycythemia, 63

Relaxation, of muscle fibers, 247

Relaxin, 488
  mammogenesis and, 507

Remastication, 401, 404, 405

Remodeling of bone, 193, 195–196
  for long bones, *197*
  osteoclastic activity preceding, *198*

Renal arteries, 313, *314*
  in horse kidney, *315*

Renal blood flow, 323–324
  for dog in normal state of hydration, *324t*

Renal clearance, 341–344
  creatinine clearance and, 343–344
  effect of tubular reabsorption and tubular secretion on, *342*
  formula for determination of, 341

Renal disease, plasma protein depletion and, 265

Renal hilus, *314*, 315
  of horse kidney, *315*

Renal pelvis, 315, *319*, *321*
  of horse kidney, *315*

Renal plasma flow, 324
  for dog in normal state of hydration, *324t*
  renal clearance and, 341, 342

Renal portal system
  avian, veins associated with, *352*
  in avian kidney, 350–353

Renal portal valve, in avian kidney, 351

Renal threshold, 329

Renal veins, 313, *314*, *320*
  in horse kidney, *315*

Renin, 172, 321, 326, 395

Repolarization, 105, 108
  of heart muscle, voltage changes and, 248–249
  recording of transmembrane potential during, *106*

Reproduction. *See* Female reproduction; Male reproduction

Reptiles, uric acid in, 353

Reptilian nephrons
  avian, location of, *351*
  in avian kidneys, 349
  within lobule, *350*

Resalivation, 401, 404, 405
Reserve cartilage, *194*
Residual volume, 280
Respiration
    defined, 269
    simultaneous recording of blood pressure,
        electrocardiogram, phonocardiogram and, *252*
Respirators, pneumothorax and use of, 285
Respiratory apparatus, 270–275
    airway to the lungs, 270–273
    lungs and pleura, 274–275
    pulmonary alveoli, 275
Respiratory bronchioles, 275
Respiratory center (brain stem)
    in birds, 304, 306
    chemosensitive area of, *295*
    components of, *292*
    four regions of, 292
Respiratory clearance, 296–300
    alveolar clearance, 297, 300
    importance of, 298
    physical forces of deposition, 297–298
    upper respiratory tract clearance, 297
Respiratory cycles, 278
Respiratory frequency, 280
    pneumogram showing effect of oxygen enrichment in,
        296
    for several animal species under different conditions,
        281*t*
Respiratory gases, diffusion of, 286
Respiratory motor pathways, *292*
Respiratory pressures, 282–284
    arterial and venous blood partial pressure, 282
    atmospheric air *vs.* alveolar air, 283–284
    partial pressure, 282
Respiratory rate index, obtaining, 488
Respiratory rates, farrowing and, 488
Respiratory surface, *274*
Respiratory system, 269–306
    acid-base balance maintenance and role of, 344, 345
    descriptive terms and pathologic conditions, 300
    nonrespiratory functions of, 298–301
    panting, 298
    purring, 300–301
Resting heart rates, animal's size and, 251
Resting membrane potential, 105
    establishment of, *105*
Rete testis, *436*, 446
Rete testis fluid, *433*
Reticlum (honeycomb), 401
Reticular connective tissue fibers, 19

Reticular groove, *402*, 403
Reticulocytes, 57
Reticulo-omasal orifice, *402*
Reticulum
    in cow, heart's location relative to, *230*
    function of, 403
Retina, 142, *142*, 143, 145–146, *147*
    ramp-shaped, 150
    tapetum's relationship to, *151*
Retinal pigment epithelium, *147*
Retractor bulbi muscle, in dog, *153*
Retractor penis, in fibroelastic penis of bull and
        musculocavernous penis of stallion, *441*
Retractor penis muscles, in bull, *433*, *443*, *444*
Retroperitoneal structures, 313
Reverberating circuit, 110, *111*
Rhinencephalon (olfactory brain), *91*
Rhodopsin, 146, 149, 150
Rhombencephalon (hindbrain), *91*
Ribosomal RNA, 11, *11*
Ribosomes, 5
Ribs, 180, 181
Right bundle branch, 246, *246*
Right cerebral hemisphere, 89
Right coronary artery, 239
Righting reflex, 113
Right kidney, *314*
Right ventricle, 232, *233*, *235*, 236
Rigor contracture, 220
Rigor mortis, 220
RNA, 4, 11
Rod protein, 149
Rods, 142, 145, 146
    black-and-white vision, 142, 147
    outer segments of, *147*
    stimulation of, 149
Rooster
    phallus of, 453
    ventral view of organs and associated structures of
        dorsal abdominal cavity of, *349*
Rooting, head movements of, 384
Roots (crura), of penis, 440
Rosette of Fürstenberg, *502*, 503
Rostral direction, 20, *21*
Roughages, 380
Round window, *134*, *140*, *141*
RPF. *See* Renal plasma flow
rRNA. *See* Ribosomal RNA
Rubriblast, 57
Ruffini corpuscles, *126*
Rumen fistula, 403

Rumen (paunch), 401
  chemistry and microbiology of, 407–408
  in cow, *230*
    uterine position in, *467*
  function of, 403
  pillars of, 403
  ventral and dorsal sacs of, *402*
Ruminant digestion
  characteristics of, 404–407
  gas production and eructation, 405–407
  rumination, 404–405
Ruminant forestomachs, 367
Ruminantia, 400
Ruminant liver, major metabolic pathways in, *409*
Ruminant metabolism, 408–411
  energy production, 409–410
  gluconeogenesis, 409
Ruminants, 365, 400
  coiled colon for, 375
  cotyledonary placenta of, 486, *486*
  ketosis and bloat in, 410–411
  relationship of ovarian artery and its branches in,
    469
  salivary secretion in, 393
  stomach in, 366, 400–404
    compartments and functions of, 403–404
    inner regions of, *368*
    structure and function of, 401–404
  vomiting in, 390
Rumination, 404–405
  tracings showing mechanism of regurgitation in,
    405
Ruminoreticular fold, *402*
Ruptured follicle, *476*

S

Saccular maculae, general structure of, *138*
Saccule, *134*, 136
Sacculus, *137*
Sacral nerves, 96
Sacral spinal cord reflex center, micturition and,
  339
Sacral (S) vertebrae, 181
Sagittal plane, 20
Saliva, 393
Salivary glands, 361, 377
  in dogs, location of, *377*
Salivation, panting in cattle and increase in, 426
Saltatory conduction, *107*, 108
Salts, inorganic, 380
Salty taste, 130

Sarcolemma, 209, *211*, *213*
Sarcomeres, 210
  contraction of, actin and myosin myofilaments
    associated with, *218*
  division of myofibrils into, *212*
Sarcoplasmic reticulum, in extracellular spaces
    between myofibrils, *214*
Sarcotubular system, 211, 213–214
Sarcotubules, of sarcoplasmic reticulum,
    213
Satellite cells, 224
Scala media, 138, *139*
Scala tympani, *134*, 138, *139*, 140, *141*
Scala vestibuli, 138, *139*, *140*, *141*
Scapula, 182, *188*
  of horse, *185*
Scapulohumeral joint, *188*
Scents, 131
Schwann cells, 86, 87
  nucleus of, *85*
Sclera, 142, *142*, *144*
  posterior, 142
Scleral venous plexus, 145
Scotopsin, 149
Scrotal hernias, 437
Scrotum, 436, 450
Seasonal breeding, photoperiod and, 478
Sebaceous glands, *425*, 426
Sebum, 426
Secondary hemostatic plug, 69
Secondary sexual characteristics, 449–450
Second heart sound, 251
Secretin, 175, 395, 396, *398*
Segmentation, 94, 387, *388*
Segmented cells, 48
Segmented neutrophil, *48*
Selectively permeable membranes, 32
Selenium, 383
Sella turcica, 162
Semen, 432, 440, 442
Semicircular duct, *137*
  structure of ampullary crista in, *137*
Semilunar valves, 231
Seminal plasma, 439, 451
  in avian male, 453
Seminal vesicle
  of bull, *433*
Seminal vesicles, 439
Seminiferous tubule
  periphery of, *435*
  spermatogenic wave and, *448*

Seminiferous tubules, 432, *433*, *436*, 446
  relationship of, to rete testis, efferent ducts,
      epididymis, and ductus deferens, *436*
  relationship of to each other and to interstitial tissue,
      434
Seminiferous tubules, in avian male, 452
Semipermeable membrane, 30–31
Sensations, 124
Sensible water losses, 39
Sensory (afferent) cranial nerves, 97
Sensory afferent (inflowing) fibers, 94
Sensory organs, 124–155
  hearing and equilibrium, 132–140
  smell, 130–132
  taste, 127–130
  vision, 140–155
Sensory pain pathway, *128*
Sensory receptors, *126*
  classification of, 124–125
  responses of, 125
Septa, 434, *436*
Septum, in fibroelastic penis of bull and
      musculocavernous penis of stallion, *441*
Serosa, 369, *370*, *371*
Serotonin, in basophil granules, 52
Serous membranes, 18
  invagination of, *22*
Serous secretion, 377
Sertoli cells, *433*, 434, 435, *435*, 446, 449, 452
Serum, 75
Sesamoid bones, 186, 187
Sex center, 477
Sex glands, accessory, 438–440
Sexual drive, testosterone and maintenance of,
      449
Sexual receptivity, 469, 476–477
Sexual stimulation, 451
Sheath of Schwann, *85*
Sheep, 401. *See also* Ewes
  adapting to lack of water by, 42
  apocrine sweat glands in, 424
  average rectal temperature in, 422*t*
  blood pressure in, 257*t*
  corpus in, 463
  critical temperature in, 427
  dental formulas and eruption times for permanent
      teeth in, 362*t*
  ejaculation of sperm in, 451
  erythrocyte size in, 59
  fundi of, *148*
  heart rates in, 253*t*

  heat loss from sweating in, 426
  lengths of intestinal parts in, 372*t*
  life span of erythrocytes in, 59–60
  mammary glands of, 506
  milk composition and, 512*t*
  normal blood values for, 521*t*
  nostrils of, *270*
  number of sperm intended for artificial insemination
      in, 440
  ovarian activity in, 479
  pancreatic duct in, 377–378
  photoperiod response in, 452, 478
  red blood cell number count in, 58
  respiratory frequency for, under different conditions,
      281*t*
  right kidney, ventral view in, *314*
  time spent on rumination by, 405
  tongue as prehensile organ in, 384
  total leukocytes per microliter of blood in and
      percentage of each leukocyte, 50*t*
  urine volumes and specific gravities for,
      341*t*
  values of some constituents of blood from,
      76*t*
  vertebral formulas of, 183*t*
Shell gland, 496
  formation of hen's egg and, 495*t*
Shell of egg, 494, *495*, 495
Shivering, 427, 429
Shorthorn cows, milk composition and, 512*t*
Short pastern bone, 186
Shoulder, 182
Shoulder slip, 224
Sickle cell anemia, 59
Sight, 124
Sigmoid flexure of penis
  of bull, *443*, *444*
  erection and, 450
  of penis, 440
Silicosis, 298
Simple circuits, 110
Simple columnar epithelium, *16*, 17
Simple cuboidal epithelium, *16*, 17
Simple diffusion, 29
Simple endothelial cells, 234
Simple epithelium, 15
Simple squamous epithelium, 15, *16*
Simple stomach, 365–367
Sinoatrial (S-A) node, 245, *246*
Sinusoids, 379, *380*, 397
  hepatic portal system, *240*

Skeletal muscle contraction, 216–221, 222
  actin and myosin myofilaments associated with
      contraction of sarcomere, *218*
  contraction *vs.* contracture, 220
  cycle of contraction followed by relaxation, *217*
  depolarization of muscle fibers, 216
  process of, 216–217, 219–220
  strength of, 220–221
    tetanus, 220
    treppe, 221
  summary of changes occurring in heads of myosin
      cross bridges in, 217, 219 –220
Skeletal muscle fiber
  longitudinal section of, *212*
  mammalian, cross section of, *213*
Skeletal muscles, 206, 207–208. *See also* Skeletal muscle
      contraction
  changes in size of, 224
  frequency of contraction in, 245
  harnessing of, 209
  hypertrophy in, 224
  longitudinal section of, *208*
  microstructure of, 210–221
  red and white fibers in, *208*
  staircase phenomenon of, *221*
Skeleton, 179. *See also* Bone(s)
  appendicular, 181–182, 184, 186–187
  axial, 180–181
  of chicken, *182*
  general features of, 180
  of horse, *180*
  of ox, *181*
Skin gland, 507
Skull, 180
Slow waves, mammalian intestinal smooth muscle and,
      387, *387*
Small colon, 375
Small intestines, *240*, 361, 367, 369–371, 373
  avian, 412
  in cow, *376*
  in dog, horse, and cattle, *360*
  lining of, three-dimensional representation of,
      373
  mechanical functions of, 391
  segmentation contractions of, *388*
Small lymphocytes, 52
Smell, 124, 130–132
  cells associated with, in dog, *132*
  odor perception, 131
  olfactory region structure, 131
  pheromones, 131–132

Smooth mouth, 363
  in horse, *364*
Smooth muscle, 206, 209
  cells of, in their longitudinal and cross-sectional
      planes, *207*
  changes in size of, 224
  in ciliary body, 143
  contraction of, 222, *223*, 245
  gastrointestinal motility and, 385
  hypertrophy in, 224
  of urinary bladder, 315
Smooth muscle sphincter, 503
Smoothness of the endothelium, 72
Sneezing, 293
Sniffing, 131, 272
Sodium, 383
  in milk, 511
  values of, in blood from mature domestic animals, 76*t*
Soft palate, 271, *386*
  of cow, *272*
  endotracheal tube in place relative to, *273*
Solar heat gain, sheep and, 42
Solutes, countercurrent exchange in vasa recta and
      passive diffusion of, *332*
Solutions
  diffusion, 29–30
  osmosis and osmotic pressure, 30–32
  physiochemical properties of, 28–34
  tone of, 32–34
Somatic nerves, 95
Somatic reflexes, 113
Somatic senses, 124
Somatomedins, 163
Somatostatin, 161, 174, 175
Somatotrope cells, 163
Somatotropin (somatotropic hormone), 163, 507
Somesthetic area, 90
Sound
  production of, 271
  range of frequencies across species, 140
Sound reception, summary of, 139–140
Sound waves, 133
  ossicles and amplification of, 134
  pathway of, into ear, *141*
  transmission patterns of, 138
Sour taste, 130
Sows
  average duration of three stages of labor in, 492*t*
  corpus in, 463
  estrous cycle in, 480
  factors related to female reproduction in, 474*t*

genital tract in, *465*
  involution of uterus in, 492–493
  location of reproductive organs relative to rectum and
      urinary bladder in, *461*
  mammogenesis in, 507
  ovaries in, 459, *463*
Space of Disse, *397*
Special senses, 124
Specific gravity, of urine, 341, *341t*
Sperm, 439
  production of, 432
Spermatic cord, 44, 436, 437, *438*
  cross section of, in mammals, *437*
  in stallion, *445*
Spermatids, 434, *435*, *447*
Spermatocytes, 434, *435*
Spermatogenesis, 12, 445–450
  epididymal transport, 446
  hormonal control and, 449
  spermatogenic wave, 446, 448
  stages of, in mammals, *447*
  temperature requirements and, 44
  testosterone and, 449–450
Spermatogenic wave, 446, 448
  12-day cycle in, *448*
Spermatogonium, 435, *435*, *447*
Spermatozoa, 12, *13*, *435*, *447*
  of farm animals, compared with other vertebrates, *448*
  motility of, 484
  pregnancy and transport of, 482–483
  reservoirs of, 482, 483
Sperm-host glands, of chicken, 494
Sperm storage, 446
Sphincter of Oddi, 397
Sphincters, 209
Sphingomyelin, 87, 382, *382*
Sphygmomanometer, 256
Spicules, 188, *190*
Spike potentials, 385
  mammalian intestinal smooth muscle and, 387, *387*
Spinal cord, 94–95
  cauda extremity of, showing cauda equina, *96*
  central canal of, 116
  of dog, transverse section of, *95*
  meninges of, 115–116, *116*
  spinal nerves and location relative to, *98*
  spinal reflex and, 113
Spinal injuries, urinary incontinence and, 340
Spinal nerves
  location of, relative to branches, roots, spinal cord,
      and vertebra, *98*

schematic of association with vertebrae in dog, *97*
  in spinal cord of dog, *95*
Spinal reflex, 112–113
Spinous process, *183*
Spiral ganglion, *141*
Spleen, 48, *240*, 242–245
  in dog, location of, *243*
  functions of, 242
  in pig, *244*
    schematic representation of, *244*
Splint bones, 186
Splints (lameness condition), 186
Spongy bone, 188, 190, *190*
Squamous endothelial cells, 234
Squamous epithelium, 15
Staircase phenomenon, skeletal muscle and, 221, *221*
Stallions
  anatomy of male reproductive organs in, *441*
  average rectal temperature in, *422t*
  double-folded prepuce in, *441*
  erectile tissue in, 440
  musculocavernous penis of, *441*
  testes in, lateral view with emphasis on pampiniform
      plexus, *445*
Standing reflex, 113
Stapedius muscle, 134, *135*
Stapes, 133, *134*, *135*
  pressure waves and, *140*
Starches, 380–381, 399
Starling's law of the heart, 253
Starvation, 359
Stem cells, in avian male, 452
Stercobilin, 60, 61
Stercobilinogen, 61
Sternum, 180, 181
Steroid hormones, 161, 450
  biosynthesis of, from cholesterol, *471*
Steroids, 469
Stethoscope, listening for lung sounds with, 280
STH. *See* Somatropin (somatotropic hormone)
Stifle (knee) joint, *189*
Stirrup, 134
Stomach, *24*, *240*, 361, 366–367, 378. *See also* Ruminant
      stomach
  canine
    dorsal view of, *369*
    parts of, *366*
  in cattle, left and right views of, *402*
  in dog, horse, and cattle, *360*
  functions of, 388
  inner regions of, in horse, pig, and ruminant, *368*

Stomach (*contd.*)
  in nonruminants, 365
  pregastric functions and, 384
  simple, 365–367
Stranguria, 340
Stratified epithelium, 15
Stratified squamous epithelium, 17
Stratified squamous keratinized tissue, 17
Stratified squamous keratinizing epithelium, *16*
Stratified squamous nonkeratinizing epithelium, *16*, 143,
    143
Streak canal, 503
Stretch receptors, pulmonary ventilation and, 297
Stretch reflex, 112, *112*, 113
Striated muscle, contraction of, 222
Stroma, 143
  of mammary gland, 502
Strychnine poisoning, third eyelid and, 15
S-T segment depression, hypoxia and, 250
Subarachnoid space, 115, 118
Subcutaneous abdominal milk vein, in cow, *505*
Subepithelial basement membrane, 143
Sublingual salivary glands, 377
  in dog, *377*
Submucosa, 369, *371*
Submucosal gland, *370*
Substantia propria, 143, *143*
Subthalamus, *90*
Sucrose, 399
  chemical structure of, *381*
Sulfonamides, 168
Sulfur, 383
Superficial (exterior) inguinal ring, 436
Superficial surface, 21
Superior canaliculus, *154*
Superior hypophyseal artery, *162*
Supine position, 21
Supraoptic nuclei, 164
Surface tension, 284
Surfactant, *274*
Surgery, external heat sources used during, 429
Suspensory apparatus, for udder, *504*, 504–505
Sustentacular cells, 131
Swallowing, 272, 364
  breathing inhibited during, 293
  displacement of structures associated with, 386
  stages of, 385
Sweat glands, types of, 424
Sweating, 424, 426
Sweeny, 224
Sweet clover poisoning, 74

Sweet taste, 130
Swine
  blood pressure in, 257*t*
  ejaculation of sperm in, 451
  heat loss from sweating in, 426
  milk composition and, 512*t*
  urine volumes and specific gravities for, 341*t*
Sympathetic efferent distribution, 102–103
Sympathetic nervous system, 98
Sympathetic stimulation, 253
Sympathetic trunk, 102
Synapses, *86*
  characteristics of, 86
  neurons and, 85–86
Synaptic gap, 86
Syncytium, 245
Synovial fluid, 199, 202
Synovial joints, 199
  blood and nerve supply of, *201*
  lubrication of, 202
Synovial membrane, 179, 200, 201
Synoviocytes, 201
Syrinx, 272, 302
Systemic circulation, 236
  canial aspects of, *239*
Systole, 247
Systolic blood pressure, 255

T
Tachypnea, 280
Tail
  of epididymis, 435, *436*, *438*
    in stallion, *445*
Tapetum, 150
  relationship of, to retina, *151*
Tarsus, *21*
Taste, 124, 127–130
  depraved appetite and, 130
  sensations with, 130
  taste reception, 128
  temperature and, 130
Taste buds, 128, *129*, 364
  association of, with papillae on dog's tongue, *129*
Taste hairs, *129*
Taste pit, 128, *129*
Taste pore, 128, *129*
TBG. *See* Thyroxine-binding globulin
TBW. *See* Total body water
T cells, 52
  life span of, *49*
  types of, 53

TCF. *See* Transcellular fluid

Tear film, 155

Tears, formation of, 154–155

Teat canal, 502

   smooth muscle around, *504*

Teats, 502, *502*, 503–504

   anatomy of, 503

   milk withdrawn from, 504

   sagittal section through, *503*

   smooth muscle encircling teat canal in, *504*

Tectorial membrane, 139, *139, 140, 141*

Teeth, 361–363

   permanent, dental formulas and eruption times for, *362t*

Telencephalon, *91*

Telodendritic zone, 85

Telophase, 9, *10,* 11

Temperature. *See also* Body temperature

   critical, 427

   spermatogenesis and, 44

   taste and, 130

Temporal bone, *135*

Tenase complex, 69, 70

Tendons, 209

Tensor tympani muscle, 134, *135*

Terminal branches, *85*

Terminal bronchioles, 272, *274*

Terminal bulb, of presynaptic neuron, *86*

Terminal bulbs, *85*

Terminal cisternae, *213*

Territoriality, pheromones and, 132

Testes

   associated structures and, 432–436

      ductus deferens, 435–436

      epididymis, 435

   cryptorchid, 438

   descended adult, *438*

   descent of, 437–438

     testosterone and, 450

   in male bird, 452

   in male chicken, *453*

   scrotum, 436

   seminiferous tubules of, 432

   skin and "dartos" of, *438*

   in stallion, with emphasis on pampiniform, *445*

Testicles

   blood supply to, 444

   of bull, *433*

   detailed structure of, *433*

Testicular arteries, 444

   in stallions, *445*

Testicular artery, vein, nerve, and lymphatics, *437*

Testicular artery and vein, *438*

Testicular fluid, *433*

Testicular function, factors affecting, 451–452

Testicular veins, 444

   in stallions, *445*

Testosterone, 164, 449, 452, *471*

   functions of, 449–450

   influence of, on spermatogenesis, 449

Tetanus, 220

Tetany, *221*

TF. *See* Tissue factor

T₄ (thyroxine), 165

   biochemistry of, 165–166

   release and transport of, 166–167

   structural formulas of, *167*

Thalamus, *90, 91,* 94

Theca externa cells, 472, *476*

Theca interna cells, 472, *472, 476*

Thecal capillaries, *472*

Thermogenesis, 427

Thermoreceptors, *126*

   pulmonary ventilation and, 297

Thermosensitive cells, in rostral hypothalamus, 424

Thick ascending limb, loop of Henle, 320

Thin ascending limb, loop of Henle, 320, 321

Thin descending limb, loop of Henle, 320

Thiocyanate, 168

Thiouracil, 168

Thiourea, 168

Third eyelid

   animals with, 15

   in dog, *155*

Third heart sounds, 251

Third ventricle, 116

Thirst

   defined, 40

   relief of, 40–41

   stimulus of, 40

Thirst center, hyperosmolality and, 334

Thirst mechanism, 40

Thoracic aorta, *233*

Thoracic cavity, 22

Thoracic girdle, *187t*

Thoracic limbs

   anatomy of bones, comparison of, *188*

   bones of pelvic limbs *vs.* bones of, *187t*

   of horse, metacarpal and phalangeal bones of, *189*

Thoracic nerves, 95–96

Thoracic (T) vertebrae, 181, *183*

Thoracic viscera, 181

Thoracic volume, in horse, *259*

Thoracolumbar origin, of nerves, 100

Thorax

    equine, schematic transverse plane of, *23*

    healthy canine, radiographs of, *277*

    during inspiration, *279*

    laboratory model of, 259, *260*

Thoroughfare channel, *236*

Three semicircular canals, 136

Three semicircular ducts, 136

Threshold, 108, 385

Thrombin, *69*

    formation of, 72

        pathways to, 69–70

Thrombocytes, 46, *48*, 67

Thrombomodulin, 67

Thromboplastin, 70, 382–383

Thrombosthenin, 71

Thromboxane A$_2$, 68, 176, *176*

Thrombus, major stages in formation of, *65*

Thryoid hormone, cold temperatures and, 427

Thymine, DNA replication and, *9*

Thyroglobulin, 165, 166

Thyroid deficiency, antithyroid compounds and,
        167–168

Thyroid gland, 165

    bovine, *165*

    canine, *165*

Thyroid hormones, 161, 165–168

    functions of, 167

    maintenance of lactation and, 509

    mammogenesis and, 507

    secretions regulated by, 167

Thyroid-stimulating hormone, 164

Thyrotrope cells, 163

Thyrotropin-releasing hormones, 167

Thyroxine-binding globulin, 167

Tidal volume, 280, *281*

    panting frequency and, 426

    pneumotaxic center modulation and increase in,
        292

Tie, 440

Tissue factor, 70

Tissue factor pathway, *69*

Tissue factor pathway (extrinsic system), 70

Tissue factor VIIa complex, *69*

Tissue plasminogen activator, 67

Tissue proteins, reversible equilibrium among plasma
        proteins, plasma amino acids and, 77

Tissues, 13–19

    connective, 14

    epithelial, 14, 15

    muscle, 14

    nervous, 14

Tissue-type plasminogen activator, 71

T lymphocytes, foreign cell destruction and, *53*

Tone

    circulatory adjustments, body heat and, 424

    of solutions, 32–34

        effect of, on erythrocytes, 32, *33*

        hypothetical example of, *33*

Tongue, 361, 363–364

    bovine, dorsal surface of, *365*

    of cow, *272*

    of dog, frenulum of, *377*

    of horse, *271*

    as prehensile organ, 384

    root of, *386*

    taste buds on, 128

Tonic receptor organ, 125

Tonsils, 48

Torr, 255

Total body water, distribution of, among fluid
        compartments, 36, *37*

Total lung capacity, 280, *281*

Touch, sense of, 124

t-PA. *See* Tissue plasminogen activator

Trabeculae (spicules), 115, 188, *190, 194, 244, 244,*
        434

Trace minerals, 383, 511

Trachea, 271, *274, 279, 386*

    in cow, *272*

    cross section of, *274*

    endotracheal tube in place relative to, *273*

    in horse, *271*

Tracheal rings, 271

    in birds, 302

    in horse, *271*

Tract, 86, 94

Transcellular fluid, 37, *37*

Transcription, 11

Transferrin, 60

Transfer RNA, 11, *11*

Transitional epithelium, *16,* 17, 315

Translation, 11

Transmembrane potential, 104

    recording of, during depolarization and repolarization,
        106

Transmission of nerve impulses, 104–108

    action potential, 108

depolarization, repolarization, and the nerve impulse, 105, 107
   resting membrane potential, 105
   saltatory conduction, 108
   transmission velocity, 108
Transmission velocity, 108
Transparency, of cornea, 143
Transport of carbon dioxide, 290
Transport of oxygen, 288, 289
Transverse colon, 24, 374
   in dog, 374
   in pig, 375
Transverse foramen, 183
Transverse plane, 20, 21
   equine thorax, schematic of, 23
Transverse process, 183
Traumatic pericarditis, 127, 229, 402
Traumatic reticuloperitonitis (hardware disease), white blood cell count in cows and, 55
Treppe, 221, 221
TRH. See Thyrotropin-releasing hormones
Triad, 214
Tricarboxylic acid cycle, 6, 410, 410
Tricuspid valve, 231, 233
Trigeminal nerve (V), 100t
   in dog, 101
Triglycerides, 382, 397, 399, 408
Tripe, 401
tRNA. See Transfer RNA
Trochlear nerve
   in dog, 101
Trochlear nerve (IV), 100t
Trophoblast, 12
Tropomyosin, 217
Troponin, 217
True capillaries, 236
True symphysis, 181
Trypsin, 396, 399
Trypsinogen, 396
TSH. See Thyroid-stimulating hormone
TSH secretion, 167
T_3 (triiodothyronine), 165
   biochemistry of, 165–166
   release and transport of, 166–167
   structural formulas of, 167
T tubules, 211, 213, 213, 214, 223
Tuber coxae, 184
Tuber ischiadicum, 184
Tubular epithelial cells, secretion of H+ associated with secretion of ammonia by, 348
Tubular epithelium, 327

Tubular fluid, 323
   countercurrent multiplier system and, 330
   mechanism for renal secretion of H+ associated with bicarbonate buffer system in, 346
   mechanism for renal secretion of H+ associated with phosphate buffer system in, 347
Tubular genital tract, 462–466
   uterine tubes, 462–463
   uterus, 463–464, 466
   vagina, 466
Tubular lumen, 327, 328
Tubular reabsorption and secretion, 323, 323, 327–329
   reabsorption of Na+, Cl-, glucose, and amino acids, 327–328
   reabsorption of water and urea, 328–329
   secretion of H+, K+, NH_3, and organic molecules, 329
   transport maximum, 329
Tubular secretion, 323, 323
Tubular transport maximum (T_M), 329
Tubulo-glomerular feedback mechanism, 326
Tunica albuginea, 434, 436, 459
   in fibroelastic penis of bull and musculocavernous penis of stallion, 441
Tunica dartos, 436
Tunics, of eyeball, 142
Turkeys
   blood pressure in, 257t
   broodiness in, 496
   digestive tract of, 412
   hydrated, urine flow for, 353
   phallus of, 453
Tusks, 361
Twain, Mark, 29
T wave, in electrocardiogram, 249
TXA_2. See Thromboxane A_2
Tylopoda, 401
Tympanic membrane, 134, 135, 139, 140
   in dog, 133
Tympanism, 406
Type I alveolar cells, 274
Tyrosine, 161, 165
   coupling of, 166
   structural formula for, 173

U
Udder
   sagittal section of, through left half, 502
   suspensory apparatus and, 504
   veinous drainage of, 505
UMNs. See Upper motor neurons
Units of measurement, interconversion of, 35–36

Unmyelinated pain fibers, 127
Unopette micro-collection system, 58
Unpleasant taste response, 130
Upper air passages, respiratory reflexes and, 293
Upper motor neurons, 109, *110*
Upper respiratory tract clearance, 296, 297
Urachus, 484
Urea, 341
    countercurrent mechanism and role of, 332–333
    countercurrent multiplication in recirculation of, *331*
    reabsorption of, 328–329
Urea excreting group of animals, 353
Urea nitrogen, values of, in blood from mature domestic
    animals, 76*t*
Ureter, *314*, 315, *321*
    avian, *454*
    in cow, *317*
    in horse, *315*
    in male chicken, *453*
    in mare, cow, sow, and bitch, *465*
Ureteral urine, avian, modification of, 353
Ureterovesicular junction, 315, *316*
Ureterovesicular valve, 339
Urethra, 316, *321*
    in cow, *317*
    in fibroelastic penis of bull and musculocavernous
        penis of stallion, *441*
    location of, on penis, 440
Urethralis, 442
Urethral muscle, around pelvic urethra, in bull, *433*
Urethral opening
    in cow, *460*
    in mare, cow, sow, and bitch, *465*
Urethral process, in ram, 440, *441*
Uric acid
    formation and excretion of, avian urinary system and,
        351–353
    in reptiles and birds, 352–353
    values of, in blood from mature domestic animals, 76*t*
Urinalysis, 340
Urinary bladder, 315, *321*
    bovine, *462*
    in cow, *317*
    in cow, sow, mare, and bitch, *461*, *465*
    gross anatomy of, 312–317
    urine transport to, 339
Urinary continence, 340
Urinary system. *See also* Kidneys; Urinary bladder; Urine
    acid-base balance and, 344–347
    aldosterone and, 337–338
    avian, 347–353

countercurrent mechanism and, 329–333
    in dog, *313*
    ECF volume regulation of, 336–337
    erythropoietin and, 338
    glomerular filtration and, 324–327
    kidneys and urinary bladder anatomy, 312–317
    mammalian urine, characteristics of, 340–341
    micturition, 339–340
    nephrons, 317–322
    parathyroid hormone and, 338
    prostaglandins and, 338–339
    renal clearance and, 341–344
    tubular reabsorption and secretion, 327–329
    urine concentration and, 333–336
    urine formation and, 323–324
Urinary urobilinogen, 61
Urine
    amount and specific gravity of, 341
    avian
        characteristics and flow of, 353
        concentration of, 353
    color of, 340
    composition of, 340
    consistency of, 341
    of horse, 341
    mammalian, characteristics of, 340–341
    nitrogenous component of, 341
    odor of, 340
    transport of, to urinary bladder, 339
    volumes and specific gravities of, 341*t*
Urine concentration, 333–336
    ADH release, other factors related to, 335
    antidiuretic hormone and osmoregulation, 333–335
    concentration failure, 335–336
Urine escape, prevention of, 316
Urine formation
    distribution of blood at glomerulus and, 323–324
    nephrons and, 323, *323*
Urine-to-plasmal osmolal ratio, 335
Urine volume, for dog in normal state of hydration, 324*t*
Urobilin, 60, 61, 340
Urobilinogen, 60, 61, 340
Urodeum, avian, *454*
Urogenital system, in male chicken, *453*
Uterine artery, 467
Uterine horn, in mare, cow, sow, and bitch, *465*
Uterine milk, 484
Uterine tubes, 459, 462
    bovine, *462*
Utero-vaginal sperm storage glands, in fowl, 453
Utero-vaginal sphincter, avian, 494

Uterus, *24*, 440, 459, 463–464, 466
  in bitch, 493
  bovine, *462*
  in cow, *317*, *460*
  in cow, position of, *467*
  in cow, sow, mare, and bitch, *461*, *465*
  involution of, in cow, 492
  life span of corpus luteum and, 473
  in mare, ewe, and sow, 492–493
  prolapsed, 116
Utricle, *134*
Utricular maculae, general structure of, *138*
Utriculus, *137*

V
Vacuoles, *5*
Vagabond nerve (vagus nerve), 103
Vagina, 450, 459, 466
  canine coitus and, *442*
  in cow, *317*
  in cow, sow, mare, and bitch, *461*
  formation of hen's egg and, 495t
  penetration of penis into, 451
Vaginal artery, *467*
Vaginal cavity, 437, *438*
Vaginal rings, 437, *438*, 442
Vaginal tunic
  parietal layer of, 436, 437, *437*
  visceral layer of, 436, 437, *437*
Vagus nerve (X), 97, 100t, 103, 160, *254*
  in dog, *101*
Vallate, 364
Vallate papillae, 128, *129*
  on bovine tongue, *365*
Valve disorders, in heart, 251
Valves, of heart, 231
Valvular endocarditis, 234
Vasa recta, *318*, 319, *320*, 330
  in avian kidney medullary cone, *351*
  countercurrent exchange in, *332*
Vascular endothelium, 66–67
Vascular system, 45
Vas deferens, 435–436
  ampulla of, in bull, *433*
  avian, terminal part of, *454*
  in avian male, 452
  in male chicken, *453*
  in stallion, *445*
Vas efferentia, in avian male, 453
Vasomotor center, 253, *254*
Vasopressin, 164, 327

Vegetative nervous system, 98
Veins, 234, 235, *235*, 237
  major, decreasing pressures from major arteries to, *237*
  mammary, *502*, 505
  pulmonary, 275
  renal, 313
  in renal portal system of birds, *352*
  testicular, 444
  valves of, showing pumping action of adjacent muscles, *237*
Velocity of transmission, 108
Venae cavae, 235, 236, *237*
Venous blood, 232, *274*
  partial pressure of, 282
  pH of, 47
Venous circle, 505
Venous drainage, for mammary glands, 505–506
Vent, of turkey, *412*
Ventilation
  defined, 283
  pressures related to, 283–286
Ventilation regulation, 292–297
  humoral control, 294–297
    braking effect, 296–297
    importance of oxygen regulation, 295–296
    influences of carbon dioxide and hydrogen ions, 294
    influences of oxygen, 294–295
  neural control, 293–294
Ventral branch, 96–97
Ventral cavity, 22
Ventral colon, 375
Ventral concha
  of cow, 272
  of horse, *271*
Ventral direction, 20, *21*
Ventral horn(s)
  of gray matter, 95
  of spinal cord, 96
  of spinal cord of dog, *95*
Ventral labial vein, *505*
Ventral meatus, 271
  of horse, *271*
Ventral oblique muscle, in dog, *153*
Ventral plane, *21*
Ventral respiratory group, 292
  in respiratory center, 292
Ventral root
  in spinal cord of dog, *95*
  in spinal nerves, 96

Ventral sac, *402*
Ventral spinocerebellar tract, 94
Ventricles
    of brain, 116–118
    in canine brain, *118*
    in canine heart, *232*
    of heart, 231, *233*
    muscle fibers of, 245
Ventricular syncytium, 245
Venules, 234, 235, *235*, *236*, 237
Vertebrae, 180
    of chicken, *182*
    of horse, *180*
    of ox, *181*
    spinal nerves and location relative to, 98
    typical, general features of, *183*
Vertebral cavity, 22
Vertebral foramen, *183*
Vertebral formulas, 181
    of common domestic animals and humans, 183*t*
Vertebral ganglions, 102
Vesicles, 223, *236*
Vesicular glands, 439
Vestibular aqueduct, *134*, *136*
Vestibular membrane, *140*, *141*
Vestibular muscle, canine coitus and, *442*
Vestibular (oval) window, 139
Vestibular portion, of inner ear, 134, *135*
Vestibular structure, function of, 136, 138
Vestibular window, 133, 140
Vestibule, *135*, 136
    of middle ear, *135*
    of vagina, 466–467
        species variations in position of, *468*
Vestibulocochlear nerve (VIII), 100*t*, 115, 134, *135*, 139
VFAs. *See* Volatile fatty acids
Vicunas, 401
Villi (villus), 370, *371*
    functional organization of, *373*
Viral infections, leukopenia and, 54
Visceral layer, of vaginal tunic, 436
Visceral nerves, 95
Visceral pain, 127
Visceral pain afferent fiber, *128*
Visceral pericardium, 229, *230*
Visceral pleura, 22, 275
    in horse, *278*
Visceral reflexes, 113
Visceral vaginal tunic, 437, *437*
Viscerocranium, 180

Vision, 140–155, *141*
    chemistry of, 146, 149
    fields of, 150–152
    vitamin A and, 149
Visual acuity, 145
Visual area, of brain, 90
Visual cycle, photochemistry of, *149*
Visual purple, 146
Visual reflex center, *90*
Visual reflexes, 150
Visual streak, 145
    in horse, 151
Vital capacity, 280, *281*
Vitamin A
    in milk, 511
    vision and, 149
Vitamin D, 161, 169
    active form of, 338
    in milk, 511
Vitamin E, in milk, 511
Vitamin K, 66
    deficiency of, 74
    in milk, 511
Vitamins, 380, 383–384
    in milk, 511
Vitreous body, 145
Vitreous chamber, *144*, 145
Volatile fatty acids, 400, 408, 409
    chemical structure of, *400*
Volkmann canals, 191, 192, 197
Voltage changes, across nerve and muscle membranes, 248–249
Volume regulation, 336
Volumes, of urine, 341*t*
Voluntary control, of respiratory movements, 294
Vomiting, 390–391
von Willebrand disease, 74
von Willebrand factor, 68, 74
Vulva, 466
    in cow, sow, mare, and bitch, *460*, *461*
vWD. *See* von Willebrand disease
vWF. *See* von Willebrand factor

W
Warm-blooded animals
    body temperature and, 421
    hibernation and, 428
Warmth-sensitive neurons, response of, in rostral hypothalamus of cat, *425*
Water, 380
    adapting to lack of, 41

countercurrent exchange in vasa recta and passive diffusion of, *332*
diffusion of, 30, 261
intestinal transport of, 392
metabolic, 269
percent of total body weight and, 28
physical properties of, 28
prehension and drinking of, 384
reabsorption of, 328–329
Water balance, 37–39
    daily, in Holstein cows eating legume hay, *39t*
    water gain and, 38–39
    water loss and, 39
    water requirements for, 39
Water deficit, hyperosmolality and, 334
Water-soluble vitamins, 383
Water vapor partial pressure value, 283
Wave forms
    in electrocardiogram, 249
    electrode placements and, in dog, *249*
Wave summation, *221*
WBCs. *See* White blood cells
Wear characteristics, tooth structure and, 363
Weeping lubrication, 202
Wettability, between cornea and tears, 155
Whales, milk composition and, *512t*
Wheezes, 282
Whey proteins, in milk, 510
White blood cells, 45
    basophils, 52
    classification and appearance of, 47–48
    diagnostic procedures related to, 54–55
    eosinophils, 52
    function of, 49

life span and numbers of, 48–49
    lymphocytes, 52–54
    monocytes, 50–52
    neutrophils, 49–50
White fat, brown fat *vs.*, 428
White lipid (sphingomyelin) substance, 87
White matter, 90, 94
    in spinal cord of dog, *95*
White (or pale) skeletal muscle cells, 207
White pulp, in spleen, 244
Wolffian ducts, 450
Wooden tongue, in cattle, 384

Y
Yellow egg yolk, 494
Yellow fibers, 19
Yolk, *495*
Yolk protein, 494
Yolk sac, 485

Z
Zinc, 383
Z lines, 210, *212*, 222
Zona fasciculata, 170, *171*
Zona glomerulosa, 170, *171*, 172
Zona pellucida, 459, *476*
Zona reticularis, 170, *171*
Zonary placenta, of dog and cat, *486*
Zones of reserve cartilage, 193
Zonular fibers, 143, *144*
    in dog, *144*
Zygomatic process, of temporal bone, *135*
Zygotes, 12, *13*, 483, 484
    mitotic division from, to blastula, *14*

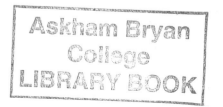